PEDIATRIC SKILLS
for Occupational Therapy Assistants

PEDIATRIC SKILLS *for* Occupational Therapy Assistants

JEAN W. SOLOMON, MHS, OTR/L

Program Coordinator and Instructor
Occupational Therapy Assistant Program
Trident Technical College
Charleston, South Carolina

JANE CLIFFORD O'BRIEN, PhD, OTR/L
Assistant Professor
Occupational Therapy Department
College of Health Professions
University of New England
Biddeford, Maine

Illustrations by Morgan Midgett
With 20 Contributing Authors

SECOND EDITION

MOSBY

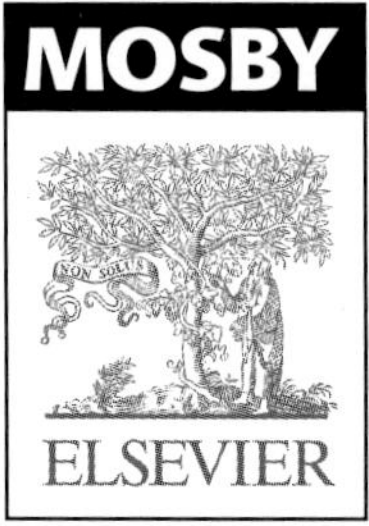

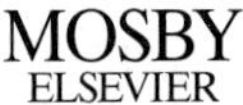

MOSBY
ELSEVIER

11830 Westline Industrial Drive
St. Louis, Missouri 63146

PEDIATRIC SKILLS FOR OCCUPATIONAL THERAPY ASSISTANTS, SECOND EDITION

ISBN-13: 978-0-323-03183-7
ISBN-10: 0-323-03183-8

Notice

Neither the Publisher nor the Authors assume any responsibility for any loss or injury and/or damage to persons or property arising out of or related to any use of the material contained in this book. It is the responsibility of the treating practitioner, relying on independent expertise and knowledge of the patient, to determine the best treatment and method of application for the patient.

The Publisher

ISBN-13: 978-0-323-03183-7
ISBN-10: 0-323-03183-8

Publishing Director: Linda Duncan
Editor: Kathy Falk
Developmental Editor: Melissa Kuster Deutsch
Publishing Services Manager: Patricia Tannian
Senior Project Manager: Anne Altepeter
Design Direction: Mark Oberkrom

Printed in the United States of America

Last digit is the print number: 9 8 7 6 5 4 3 2 1

Contributors

Diana Bal, MHS, OTR/L, BCP
Summerville, South Carolina

Gilson J. Capilouto, PhD
Assistant Professor, Rehabilitation Sciences
University of Kentucky
Lexington, Kentucky

Ricardo C. Carrasco, PhD, OTR/L, FAOTA
Chairman, FiestaJoy Foundation, Inc.
Winter Park, Florida

Melissa A. Fullerton, MSOT
Occupational Therapist (graduate)
University of New England
Biddeford, Maine

Nadine Kuzyk Hanner, AHS COTA, MSOT OTR/L
Occupational Therapist, Special Education Department
Charleston County School District
Charleston, South Carolina

Lise M.W. Jones, MA, OTR, SIPT Certified
Occupational Therapy Coordinator, Clinical Department,
The Reece School for Special Teaching
New York, New York
Private Practice, Occupational Therapy Consultant
New York, New York

Allyson LaChance, MSOT
Occupational Therapist (graduate)
University of New England
Biddeford, Maine

Kathleen Logan-Bauer, MA, OTR
Senior Occupational Therapist
St. Mary's Hospital for Children
Bayside, New York

Dianne Koontz Lowman, EdD
Associate Professor, Director of Distance Education and Academic Performance, Occupational Therapy
Virginia Commonwealth University
Richmond, Virginia

Peggy Zaks Machover, MA (Psychology)
Consultant, Life Span Development
Long Island, New York

Melissa A. Mailhot, MSOT
Occupational Therapist (graduate)
University of New England
Biddeford, Maine

Angela Chinners Marsh, AHS COTA/L
Occupational Therapy Assistant, Special Education Department, Charleston County School District
Charleston, South Carolina

Randi Carlson Neideffer, AA, AHS COTA, MSOT OTR/L
Occupational Therapist, Special Education Department,
Charleston County School District
Charleston, South Carolina

Dawn B. Oakley, MS, OTR
Director of Rehabilitation
St. Mary's Hospital for Children
Bayside, New York

Gretchen Evans Parker, BS, OTR/L
Owner, Gretchen Evans Parker Neuro Developmental Therapy
Lexington, South Carolina

Susan Stallings-Sahler, PhD, OTR/L, FAOTA
Professor, School of Allied Health Sciences
The Medical College of Georgia
Augusta, Georgia

Kerryellen G. Vroman, MHSc, OTR/L
Associate Professor, Occupational Therapy
University of New Hampshire
Durham, New Hampshire

Harriet G. Williams, PhD
Professor, Exercise Science
Arnold School of Public Health
University of South Carolina
Columbia, South Carolina

Pamela J. Winton, PhD
Senior Scientist and Director of Outreach,
FPG Child Development Institute
Research Professor, School of Education
University of North Carolina—Chapel Hill
Chapel Hill, North Carolina

Robert E. Winton, MD
Psychiatrist
Durham, North Carolina

Previous Edition Contributors

Paula Kramer, PhD, OTR, FAOTA
Professor and Chair
Department of Occupational Therapy
Kean University
Union, New Jersey

Angela M. Peralta, AS, COTA
Toddler and Infant Programs for Special Education (TIPSE)
Staten Island, New York
Adjunct Instructor
Touro College
New York, New York

Sharon Kalscheuer Suchomel, OTR
Positioning and Mobility Specialist
Morton Medical
Neenah, Wisconsin

Joyce A. Wandel, MS, OTR/L
Director
Occupational Therapy Assistant Program
Wright College
Chicago, Illinois

Reviewers

Rebecca Ashe, MSOT
Occupational Therapist (graduate)
University of New England
Biddeford, Maine

Kilian James Garvey, PhD
Assistant Professor
Psychology Department
University of New England
Biddeford, Maine

Kathryn M. Loukas, MS, OTR/L, FAOTA
Assistant Clinical Professor
Occupational Therapy
University of New England
Biddeford, Maine

Nancy MacRae, MS, OTR/L, FAOTA
Director and Associate Professor
Occupational Therapy
University of New England
Biddeford, Maine

Julie Savoyski, MSOTR
Occupational Therapist (graduate)
University of New England
Biddeford, Maine

To my **family** *and* **dearest friends**
I thank you for your love and encouragement,
which gave me the serenity to write this book.
JWS

To my husband, **Mike,**
and my children, **Scott, Alison,** *and* **Molly**
You are my support, inspiration, and love.
JCO

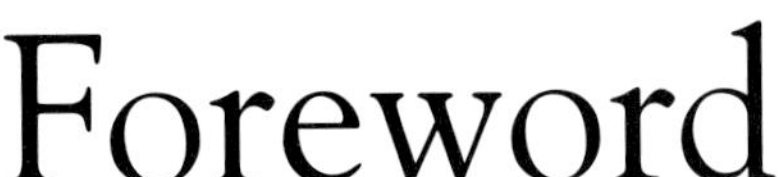

Foreword

Educators and students will welcome the second edition of *Pediatric Skills for Occupational Therapy Assistants*, with its expanded foundation for pediatric practice and broader coverage of material mandated under the standards of the Accreditation Council for Occupational Therapy Education. Student-friendly features and clear organization make this a useful basic textbook for occupational therapy assistant (OTA) education; beyond that, it will quickly become a resource for the practitioner new to pediatric practice.

Important new features include expanded practice models and frames of reference. Separate chapters are devoted to development, sensory integration, and motor control. The practitioner's role with the family is well delineated and supported with an explanation of family systems theory. Recent legislation is explained in the context of occupational therapy interventions.

The adolescent receives additional emphasis; discussion of instrumental activities of daily living is expanded, featuring those important to adolescents. New chapters give ample detail on handwriting, and on splinting of the child and adolescent.

Greater detail and broader range is provided on pediatric health conditions, with many diagnoses newly included. The assistive technology chapter has been updated. A new chapter discusses use of therapeutic media and selecting and adapting activities for different age groups. Even animal-assisted services have been included! This is an occupation-based, client-centered text.

The authors and their many distinguished contributors present complex material in an engaging way. Throughout the text, case examples illustrate principles. Samples of documentation are interwoven with the cases, making the connection explicit. The separate and complementary roles of the occupational therapist (OT) and the OTA become clear through the multiple detailed examples. Respect for the family, child, and adolescent as co-partners in the occupational therapy process provides students with an excellent model for beginning practice in pediatrics.

Pediatric practice is expanding for the OTA even while basic entry-level education for the OT has moved to the master's degree level. Different and complementary texts are needed for the two levels of practitioner. This book delivers the required foundation content for the OTA with great depth and breadth, preparing the OTA to work as a partner with the OT. The arrival of the second edition of *Pediatric Skills for Occupational Therapy Assistants* will be an occasion for joyful celebration by the faculty and students of OTA education programs.

Mary Beth Early, MS, OTR/L
Professor, Occupational Therapy Assistant Program
Department of Natural and Applied Sciences
LaGuardia Community College
City University of New York
Long Island City, New York

Preface

This book has been written for the occupational therapy assistant (OTA) student and the certified occupational therapy assistant (COTA) working in the pediatric practice arena. The language is consistent with the *Occupational Therapy Practice Framework*. Emphasis is on concrete, practical information that may readily be used by students, COTAs, and entry-level registered occupational therapists (OTRs) who work with children and adolescents. Theories, frames of reference, and practice models are introduced and integrated into the content so that they can be easily applied. When possible, the text differentiates between the roles of the COTA and the OTR. The term *occupational therapy practitioner* generally refers to OTRs and COTAs, and is used during discussions of procedures that can be performed by either professional.

All of the chapters contain the following elements: outline, key terms, objectives, summary, review questions, and suggested activities. The chapter outlines provide readers with information about the specific topics that are discussed in each chapter. The list of key terms contains important words appearing in the chapter that the author(s) want to emphasize for readers before they begin the chapter. The key terms are listed in the order in which they appear in the chapter. The chapter objectives concisely outline the material readers will learn after studying a specific chapter. Each chapter has a summary that reemphasizes the key points of the chapter. Review questions included at the end of each chapter help readers synthesize the information presented. Suggested activities, also found at the end of each chapter, are designed to be performed by individuals or small groups of students. Engaging in the suggested activities helps reinforce information presented in the chapter.

Boxes, case studies, vignettes, tables, and figures have been used to reiterate, exemplify, or illustrate specific points. "Clinical Pearls," which are words of wisdom based on the clinical expertise of the chapter author(s), are also included. The Clinical Pearls contain helpful hints or reminders that have been consistently useful for pediatric occupational therapy practitioners. Appendixes are included at the end of several chapters of the book.

The first four chapters present an overall framework for the book. Chapter 1 presents information about recommended pediatric curriculum content, selected practice models, and COTA supervision and service competency. The next three chapters present information about the systems—family, medical, and educational—in which a pediatric occupational therapy practitioner may work.

The next part of the book discusses normal, or typical, development. Chapter 5 presents an overview of the periods and principles of normal development and also discusses the occupational performance contexts. The next two chapters present information about normal development in the occupational performance skills and areas of occupation. Chapter 8 discusses the uniqueness of adolescence.

Chapters 9 through 15 present information about specific pediatric disorders that a pediatric occupational therapy practitioner may encounter. Chapter 9 provides general considerations for intervention and is followed by a review of pediatric health conditions. The next three chapters discuss single diagnoses, intellectual disabilities, and cerebral palsy. A chapter on positioning and handling techniques follows the chapter on cerebral palsy, since much of the information is specific to this diagnosis. Chapter 14 discusses psychosocial and behavioral disorders, and Chapter 15 describes other common pediatric disorders. Case studies are included throughout the chapters to help readers apply the presented information.

The final nine chapters contain specific program planning and intervention information. Chapter 16 provides readers with an overview of the use of therapeutic media, including a variety of specific activities to use with children and adolescents. Chapter 17 focuses on play and playfulness, while Chapter 18 examines daily living and work/productive occupations in children and adolescents. Chapter 19 describes handwriting intervention, and

Chapter 20 explores the motor control aspects of fine motor skills. Each chapter provides readers with intervention techniques and case studies to make application clear.

The final chapters explore more specialized areas of pediatric practice. Chapter 21 explores sensory processing and integration. Chapter 22 describes the process of assistive technology, and Chapter 23 reviews splinting for the child and adolescent. The final chapter examines the use of animals in therapy.

This book has evolved from many years of teaching pediatric skills to students. The second edition includes seven new chapters, and all chapters have been revised and updated to reflect current practice. The talent of the contributing authors is impressive and reflects expertise from many areas. We are grateful to the authors, reviewers, and contributors for their wisdom and skill.

Jean W. Solomon
Jane Clifford O'Brien

Acknowledgments

We have had the opportunity to work with many talented people on this second edition. The authors come from various areas of the country and represent a wide range of disciplines and practice areas. They are talented and dedicated professionals who are passionate about the care of children with special needs. The authors have extensive clinical experience and knowledge that they have shared with the readers. It was fun and exciting reconnecting with colleagues and friends to participate in this project.

We acknowledge Joyce Wandel, Angela Peralta, and Paula Kramer, whose contributions from the first edition were revised for this edition. Melissa Fullerton, Melissa Mailhot, and Allyson LaChance should be applauded as first-time authors who agreed to work quickly to meet the deadline.

We thank the professionals who reviewed specific chapters in preparation for the final draft of the manuscript: Rebecca Ashe, Melissa Fullerton, Kilian Garvey, Kate Loukas, Nancy MacRae, and Julie Savoyski. Their feedback and comments were invaluable and helped strengthen the content of the chapters.

We also thank and acknowledge the talents of Morgan Midgett, a children's book illustrator, who illustrated this text and was a wonderful support for us. We appreciate all the photographs contributed from family, friends, and colleagues, including Cheryl Joyce, a wonderful friend and photographer; Chloe Troia, an aspiring photographer; and Scott O'Brien, who takes wonderful family photos.

We appreciate the hard work of the Elsevier editorial and production staff—Kathy Falk, Melissa Kuster, and Anne Altepeter. They have been very helpful and supportive throughout the process.

A special thank you goes to our friends and family, who allowed us to present ideas to them (often while running or horseback riding) and unofficially collaborated with us throughout this process.

JWS & JCO

I thank my family, Mike, Scott, Alison, and Molly, who have continually supported me through this book and in all my other endeavors. My family provides me with inspiration. I thank my family for letting me relearn daily about the beauty of being a child.

In closing, I would like to thank Jeannie Solomon, for her friendship and for inviting me to join her. I am really honored to have worked with her on this book. She has made this process fun and rewarding.

JCO

Finally, I would like to recognize my friend and colleague, Jane Clifford O'Brien, for her dedication and enthusiasm throughout this project. I knew that writing the second edition was a task greater than one person. The honor is mutually shared.

JWS

Contents

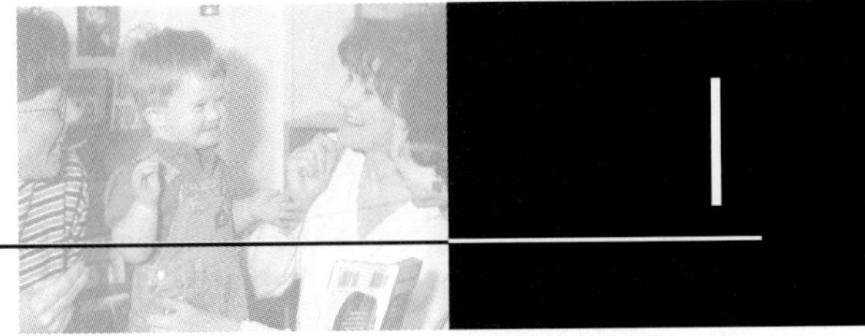

1

Scope of Practice

JANE CLIFFORD O'BRIEN
JEAN W. SOLOMON

CHAPTER *Objectives*

After studying this chapter, the reader will be able to accomplish the following:

- Describe the basics of the Occupational Therapy Practice Framework and its relationship to clinical practice
- Recognize eight subject areas in which entry-level certified occupational therapy assistants should have general knowledge
- Define models of practice and frames of reference
- Describe selected models of practice
- Describe the developmental, sensory integrative, biomechanical, sensorimotor, motor control, and rehabilitative frames of reference
- Describe the four levels at which registered occupational therapists supervise certified occupational therapy assistants
- Define service competency and give examples of the way it may be obtained

KEY TERMS

Occupational Therapy Practice Framework
American Occupational Therapy Association's "Uniform Terminology for Occupational Therapy"
Model of practice
Frame of reference
Developmental frame of reference
Sensory integration frame of reference
Biomechanical integration frame of reference
Sensorimotor frame of reference
Motor control frame of reference
Rehabilitative frame of reference
Levels of supervision
Service competency

CHAPTER OUTLINE

During the past 20 years, significant changes have occurred in the provision of pediatric occupational therapy (OT) services.[13] Numerous federal laws have been implemented that expand the services available to infants, children, and adolescents who have special needs or disabilities. Approximately 20% of all certified occupational therapy assistants (COTAs) work in pediatric settings. OT practitioners also provide pediatric services in medical settings such as outpatient clinics and community settings such as schools, homes, and daycare centers.[14] Because numerous practitioners work with infants, children, and adolescents, both entry-level registered occupational therapists (OTRs) and COTAs must have a solid foundation in pediatrics.

The American Occupational Therapy Association (AOTA) has identified eight subject areas that should be included in any pediatric OT curriculum.[3,6] An entry-level OT practitioner should have knowledge in the following areas:

Normal development: Children with special needs or atypical development patterns should be recognized and treated.

Importance of families in the OT process: Families are the most consistent participants on the pediatric team.

Specific pediatric diagnoses: Pediatric OT practitioners must determine which tools and methods are the most appropriate for assessment and intervention.

OT practice models (i.e., frames of reference): Assessment and intervention information should be organized into a meaningful plan.

Assessments appropriate for a specific child with a specific disability or diagnosis: Practitioners must be able to accommodate numerous types of diagnosis.

Age-appropriate activities: Pediatric OT practitioners should be able to vary therapy activities to suit the age of the child.

Differences among systems in which OT services are provided: Therapy is tailored to specific settings. For example, a child who is receiving services in a public school system has therapy goals and objectives that are educationally relevant, whereas a child who is receiving services as an inpatient in a hospital has medically necessary goals.

Assistive technology: Pediatric OT practitioners should be able to work effectively with infants, children, and adolescents who have disabilities or special needs and provide assistive technology that promotes safe and independent living.

OCCUPATIONAL THERAPY PRACTICE FRAMEWORK

The Occupational Therapy Practice Framework (OTPF) was developed to assist practitioners in defining the process and domains of OT.[4] Although **AOTA's "Uniform Terminology for Occupational Therapy"**[8] gave OT practitioners a common language, the terminology did not provide consumers and practitioners with an understanding of the breadth of OT practice.

OTPF is designed to be used by occupational therapists, certified occupational therapists, consumers, and health care providers. Figure 1-1 illustrates the framework. It defines the process of OT as a dynamic, ongoing process that includes evaluation, intervention, and outcome. Evaluation provides an understanding of the clients' problems, occupational history, patterns, and assets.[4] Intervention includes the plan (based on selected theories, frames of reference, and evidence), implementation, and review. Outcome refers to how well the goals are achieved. The domain of OT practice is occupation, which is defined as "activities...of everyday life, named, organized, and given value and meaning by individuals and a culture. Occupation is everything people do to occupy themselves, including looking after themselves, enjoying life, and contributing to the social and economic fabric of their communities."[11] Occupation is viewed as a means and an end.[4] Using occupation as a means includes such things as participating in school activities to improve the ability to function in the school; it follows the "learning by doing" philosophy. Occupation is also viewed as an end in that the goal of therapy sessions is to enable the child to function in his or her occupations. For example, therapy sessions focusing on handwriting skills are intended to improve the child's ability to function in an academic occupation.

The OTPF defines the areas of occupation as activities of daily living (ADLs), instrumental activities of daily living (IADLs), education, work, play, leisure, and social participation.[4] Clinicians examine performance skills (motor, processing and communication) and patterns (habits, routines, roles) associated with the areas of occupation. Clinicians analyze the demands of activities and client factors required for the occupation in order to develop intervention plans. Client factors include all the body structures and functions and include many of the components from Uniform Terminology. However, the OTPF emphasizes the focus of the occupation instead of its components. Equally important is an examination of the contexts in which the occupation occurs. The OTPF identifies these contexts as cultural, physical, social, personal, spiritual, temporal, and virtual.

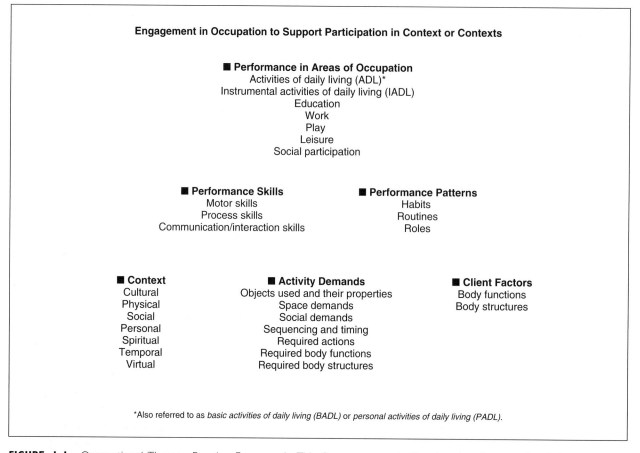

Engagement in Occupation to Support Participation in Context or Contexts

■ Performance in Areas of Occupation
Activities of daily living (ADL)*
Instrumental activities of daily living (IADL)
Education
Work
Play
Leisure
Social participation

■ Performance Skills
Motor skills
Process skills
Communication/interaction skills

■ Performance Patterns
Habits
Routines
Roles

■ Context
Cultural
Physical
Social
Personal
Spiritual
Temporal
Virtual

■ Activity Demands
Objects used and their properties
Space demands
Social demands
Sequencing and timing
Required actions
Required body functions
Required body structures

■ Client Factors
Body functions
Body structures

*Also referred to as *basic activities of daily living (BADL)* or *personal activities of daily living (PADL).*

FIGURE 1-1 Occupational Therapy Practice Framework. This figure represents the domain of occupational therapy and is included to allow readers to visualize it with all of its various aspects. No one aspect is intended to be perceived as more important than another. (From the American Occupational Therapy Association: *Occupational therapy practice framework: domain and process,* Bethesda, Md, 2002, The Association.)

See Table 1-1 for definitions of the terms. Contexts influence how the occupation is viewed, performed, and evaluated. For example, when considering the temporal context, practitioners would expect differences in social behavior between 2- and 16-year-old children.

OCCUPATIONAL THERAPY MODELS OF PRACTICE

A **model of practice** helps OT practitioners organize their thinking.[12] For example, practitioners using the Model of Human Occupation know that they must find out information concerning volition (e.g., the child's or parents' goals), habituation (e.g., how the child spends the day), performance (e.g., the physical skills and abilities of the child), and environment (e.g., the physical layout of the home). Therapists using the Person-Environment Occupational Performance model will organize their thinking into information about the child (e.g., the child's physical abilities), the environment (e.g., where the child attends school) and occupational performance (e.g., how the child is performing his/her daily occupations). Other commonly used pediatric models of practice include Occupational Adaptation, Spatiotemporal Adaptation, and Canadian Occupational Performance.

Models of practice provide practitioners with a framework for thinking and arranging their materials. They help practitioners focus on factors that influence functioning. Models of practice are developed from OT theory and philosophy. As such they fit with the OTPF in their emphasis on occupation. See Table 1-2 for an overview of selected models of practice.

SELECTED OCCUPATIONAL THERAPY FRAMES OF REFERENCE

Once practitioners have gained information by using a model of practice, they must decide how to intervene. **Frames of reference** (FORs) are used to direct OT intervention. They inform practitioners on what to do[12] and are based on theory, research, and clinical experience. FORs define populations for which they are suitable,

TABLE 1-1

*Definitions of Contexts**

CONTEXT	DEFINITION	EXAMPLE
Cultural	Customs, beliefs, activity patterns, behavior standards, and expectations accepted by the society of which the individual is a member. Includes political aspects, such as laws that affect access to resources and affirm personal rights. Also includes opportunities for education, employment, and economic support.	Ethnicity, family attitude, beliefs, values
Physical	Nonhuman aspects of contexts. Includes accessibility to and performance within environments having natural terrain, plants, animals, buildings, furniture, objects, tools, or devices.	Objects, built environment, natural environment, geographic terrain, sensory qualities of environment
Social	Availability and expectations of significant individuals, such as spouse, friends, and caregivers. Also includes larger social groups that are influential in establishing norms, role expectations, and social routines.	Relationships with individuals, groups, or organizations; relationships with systems (political, economic, institutional)
Personal	"[F]eatures of the individual that are not part of a health condition or health status" (WHO, 2001, p 17). Personal context includes age, gender, socioeconomic status, and educational status.	25-year-old unemployed
Spiritual	The fundamental orientation of a person's life; that which inspires and motivates the individual.	Essence of a person, greater or higher purpose, meaning, substance
Temporal	"Location of occupational performance in time" (Neistadt and Crepeau, 1998, p 292).	Stages of life, time of day, time of year, duration
Virtual	Environment in which communication occurs by means of airways or computers and an absence of physical contact.	Realistic simulation of an environment, chat rooms, radio transmissions

*Context (including cultural, physical, social, personal, spiritual, temporal, and virtual) refers to a variety of interrelated conditions within and surrounding the client that influence performance. Some of the definitions for areas of context or contexts are from the rescinded *Uniform terminology for occupational therapy*, ed 3, Bethesda, Md, 1994, The Association.
From the American Occupational Therapy Association: *Occupational therapy practice framework: domain and process*, Bethesda, Md, 2002, The Association.

describe the continuum of function and dysfunction, provide assessment tools, describe treatment modalities and intervention techniques, define the role of the practitioner, and suggest outcome measures. A FOR helps the OT practitioner identify problems and develop solutions.[10] Common pediatric FORs in OT are developmental, sensory integration, biomechanical, sensorimotor, motor control, and rehabilitative. See Table 1-3 for an overview.

Practitioners may choose to use a variety of FORs. However, they should be cautious in choosing an appropriate one and be clear about the theories and methodologies used with the given FOR. In cases when intervention does not progress as planned, practitioners adhering to one FOR may explore other suggested intervention techniques or change to another FOR. Intervention techniques are based on evidence from research. Given the need for evidence-based intervention, clinicians adhering to an FOR are using techniques investigated through research. Therefore, practitioners must keep themselves informed by reading and critically analyzing current research literature.

Developmental Approach

Corey is a 2-year-old boy diagnosed with global developmental delays. Corey attends an early intervention center twice weekly for 2 hours of "group" time and 1 hour weekly for direct OT services. Roanna, the COTA, works with Corey and provides activities for the family to continue at home. The OT evaluation, which is based on the Hawaii Early Learning Profile (HELP), revealed that Corey functions at a level between 16 and 20 months for most skills, with gross motor skills as a strength and fine motor and language skills as weak areas. Cognitively, he recognizes and points to four animal pictures (16-21), identifies himself in a mirror (15-16), identifies one body part (15-19), and searches for a

TABLE 1-2

Models of Practice

MODEL	AUTHOR(S)	COMPONENTS	PREMISES
Model of Human Occupation	Kielhofner	Volition Habituation Performance Environment	The human is an open system. Volition drives the system. The clinician's role is to understand the client in terms of these systems (and subsystems) and intervene to facilitate engagement in occupations.
Canadian Occupational Performance Model	Canadian Occupational Therapy Association (Townsend et al)	Spirituality Occupation Context (institutional included)	The worth of the individual is central to this model. Spirituality is the core of a person. Thus, occupational therapy practitioners must understand the client's spirituality to facilitate engagement in occupations. Performance of occupations takes place within social, physical, and cultural environments.
Occupational Adaptation	Schkade and Schultz	Occupations Physical and emotional affords and presses	Helps people participate in their desired occupations by adapting the occupations or using other methods to perform them.
Person-Environment-Occupation	Law et al	Person Environment Occupation	Looks at the person in terms of physical, social, and emotional factors. The environment (context) influences the person and occupations. The environment includes culture. Occupations are the everyday things people do.

Kielhofner G: *A model of human occupation: theory and application,* ed 2, Baltimore, 1985, Williams & Wilkins; Law M, Cooper B, Stewart D, et al: The person-environment-occupation model: a transactive approach to occupational performance, *Can J Occup Ther* 63:9, 1996; Schkade JK, Schultz S: Occupational adaptation: toward a holistic approach in contemporary practice, Part I, *Am J Occup Ther* 46:829, 1992; Townsend E, Brintnell S, Staisey N: Developing guidelines for client-centered occupational therapy practice, *Can J Occup Ther* 57:69, 1990.

hidden object (17-18). Expressive language skills include saying no meaningfully (13-15), naming one or two familiar objects (13-18), and using 10 to 15 words spontaneously (15-17). Gross motor skills are solid to 20 months: Corey picks up a toy from the floor without falling (19-24), runs fairly well (18-24), and squats when playing (20-21). He does not walk upstairs independently (22-24) or jump in place (22-30). Fine motor skills include scattered ones to 18 months. Corey builds a tower with two cubes (12-16) and scribbles spontaneously (13-18). He uses both hands at midline (16-18) but has difficulty pointing with his index finger (12-16) and placing one round peg in a pegboard (12-15). Social-emotional skills included enjoying rough-and-tumble play (18-24), expressing affection (18-24), and showing toy preferences (12-18). Corey has developed self-help skills to 12 months. He holds a spoon and finger-feeds himself (9-12), naps once or twice each day (9-12), cooperates with dressing (10-12), and removes a hat (15-16).

The COTA designed intervention based on this developmental picture of Corey and the parents' concern that Corey is not "playing like his 30-month-old cousin." The overall goal of the intervention based on the developmental FOR is to facilitate the child's ability to perform age-appropriate tasks in the areas of self-care, play/leisure, education/work, and social participation. The developmental FOR approaches intervention at the level at which the child is currently functioning and requires that the clinician provide a slightly advanced challenge. Clinicians using the developmental FOR need a clear understanding of the logical progression of skills. A typical therapy session is illustrated by the following SOAP note. See Box 1-1 and Chapter 3 for additional information on SOAP notes.

S

His mother stated that Corey draws a line now.

O

Corey scribbled spontaneously, holding the crayon in a palmer grasp. He imitated a vertical stroke (18-24) consistently and a circular stroke 1 out of 5 times (20-24). Corey built a tower of 4 cubes (18-22). He pointed with his index finger on command (2 out of 5 times). Corey had difficulty isolating his index finger for finger games. Corey removed his socks (15-18), placed a hat on his

TABLE 1-3

Pediatric Frames of Reference

FRAME OF REFERENCE	REFERENCE(S)	PRINCIPLES	SAMPLE POPULATIONS	TREATMENT MODALITIES
Developmental	Llorens	Development occurs over time and between skills (e.g., gross and fine motor). Some children experience a gap in their development due to physical, emotional, and/or social trauma. The role of occupational therapy is to fill in this gap.	Down syndrome Mental retardation Failure to thrive Cerebral palsy Pervasive developmental disorder	Identify current level of functioning. Work on the next step to achieve the skill. Intervention includes practice, repetition, education, and modeling of skills.
Biomechanical	Pedretti and Paszuinielli	Improve strength, endurance, range of motion	Children with cardiac concerns Brachial plexus Cerebral palsy Juvenile rheumatoid arthritis Down syndrome	Strength: Increase weight of toys or repetitive use of objects. Endurance: Increase time engaged in occupatio Range of motion: Repetitively provide slow, sustained stretch to increase end range.
Sensory integration	Ayres	Children with sensory integration dysfunction have difficulty processing sensory information (vestibular, proprioceptive, tactile). Improvements in sensory processing lead to improved engagement in occupations.	Sensory integrative dysfunction Developmental coordination disorder Sensory modulation disorder Pervasive developmental disorder	Provide controlled sensory input to improve the child's ability to process sensory stimuli. Use of suspension equipment and the "just right challenge." Activities are child directed

head (16-18), and held a cup handle (12-15). He showed difficulty scooping food with a spoon (15-24) and continues to drink from a bottle (18-24).

A

Corey exhibits fine motor and self-care skills consistently to 18 months. He shows many emerging self-care skills. Corey is making progress in achieving age-appropriate skills for play, self-care, and academics.

P

At the clinic, Corey participates in group sessions, which are designed to facilitate social-emotional and play skills.

The parents were provided with developmental activities to engage in at home.

Corey will continue to receive weekly OT services to improve fine motor and self-care skills for play, self-care, and academics.

Roanna used the **developmental FOR** to treat Corey. She focused on fine motor and self-care skills because he was receiving group sessions to focus on social-emotional and play skills. Roanna designed the intervention sessions to be fun and playful and begin at the level at which Corey was functioning. She gradually increased the level

TABLE 1-3

Pediatric Frames of Reference—cont'd

FRAME OF REFERENCE	REFERENCE(S)	PRINCIPLES	SAMPLE POPULATIONS	TREATMENT MODALITIES
Motor control	*Shumway-Cooke*	Acquisition of motor skills is based on dynamic systems theory. (All systems, including sensory, motor, and cognitive, work on each other for movement to occur.)	Cerebral palsy Developmental coordination disorder Down syndrome	Task-oriented approach: Children learn motor skills best by repeating the occupations in the most natural settings, varying the requirements. They learn from their motor mistakes.
Neuro-developmental	Bobath Schoen and Anderson	Children learn motor patterns when they "feel" normal movement patterns.	Cerebral palsy Traumatic brain injury	Clinician uses handling techniques and key points of control to inhibit abnormal muscle tone and facilitate normal movement patterns. Children learn through "feeling" normal patterns and thus should not make motor mistakes.
Sensorimotor	Trombly (Rood)	Sensory input to change the muscle tone or promote a muscle contraction.	Cerebral palsy	Icing techniques, neutral warmth, slow stroking, and vibration are all techniques used in this approach.

Ayres AJ: *Sensory integration for the child,* Los Angeles, 1979, Western Psychological Services; Bobath B: Sensorimotor development, NDT Newsletter 7:1, 1975; Llorens LA: *Application of a developmental theory for health and rehabilitation,* Rockville, Md, 1976, The Association; Pedretti LW, Paszuinielli S: A frame of reference for occupational therapy in physical dysfunction. In Pedretti LW, Zoltan B, editors: *Occupational therapy: practice skills for physical dysfunction,* ed 3, St Louis, 1990, Mosby; Schoen S, Anderson J: Neurodevelopmental treatment frame of reference. In Kramer P, Hinojosa J, editors: *Frames of reference for pediatric occupational therapy,* Baltimore, 1973, Williams & Wilkins; Shumway-Cook A, Woolacott M: Motor control: issues and theories. In Shumway-Cook A, Woolacott M, editors: *Motor control: theory an practical applications,* ed 2, Baltimore, 2002, Lippincott Williams & Wilkins; Trombly CA: Rood approach. In Trombly CA, editor: *Occupational therapy for physical dysfunction,* ed 4, Baltimore, 1994, Williams & Wilkins.

of difficulty and provided developmentally appropriate activities for the parents to use at home.

CLINICAL *Pearl*

Parents love to receive developmental checklists. Clinicians may help the parents of children with special needs by developing simple checklists without age ranges, providing parents with activities and goals without the reminder that their child is behind the "typical" child. It is important that parents enjoy their children. Activities that are fun and successful are more likely to be practiced at home.

Sensory Integration Approach

Jamar is a 13-year-old boy with sensory integration dysfunction. His movements are awkward, and he has poor balance and coordination; associated reactions with effort are noted (such as both hands moving when he writes). Jamar shows poor eye-hand coordination, poor rhythmic skills, and poor body awareness. He also shows signs of poor tactile, vestibular, and proprioceptive processing. The OTR classified Jamar's dysfunction as poor motor planning and body awareness due to inadequate processing of vestibular input (vestibule-based somatodyspraxia).

Jamar is an intelligent child who has expressed the desire to "be smoother, learn to dance, and not be the last one in every

BOX 1-1

The SOAP Note Format of Documentation

S (SUBJECTIVE)
Information from client or family concerning feelings or beliefs

O (OBJECTIVE)
Therapist's observations or evaluations of client's performance

A (ASSESSMENT)
Summary of therapist's interpretation of client's progress and analysis of current treatment plan

P (PLAN)
Plan of action for continued treatment, including any modifications to current treatment plan

sport in gym." He has also described handwriting difficulties leading to lower grades in school.

Jamar is treated in OT by Jackie, a COTA with 10 years of experience in a community-based sports injury clinic. The following SOAP note describes a therapy session. The goal of Jamar's treatment sessions is to improve body awareness, vestibular processing, and overall quality of movement so that he will be more confident in his body. Sensory integration theory postulates that by improving the ability to process sensory information, the body's ability to plan and execute movements will improve. Ayres emphasized movement-related activities with the use of suspended equipment (to get the intensity needed) and the "just-right challenge."[9]

S

Jamar stated that there is a dance at school in 2 weeks.

O

Jamar was reluctant but participated in the fast-moving tire swing activity. He quickly became dizzy with the spinning and enjoyed bouncing into objects. Jamar had difficulty getting on new pieces of equipment. He "talked" his way through a difficult 5-step obstacle course. Jamar showed difficulty clapping to the rhythm (five beats before an error) while on the trampoline but was able to clap to the rhythm (20 beats without an error) when sitting on the platform swing. On hearing a noise he jumped into hoops placed randomly on the floor, showing some difficulty in sequencing and planning. Jamar was able to sequence and plan a difficult 3-step obstacle course that involved crawling, swinging, and throwing a ball at a target. He completed 10 minutes of the *Mavis* typing program with a 70% success rate and was able to imitate simple dance moves from song 1 of the *Twister Moves* game. Jamar was not able to successfully complete the dance moves and could not stay with the music after song 1.

A

Jamar exhibits difficulty with motor planning, sequencing, and timing of movements, interfering with his leisure activities (dancing) and academics (writing).

P

Jamar will continue with intensive sensory integration therapy to improve his processing of vestibular, proprioceptive, and tactile information for quality of movements and educational and leisure activities.

Jamar was provided with a homework assignment to select one song from *Twister Moves* and complete the dance steps from the game.

Jamar will complete a *Mavis* typing program at the eighth-grade level and use a laptop computer for writing assignments. He will discuss these activities with his parents and teacher.

Jackie, the COTA, used a **sensory integration frame of reference** to improve the motor planning, sequencing, and timing of movements. Jamar chose the activities, and the session was tailored to address his concern about looking good at the dance. Using goals that children pick themselves is empowering and gratifying to them. Furthermore, the child will work very hard to achieve these goals, making the likelihood of success greater. In this example, Jackie used suspended equipment to provide the intensity of input needed for a 13 year old. She also challenged Jamar to participate in a slightly uncomfortable activity. Children gain confidence when they succeed in activities they deem to be slightly "tougher." In this way, Jackie worked on Jamar's self-concept as well. Recommending the use of a laptop is not necessarily a sensory integration technique. However, Jamar is 13 years old and needs to be able to communicate in writing for success in school. Therefore, Jackie decided that it was time to move away from teaching writing skills and help Jamar perform his occupation.

CLINICAL *Pearl*

Ask children what they want to learn in therapy. This provides insight into intervention goals and shows them you are listening.

Biomechanical Approach

Abigail is a 14-month-old infant who suffered a left brachial plexus injury (i.e., damage to the nerves that control arm movement) during birth. She is treated by an OTR once every 2 weeks. Teresa, a COTA, visits Abigail twice a week to work on the goals that have been established by the OTR in collabora-

tion with the child's family. Abigail's long-term OT goals include (1) increasing active range of motion (AROM) in her left arm, (2) increasing the functional strength in her left arm, and (3) increasing her ability to use her left arm during age-appropriate activities such as playing with a toy and self-feeding. Abigail's treatment sessions with Teresa last 30 minutes. A typical therapy session is shown in the following daily progress note.

The goals of therapy sessions using a biomechanical FOR are to increase strength, endurance, and range of motion for occupations (e.g., play and self-care).

S

Her mother stated that Abigail enjoys the range-of-motion (ROM) exercises she does each day. She especially enjoys singing "Row, row, row your boat" during stretching exercises.

O

Abigail received a 30-minute therapy session in her home. Her mother and older brother were present for the entire session. AROM and passive range of motion (PROM) of Abigail's left arm were performed. Left shoulder AROM was 0° to 105° and PROM 0° to 180°. Activities included weight bearing on her extended (straightened) left arm for 1 minute while reaching for toys with her right arm. Abigail also reached for toys with her left arm while bearing weight on her right arm. Abigail spontaneously used her left arm as an assist while playing with a shape sorter.

A

Abigail actively participated in the activities throughout the session. Her ability to sustain weight on her left arm with minimum physical assistance has improved from 20-second to 1-minute intervals. Left shoulder AROM from 0° to 105° has shown an increase of 5° since last month.

P

Abigail will participate in OT twice weekly to work on improving left upper extremity functioning for play, self-care, and academic work. Specifically, her goals include (1) achieving full AROM for the left upper extremity, (2) strengthening her left arm to lift objects, and (3) spontaneously using the left upper extremity as an assist.

Teresa used the **biomechanical frame of reference** to treat Abigail. It is used with children who have orthopedic (i.e., bone, joint, or muscle) problems such as hand injuries or lower motor neuron disorders (affecting the nerve connections outside the central nervous system [CNS]) such as brachial plexus injuries. The goals of the biomechanical approach are to (1) assess physical limitations on the client's ROM, muscle strength, and endurance; (2) improve ROM, strength, and endurance; and (3) prevent or reduce contracture and deformities.[10] This approach focuses on the specific physical limitations that interfere with the client's ability to engage in the occupational performance areas of ADLs, play and leisure activities, and work and productive activities. Teresa will work on the overall goal of improving Abigail's ability to use both arms for play, self-care, and academics.

CLINICAL *Pearl*

Biomechanical techniques such as ROM, strength, and endurance can be easily integrated into play sessions. Singing songs is a great technique in making the sessions playful while working on biomechanical goals to improve occupational performance.

Sensorimotor Approach

Raja is a 4-year-old child who has been diagnosed with spastic right hemiplegia cerebral palsy. A brain lesion caused abnormal muscle tone on the right side of her body, which prevents her from properly using the right arm and leg. She is receiving outpatient OT services at the local hospital; her mother usually brings her to the clinic. Raja recently had a phenol alcohol nerve block—an injection into the nerves that innervate the arm—to help reduce the increased flexor tone in her right arm. Because of the recent changes in Raja's right arm, Alejandro, the OTR, is currently providing all of the direct OT services. His sessions with Raja usually last 45 minutes. A typical therapy session is shown in the following daily SOAP note.

The goal of therapy sessions with a sensorimotor FOR is to improve movement patterns for occupations (e.g., academics, self-care, and play).

S

Her mother stated that Raja's right arm is easier to wash and the elbow is straighter since the nerve block.

O

Raja arrived this morning eager to work on the therapy ball. She performed activities on the therapy ball while lying on her stomach and bearing weight on her elbows, followed by bearing weight on her extended arms. Alejandro performed tapping—using the fingertips to deliver successive light blows to the muscle belly—over the triceps to facilitate full extension (straightening) of Raja's elbow. (The triceps muscle is primarily responsible for elbow extension.) Raja participated in bilateral hand activities, such as fastening large buttons and creating pictures using finger paint. When necessary, the wrist extensor muscles were stroked to encourage maintenance of a functional wrist position (e.g., wrist extension while grasping) during the bilateral tasks. Raja fastened five large buttons in 2 minutes.

A
Raja's ability to use her right arm has improved, as shown by her ability to fasten five large buttons while her wrist is extended.
P
Raja will receive OT weekly to work on increasing right arm functioning for self-care, academics, and play.

Alejandro is using a **sensorimotor frame of reference** to treat Raja. This type of approach involves the use of sensory input to change muscle tone and movement patterns in infants, children, and adolescents who have CNS damage.[10] Several types of sensorimotor approach are used by OT practitioners. Because their use requires skill and experience, entry-level OTRs and COTAs should be closely supervised while using them.

Motor Control Approach

Talasi is a 6-year-old child who shows a slight intention tremor in her right arm and walks with a wide-based gait. She performs the skills expected of her age, yet the quality of the movement is poor and she falls often. She is unable to keep up with her peers on the playground, is slow in getting dressed/undressed, frequently has her clothes on backwards, and spills food and drink during mealtimes. Her parents are concerned that she is "falling behind" in school because she is forgetful and disorganized. Brian is the COTA responsible for treating Talasi at school. The following SOAP note describes a therapy session with a motor control FOR to improve Talasi's quality of movement for play, academics, and self-care.

S
Talasi stated that she is having a bad day. She forgot her "show and tell" book from her Grammy.
O
Talasi participated in a game of "dress-up." She put on a sweater and pants, buttoned them, and then removed them. Talasi dressed her doll and played a timed game of dress-up. She played eye-hand games using beanbags, targets, and catching a ball. The placement of the targets, the speed, and her position in relation to the target varied. Talasi balanced herself for 1 minute on the right foot with eyes open and 5 seconds with eyes closed. She drank her juice without spilling it but did spill applesauce from a spoon. An intention tremor was noted in her right arm during spoon feeding. Talasi was instructed to hold the spoon closer to the bowl. A weighted spoon eased some of the tremor and resulted in less spilling.
A
Talasi demonstrates poor quality of movement, an intention tremor in her right arm, and slow movements interfering with her functioning in school, play, and self-care.
P
Talasi will receive OT weekly to work on increasing the quality of movement for self-care, academics, and play.

Brian used the **motor control frame of reference** to improve Talasi's quality of movement. This FOR follows a task-oriented approach that encourages the repetition of desired movements in a variety of settings and circumstances. For example, Talasi practiced dressing herself with large clothing and a small doll. Both of these tasks work on dressing/undressing skills. Motor control theory promotes a practice approach. The clinician provides verbal feedback but allows the child to perform the task and learn from his or her mistakes. For example, Brian allowed Talasi to feed herself; then he instructed her on a different technique, which she practiced. Finally, Brian used a weighted spoon to see if this would decrease the tremor and thus the spilling.

Motor control theories support using activities that motivate the child and resemble the actual task as close as possible. Imagery and practice are intervention techniques used in a motor control approach.

CLINICAL *Pearl*

Motor control refers to the study of movements. Current studies suggest that participating in the actual task in a variety of situations that require adapted responses results in the best motor learning, which is consistent with OT practice. Furthermore, research supports the use of "meaningful" activity over rote exercise. Imagery has also been found to be effective in motor learning. The intervention techniques support OT philosophy and practice, focusing on occupation.

Rehabilitative Approach

Dewayne is a 6-year-old child whose left arm is amputated below the elbow as the result of a car accident 2 years ago. Dewayne goes to a Shriner hospital in another town for the fitting of his prosthesis, or artificial limb, and training in its use. He has outgrown his old prosthesis and is meeting with Missy, a COTA, to work on using and caring for his new artificial arm and learn activities that will improve his ability to use it functionally. A typical therapy session is shown in the following daily SOAP note.

S
Dewayne said that his new arm feels good.
O
Dewayne was treated in the OT department for prosthetic training and home and family instruction on its care. The department's Prosthetic Checklist was completed during

the session. No red areas were noted. Dewayne's father was shown how to don and doff the stump sock and new artificial arm; he demonstrated the process as well. Dewayne dressed and undressed himself using the artificial arm. He stabilized a paper with the prosthetic arm and wrote with his right hand.

A

The new artificial arm fits well. Dewayne and his father demonstrated knowledge of care and fitting of the prosthesis. Dewayne is able to engage in age-appropriate self-care and writing activities while using his prosthesis.

P

Dewayne is discharged from Shriner's Hospital. He will be followed by an OTR at school.

Missy used the **rehabilitative frame of reference** to treat Dewayne. This FOR is used after an injury or illness to return a person to the highest possible level of functional independence as well as teach any compensatory methods that may be needed to perform certain activities.[10] Because many children are born with disabilities, OT practitioners are required in some cases to teach new skills (habilitate) instead of teach previously known skills (rehabilitate). However, for cases in which a child acquires a disability after birth, a rehabilitative approach is appropriate. The methods used during rehabilitation and habilitation include the following:

- Self-care evaluation and training
- Acquisition and training in the use of assistive devices
- Prosthetic use training
- Wheelchair management training
- Architectural and environmental adaptation training
- Acquisition and training in the use of augmentative communication devices and assistive technology
- Play assessment and intervention

An OT practitioner who is using a rehabilitative or habilitative approach focuses on skill acquisition in the occupational performance areas of ADLs, play and leisure skills, and work and productive activities.

THE OCCUPATIONAL THERAPY PROCESS

The OT practitioner uses a model of practice to organize thinking and chooses a FOR to design intervention based on the child's and family's needs. The FOR helps the practitioner decide what to do during the therapy sessions. The OT process begins when a referral for OT services is made by a parent, physician, teacher, or other concerned professional. The OTR decides whether the referred client should be screened, which helps him or her determine whether the client will benefit from OT services. If the screening shows that the client is likely to benefit from OT services, then an evaluation is done. The OTR decides the areas to be evaluated and assigns portions of the evaluation to the COTA. The evaluation process helps the OTR identify the client's strengths and weaknesses. Long-term goals and short-term objectives are established based on the OTR's interpretation of the assessment. In collaboration with the COTA, the OTR develops an intervention plan based on these goals and objectives. The plan is implemented and modified based on the client's progress and periodic reassessments. Intervention is designed to address the goals and objectives based on a selected FOR. There may be more than one FOR that works with a client. It is the responsibility of the practitioner to determine which FOR is the best match for the client. When deciding on a FOR, clinicians consider the diagnosis, time period, setting, their clinical expertise, and current evidence-based research as well as the client's goals. Clinicians must keep informed on the current research and intervention strategies to develop effective intervention for the children they serve. The client is discharged when all of the goals and objectives are met or the OTR determines that services should be discontinued. (For a more detailed discussion of the occupational therapy process, see Chapter 9.)

ROLES OF THE REGISTERED OCCUPATIONAL THERAPIST AND CERTIFIED OCCUPATIONAL THERAPY ASSISTANT

The OTR is responsible for all aspects of the OT process and supervises the COTA. The extent to which the COTA is supervised by the OTR depends on a variety of factors, including the knowledge, skill, and experience of the COTA. In any case, OTRs and COTAs are both considered OT practitioners, and therefore they share the responsibility of communicating with each other about their clients.[1,7]

QUALIFICATIONS, SUPERVISION, AND SERVICE COMPETENCY

Entry-level COTAs must meet basic qualifications to practice in the field of OT. As they gain experience by working with OTRs, COTAs require less supervision and gradually become more competent at providing occupational therapy services.

Qualifications

Entry-level COTAs meet specific qualifications, which include having successfully completed course work in an AOTA-accredited school and having passed the certification examination administered by the National

Board for Certification in Occupational Therapy (NBCOT). In addition, COTAs must meet specific requirements established by OT regulatory boards in their respective states and obtain a license if required by state law.

Supervision

Four **levels of supervision** have been delineated by AOTA: close, routine, general, and minimal. Close supervision is direct, daily contact between the COTA and OTR at the work site. Routine supervision is direct contact between the COTA and OTR at the work site at least every 2 weeks and interim contact through other means, such as telephone conversations or e-mail messages. General supervision is minimum direct contact of 1 day per month and interim supervision as needed. Minimum supervision is that provided on an "as needed" basis. It is important to note that individual state OT regulatory agencies may require stricter guidelines than those established by AOTA. Stricter state guidelines supersede those of the AOTA.[1,2,5,7]

The level of supervision that COTAs require varies with their level of expertise. AOTA defines three levels of expertise: entry, intermediate, and advanced. COTAs' progress from one level to another is based on their acquisition of skills, knowledge, and proficiency and not on their years of experience. Entry-level COTAs are typically new graduates or those entering into a new practice setting. Intermediate-level COTAs have acquired a higher level of skill through experience, continuing education, and involvement in professional activities. Advanced-level COTAs have specialized skills and may be recognized as experts in particular areas of practice. Although the extent to which a particular COTA is supervised varies according to the individual, the level of supervision generally falls into one defined by AOTA based on the COTA's expertise. An entry-level COTA requires close supervision, an intermediate-level COTA requires routine or general supervision, and an advanced-level COTA requires minimum supervision (see Table 1-4).[12]

Service Competency

Levels of supervision are closely related to establishing **service competency.** AOTA's definition of service competency is "the determination, made by various methods, that two people performing the same or equivalent procedures will obtain the same or equivalent results."[1,2,5,7] Service competency is a means of ensuring that two individual OT practitioners will have the same results when administering a specific assessment, observing a specific performance area or component, or providing treatment. Communication between COTAs and OTRs is an essential part of the entire OT process but is especially important when establishing service competency. OTRs must be sure that they and the COTAs are performing assessments and treatment procedures in the same way. Once an OTR has determined that a particular COTA has established service competency in a certain area, the COTA may be allowed to perform an assessment or treatment procedure (within the parameters of that particular area) without close OTR supervision. Ensuring service competency is an ongoing mutual learning experience.

AOTA has specific guidelines for establishing service competency. For standardized assessments and treatment procedures that require no specific training to administer, the OTR and COTA both perform the procedure. If they obtain equivalent results, the COTA can be allowed to administer subsequent procedures independently. For assessments and treatment procedures requiring more subjective interpretations, direct observation and videotaping are valuable tools that can be used to establish service competency. These tools allow practitioners to observe a client performing a particular task and compare their individual interpretations of the performance. Likewise, an OTR can videotape a client, have a COTA watch the tape, and compare and contrast the observations that have been made. If the OTR and COTA consistently have similar interpretations, the COTA has established competency in observing and interpreting the particular area of performance.[1,2,5,7] Specific examples of establishing service competency are provided below.

Videotaping

Teresa is the previously mentioned COTA who used the biomechanical approach to treat Abigail's brachial plexus injury. Before working with Abigail, Teresa watched a videotape of her supervising OTR treating another child who had a brachial plexus injury. She discussed the tape with the OTR, which revealed that she understood the treatment procedures used. Abigail's next therapy session, which was led by Teresa, was videotaped. The OTR watched the tape and observed that Teresa carefully positioned the child and successfully carried out the treatment plan. The OTR determined that Teresa had established the service competency needed to treat Abigail. The OTR and Teresa agreed that as part of the ongoing learning process they would videotape one of Abigail's treatment sessions each month.

Cotreatment

Raja is the previously mentioned 4 year old who was diagnosed with cerebral palsy and recently received a nerve block to decrease flexor tone in her right arm. Alejandro, the OTR, has been treating him since the nerve block was performed. Alejandro recently asked Richard, a COTA, to assist him in treating Raja. Richard prepared for cotreatment by reading about nerve blocks and carefully observing Alejandro's one-on-one treatment session with Raja.

TABLE 1-4

Supervision of the Certified Occupational Therapy Assistant

LEVEL OF SUPERVISION	TYPE OF SUPERVISION
Close	Direct and daily contact; on-site supervision
Routine	Direct and regularly scheduled contact; on-site supervision
General	Indirect supervision as needed and direct contact once per month or as mandated by state regulatory board
Minimum	Direct and indirect supervision as needed or as mandated by state regulatory board

Richard asked pertinent questions and expressed a keen interest in working with Raja. After several successful cotreatment sessions in which Alejandro and Richard obtained equivalent outcomes from the treatment procedures used, Alejandro assigned Raja's case to Richard. Richard now receives only general supervision from Alejandro because he demonstrated service competency while working with Raja.

Observation

Missy, a COTA, used the rehabilitative approach to treat Dewayne, the 6 year old who sustained an amputation below the elbow. Before becoming a COTA, Missy volunteered regularly at the Shriner hospital. She observed many clients being fitted with prostheses. After graduation she was hired to work in the OT department at the hospital. As a COTA she worked closely with the OTR, who developed treatment plans for clients with injuries similar to those of Dewayne. Missy also observed and assisted in administering the department's Prosthetic Checklist, which is designed to assess prosthetic care, application and use. Missy began working with Dewayne when the child was fitted for his first prosthesis at the age of 3. The OTR observed Missy administering the Prosthetic Checklist; the findings were equivalent. When Dewayne was fitted with a new prosthesis, the OTR was confident Missy could independently complete the checklist accurately. Missy demonstrated service competency in administering the assessment.

SUMMARY

This chapter presented an overview of pediatric OT practice, with particular focus on the COTA. An overview of the OT practice framework and models is followed by a discussion of the developmental, sensory integration, biomechanical, motor control, sensorimotor, and rehabilitative FORs. The areas of proficiency for the entry-level COTA are followed by a discussion of his or her qualifications and levels of supervision. The roles of the OTR and COTA are defined, and service competency and the means of establishing it are presented. Finally, specific examples illustrate how the FORs, levels of supervision, and service competency are used in the delivery of OT services within the realm of the OT Practice Framework.

References

1. American Occupational Therapy Association: Entry-level role delineation for registered occupational therapists (OTRs) and certified occupational therapy assistants (COTAs), *Am J Occup Ther* 44:1091, 1990.
2. American Occupational Therapy Association: Guide for supervision of occupational therapy personnel, *Am J Occup Ther* 48:1045, 1994.
3. American Occupational Therapy Association: *Guidelines for curriculum content in pediatrics*, Bethesda, Md, 1991, The Association.
4. American Occupational Therapy Association: *Occupational therapy practice framework: domain and process*, Bethesda, Md, 2002, The Association.
5. American Occupational Therapy Association: Occupational therapy roles, *Am J Occup Ther* 47:1087, 1993.
6. American Occupational Therapy Association: *Revision of guidelines for pediatric curriculum content for occupational therapy*, Bethesda, Md, 1998, The Association.
7. American Occupational Therapy Association: Supervision guidelines for certified occupational therapy assistants, *Am J Occup Ther* 44:1089, 1990.
8. American Occupational Therapy Association: Uniform terminology for occupational therapy, *Am J Occup Ther* 48:1047, 1994.
9. Ayres AJ: *Sensory integration for the child*, Los Angeles, 1979, Western Psychological Services.
10. Early MB: *Physical dysfunction skills for the occupational therapy assistant*, St Louis, 1998, Mosby.
11. Law M, Baptiste S, McColl M, et al: The Canadian occupational performance measure: an outcome measure for occupational therapy, *Can J Occup Ther* 57:82, 1990.
12. MacRae N: *OT 301: Foundations of occupational therapy*, Unpublished lecture notes, 2001, University of New England.
13. Rainville EB, Cermack SA, Murray EA: Supervision and consultation for pediatric occupational therapists, *Am J Occup Ther* 50:725, 1996.
14. Steib PA: Top employment settings for COTAs, *OT Week* 10:18, 1996.

15. World Health Organization: *International classification of functioning disability and health* (ICF), Geneva, Switzerland, 2001.
16. Neistadt ME, Crepeau EB, editors: *Willard & Spackman's occupational therapy*, ed 9, Philadelphia 1998, Lippincott Williams & Wilkins.

Recommended Reading

Kramer P, Hinojosa J, editors: *Frames of reference for pediatric occupational therapy*, ed 2, Philadelphia, 1999, Lippincott Williams & Wilkins.

Crepeau EB, Cohn ES, Boyt Schell BA, editors: *Willard & Spackman's occupational therapy*, ed 10, Philadelphia, 2003, Lippincott Williams & Wilkins.

REVIEW *Questions*

1. List and describe five content areas in which a pediatric OT practitioner needs to have knowledge while working with children and adolescents.
2. Describe the guidelines for evaluation and intervention discussed in the OTPF.
3. What is a model of practice? Why are models of practice useful to OT practitioners?
4. What is a FOR? What information does it provide?
5. What are the primary concerns that OT practitioners have while using the developmental, biomechanical, sensorimotor, motor learning, and rehabilitation FORs?
6. What is service competency? How is it established?

SUGGESTED *Activities*

1. In small groups, list and discuss daily living and play activities that you think would be appropriate while working with Abigail, Raja, and Dewayne. How do the chosen activities relate to the biomechanical, sensorimotor, and/or rehabilitative frame(s) of reference?
2. Interview a COTA or OTR who works in pediatrics. The focus of the interview should be supervision and service competency. Questions might include the following.
   (a) Which courses in school have been the most useful to you as a pediatric OT practitioner?
   (b) How many years of clinical experience do you have?
   (c) What is the level of supervision that you receive (COTA) or give (OTR)? What are the means by which this occurs?
   (d) How is service competency established between the OTR and the COTA in your workplace?

2

Family Systems

PAMELA J. WINTON
ROBERT E. WINTON

CHAPTER *Objectives*

After studying this chapter, the reader will be able to accomplish the following:

- Describe the reason it is important for an occupational therapy practitioner to have knowledge of and skills related to working with families
- Describe the differences between the prescriptive and consultative professional roles
- Understand the way a therapy program for a child always has an impact on the family unit
- Describe the key concepts of family systems and life cycle theories and the roles of these concepts in intervention with children
- Recognize and appreciate that all families have unique ways of adapting and coping with life events and that effective therapy builds on these existing coping strategies
- Describe several communication strategies that an occupational therapy practitioner can use to promote familial-professional partnerships

KEY TERMS

- Domain
- Client-centered
- Prescriptive
- Consultative
- Morphostatic principle
- Morphogenetic principle
- Equifinality
- Consultative and prescriptive professional roles
- Life cycle
- Normative life cycle events
- Non-normative life cycle events
- Adaptation
- Resources
- Perceptual coping strategies
- Acknowledgment

CHAPTER OUTLINE

Margarita Sanchez is a 3-year-old child who has been diagnosed with pervasive developmental delays and mild to moderate cerebral palsy. She lives in a small apartment with her paternal grandmother, great aunt, parents, and three siblings who are 11 months, 5 years, and 6 years of age. When Heather McFall, the occupational therapy (OT) practitioner, arrives for a routine visit, she learns that Margarita's mother has not been working with Margarita on the toilet training program that was discussed during the last visit. Heather had recommended that they start the program because she thought it was important that Margarita be toilet trained in time to begin a public school prekindergarten program in the fall. After some discussion, it becomes apparent that in the winter Mrs. Sanchez is unable to deal with the wet, soiled clothes that invariably accompany a toilet training program. After further discussion, Heather and Mrs. Sanchez agree to wait until the weather gets warmer to begin toilet training. During their conversation, Heather also realizes that she needs to plan a time for the Sanchez family to visit the prekindergarten classroom and see what they think of the program. Although Heather is enthusiastic about the academic and social experiences that Margarita would have in the classroom, Mrs. Sanchez seems hesitant and uncharacteristically quiet when they talk about the program. Heather has learned that Mrs. Sanchez becomes quiet when she has reservations about an idea.

As Heather leaves the apartment, she thinks about her relationship with the family and how it has developed during the 2 years she has been working with Margarita. At the beginning of the relationship, Heather was often frustrated by Mrs. Sanchez's seeming disinterest in or inability to follow through with some of the home program ideas that Heather introduced. She had fretted and fumed and tried to help Mrs. Sanchez see the importance of taking Margarita's needs seriously and devoting the necessary time to therapy. It was only after discussing the case with a colleague that Heather realized she had departed from the guidelines of the Occupational Therapy Practice Framework published in 2002.[2] *She had gotten caught up in her own expertise in the* **domain** *of occupational therapy and had strayed from a* **client-centered*** *consultative process. As she remembered this, she laughed to herself as she recognized that she had "done it again" with the toilet training directive. She was also happy that she had recovered her client-centered role and had helped Mrs. Sanchez develop a plan that incorporated some of her ideas into the family routines. Mrs. Sanchez's quiet response also clued her in to the fact that she had departed from the client-centered consultative role related to the preschool issue. She resolved that on the next visit she would attempt to remain client centered as she revisited the idea of preschool.*

BOX 2-1

Reasons Families Are Important

- A family has a significant environmental influence on a young child's life and development.
- Interventions with children inevitably affect the family.
- Laws and current service delivery models promote a family-centered approach.
- Professional organizations, including the American Occupational Therapy Association, have identified the areas of competency and created recommended guidelines for working with families.

THE IMPORTANCE OF FAMILIES

The vignette of Margarita and her family underscores the reason it is important for OT practitioners to understand family systems. Box 2-1 contains the key reasons why using a family-centered approach is recommended in early intervention when working with young children who have disabilities.

Families have the most *significant* environmental influence on a young child's life and development. As evident in the previous story, the majority of Margarita's time is spent with her family. If the family members are not convinced of the benefits of therapy or are unable to find time to carry out the intervention plan, Margarita is unlikely to improve optimally. As interventionists, OT practitioners enter children's lives for relatively brief periods of time. Family members are the "constants" in most children's lives.

The OT practitioner may function in two distinct roles in his/her involvement with a family. They may be called **prescriptive** and **consultative**: When working directly with the child, s/he is primarily in the prescriptive and directive role; when working with the family, s/he is primarily in the consultative role. Consulting with the family on the possibility of achieving the desired goals for the child and family builds the collaboration and trust that are key ingredients for intervention success with families.

CLINICAL *Pearl*

Developing a trusting and collaborative relationship with families is a key ingredient for intervention success.

Interventions with children have an inevitable impact on family life; therefore, they are the most effective when the family is consulted and invests in the development of the treatment plan. Margarita's story reveals the

* The *Occupational Therapy Practice Framework: Domain and Process*[2] defines the term "client" as the individual or the individual within the context of a group (i.e., a family). The terms "client-centered" and "family-centered" are used interchangeably in this manuscript.

importance of thinking about the family as a whole. It also illustrates the advantages of the occupational therapist being in a family-centered, consultative role, one that acknowledges and supports a family's central function in the design and implementation of intervention plans. Margarita's therapist learned the importance of this concept when she struggled with getting the family to use the adaptive high chair. She was also reminded of its importance in her initial failed attempt to help the family institute a toilet training program and again with the idea of preschool for Margarita.

The family-centered approach is also the focus of many current laws and health care delivery models. The passage of Public Law 99-457 in 1986 (IDEA, Part C) is considered revolutionary because of its emphasis on the central role a family plays in interventions with young children. This law and its subsequent interpretations have altered the way in which services for young children are planned and delivered. Some of the highlights of the early intervention component of the law include the following: (1) families are mandated co-leaders on state-level advisory boards that make recommendations about the way in which service systems are designed; (2) family concerns, resources, and priorities guide the development of individual intervention plans; (3) families play an important role in children's assessments and evaluations; and (4) families have certain rights to confidentiality, record keeping, notification, and other procedures related to the programs and agencies that serve their children. The law ushered in additional changes that ultimately benefit families, such as promoting interdisciplinary and interagency collaboration. It was clear that collaboration among agencies and disciplines was needed when numerous stories surfaced about families receiving conflicting advice and recommendations from various health care professionals about their children's disabilities.[6]

BOX 2-2

American Occupational Therapy Association Guidelines for Curriculum Content in Pediatrics

ACADEMIC AND LEVEL I FIELDWORK

Family Systems Theory
The way families operate as units, the impact of diverse cultures and child-rearing patterns on family life, and differences in child rearing

Family Life Cycle
Critical stages of family life and parenting

Family Ecology
The way family systems operate in society, including the immediate community and the state and federal systems

Effects of Disabilities on Families
The emotional and social impact of an infant, toddler, child, or youth with disabilities on the parents' and family's life

Effects of Family and Environment on Children with Disabilities
The impact of different family styles and environments on an infant, toddler, child, or youth with disabilities

Role of Occupational Therapy
The role of the occupational therapist in helping a family assess their concerns and priorities for intervention; the use of self-reporting instruments in OT

LEVEL II PEDIATRIC FIELDWORK (FOR ENTRY-LEVEL PRACTICE)

Rapport
The way to establish rapport with caregivers; the role of the occupational therapist as a partner in treatment planning

Collaboration
Strategies for having collaborative consultations with infants, toddlers, children, or youths with disabilities and their caregivers

Adapted from the American Occupational Therapy Association Commission on Education: *Guidelines for curriculum content in pediatrics,* Bethesda, Md, 1991, The Association.

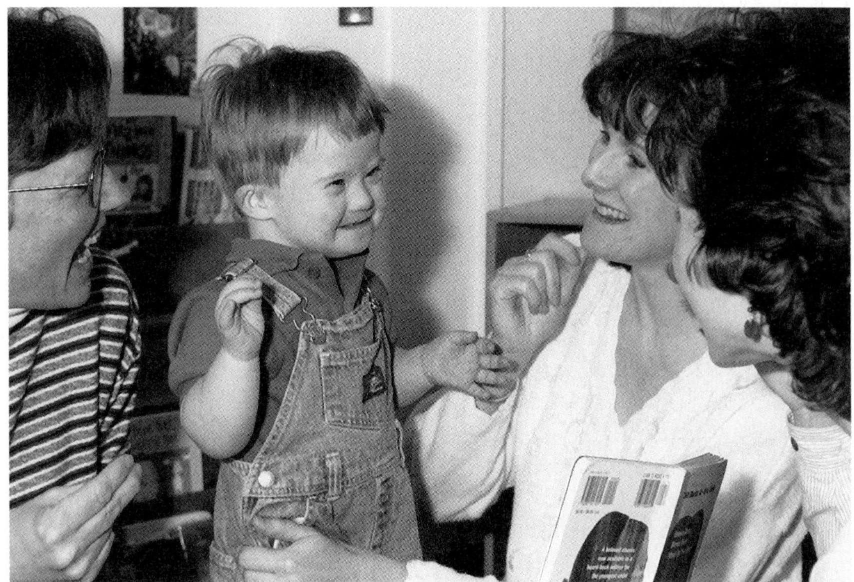

FIGURE 2-1 Therapist working with the mother, child, and early-childhood teacher at a daycare center. This is an example of interdisciplinary collaboration and embedding therapy into the daily routine. (Courtesy Don Trull, FPG Child Development Institute, University of North Carolina—Chapel Hill, Chapel Hill, NC.)

Professional organizations, including the American Occupational Therapy Association (AOTA), have identified particular areas of competency and recommended certain guidelines to emphasize the importance of practitioners having the skills and knowledge necessary to work effectively with families.[1] The dramatic changes in the relationship between families and professionals catalyzed by Public Law 99–457 and the increased focus on the importance of families in all human service organizations have not developed overnight. The existing workforce has had to develop new collaboration and communication skills. University and community college training programs have had to retrain their faculties and upgrade their curricula to prepare students adequately for the newly defined pediatric roles (Box 2-2).[3] Professional organizations have supported the changes by creating recommended practice guidelines and areas of competency.

CURRENT ISSUES AFFECTING OCCUPATIONAL THERAPY PRACTITIONERS AND FAMILIES

Changes in Policies and Service Delivery Models

As mentioned previously, policies and legislation passed during the last 15 years have affected service delivery models and recommended OT practices. The resulting changes have included emphasis on the following approaches to service delivery.

- Interdisciplinary and family-centered approaches are used when planning and implementing interventions.
- Children who have disabilities are included in regular educational settings.
- Therapists act as consultants, providing pediatric treatment that is integrated into the children's regular routines and natural environments instead of using "pull out therapy"* (Figure 2-1).

Expansion of Practitioners' Roles

Recent changes in service delivery and implementation have resulted in an expansion of the OT practitioners' roles. Their duties now also include the following:

- Assessing family interests, priorities, and concerns
- Observing and gathering information about the daily routines of the child and family and in the classrooms
- Gathering and sharing information with families about development and intervention strategies
- Implementing therapy in collaboration with parents, caregivers, and general educators

Demographic Changes in the U.S. Population

In addition to changes in laws, policies, and recommended practices, the demographic makeup of the children being

* "Pull out therapy" is therapy not provided in the context of a child's daily routine.

served has also changed. It is estimated that by the year 2080, the majority of Americans will be persons of color.[5] In contrast, although the U.S. population is becoming more diverse, the members of professional organizations such as AOTA and the American Speech and Hearing Association (ASHA) are predominantly Caucasian.[1,4]

Implications for Practice

The myriad changes taking place in the OT environment affect service delivery and implementation in numerous ways, including the following:

- OT practitioners are more likely than ever to be working with children and families whose cultural background and native language are different from their own. They may need to use translators or interpreters. They must develop the ability to appreciate and respect cultural differences, which may mean developing an awareness of their own cultural identity, the acknowledgment of inherent biases and values, and knowledge of other cultures.
- Young children who have disabilities are more likely than ever to be in regular early childhood and educational programs. OT practitioners must be able to embed therapy into the daily routines of the home, child care setting, and regular educational setting and must develop expertise in consulting with early-childhood teachers, families, and other specialists.
- OT practitioners need the knowledge and skill to work as members of interdisciplinary teams, which requires interpersonal, communicative, and collaborative skills.
- OT practitioners must obtain information on a wide range of community-based programs and services, both specialized and generic, to meet the individual needs of the various families and children with whom they work.

BOX 2-3

Family Systems Theory Concepts

MORPHOSTATIC PRINCIPLE

Like all systems, family systems are organized with recognizable feedback loops and "rules." These "rules" may be ones that are consciously recognized and spoken by family members but most are nonverbal and shared assumptions of family functioning. An example of a *spoken* "rule" is "In our family, parents always inquire about his or her child's day and the child always responds," responding. An example of a nonverbal "rules" is a parent expressing anger at a child and the child withdrawing to avoid conflict. Deviation from either pattern by the parent or child would be met with corrective (morphostatic) action. Failure of the parent to inquire or the child to respond in the first instance would draw the immediate attention of the other, wondering if there was a problem. In the second example, an arguing response could be met with increasing anger from the parent until the child finally withdraws; if the parent fails to respond angrily to an "infraction," the child might escalate the misbehavior until the angry response occurs.

MORPHOGENETIC PRINCIPLE

Families do evolve; that is, they change. Just as a child grows and develops, families can be thought of in the same way. In the examples above, the parent who asks how his or her child's day was might get caught up in work or a younger sibling and not be available when the now older and more independent child arrives home. S/he might start volunteering more about his or her activities. In the latter example the child, as s/he ages and gains experience outside the family, may see this as undesirable and no longer be willing to continue the sequence. Either the parent or child will initiate a conversation that leads to an agreement to make changes in the sequence.

EQUIFINALITY

This concept is in many ways a subset of the morphogenetic principle. Simply stated, it says that any system can change in an infinite number of ways. If we again take the second example above, a positive change was described. Another version might be that the now 16-year-old boy becomes increasingly belligerent, gets into a physical fight with his dad, and either runs away or is kicked out of the house. Even in this extreme example, it is important to recognize that the "family" continues and the notion of *equifinality* still applies. The child could become addicted to drugs, with the parents forever grieving, or he could eventually get into the military, receive the GI bill, do well in college for a couple of years, and be reunited with his family, who then support him through graduate school and he subsequently wins the Nobel prize. Equifinality does not imply an endpoint but rather a series of way stations in the life of a family. For the OT practitioner it is the most important idea, one of hope and optimism.

FAMILY SYSTEMS THEORY

Description

Family systems theory is a core framework for guiding interactions with families. It is a group of ideas that describe the many ways that individuals in families are connected across time and space,* and its implications for the families with whom practitioners work are far reaching. Developing and increasing an understanding of the family as a system significantly affects the way practitioners working with families perceive their own roles, determine which potential outcomes are positive, and perceive family changes. The core concepts of family systems theory are provided in Box 2-3.

General Systems Theory Concepts

Each living (including family) system, to be recognizable as such, must have some order no matter how undesirable or chaotic it appears to an outside observer. The maintenance of this order has been named the **morphostatic** (form maintenance) **principle.** Examples for families include daily family rhythms such as meals, bedtime, expectations for bathing, greetings or departures, and affectionate naming. At the same time these systems have a capacity for change, which has been named the **morphogenetic** (form-evolving) **principle.** Examples for families include gaining or losing a member through marriage, divorce, birth and death, and the shifting roles of members through marriage, school progression, or aging. Change is possible only through the introduction and assimilation of new information into the system, such as gaining or losing members.

A feature of the form-evolving (morphogenetic) aspect of living systems is their capacity to evolve along different paths and yet arrive at a given "destination." It implies that no single past event predicts a system's current form, nor does any specific current event specifically predict a future form. This has been named **equifinality.** The practitioner will see families that are similar in many ways but whose lives have been affected in dramatically different ways by the introduction of a child with special needs. A clear example is one in which the family seems to have been drawn closer together, in contrast with that in which the family has become emotionally disconnected.

* The definition of *family* in this chapter is inclusive: ". . . two or more people who regard themselves as a family and who perform some of the functions that families typically perform. These people may or may not be related by blood or marriage and may or may not usually live together."[8]

Implications for Practice

The OT practitioner is an agent for bringing new information into the system. In addition to the core knowledge (the domain of the profession) the practitioner brings, s/he must develop communication skills to help the family assimilate this new information. To do so, the OT practitioner is guided by these two basic ideas: "*I must acknowledge and accept current family form and function (support the current form)*," *and* "*I must ally myself with the system's capacity for change*" *(support the assimilation of the new knowledge I bring)*. These ideas form the basis for the consultative role.

The OT practitioner leverages his or her ability to support change by eliciting from the family its desired outcomes and integrating his or her ideas into a collaborative plan aimed first and foremost at achieving the family's goals. This is truly family-centered practice, with the client being the family and the OT practitioner's role being one of a consultant rather than prescriptive interventionist.

A major goal in working with families is establishing a trusting relationship, particularly with key members. One of the first steps in establishing trust is to identify the outcomes family members desire. Given that different family members have different priorities, helping them find verbal expression for outcomes that everyone can endorse powerfully builds that trust. Families sometimes simply have the basic desire of helping their children grow and develop. Regardless of whether a family's goals are vague, it is important to acknowledge the ways each member perceives the current situation and priorities while helping them agree on goals.

CLINICAL *Pearl*

The first step in a successful intervention is identifying what the family hopes to accomplish.

CLINICAL *Pearl*

Intervention efforts should begin with a clarification and acknowledgment of the way in which family members perceive their situation and define their priorities, regardless of how unfocused their goals may seem.

The second step in building a trusting relationship is developing strategies for accomplishing the family's agreed-upon goals. The strategies should be developed in collaboration with the family to ensure adherence to its beliefs and daily living patterns. In the case of Margarita, Heather began the intervention process by working with the mother, which, given her key role, was the appropriate way to begin establishing a trusting relationship. However, even if she had successfully consulted with the mother at the previous visit to determine that toilet training or the high chair were desirable for the family, she departed from the consultative role when *she* determined the timeline for Margarita's toilet training and *she* determined that a high chair should be used during meals. Instead, once the family had endorsed these ideas, Heather could have consulted with Mrs. Sanchez about the practical realities and timing of implementing these ideas. Even more powerfully, she could have included the father, grandmother, and aunt in developing implementation strategies once they had endorsed these ideas as goals. This would bypass some of the constraints created by Mrs. Sanchez's already complex life. Because Heather had failed to include them in the planning process, she missed some opportunities to support the intervention/change process. Fortunately, Heather was able to shift out of the prescriptive and directive role, which had led to a useless high chair and frustration.

Margarita's story illustrates a common occurrence—the professional role as the prescriber of intervention, clashing with existing family functioning. This can significantly reduce the efficiency and effectiveness of any intervention. The paradox is that families desire professional expertise and assistance. It is hard to resist the temptation to take such a directive role and tell a family exactly what to do. Although some families can creatively take a prescribed intervention and weave it into existing family routines, beliefs, and daily living patterns, many will do less well or discard the intervention altogether. Staying in a consultative role is key. The OT practitioner helps the family integrate the interventions that move them toward the agreed-upon goals and into the daily living patterns as best they can. As the consultant the OT practitioner not only helps the family integrate new intervention strategies but also helps them troubleshoot those aspects of the plan that they were unable to actually accomplish. Rarely does it work to "try harder." Changing the process, the goals, and the timeline are all reasonable adaptations to current family functioning. With this approach, the family is more likely to take full advantage of the practitioner's expertise. Those who are able to relinquish their felt professional power as experts and provide consultation in a truly family-centered fashion are often able to make the most of their professional skills and expertise.

CLINICAL *Pearl*

The likelihood that families will follow through with intervention plans depends on the extent to which those plans are constructed to fit within families' existing routines, beliefs, and patterns of family life.

OT practitioners should also be aware that success with a family is an evolving process. As with Heather, the only real mistake is the one which is not recognized. An easy way to enhance family trust is to consult with them on intervention plans gone awry. Being truly curious and collaborating with the family about what elements in a plan might be added or changed to improve the chances for success not only improve the odds of success but also furthers their acceptance of the therapist. Developing a trusting relationship with families takes time. Differences in cultural and linguistic backgrounds and heritages also influence how quickly and easily relationships are formed, but adhering to the consultative role accelerates the process.

FAMILY LIFE CYCLE

Description

Another concept covered in AOTA's guidelines is the family **life cycle.** Like individuals, families go through normal or typical developmental phases. No consensus exists on the number of phases that should be considered, which is not surprising considering that family development is a fluid process and not a discontinuous series of steps. Critical stages of the family life cycle are those involving life transitions: birth, marriage, leaving home, and death.

Perhaps one of the most important points about the phases of the life cycle is the fact that moving from one phase to another causes stress and requires the family to adapt. Stress is completely normal and necessary for the family system's evolution (morphogenesis). Life cycle changes bring about changes in the needs, interests, roles, and responsibilities of each family member. For instance, becoming a parent entails learning a whole new set of skills and alters the relationships between the parents and among the parents and their extended family and friends. Families can often benefit from the extra support of friends, neighbors, or extended family members during life cycle transitions.

Children who have disabilities often have special needs and undergo numerous stressful life cycle events. These events may include being unexpectedly hospitalized for a lengthy period, undergoing unusual and sometimes painful treatments, and becoming involved in special education and early intervention programs. They often involve new relationships with numerous different professionals. Forming new relationships, especially when individual choice is not involved (which is what happens when a practitioner is assigned a case), can be stressful. In the case of Margarita, the arrival of an OT practitioner in the Sanchez household created a certain degree of stress. As Heather shifted into a more consultative role, the stress of intervention was no longer dealt with by dropping the prescribed intervention (the high chair) and changing nothing (morphostatic principle) but rather was integrated into a family plan for change (toilet training) that was endorsed, at least in its timing, by Mrs. Sanchez and was therefore more likely to succeed (adhering to the morphogenetic principle).

Watching a child miss the typical milestones that usually take place in his or her life can create stress for a family. For instance, the realization that a child has not started walking or talking by the appropriate age can be very stressful. In Margarita's case, the fact that her younger 11-month-old sister had begun to walk while the 3-year-old Margarita had not clearly highlighted the ongoing and unexpected stress of extended dependency for basic functions such as feeding and toileting.

Because certain events, such as frequent hospitalization and participating in OT intervention or not reaching important milestones, are not **normative life cycle events** (i.e., the usual or expected transition events), families have fewer people with whom to share their experiences. For instance, the parents of adolescents often find it helpful to share "war stories" with other parents about transition events such as teaching the adolescent to drive. The majority of the parents of adolescents can relate to the challenges and triumphs associated with this event. Research has shown that sharing experiences and getting support from family, friends, and neighbors are effective strategies for dealing with stress.[6] However, few parents can relate to **non-normative life cycle events** (not the usual or expected transition events), such as the experience of raising a child who will never be able to walk.

Implications for Practice

The life events that have been described are somewhat arbitrary and obviously overlap and are grossly inadequate representations of the wide range of family experiences that exist. Cultural factors can also affect how these events and life stages are perceived and experienced. For example, is it acceptable for an adult child to be living with his or her parents? For many Caucasian families this situation would be considered a failure, whereas for many Latino families this may be normal. It is the tendency of practitioners to attach meaning to the phases of the family life cycle, and the meanings are usually rooted in our own backgrounds, beliefs, and experiences. This tendency can potentially put practitioners at odds with certain families. An example of this is shown in the previously mentioned case of Margarita. Heather, with her Anglo values, wanted Margarita to attend the prekindergarten program connected with the public schools because she thought it would enhance her social and cognitive development. Mrs. Sanchez became quiet, a sign which Heather recognized. Perhaps the Sanchez family considered it unusual for children to attend any school at such a young age, or they may have preferred a neighborhood parochial school with several bilingual nuns on the staff.

Being sensitive to family transition events (normative and non-normative) is also important. Events such as the death of a parent, an older child leaving home, and job transition can all take time and attention away from intervention efforts. Consider the big picture when working with a family. Family-centered consultation is clearly preferred under such circumstances.

During non-normative transition events, the families of children who have disabilities sometimes find it extremely helpful to be connected with each other. They can share information, similar experiences, and methods of coping. Parent-to-parent programs exist in many communities, and research has demonstrated their helpfulness.[7]

FAMILY ADAPTATION

Description

In what ways do families adapt to unexpected events, such as the birth of a child who has developmental delays? Crises, which are brought on by overwhelming stress, are not *always* negative. Families are living systems that evolve in response to internal events (e.g., illness, death, birth, emancipation) and external events (e.g., the loss of a job, a move to another city, the involvement of the OT practitioner). Like all living things, families are generally adaptive (the morphogenetic principle) by nature. Although serious crises can precipitate alcoholism, separation or divorce, or family violence, in some cases they can enable rapid positive changes, such as recommitment to a marriage or resolution of a long-standing conflict. For many years, research on the families of children with disabilities was focused on family dysfunction, stress, and pathology. However, in recent years research has revealed what some families had been saying for years: despite the stress caused by their child's disability, dealing with the disability strengthened the family or changed it in some positive way.[8]

Families react and adapt to crises in individualized and unique ways. Family **adaptation** is affected by the interaction of family **resources** (e.g., time, money, and friends) and perceptions (the way events are defined). Social support plays an extremely important role in family and individual well-being. For the families of children with disabilities, the informal support of the extended family, friends, and neighbors appears to be more important than the formal support received from professionals and institutions. Of course, an important factor is the way families define their resources. In the previously mentioned Sanchez family the extended family is a source of positive support for Margarita's parents, whereas in other

BOX 2-4

Perceptual Coping Strategies

PASSIVE APPRAISAL
Ignoring a problem and hoping it will go away

REFRAMING
Redefining a situation in ways that make it more manageable

DOWNWARD COMPARISON
Identifying a situation that is worse than your own

USE OF SPIRITUAL BELIEFS
Using philosophical or spiritual beliefs to make sense of and find meaning in a situation

families a mother-in-law and aunt living in the home could be a source of additional stress.

In addition, the way families define and understand a particular event, such as the birth of a child with a disability, is an important component of family adaptation. Specific **perceptual coping strategies** are listed in Box 2-4.

At times therapists get impatient with families who seem to be ignoring or minimizing problems. Although being judgmental in these situations is tempting, these families are using their own coping strategies. Families adapt as a whole, and this adaptive capacity should be supported. OT practitioners should not assess a given situation and assign direct responsibility to any specific factor. For example, a practitioner cannot accurately assume that George, a 6 year old who cannot tie his shoes, would be able to if only he had started OT work at age 3. Too many other variables are relevant. For example, family financial demands, time constraints, and emotional strain may have been significant when George was 3. Beginning OT at that age could have forced George's father, who had overcome drinking and spousal abuse problems, to regress. In turn, this could have caused George to regress and lose his toileting skills. No individual, not even an OT practitioner, can conceive of all the potential positive outcomes and all the ways to achieve those outcomes (equifinality). Families and OT practitioners have attitudes and biases about the causes of problems and the possibilities of overcoming them. Regardless, the adaptive potential of a family as a whole is unlimited, and remembering this can help families and OT practitioners achieve the best possible outcomes.

Implications for Practice

When meeting a family for the first time, it is important to be curious and interested in the unique ways that the parents have been adapting to their child's disability—the ingenious ways that they cope in their daily lives. In the previously mentioned story about Margarita Sanchez, Heather regained this curiosity and interest as she recognized Mrs. Sanchez's indirect feedback of being quiet as evidence that she had departed from the consultative role.

CLINICAL *Pearl*

When meeting a family for the first time, it is important to express curiosity and interest in the unique ways that they are adapting to their child's disability without judging and evaluating.

It is also important to use and support existing resources in families' lives. OT practitioners sometimes get so excited about specialized support services that they forget about generic support services such as churches, neighborhood playgrounds, and community recreation centers that are closer to home. If OT practitioners are not careful, their clients may suddenly realize that they have lost touch with neighbors and friends because of the time spent taking their children to specialized programs far from home. They could end up as part of a specialized world inhabited mainly by professionals.

Families must carry out daily tasks to perform their basic functions.* Family routines must be considered when home therapy programs are developed or else time-consuming programs may be prescribed that simply cannot be done within the parameters of the daily household routines and time schedule:

ESSENTIAL SKILLS FOR SUCCESSFUL INTERVENTION WITH FAMILIES

For OT practitioners, having good communication skills is just as important as having the proper knowledge to treat a client. Some essential communication skills include the following:

- *Solution-focused curiosity and interest:* People generally have an extremely positive response to practitioners who are nonjudgmentally interested in them and their situations. The focus should be on strengths, achievements, and desires rather than on the traditional problems and deficits. This "solution focus" allows the practitioner to support the adaptive (morphogenetic) potential of the family while not

* Family functions include activities related to education, recreation, daily care, affection, economics, and self-identity.[8]

challenging or criticizing its current status. If we use the previous story about the Sanchez family as an example, Heather could have asked Mrs. Sanchez, "What have you found that works best for feeding Margarita?" rather than "What problems do you encounter when feeding Margarita?"

- *Collaborative goal setting:* A family who has requested or been referred for OT services has some goal, even if only a vague one, that they hope the services will help achieve. The practitioner may have a very different idea of what the goal should be. Collaborating with the family to clarify and develop a common set of goals helps practitioners efficiently and effectively manage the treatment planning process. Staying close to the agreed-upon plan while being willing to change the plan as family needs evolve builds trust as the family members experience the therapist as interested in helping them achieve *their* goals. For example, after introducing herself, Heather could have asked Mrs. Sanchez about Margarita and what she hoped to accomplish by getting involved in the early intervention program. Asking "What are Margarita's biggest problems?" is a deficit-oriented approach. Stating "I think we should work on toileting so that Margarita is ready for kindergarten" could slow the development of a relationship between Heather and the Sanchez family. Carefully eliciting and acknowledging the family's wishes would create a solid basis for working with them. Starting with the family's hopes, dreams, and moments of pride reinforces its members as being capable and competent. After listening carefully to Mrs. Sanchez's expressed wishes for Margarita, Heather could say something like "So, you aren't sure about what you want to accomplish, but no matter what we do, Mrs. Sanchez, you want Margarita to feel like she is a part of the whole family." If Mrs. Sanchez nodded and smiled, Heather would know that she had identified a primary goal to be reached with the Sanchez family. She would keep that as a major feature of the treatment planning process.
- *Acknowledgment*: "Solution-focused curiosity and interest" and "collaborative goal setting" are skills that are grounded in the central communicative tool known as **acknowledgment,** which practitioners can use to assure their clients that what they are saying is being heard and understood. OT practitioners can acknowledge the clients with whom they are speaking by providing appropriate feedback. This feedback can be in the form of verbal repetition or confirmation of the clients' statements (e.g., "So you have lived here for 5 years" or "I see"), nonverbal body movements (e.g., nodding the head, sitting forward with an interested expression), or paraverbal cues (e.g., "uh-huh" or "mm-hmm").
- *Continuity*: An OT practitioner's arrival and departure are the most important moments of contact with a family. At both times the practitioner should be solution focused or future oriented. When arriving at the home, the practitioner is attempting to establish or reestablish positive rapport with the family. After discussing any relevant events that have taken place since the previous visit, the practitioner elicits from the family a desired outcome for that visit or restates an agreed-upon goal to guide activities during the current visit. When departing from the home, the practitioner and family identify events that will or may take place before the next visit as well as discuss a potential goal for the next visit. It can be difficult and frustrating for a practitioner to leave after a visit in which little progress has been made. In such a case, it is often helpful to leave the family with some "homework" related to their goal—to look for and note circumstances that relate to it—so that the practitioner can use the information as a stepping stone for the next session. For example, imagine that the parents want their daughter to be able to be more independent in dressing and have identified the goal of using a zipper; however, the goal seems unreachable and little progress is being made. Their OT practitioner could ask them to pay attention to the circumstances under which their daughter attempts to touch or play with the zipper. The visit can then end on a more positive note, with the family having a smaller goal on which to focus.

CLINICAL *Pearl*

Build on family strengths, dreams, and hopes. When talking with families, ask "how" rather than "why" questions. Ask them to describe rather than explain situations. Instead of trying to establish some sort of linear cause and effect relationship among different factors, try simply to understand the relationships among events, people, and situations.

SUMMARY

Family systems theory provides a useful framework for thinking about families and the ways in which they operate. The challenges and triumphs of parenting a child who has disabilities are similar to others that all families face regardless of whether they have children with disabilities. An important factor in determining whether families can successfully adapt to these challenges is the strength and support of their relationships with other key individuals. An OT practitioner is one of these key players—a person who has the opportunity to make a difference in the life of a family through a sensitive, individualized intervention approach.

References

1. American Occupational Therapy Association: AOTA *1995-96 member update*, Bethesda, Md, 1996, The Association.
2. American Occupational Therapy Association: *Occupational therapy practice framework: domain and process*, Bethesda, Md, 2002, The Association.
3. American Occupational Therapy Association Commission on Education: *Guidelines for curriculum content in pediatrics*, Bethesda, Md, 1991, The Association.
4. American Speech-Language-Hearing Association: *We can do better: recruiting, retaining, and graduating African-American students*, Rockville, Md, 1995, ASHA.
5. Bacharach S: *Education reform: making sense of it all*, New York, 1990, Medina.
6. Simons R: *After the tears: parents talk about raising a child with a disability*, San Diego, 1987, Harcourt Brace.
7. Singer GH, Marquis J, Powers L, et al: A multi-site evaluation of parent-to-parent programs, *J Early Intervention* 22:217, 1999.
8. Turnbull AP, Turnbull HR: *Families, professionals, and exceptionality: a special partnership*, ed 4, Upper Saddle River, NJ, 2001, Merrill–Prentice Hall.

Recommended Reading

Buysse V, Wesley P: *Consultation in early childhood settings*, Baltimore, Md, 2004, Paul Brookes.

Dunst C, Trivette C, Deal A: *Enabling and empowering families: principles and guidelines for practice*, Cambridge, Mass, 1988, Brookline Books.

Turnbull AP, Turnbull HR: *Families, professionals, and exceptionality: a special partnership*, ed 4, Upper Saddle River, NJ, 2001, Merrill–Prentice Hall.

REVIEW *Questions*

1. What are three current societal trends that impact the work of the OT practitioner? Describe the impact of these trends on OT pediatric practice.
2. Describe three key concepts related to family systems theory and the implications of these concepts for OT practitioners.
3. Explain the reason why non-normative transition events may be more stressful than normative transition events.
4. With the information provided on family systems and family adaptation, explain the reason why it is important to individualize therapy programs for children and families.
5. What are four communication strategies that could be used during the initial home visit with a family?

SUGGESTED *Activities*

1. Spend some time with a child with special needs in his or her natural environment (e.g., home, neighborhood). Observe the various activities taking place. Keep a list of the ways different therapy activities could be embedded in these routines. Imagine the way therapy concepts could be introduced to the parents and then implemented. Write these ideas down.
2. Talk with the families of children with disabilities and with OT practitioners. Ask each group to describe the characteristics of an OT practitioner that they think are important. Take notes and summarize their comments. Compare the comments of the two groups. Create a personal list of the skills and competencies of an effective OT practitioner.

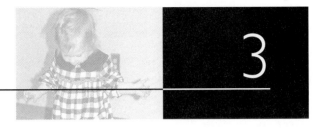

3

Medical System

DAWN B. OAKLEY

KATHLEEN LOGAN-BAUER

CHAPTER *Objectives*

After studying this chapter, the reader will be able to accomplish the following:

- Identify and discuss the key components (i.e., settings and key members) of a pediatric medical system
- Differentiate among pediatric acute care, subacute care, long-term care, and home care medical settings
- List five commonly assessed areas of function in a pediatric medical-based occupational therapy evaluation
- Differentiate among the multidisciplinary, transdisciplinary, and interdisciplinary styles of collaboration
- Discuss the roles of treatment and documentation in a pediatric medical system
- Discuss medical reimbursement issues and payment options for pediatric medical services
- Identify three important challenges faced by a medical-based pediatric practice

KEY TERMS

Pediatric medical care system
Acute
Subacute
Home care
Long-term care
Screening
Evaluation
Multidisciplinary
Interdisciplinary
Transdisciplinary
SOAP note

CHAPTER OUTLINE

MEDICAL CARE SETTINGS

A medical system includes many team members, including children, families, specialists, generalists, nurses, physicians, physical therapists, recreational therapists, speech and language pathologists, and occupational therapists. A *pediatric medical care system* comprises a group of individuals (professional, paraprofessional, and nonprofessional) who form a complex and unified whole dedicated to caring for children who are ill (Box 3-1).[11] To a beginning allied health care professional, this environment may seem overwhelming at first.

Comprehensive pediatric medical care includes a continuum of various settings. Pediatric medical care is provided in one of five settings: a neonatal intensive care unit (NICU), a step-down nursery or pediatric intensive care unit (PICU), a subacute setting, the home, or a residential (long-term care) facility.

BOX 3-1

Key Pediatric Medical Terms

CARDIOLOGIST
A physician specializing in the treatment of heart disease

CIVILIAN HEALTH AND MEDICAL PROGRAM OF THE UNIFORMED SERVICES (CHAMPUS)
CHAMPUS provides supplemental benefits to those in the uniform services direct medical care system. The program pays for medical care given by civilian providers to eligible persons, who include the retired members of the United States uniformed services and their dependents, the dependents of deceased members of the military, and the dependents of members of the North Atlantic Treaty Organization (NATO) when the NATO member is stationed in or passing through the United States on official business. The CHAMPUS program is spelled out in 32 CFR, section 199. The program is administered by the Department of Defense.

CIVILIAN HEALTH AND MEDICAL PROGRAM OF THE VETERANS ADMINISTRATION (CHAMPVA)
The federal program administered by the Defense Department for the Veterans Administration that provides care for the dependents of totally disabled veterans. Care is given by civilian providers.

DEVELOPMENTAL PEDIATRICIAN
A pediatrician with specialized training in the developmental milestones of typical childhood development

GENETICIST
A person who specializes in genetics

HMO/PPO
Health maintenance organization/preferred provider organization

MEDICAID
The federal program that provides health care to indigent and medically indigent persons (i.e., those who cannot afford to pay their medical bills and qualify for Medicaid for medically related services). Although it is partially federally funded, the Medicaid program is administered by the states, in contrast to Medicare, which is funded and administered at the federal level by the Health Care Financing Administration (HCFA). The Medicaid program was established in 1965 by an amendment to the Social Security Act under a provision entitled *Title XIX—Medical Assistance.*

NEONATOLOGIST
A pediatrician with 3 years of advanced education who specializes in the treatment of neonates and premature infants

NEUROLOGIST
A physician who specializes in nervous system diseases

OPHTHALMOLOGIST
A physician who specializes in the treatment of eye disorders

Adapted from Slee V, Slee D: *Slee's health care terms,* ed 3, St Paul, Minn, 1996, Tringa Press; Thomas CL, editor: *Taber's cyclopedic medical dictionary,* ed 18, Philadelphia, 1997, FA Davis.

BOX 3-1

Key Pediatric Medical Terms—cont'd

ORTHOPEDIST
A specialist in orthopedics

PEDIATRICIAN
A physician who specializes in the diagnosis and treatment of illnesses and dysfunctions in children

PEDIATRIC NURSE PRACTITIONER
A registered nurse who provides primary health care to children (e.g., Jane Grey, R.N., P.N.P.). Special preparation is required.

PHYSIATRIST
A physician who specializes in physical medicine

PHYSICAL THERAPY ASSISTANT
A technical health care worker trained to carry out physical therapy procedures under the supervision of a physical therapist

PULMONOLOGIST
A physician who is trained and certified to treat pulmonary diseases

RADIOLOGIST
A physician who uses x-rays or other sources of radiation for diagnosis and treatment

REGISTERED PHYSICAL THERAPIST
A health care worker who has successfully completed an accredited physical therapy education program and passed a licensing examination. A registered physical therapist is legally responsible for evaluating, planning, conducting, and supervising a physical therapy program using rehabilitative and therapeutic exercise techniques and physical modalities.

SPEECH AND LANGUAGE PATHOLOGIST
An individual who is educated and trained to plan, direct, and conduct programs to improve the communication skills of children and adults with language and speech impairments caused by physiological factors, articulation problems, or dialect. A speech and language pathologist can evaluate programs and may perform research related to speech and language problems.

Adapted from Slee V, Slee D: *Slee's health care terms,* ed 3, St Paul, Minn, 1996, Tringa Press; Thomas CL, editor: *Taber's cyclopedic medical dictionary,* ed 18, Philadelphia, 1997, FA Davis.

Neonatal Intensive Care Unit

The NICU is needed for infants who have complicated births. The goal of the NICU team is to address the **acute,** or extremely severe, symptoms or conditions of an infant so that the infant can become physiologically stable (i.e., maintain a stable body temperature, heart rate, and respiratory rate).

The medical team closely monitors the medical status of NICU clients. A neonatologist serves as the leader of the NICU team (Figure 3-1). In addition to conducting a neonatal assessment, the neonatologist consults with the other medical team professionals about the specific needs of the infant. The following conditions may indicate that an infant should be admitted to the NICU: cyanosis—an infant who turns blue because of insufficient oxygen; bradycardia—a heart rate of less than 100 beats per minute (bpm); low birth weight (LBW)—a weight of less than 2500 g; very low birth weight (VLBW)—a weight of less than 1500 g; or extremely low birth weight (ELBW)—a weight of less than 750 g. When presented with an infant who has one or more of these conditions, additional medical team members should take part in consultations and provide additional examinations. Pulmonologists (lung specialists), cardiologists (heart specialists), gastroenterologists (digestive specialists), and respiratory therapists are examples of the additional medical team members who may be needed to address the needs of infants in the NICU.

Pediatric Intensive Care Unit

After meeting certain physiological requirements, the infant is moved out of the NICU. If the medical team determines that the infant still requires some form of hospital-based medical care, the infant can be transferred to a

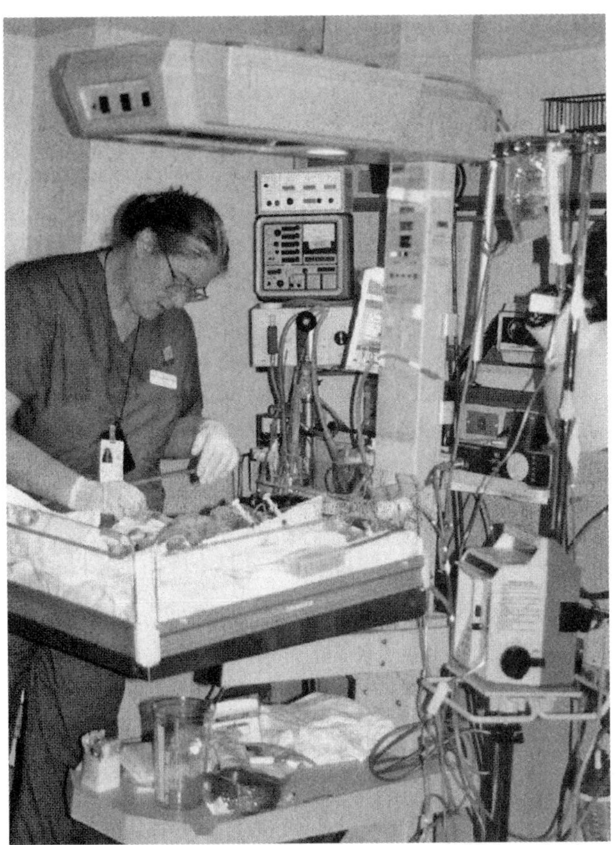

FIGURE 3-1 The neonatal intensive care unit can be an overwhelming environment. (From Parham LD, Fazio LS: *Play in occupational therapy for children,* St Louis, 1997, Mosby.)

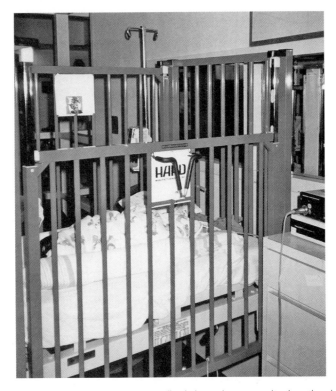

FIGURE 3-2 Infants are transferred to a step-down nursery or pediatric intensive care unit when they have the ability to maintain satisfactory physiological functioning. (Courtesy Dawn B. Oakley and Kathleen Logan-Bauer, Bayside, NY.)

step-down nursery or pediatric intensive care unit (PICU) (Figure 3-2). In addition to continuing to address the infant's acute symptoms, the goals of the PICU team are to attempt to wean the infant from external sources of medical support and, when applicable, provide sensorimotor stimulation. As the infant is moved from one unit to another, certain additional team members may be required, whereas the services of certain other members may no longer be needed. For example, in the PICU the infant's medical team leader is no longer a neonatologist; it is a pediatrician.

Subacute Setting

After being released from a step-down nursery or PICU, an infant may be able to go home but may be required to move to a **subacute** (Figure 3-3) setting. The medical needs of a given infant, as well as the desires of the infant's primary caregivers, affect this decision. The goals of the subacute team are to provide appropriate medical treatment while continuing to wean the infant off medical supports and continue carrying out developmentally based therapeutic interventions.

Home

As an infant's status improves, discharge plans are formulated. The issue of where the infant goes after being discharged is discussed with the infant's primary caregivers. Going home is the ultimate goal for infants in acute, step-down nursery, and subacute settings. Once at home, the goals are to facilitate caregiver and infant bonding and promote the continued acquisition of developmentally appropriate skills.

The medical needs of infants who have been discharged home are handled on an outpatient basis. They receive medical care through scheduled clinic and outpatient hospital-based visits (Figure 3-4). The infant's nursing, therapy, and equipment needs are coordinated by a

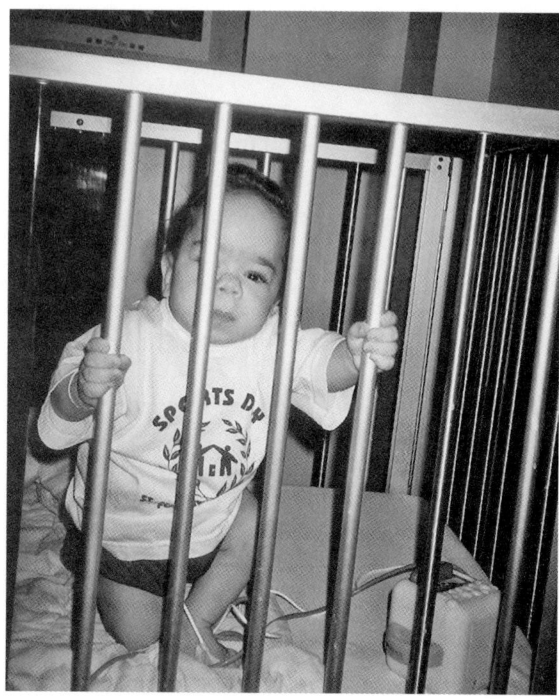

FIGURE 3-3 As infants become medically stable, they are discharged and transferred to a subacute or home care setting. A commercially available device is often all that is necessary to monitor the infants when they are alone. (Courtesy Dawn B. Oakley and Kathleen Logan-Bauer, Bayside, NY.)

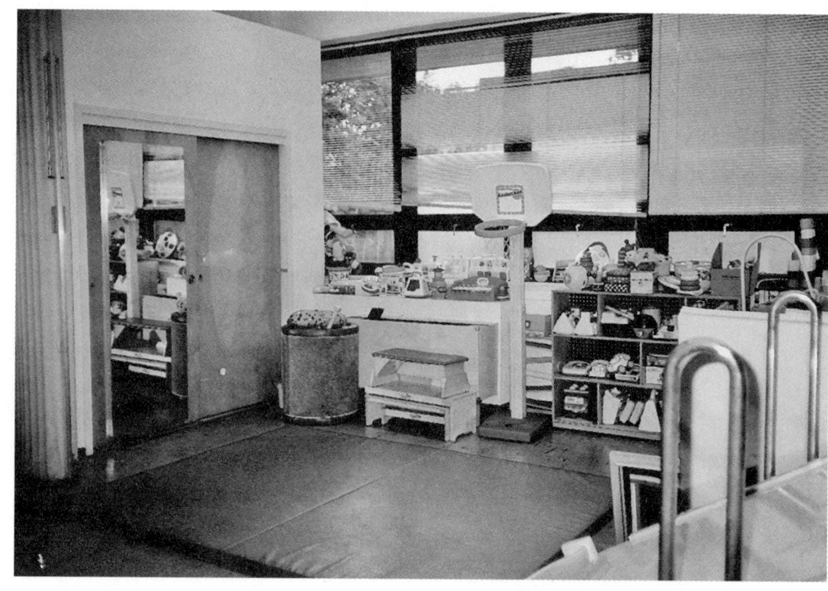

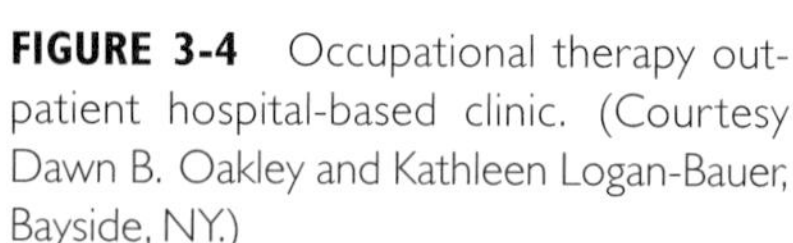

FIGURE 3-4 Occupational therapy outpatient hospital-based clinic. (Courtesy Dawn B. Oakley and Kathleen Logan-Bauer, Bayside, NY.)

community **home care** agency. These agencies monitor their clients' medical needs and provide and coordinate home-based therapeutic services. The age of the client determines where the services are provided. Infants and young children usually receive home-based services. As children mature, any additional needed therapy services may be provided in an outpatient clinic or community-based school setting.

CLINICAL *Pearl*

Practitioners must respect the families' values, beliefs, and customs while providing home-based occupational therapy (OT) services for children.

Long-Term Care Facility

During discharge planning, some primary caregivers decide that they are unable to handle their child's specific medical needs. In these cases, residential **(long-term care)** facilities are options. The goals of the long-term care team are to provide appropriate medical care and carry out appropriate therapeutic interventions. An example of a therapeutic intervention is providing sensorimotor stimulation to prevent the development of contractures and prevent or minimize losses in range of motion.

MODELS OF MEDICAL CARE

In addition to the practice setting, a clinician needs to be aware of the model of medical care under which services are being provided. The increased number of uninsured or underinsured children and families has resulted in the expansion of medical care practice outside of the more traditional arena (i.e., inpatient, center-based care). The models of pediatric service delivery have been broadened to include the stages of medical service provision. Federal programs such as early intervention involve the primary physician as a vital member of the treatment team. In addition, therapy, nutrition, social work, and other services are provided under this federally mandated (state-governed) program to assist with meeting first-level (primary) medical care needs. One of the components of a primary medical care model is education. Pediatric primary care is strongly grounded in the understanding that caregivers must receive assistance in order to recognize the need for routine and follow-up medical care. Practices such as immunizations, vaccinations, regularly scheduled checkups, and ongoing monitoring of chronic conditions are all examples of strategies that are used under the primary care model to promote and support good health in children. All medical personnel who provide services under this model of care are responsible for participating in the educational process.

The second-level (secondary) medical care model involves the follow-up that occurs once a child has become ill. In these instances, the caregiver is provided with guidelines to prevent the further contamination of the child or others within the household or community. This level of medical care involves caregiver education, specifically focusing on caregiver recognition of the importance of adherence to guidelines regarding care, sanitation, dispensing medication, and observation for signs of improvement or worsening of a condition. This level of care is intensified compared with that of the primary care model. The increased level of medical care is provided to prevent the necessity of tertiary medical care.

The third-level (tertiary) medical care model involves the need for hospitalization. At this point in the medical care continuum, serious concerns have arisen regarding involvement of the child's body system(s). A concern also exists that additional body systems will be affected by primary or secondary causes associated with the child's illness. This model continues to involve caregiver education; however, a greater level of responsibility for the child's recuperation is dependent on interventions provided by the medical personnel.

The next section of this chapter focuses on a discussion of the continuum of medical care service options. The information gained from medical care models aids in the development of the pediatric knowledge base necessary to provide medical-based treatment.

MOVING THROUGH THE MEDICAL SYSTEM CONTINUUM

The extent to which a child is involved in the medical system continuum can change significantly as the child's circumstances change. For example, a child may be admitted to an acute care facility because of an acute illness. The child may be subsequently discharged and return home but then be admitted to a long-term care facility because of extenuating circumstances at home. This is just one example of the way a child's involvement in the pediatric medical care system can change. The following case study follows the progression of one child through the pediatric medical care settings.

CASE *Study*

Daniel was born after 33 weeks of gestation by a cesarean section with vacuum extraction because of fetal distress. At birth he was limp and cyanotic, with a heart rate of less than 100 bpm. No respiratory effort was noted at birth. Daniel's birth weight was 2900 g. He required mechanical ventilation for the first 3 days of life. Daniel was weaned to nasal continuous positive airway pressure (CPAP) from days 3 to 18. He was reintubated on day 25 for gastrostomy tube placement.

Three days after his gastrostomy tube placement, Daniel was transferred to a step-down nursery. After the transfer, consultation requests were made to the staff geneticist, a physiatrist, and rehabilitation services.

After Daniel had spent 30 days in the step-down nursery, the medical team and his parents determined that he should be discharged and transferred to a subacute facility. The responsibility for Daniel's treatment was assumed by the subacute facility.

The medical team and Daniel's parents decided that he was ready to be discharged and return home after he spent 1 year as an inpatient at the subacute facility. Daniel was transferred from inpatient, medical-based care to outpatient, home-based care.

As noted in the case study, when a pregnant mother has an emergency delivery, some degree of pediatric medical care is often required to treat birth-related trauma. In addition, children may need pediatric medical care for accidental injuries, neurological and musculoskeletal traumas, and complications resulting from genetic defects.

ROLE OF OCCUPATIONAL THERAPY IN THE PEDIATRIC MEDICAL SYSTEM

CLINICAL *Pearl*

Childhood is filled with many typical developmental stages and events. The normal developmental progression can be negatively affected by atypical experiences and events, such as a prolonged hospitalization.

The prolonged hospitalization of an infant or child is not a normally occurring event. A hospitalization of more than a few days puts a typical child at risk for some degree of developmental delay. For example, to develop meaningful social and emotional bonds, infants and children need to be comforted and held by other human beings. Children and infants who are hospitalized typically are not held as often as those who are not in a hospital. These children and infants may have difficulty developing the social and emotional skills needed for successful interactions with members of their families and schools.

The perceived or actual presence of developmental deficits warrants the provision of OT and other rehabilitative services. Perceived deficits are those that may not yet be present but are known to be associated with a particular condition, such as Down syndrome. Perceived deficits can also be temporary developmental delays resulting from atypical experiences and events. The fundamental principle of OT is to promote optimum performance in each of the areas of occupation: play/leisure, activities of daily living (ADLs), instrumental activities of daily living (IADLs), social participation, and education. Pediatric medical-based OT practitioners use play activities to facilitate the acquisition of age-appropriate developmental skills (e.g., gross motor, fine motor, cognitive).

Role of the Occupational Therapy Practitioner

Medical-based occupational therapy practitioners are either registered occupational therapists (OTRs) or certified occupational therapy assistants (COTAs). OTRs are responsible for providing the overall framework for medical-based services. Collaboration between the two types of OT practitioner is essential and is facilitated by the COTA's knowledge of the OTR's responsibilities, which include conducting **screenings** and **evaluations,** formulating and carrying out daily treatment plans, and documentation. The COTA's responsibilities include formulating and carrying out daily treatment plans and documentation. COTAs also assist with or conduct portions of the pediatric medical-based screening and contribute to the pediatric medical-based evaluation.

After receiving a referral from a physician, the medical-based pediatric screening and evaluation are usually completed by the OTR within 24 and 72 hours, respectively. The screening and evaluation are conducted by means of formal and informal measurement tools as well as clinical and parental observations. Throughout the assessment process, a medical-based practitioner should be aware that factors such as time, the severity of the illness, and the overall stress associated with being in a hospital environment may mask a child's true abilities in a given performance area.

The deficits that are identified during the screening and evaluation are addressed in a medical treatment plan. An OTR usually formulates the long-term goals and short-term objectives that guide the treatment plan. The medical treatment plan is developed either solely by an OTR or jointly by an OTR and COTA. The medical treatment plan is an outline of the activities and tasks that are used during treatment sessions.

The OT practitioner initiates OT treatment only when the medical stability of a child has been determined. Medical stability is used to determine the manner in which services are provided and how often they are provided. The goals of the treatment plan should be gradually integrated into the child's environment. Treatment strategies should increase, not decrease, the child's functional level.

Role of the Certified Occupational Therapy Assistant

As mentioned previously, medical-based pediatric OT services are provided to promote the optimum function of hospitalized children. COTAs are prepared to play a role in the provision of these services. The responsibilities of the COTA are dictated by the facility in which the services are being provided. The typical responsibilities of a COTA include conducting an initial developmental screening, collaborating with another practitioner on an evaluation, planning treatment, updating goals, and collaborating with another practitioner on developing a discharge plan.

COTAs working in the pediatric medical setting should be aware of client factors that will impact their provision of services. The plan of care developed for a child admitted to a medical setting incorporates information reflecting a child's preadmission as well as his or her current status. This information, along with the child's medical diagnosis and medical course, is used to develop goals that will lead to discharge. Clinicians gather information regarding preadmission status to develop an understanding of a child's baseline performance in the following areas:

- Cognitive (level of alertness, orientation, behavior, moods, activity level, memory, attention to task)
- Sensory (visual, auditory, oral, tactile, vestibular, gustatory, pain)
- Neuromuscular system (extremity movements and limitations, strengths, weaknesses, prior injuries/surgeries, presence or absence of age-appropriate reflexes)
- Cardiovascular and respiratory systems (blood pressure, breathing patterns, prior activity and fatigue levels)
- Voice/speech/respiration (verbal or nonverbal communication, quality of voice, ability to sustain conversation)
- Digestive/metabolic (eating, absorption, energy return on caloric intake), skin (intact, abrasions, cuts, wounds, injection or access sites)
- Elimination function (output schedule, level of independence)[2]

Experienced COTAs will be able to evaluate this information based on their understanding of the connections that exist among body systems, body structures, and function. Their knowledge surrounding the interrelatedness of the body systems and how strengths or deficits in one system affect the performance of another will assist in the development of the most appropriate plan of care (inclusive of objectives and goals that maximize a child's optimum level of function).

The following discussion of the role of the COTA in a pediatric medical care setting follows the course outlined in the previous case study. Daniel's medical care was initiated in the hospital and continued after he was discharged and sent home.

Neonatal Intensive Care Unit

Only highly qualified allied health professionals perform NICU-based treatment. The therapists who work in the NICU are required to have advanced education and certification in NICU-based treatment. For example, therapists in the NICU must have a thorough knowledge of life signs, which are key indicators of the infant's status (e.g., color, respiration rate, body temperature, extremity movement). Changes in these indicators are noted by the therapist through sight, hearing, and touch.[9] A role for the COTA in the provision of NICU services has not been identified.[1] If a practitioner would like to work with this special client population, s/he should obtain the necessary education and certification required to ensure that treatment is provided safely and appropriately.

Step-Down Nursery, Pediatric Intensive Care Unit, and Subacute Settings

Providing treatment in a step-down nursery or PICU also requires related experience to ensure the provision of the most appropriate treatment. However, unlike the situation in the NICU, COTAs with appropriate educational training may be able to receive on-the-job training, which qualifies them to assume a role in providing medical services in the step-down nursery and PICU.[1]

Additional education and on-the-job training are necessities for COTAs in the step-down nursery and PICU because the infants and children admitted to these units may still have significant medical problems. A COTA working in one or both of these settings usually participates in the screening, evaluation, and treatment of the clients. COTAs should be aware that the initiation of screening or treatment might distress a step-down nursery or PICU client. During the initiation of any screening or treatment procedure, COTAs should be sensitive to indications of distress and prepared to respond appropriately.

During the initial screening and assessment, the COTA is introduced (oriented) to the client's case. Each client is evaluated to establish a functional physiological baseline (e.g., respiratory rate, heart rate, oxygen saturation level). Clients must be constantly evaluated during daily treatment sessions to ensure that they remain within the physiological range that was established according to their baseline functioning levels.

The NICU, PICU, and subacute pediatric care settings can be intimidating secondary to the intricacies associated with these settings. The provision of services in these areas is typically reserved for the experienced clinician. As noted previously, the NICU and PICU are not traditionally entry-level placements for the beginning COTA. However, also as previously stated, an experienced COTA can provide services in a PICU or subacute setting with the appropriate OTR supervision. One of the steps that lead toward becoming an experienced COTA is the development of a pediatric medical knowledge base.

The knowledge necessary to work in these areas is made up of three components: an understanding of the equipment, an understanding of the standards of care that govern operations in these settings, and an understanding of medical status signs that will guide the provision of therapeutic services. The level of care required by the children admitted to one of these settings is high. In response to the increased level of care, the status of these children is monitored regularly. They may also have a need for the administration of scheduled medication(s). The equipment found in these settings will vary based on the population of children being served. Some examples of the equipment found in these settings are shown in Box 3-2.

BOX 3-2

Equipment Examples

APNEA MONITORS
Monitor respiration

INTRAVENOUS LINES/TUBES
Tubes that pass through the skin and into the veins

PULSE OXIMETER
Measures pulse and oxygen saturation levels, that is, the amount of oxygen found in the blood

FEEDING TUBES
Oral can be placed in the mouth and empty into the stomach; nasal can be placed in the nose and empty into the stomach; and gastro can be placed in the abdomen and empty into the stomach.

ULTRAVIOLET LIGHTS
Light ray frequencies used to treat illness

WARMING BLANKETS/LIGHTS
Temperature control coverings (may be placed directly over a protective covering on the body or above a bed) used to assist in the maintenance of body temperature

Adapted from Thomas CL, editor: *Taber's cyclopedic medical dictionary,* ed 18, Philadelphia, 1997, FA Davis.

Some examples of standards of care include adherence to treatment guidelines (where and when treatment can occur), sign-out practices (children's locations must be recorded at all times), medical supervision (treatment must be provided in accordance with medical orders), and caregiver/parental expectations (guardian expectations and goals are included in the development of a comprehensive plan of care). Clinicians providing services in these settings must accommodate all of these factors.

In addition to the equipment that monitors the children's status, a clinician needs to perform ongoing monitoring to assess their readiness to receive therapy services or their ability to tolerate specific therapeutic interven-

BOX 3-3

Medical Status Checklist

HEALTH STATUS
Should be well enough to receive therapy services

HEART RATE
Should be within child-specific, established guidelines

OXYGEN SATURATION

Levels
Should be within child-specific, established guidelines

Color
Should be within typical shading, as demonstrated by the child when not in distress

SKIN TEMPERATURE
Should be warm to the touch unless child presents with a condition that affects internal temperature regulation

BREATHING PATTERN
Should be typical of the child when not in distress (i.e., based on either age-appropriate or diagnosis-related breathing patterns)

AFFECT
Should verify that presenting behavior is typical of a child

SLEEP–WAKE CYCLE
Should verify that existing patterns have not been interrupted

MOVEMENT PATTERNS
Should demonstrate movement patterns that are part of the child's repertoire and those that are fostered by the introduction of therapeutic interventions

tions. Once a clinician has the opportunity to develop a level of comfort for service provision in the medical setting, s/he will develop a site-specific medical status checklist. Box 3-3 shows a medical status checklist provided as a guideline for the entry-level clinician used before working with a child.

The checklist can serve only as a general guideline. The clinician and child will share the ultimate responsibility of determining whether a therapeutic intervention is being tolerated. Since it is not uncommon for medically fragile children to experience distress when they are moved or touched, a clinician may need to develop monitoring ranges that are acceptable for treatment.

Subacute, Long-Term, and Home Care Settings

COTAs must be trained in medical-based pediatric therapy to provide services in the PICU, subacute, long-term, and home care settings. Working in a subacute, long-term, or home care setting is different from working in a step-down nursery or PICU setting in that an experienced COTA practitioner may not be required to work under the direct supervision of an OTR. The clients in these settings are typically more medically stable than those in the NICU, step-down nursery, or PICU. However, COTAs working in these settings should be familiar with the signs of physiological distress and prepared to respond properly.

TEAM COLLABORATION

Team collaboration is important in any medical setting, but it plays a particularly essential and integral part of medical and therapeutic intervention in pediatric care. Before the initiation of a therapeutic intervention, practitioners consult with the physicians and nurses assigned to the client's care. They frequently obtain updates on the status of their clients. Areas of particular importance include medications, physiological stability, nutritional sta-

TABLE 3-1

Methods of Team Collaboration

APPROACH	DESCRIPTION
Multidisciplinary	The multidisciplinary approach evolved from a medical model in which multiple professionals evaluated the child and made recommendations.[2] Professionals who use this type of approach may be directly or indirectly involved with the child and family but do not necessarily consult or interact with each other. Assessment, goal setting, and direct intervention may be carried out by each professional with a minimum of integration across disciplines.[4]
Interdisciplinary	The interdisciplinary approach to treatment is cooperative and interactive. A team comprising professionals from several disciplines (who are often at the same location) have frequent direct involvement with the child and collaborate with each other on the child's program. Although the evaluations are performed independently by each discipline, program planning is carried out by group consensus, and the goals are set collaboratively between the professionals and parents. This approach allows the child and family to receive coordinated services and benefit from the expertise of professionals from several disciplines.[6]
Transdisciplinary	Although the transdisciplinary approach involves collaboration among various disciplines, one team member is usually designated to intervene directly and the other team members act as consultants. This approach was developed on the assumption that families benefit more from having their intervention programs provided by one primary professional than multiple professionals. All team members contribute to the assessment and program planning, and then the designated person implements the plan while consulting with other members of the team. Therefore, the transdisciplinary model enables health care professionals to perform tasks that are normally outside the scope of practice of their discipline. Implementation of this model requires professionals to be comfortable with role release, or relinquishing some or all of their professional duties to another professional. During this process the team members must share information and exchange responsibilities.[8]
"Individual versus group" sessions	The "individual versus group" session approach is used to encourage frequent team member collaboration. It allows for informal and impromptu communication between two or three team members. During team collaboration, information is exchanged about the child's status. Specific information is shared so that members can compare notes, which in turn serves to improve the treatment approaches of the members of the individual disciplines.[10]

Adapted from Case-Smith J, Allen AS, Pratt PN: Arenas of occupational therapy services. In Case-Smith J, Allen AS, Pratt PN, editors: *Occupational therapy for children*, ed 3, St Louis, 1996, Mosby.

tus, and sleep patterns. Practitioners can obtain this information from written reports and during rounds and medical team meetings.

Consultations among medical team members facilitate collaboration. Team members may use one of the four types of collaborative style: **multidisciplinary, interdisciplinary, transdisciplinary,** or **"individual versus group"** sessions[10] (Table 3-1).[5]

CLINICAL *Pearl*

For a transdisciplinary team to be effective, the team members must trust and respect each other so that they are comfortable with role release (i.e., relinquishing certain professional duties to other team members).

DOCUMENTATION

The ability to clearly document the events that occur in a pediatric medical setting is crucially important. Documentation is used for many purposes, including updating others on client status, justifying the necessity of services, and explaining requests for supplies and reimbursements.

A practitioner who works in a pediatric medical care system should know the types of documentation that exist and the reasons these documents are necessary. A medical-based screening or assessment is usually the first type of document a practitioner is required to complete. An initial screening may be used to determine whether a thorough evaluation is needed. In some medical care settings, a more detailed assessment is the second step in the

BOX 3-4

Medical-Based Occupational Therapy Education

ST. MARY'S HOSPITAL FOR CHILDREN INITIAL OCCUPATIONAL THERAPY EVALUATION

Name: Kevin Unit CUW
DOB 7/13/80 Sex: Male
Medical Record # 12345
Diagnosis: Duchenne muscular dystrophy
2/28/98: Doctor's orders received. Full evaluation with recommendations to follow.

MEDICAL HISTORY

Kevin is a 7 year 8 month old male with Duchenne muscle dystrophy. On 3/.21/96, he underwent a spinal fusion and multiple tendon releases. Hw was subsequently placed in two long-leg casts with bars. Kevin was born at 36 weeks' gestation and weighed 5 lb 5 oz. Kevin was a healthy child until he was diagnosed with Duchenne muscular dystrophy at age 5.

GENERAL OBSERVATIONS

Kevin is a thin, frail male who has an overall decreased affect. He has a scar from spinal surgery that extends from approximately T1/T2 to his coccyx. He is able to verbalize his needs by speaking in a soft, high-pitched voice, Kevin is able to visually track objects in all planes. He is seated in a reclined wheelchair with his lower extremities elevated and in a spica cast.

GROSS MOTOR FUNCTION

Kevin has hypotoniicty throughout his trunk and upper extremities. He is able to transition from a prone to a supine position or a supine to a prone position. Kevin requires significant assistance to maintain a sitting posture. He exhibits pectus excavation, bilateral scapular winging, a kyphotic posture, and bilateral rib flaring.

UPPER EXTREMITY FUNCTION

Passive range of motion (PROM) is WNL. Gonometric active range of motion (AROM) measurements are as follows: (WNL with normal limits)

	R	L
Shoulder flexion	No ROM at either shoulder; uses compensatory techniques (e.g., climb arms on chest)	
Elbow flexion	Flexes both elbows in a gravity-eliminated plane	
Wrist extension	0-30 degrees	0-25 degrees
Wrist flexion	0-60 degrees	0-55 degrees
Ulnar deviation	0-30 degrees	WNL
Radial deviation	0-20 degrees	WNL
Supination	WNL	WNL
Pronation	WNL	WNL

(Courtesy Kathleen Logan-Baucer, Bayside, NY.)

documentation process. In other medical care settings the assessment is the first document completed by a practitioner. Screenings and evaluations usually comprise some if not all of the following sections: medical history, general observations, gross motor function, fine motor function, visual and perceptual function, cognitive function, sensory function (when applicable), ADL function, summary and recommendations, frequency, and long- and short-term goals. Box 3-4 contains an example of a medical evaluation that outlines a client's strengths and weaknesses. The information is used to establish baseline functioning, thereby delineating the parameters for improvement.

A specific example of a standardized pediatric assessment is the WeeFIM (UB Foundation Activities, Inc, Queens, NY).[13] The WeeFIM is a functional assessment that is used to describe a child's performance during essential activities; it is used to measure those activities that children can actually carry out and not what they may merely be capable of doing. The assessment can be used to clarify a child's functional status, provide information for team conferences, facilitate goal planning, and provide information on burden-of-care issues, which are those issues related to the person who is meeting the child's basic needs (i.e., eating, bathing, dressing, grooming, transferring, moving, and toileting).[12,13] The WeeFIM also provides a uniform language for practitioners to use when measuring and documenting the severity of disabilities and outcomes of pediatric rehabilitation and habilitation. It allows practitioners to measure disability types as well as determine the amount of help a certain child needs to perform basic skills. The assessment is conducted by means of direct observations or interviews of the caregiver and can be used for pediatric inpatients and outpatients (Box 3-5); however, it is not meant to be used as the only diagnostic tool.

BOX 3-5

WeeFIM Instrument Rating Guidelines

INPATIENT

Within 72 Hours of Admission
WeeFIM admission assessment must be completed.

Within 72 Hours of Discharge
WeeFIM discharge assessment must be completed.

Within 80 to 180 Days of Discharge
WeeFIM follow-up assessment must be completed. Interim WeeFIM assessments (between admission and discharge) may be performed at the facility's discretion.

OUTPATIENT

During Initial Contact
WeeFIM admission assessment must be completed. Additional WeeFIM assessments may be performed at the facility's discretion.

At Time of Discharge
WeeFIM discharge assessment must be completed.

Adapted from Uniform Data Systems for Medical Rehabilitation: *WeeFIM system workshop,* Queens, NY, 1988, UB Foundation Activities, Inc.

After the initial screening or assessment has been completed, the practitioner notes the child's progress and changes in the status over time. The progress is recorded in the form of a daily note, weekly progress note, or monthly progress note in a narrative or **SOAP note** format (see Chapter 1). SOAP stands for **s**ubjective information (general statements concerning the child by the caregiver or child), **o**bjective information (what is done), **a**ssessment (effect of treatment), and **p**lan (what will be done). (See *Physical Dysfunction: Practice Skills for the Occupational Therapy Assistant* for a clear, concise description of common medical documentation.[6]) An example discharge SOAP note that corresponds to the previously cited case study might be as follows.

S

Nursing reports that Daniel is in a "great mood" today and drank 8 ounces of formula this morning.

O

Daniel is a 14-month-old male who presents with a diagnosis of prematurity, bronchopulmonary dysplasia, and a gastrointestinal tube (GT) placement. Daniel receives OT, PT, and ST services twice weekly for 30 minutes each. He is medically stable and receives his nutrition by way of a combination of oral and overnight GT feedings.

At present Daniel is alert and oriented to person and place. He is able to cruise with contact guard. He demonstrates right and left unilateral hand skills (active grasp and release in response to verbal prompts). Daniel is able to attend to light-up/auditory toys for approximately 45 seconds with moderate cueing. He tolerates hand-over-hand assistance to participate in cause-and-effect activities in approximately 75% of the trials.

A

Daniel presents with developmental delays in the areas of advancing postural control, bilateral hand function, eye-hand coordination, and attention to a task interfering with his ability to engage in self-care, social participation, and play.

CLINICAL *Pearl*

The WeeFIM is a tool that can be used for the efficient assessment and documentation of progress.

P

Daniel would benefit from home-based OT services to address his continued improvement in the areas of independent mobility/transition, in-hand manipulation, visual perception, and sustained attention skills needed for engagement in self-care, play, and social participation. Daniel was referred to the early intervention (EI program).

Progress notes are important for justifying service implementation and the continuation of services and for discharge planning. A practitioner should record clearly and concisely the therapeutic interventions and the child's responses to them.

When a child's therapy program includes a piece of specialized medical equipment, the practitioner must document the reason. Insurance sources may be reluctant to provide equipment for children in inpatient medical care settings. A child's insurance source may approve or deny a request based on a practitioner's ability to justify the necessity of the requested item. The necessity of a certain piece of equipment can be justified by identifying the ways in which it will benefit the child's level of functioning. Some examples of functions that should be discussed include respiratory, cardiac, musculoskeletal, esophageal, and gastrointestinal; the benefits related to the child's safety should be discussed as well. An example of a letter of justification is shown in Box 3-6. The letter includes information on the way the requested equipment will improve the child's ability to function in the areas of respiration, trunk control (musculoskeletal), endurance (cardiac and respiratory), and swallowing and digestion (physiological).

REIMBURSEMENT

Medical-based treatment is reimbursed by a variety of sources, including private insurance companies, Medicaid, the Civilian Health and Medical Program of the Uniformed Services (CHAMPUS), the Civilian Health and Medical Program of the Veterans Administration (CHAMPVA), health maintenance organizations (HMOs), and preferred provider organizations (PPOs) (see Box 3-1). Many of these sources require specific documentation to justify the services rendered. An OT practitioner should be aware of the general billing requirements and documentation for each source. For example, private insurance companies, HMOs, and PPOs require frequent docu-

BOX 3-6

Letter of Equipment Justification

RE: FRANKIE
DIAGNOSIS: SEVERE TRACHEOMALACIA, GASTROESOPHAGEAL REFLEX, AND SUPRAVENTRICULAR TACHYCARDIA MEDICAID #: GF12345U
DOB: 7/12/96

To whom it may concern:

Frankie is a 10-month-old male who had severe tracheomalacia, gastroesophageal reflex, and supraventricular tachycardia at birth. He has decreased head and postural control as well as tracheotomy.

Current equipment: Currently Frankie does not have any equipment.

Equipment ordered: One Panda stroller with swivel-front wheels, a combined sun/rain hood, and foot straps.

Justification: Frankie is an active, alert, and oriented 10-month-old male with decreased head and trunk control, affecting his ability to assume and maintain independent, upright postural sets. Frankie's inability to maintain an upright and erect posture places him at risk for occluding his tracheostomy and limits his ability to achieve his full respiratory capacity. These limitations affect his endurance and gas exchange.

A Panda stroller will assist Frankie with maintaining a neutral posture, which will facilitate his mechanical efficiency and therefore improve his endrance for maintaining an upright position. Improving his endurance will increase his upper extremity usage, which will foster the acquisition of age-appropriate fine motor skills. The stroller will help prevent bony deformities and joint contractures, thereby preventing the need for future surgeries. Frankie's ability to swallow and digest will also be improved if he can maintain a neutral position. A neutral position allows Frankie to use gravity to help him carry out the previously stated functions.

Thank you in advance for your assistance with this matter.

____
Therapist's signature

____
Therapist's signature

____
Physiatrist's signature

(Courtesy Nechama Karman, Dawn B. Oakley, Queens, NY, 1996.)

mentation to justify the initiation and continuation of services. In certain instances, specific clinics and vendors must be used. A hospital social worker or case manager is the best source of information regarding insurance requirements and coverage.

Another reimbursement source is charitable organizations. Many of these organizations do not give money to a particular child. They are usually nonprofit companies or organizations that raise funds to be given to other nonprofit organizations. A charitable organization makes a donation to a pediatric institution or agency that then deposits the donation into an appropriate general fund. The agency then determines the way to distribute these funds to pay for the specific expenses of individual children.

CHALLENGES FOR OCCUPATIONAL THERAPY PRACTITIONERS WORKING IN THE MEDICAL SYSTEM

Five major areas present unique challenges for OT practitioners in medical care system settings. The first is the number of specialties that are included in the pediatric medical care system. In addition to rehabilitative services (e.g., OT, physical therapy, speech therapy), a variety of specialized services constitute the system, including radiology technicians, medical laboratory technicians, audiologists, pharmacists, dietitians, orthotists, and recreational therapists. A medical-based OT practitioner has to become familiar with the specific pediatric disciplines and their roles in the medical institution. This knowledge will further facilitate the team collaboration process that was discussed previously.

The second challenging area is medical terminology. A medical-based OT practitioner has to be familiar with the extensive medical terminology typically used in pediatric medical settings. The terminology can initially seem overwhelming. However, the study of the basic word roots and common diagnoses used in pediatric medical practice can help practitioners develop this much-needed knowledge base. A good reference source for medical terminology is *Mosby's Medical, Nursing, and Allied Health Dictionary*.[3]

The third challenging area, which is related to that of learning medical terminology, is continuing education. A medical-based practitioner should obtain additional education and become certified in advanced pediatric practice skills such as sensory integration and neurodevelopmental treatment. The medical field is a dynamic system, and practitioners who would like to maintain a role within this system must keep up with developments in current assessment techniques, treatments, and medical equipment.

The fourth challenging area is frequent readmissions. Certain conditions, such as pneumonia, asthma, diabetes, and cerebral palsy, may result in children undergoing recurrent hospital admissions. The development of episodes of acute illness or the need for corrective surgery is often associated with chronic conditions similar to those previously listed. Children who are frequently hospitalized will require a different approach to treatment if they are to receive assistance in order to maintain some sense of continuity with the aspects of their lives outside the hospital. The COTA should draw upon the components of the OT practice framework to assist in the development of therapeutic plans of care that will integrate the children's preadmission habits, routines, and roles with their current levels of performance. The integration of all performance patterns will work toward the achievement of two goals: It motivates the child to work toward goals that will lead to discharge, and it aids the child in resuming prior admission status on discharge from the hospital setting.

The fifth challenging area is palliative care. Children who have been diagnosed with a terminal illness may be treated in a medical or home-based setting. Either one may require the provision of therapy services. The focus of the services provided for children diagnosed with a terminal illness will vary in accordance with changes in their status. A child's services may initially focus on the restoration or maintenance of function related to the child's or caregiver's ability to carry out prediagnosis performance skills. In response to a decline in the child's status, the focus of therapy services will shift to the maintenance and integration of energy conservation techniques that will assist in easing the performance of independent or assisted performance skills. The clinician may also integrate the use of treatment modalities that will allow the caregiver's and child's memories to be recorded in a permanent manner as a source of future comfort for the family once the child dies. As a child enters the final stages of life, the focus of intervention shifts to the provision of comfort measures for him or her in order to achieve optimum positioning and interactions with his or her environment. The clinician providing services will work closely with the caregiver and child to provide opportunities for meaningful interactions.

Infection Control

Infection control is the responsibility of every practitioner. OT practitioners must follow universal precautions when working with any client. They are expressed as a set of rules put forth by the Centers for Disease Control in 1985 to address concerns regarding the transmission of the human immunodeficiency virus (HIV) and the hepatitis B virus (HBV) to health care and public safety workers. When a health care worker has the potential to be exposed to blood, certain other body fluids, or any other fluid visibly contaminated by blood, s/he must assume that all persons may be infected with HIV or HBV and follow these precautions at all times.

All professionals working within the medical setting must adhere to infection control practices. One of the first lines of defense against the spread of infection is that of proper hand washing. Most if not all medical settings provide a detailed orientation that discusses the practices that have been implemented to prevent the spread of infection. Some medical facilities employ a nurse who is responsible for overseeing infection control. The nurse monitors the status of communicable infections and assists in the quarantine of an infected child, caregivers, or medical personnel to prevent the spread of contagious infections to other medically compromised children. The use of personal protective equipment is another method used by health care facilities to prevent the spread of disease. Masks, eye shields, gloves, and gowns are all examples of protective equipment that can be used to prevent the spread of infection. The appropriate disposal of waste materials (i.e., diapers, soiled linens, blood, or other bodily fluid spills) is another area that is covered during the orientation of new staff and frequently on an annual basis to foster compliance with infection control policies and procedures.

Hand washing

Hand washing is the single most important component of infection control. Hands should be washed before and immediately after working with a client or whenever a person comes into contact with any type of body fluid. Hands should be washed when gloves are removed.

Use of gloves

Gloves should be used by OT practitioners when the possibility exists of coming into contact with infected material, providing oral motor intervention which requires that the practitioners' fingers enter the oral cavity, and changing diapers. Gloves should also be worn by OT practitioners who have scratches on or breaks in their skin.

Cleaning of equipment and toys

OT practitioners need to maintain equipment and toys in good, clean working order. Although they do not sterilize equipment and toys after children use them, all of these items should be properly cleaned. The OT practitioner can also require that families provide the child's favorite toys for use during therapy. S/he can educate the families about the safest and most effective methods of cleaning their children's toys.

According to the U.S. Department of Labor, Occupational Safety and Health Administration (OSHA), facilities and agencies must provide their workers with policies and procedures for cleaning and disinfecting.[14] These specific procedures are beyond the scope of this chapter. It is the responsibility of practitioners to become familiar with their facilities' policies and procedures for disinfecting.

Hepatitis B vaccination

The OSHA standard regarding blood-borne pathogens requires employers to offer a free three-injection hepatitis B vaccination series to all employees who are exposed to blood or any other potentially infectious material as part of their job duties. This policy includes OT practitioners and other health care workers. Vaccinations must be offered within 10 days of initial assignment to a job in which exposure to blood or other potentially infectious materials can be "reasonably anticipated."[14]

SUMMARY

The pediatric medical care system is composed of individuals dedicated to caring for ill children. The five major settings in the pediatric medical care system are the NICU, step-down nursery or PICU, subacute, residential or long-term care, and home-based care settings. Specific goals are addressed for each of these settings. Depending on their needs, infants or children are transferred from one setting to another for treatment.

Because a long-term hospitalization is not a typical event in an infant's or child's life, it can hinder their development. As early as 1947, this fact prompted members of the medical community to identify a role for hospital-based OT services. Although their practice in certain settings requires an advanced level of skill, medical-based OT services can generally be carried out by competent OTRs or COTAs.

Medical-based OT services should be provided in a way that promotes team collaboration, whether it be specific to an institution or facility. The four most common team collaboration approaches are multidisciplinary, transdisciplinary, interdisciplinary, and "individual versus group" sessions.

Appropriate documentation facilitates the collaboration process. Although documentation requirements vary based on the regulations of each institution, they commonly include screenings, evaluations, treatment plans, progress notes, letters of justification, and discharge summaries. An OT practitioner may be required to complete one or more of these documents. His or her ability to clearly document medical-based objectives and progress has a direct impact on an institution's reimbursement rate and the client's ability to receive requested services and equipment.

The complex nature of the pediatric medical system poses a unique challenge for medical-based OT practitioners because they must possess more than the basic

OT skills. In addition, they need to have a working knowledge of the pediatric medical specialties, be able to use and interpret pediatric medical terminology, and stay informed about the frequent changes in the pediatric health care environment.

References

1. American Occupational Therapy Association: *COTA information packet (a guide for supervision)*, Bethesda, Md, 1995, The Association.
2. American Occupational Therapy Association: Occupational therapy practice framework: domain and process, *Am J Occup Ther* 56:609, 2002.
3. Anderson KN: *Mosby's medical, nursing, and allied health dictionary*, ed 6, St Louis, 2002, Mosby.
4. Bruder M, Bologna T: Collaboration and service coordination for effective early intervention. In Brown W, Thurman SK, Pearls LK, editors: *Family-centered early intervention with infants and toddlers: innovative cross-disciplinary approaches*, Baltimore, 1993, Brookes.
5. Case-Smith J, Allen AS, Pratt PN: Arenas of occupational therapy services. In Case-Smith J, Allen AS, Pratt PN, editors: *Occupational therapy for children*, ed 3, St Louis, 1996, Mosby.
6. Case-Smith J, Wavrek B: Models of service delivery and team interaction. In Case-Smith J, editor: *Pediatric occupational therapy and early intervention*, Boston, 1993, Andover Medical.
7. Jabri J, Dreher JM: Documentation of occupational therapy services. In Early MB, editor: *Physical dysfunction: practice skills for the occupational therapy assistant*, Baltimore, 1998, Mosby.
8. Lyon S, Lyon G: Team functioning and staff development: a role release approach to providing integrated educational services for severely handicapped students, *J Assoc Severely Handicapped* 5:250, 1980.
9. Oakley D, Bauer-Logan K: *Early intervention symposium*, St. Mary's Hospital for Children, Queens, NY, 1996.
10. Oakley D, Bauer-Logan K: *Traumatic brain lecture series*, St. Mary's Hospital for Children, Queens, NY, 1995.
11. Slee V, Slee D: *Slee's health care terms*, ed 3, St Paul, Minn, 1996, Tringa Press.
12. Thomas CL, editor: *Taber's cyclopedic medical dictionary*, ed 19, Philadelphia, 2001, FA Davis.
13. Uniform Data System for Medical Rehabilitation: *WeeFIM system workshop*, Queens, NY, 1988, UB Foundation Activities.
14. United States Department of Labor, Occupational Safety and Health Administration: *Bloodborne facts: hepatitis B vaccination for you*, Washington, DC, The Administration.

Recommended Reading

Peterson NL: *Early intervention for handicapped and at-risk children*, Denver, 1987, Love.

REVIEW *Questions*

1. When might a child be transferred from one medical setting to another?
2. Which functional areas are assessed in a pediatric medical-based OT evaluation?
3. In what ways do the multidisciplinary, transdisciplinary, and interdisciplinary models of collaboration differ?
4. In what ways could a medical practitioner's documentation have an impact on the treatment and equipment needs of a child?
5. Why is continuing education an important aspect of medical-based practice?

SUGGESTED *Activities*

1. Create three examples of a narrative or SOAP note based on three observations of children in a natural setting (e.g., schoolyard, playground).
2. Purchase and review flash cards of common roots of medical terms.

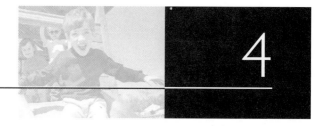

4

Educational System

DIANA BAL

CHAPTER *Objectives*

After studying this chapter, the reader will be able to accomplish the following:

- Identify the federal laws that govern the provision of educational services to children with disabilities
- Explain the formation and function of an individual educational program team
- Explain the process involved in an individual educational program
- Compare and contrast the roles of the occupational therapist and certified occupational therapy assistant in the school setting
- Discriminate between the medical and educational models for occupational therapy service delivery
- Describe the techniques for working with teachers and parents in schools
- Differentiate between the direct, monitoring, and consultation levels of occupational therapy service delivery

KEY TERMS

Free appropriate public education
Least restrictive environment
Due process
Inclusion model
Related services
Individuals with Disabilities Education Act
Individual educational program
No Child Left Behind Act
Individual educational program team
Exceptional educational need
Individual family service plan
Role delineation

CHAPTER OUTLINE

PRACTICE SETTINGS

FEDERAL LAWS

Education of Handicapped Act (Public Law 94–142)
Rehabilitation Act and the Americans with Disabilities Act
Public Law 99–457
Individuals with Disabilities Education Act
No Child Left Behind Act

RIGHTS OF PARENTS AND CHILDREN

IDENTIFICATION AND REFERRAL

EVALUATION

ELIGIBILITY

INDIVIDUAL EDUCATIONAL PROGRAM

Tips for working with parents
Tips for working with teachers
Tips for providing intervention in the classroom

TRANSITIONS

ROLES OF THE REGISTERED OCCUPATIONAL THERAPIST AND CERTIFIED OCCUPATIONAL THERAPY ASSISTANT

CLINICAL MODELS VERSUS EDUCATIONAL MODELS

LEVELS OF SERVICE

Direct service
Monitoring service
Consultation services

DISCONTINUING THERAPY SERVICES

SUMMARY

It is estimated that one third to one half of the practicing occupational therapists work with children and that public school systems are their second largest employers.[4] Despite these statistics, occupational therapy (OT) practitioners in the public schools often find that they work alone with a limited support network. This is especially true in rural areas, where one practitioner may provide therapy services to several small school districts or a cooperative educational service area. Being a member of an educational team requires practitioners to broaden their focus on the ways children function in their families, communities, and schools. This mode of thinking contrasts significantly with the traditional medical model of "evaluate and treat," which focuses on the disabilities or limitations of children.[7] When serving as a multidisciplinary educational team member, a practitioner interacts with a variety of people and must possess specialized technical skills as well as have knowledge of the educational system, current special education laws, and regulations.[3,9] Practitioners must also apply their OT knowledge and intervention skills in the context of a school setting while communicating effectively with parents* and educators.

PRACTICE SETTINGS

Therapists working in the public school setting must collaborate with teachers and special educators. Therapy should be integrated by working with the student in the classroom whenever possible. Sometimes taking the student to a separate room might be the optimum learning situation for the student (Figure 4-1). OT practitioners develop strategies to facilitate educational goals. Strategies and suggestions may be provided to the teacher to better enhance the student's learning.

FEDERAL LAWS

Pediatrics is the only area of practice in which OT services are mandated by law.[4] Box 4-1 summarizes the laws that have an impact on OT services in public school systems. Education is an important occupation of children. As such, clinicians working in school systems are allowed the opportunity to have a direct impact on this occupation. Clinicians working in the school system are afforded the luxury of seeing the results of their intervention daily within the context for which it is intended. The role of the OT clinician working in an educational setting is to improve the child's ability to function within that environment. Practitioners working in school systems must become skillful in advocating the needs of the children within the contexts of the setting and laws.

Education of Handicapped Act (Public Law 94–142)

Before 1975 school-age children with moderate to severe disabilities did not receive adequate services in public schools. In 1975 Congress passed the Education of the Handicapped Act (EHA) (Public Law 94–142) requiring schools to provide **free appropriate public education** (FAPE) to all children from 5 to 21 years of age.[5,9,10] Children with special needs have the right to have their educational programs geared toward their unique needs regardless of the nature, extent, or severity of their disabilities. In 1986 the law was amended so that public schools could be responsible for providing educational services to children at 3 years of age.

Provisions under this law guarantee children the right to be educated in the **least restrictive environment** (LRE) and receive other services that may be required for them to benefit from their educational program. The law also outlines parents' and children's rights and explains their legal course of action. Parents have a right to **due process,** or voluntary mediation and an impartial hearing, to resolve differences with the school that cannot be resolved informally when the right to a free, appropriate public education is hindered.

Least restrictive environment

The right to be educated in the LRE requires a student with special needs to be educated in a regular classroom whenever possible.[4,10] S/he is entitled to interact with peers who do not have disabilities. Before this law students with disabilities were placed in special schools with other students who had disabilities, or they were placed in self-contained classrooms in a separate school building with no opportunity to interact with other peers.

The LRE guidelines provided the impetus for the development of mainstreaming and **inclusion models** (i.e., models in which children with disabilities are able to spend time in regular classrooms). School personnel determine whether a student with disabilities can receive an appropriate education in a regular classroom with the aid of support services and necessary modifications. The team must consider whether the child can benefit from any time in a regular classroom. The spirit of the EHA is to require schools to provide an entire continuum of services to those students with special needs.[2,6,10] For some students this may mean placement in a regular classroom that has been modified to meet their needs (e.g., one that has been equipped with positioning devices). For other students it may mean placement in a regular classroom

* In the chapter the term *parents* is used generally and refers to the legal guardian who is the child's primary caregiver and is responsible for the child's well-being. For example, the parent may be a grandparent, aunt, or uncle or even a friend of the family.

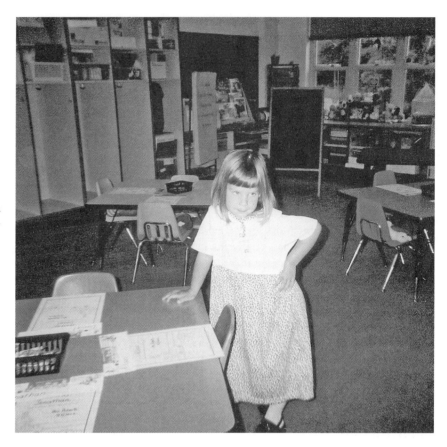

FIGURE 4-1 Working with a child in a separate room may help facilitate educational goals.

BOX 4-1

Summary of Federal Laws That Affect Occupational Therapy in Educational Settings

1973

Public Law 93–112, Section 504 of the Rehabilitation Act

- Discrimination against people with disabilities when offering services is prohibited.

1975

Public Law 94–142: Education for All Handicapped Children Act (renamed Education of the Handicapped Act [EHA])

- All children have the right to free and appropriate public education.

1986

Public Law 99–457, Part H (added to EHA)

- Birth to Three services should be equal in all states and counties.

1990

Americans with Disabilities Education Act

- In areas of public services, discriminatory practices against individuals with disabilities by employers are prohibited.
- EHA is renamed Individuals with Disabilities Education Act (IDEA).

1997

- IDEA is revised (IDEA-R).
- Part H of IDEA-R is renamed Part C.

2001

- No Child Left Behind stresses the use of scientifically or evidence-based programs and practices.

that allows them to go to a resource room for assistance from a special education or resource teacher. Some students need specialized instruction from a special education teacher, and they spend most of the day in the self-contained classroom but are integrated into a regular classroom for certain classes or activities. Students who have difficulty with the transition from one area to another can benefit from reverse mainstreaming, where the regular education students come into the special education classroom during certain courses.

Related services

According to the EHA, schools are required to provide special, or **related,** services as necessary for the student to benefit from the educational program. These services include transportation, physical therapy, OT, speech therapy, assistive technology services, psychological services, school health services, social work services, and parent counseling and training.[5,10] Except for speech therapy, they are available only to a student classified as a special education student. Speech therapy is a "stand-alone" service, which means that a student who does not receive special education services may receive speech therapy.

Rehabilitation Act and Americans with Disabilities Act

The educational rights of children with disabilities are protected by two additional federal laws: Section 504 of the Rehabilitation Act (1973) and the Americans with Disabilities Act (ADA)(1990).[2,10-12] Section 504 of the Rehabilitation Act stipulates that any recipient of federal aid (including a school) cannot discriminate when offering services to people with disabilities. The ADA prohibits discriminatory practices in areas related to employment, transportation, accessibility, and telecommunications. A student with a disability who is not eligible for special education services but requires reasonable accommodation in his or her regular educational program may be eligible to receive related services under these laws. To be eligible the student must have a condition that "substantially limits one or more major life activities," with learning being a major life activity.[2]

Jack is a 5 year old with spina bifida. He attends a regular kindergarten class and is able to perform academic skills in a manner equal to his peers. Jack comprehends the information but has diminished strength and endurance due to his disability, and he is slower in completing his work. Jack needs to be catheterized twice daily by the nurse. Jack qualifies for related services under section 504 of the Rehabilitation Act. Specifically, the following accommodations will allow Jack to use educational services:

1. *He must complete 50% of his work in class; other work will be sent home.*
2. *He will have extra class time to complete work whenever possible.*
3. *Classroom supplies will be readily available and placed in front of him before the task begins.*
4. *OT will be provided to increase strength and endurance for academics.*
5. *A peer or an adult will walk with him when he leaves the classroom.*

Public Law 99–457

Public Law 99–457, which was passed in 1986, added Part H (which is now known as Part C) to the EHA. The law mandates services for preschoolers with disabilities and provided the impetus for the development of early-intervention services for infants and toddlers from birth to 3 years of age.[13]

Although the specific policies, procedures, and timelines for Birth to Three programs vary from those of the public school setting, both systems follow a similar framework that includes identification and referral, evaluation, determination of eligibility, development of the **individual educational program** (IEP) or **individual family service plan** (IFSP), and transitions.

Individuals with Disabilities Education Act

EHA was renamed the **Individuals with Disabilities Education Act** (IDEA) in 1990; it was revised in 1997 and is now known as IDEA-R. This act encourages OT practitioners to work with children in their classroom environment (inclusion) and provide support to the regular eduation teacher (integration). It also encourages schools to allow students with disabilities to meet the same educational standards as their peers.[14] IDEA-R changed the process for the identification, evaluation, and implementation of IEPs. Table 4-1 contains a comparison of the IDEA and the IDEA-R. For example, the registered occupational therapist (OTR) and certified occupational therapy assistant (COTA) can assist in the evaluation of the student to determine the need for acquisition of the device that allows the child to remain in a regular classroom. The practitioner may consult with others on positioning, train team members, and consult with others on strategies to increase the likelihood of success in the classroom. The role of OT under IDEA-R is to assist children with special needs so that they can participate in educational activities.

No Child Left Behind Act

The **No Child Left Behind Act** (NCLB) of 2001 was established to increase the standards for teaching and

TABLE 4-1

Comparison of IDEA and IDEA-R

FORMER IDEA	IDEA-R
TEAM NAMES	
M-team (multidisciplinary team)	IEP team
REGULAR EDUCATION TEACHERS	
Works with students other than those with learning disabilities; not involved with special education students	Participation on IEP team
MEETINGS	
Number of Meetings	
Two meetings: (1) an M-team meeting to determine eligibility and (2) a separate IEP and placement meeting to determine services and program	One meeting
Placement Meeting	
Possible parental involvement	Required parental involvement
REPORTS	
M-team summary with minority report (If a member of the team disagrees with the eligibility findings, that member can submit a dissenting report.)	Single report of IEP team's determination of eligibility; no minority report
CONSENT	
Not required for reevaluation	Parental consent for reevaluation
MEDIATION	
Not available	Mediation (A voluntary process in which an impartial person helps schools and families reach agreement on issues related to the identification, evaluation, and educational placement of the child and provision of a free, appropriate public education without going through a due process hearing)
SPECIAL NEEDS TERMINOLOGY	
Handicapping condition, or handicap	Disability
PARENTS' RIGHTS	
Sent six times	Sent three times

IEP, Individual educational plan; *IDEA,* Individuals with Disabilities Education Act; *IDEA-R,* IDEA, revised.

improve the student's learning results. NCLB supports the use of scientifically based practices by professionals working in the educational setting. Therefore, educators and OT practitioners are required to consider research when selecting instructional or interventional practices. Schools must report "Adequate Yearly Progress" through a single accountability system that applies the same standards to all students. These standards are based on each state's academic achievement standards. Teacher quality and paraprofessional competencies are also parts of this act, yet it does not specifically address the competencies of related services such as OT.[15] OT practitioners need to collaborate and consult with the team to prioritize the student's needs. Therapy is integrated into the classroom and provides consistent follow-through. Student-centered IEP goals and objectives enhance success in the educational environment (Figure 4-2).[15]

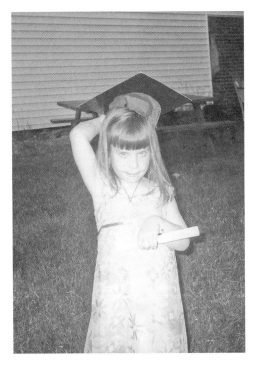

FIGURE 4-2 Education is an important occupation.

RIGHTS OF PARENTS AND CHILDREN

The IDEA-R outlines several procedural safeguards for children with disabilities and their parents. These procedures are detailed in the United States Code of Federal Regulations, Title 34, Subtitle B, Chapter III, Part 300. In brief, the safeguards include notifying parents of all proposed actions, obtaining consent to evaluate, allowing parents to attend IEP team meetings, and providing the right to an independent evaluation and the right to appeal school decisions in front of an impartial hearing officer.[10,17,18] The IDEA-R requires that school districts inform parents of their rights in a written format.

IDENTIFICATION AND REFERRAL

Children are frequently identified and referred for special programs by physicians and health care professionals. Screening clinics offered by agencies, schools, and early-intervention programs aid in identifying children who may be eligible for special education services. Referrals are made to the appropriate agency (e.g., Child Find, an early-intervention clinic, or a public school system). Once a referral is made, the responsible agency determines whether screening or an evaluation is needed.

Once children enter the school system, teachers frequently identify those who experience difficulty with educational expectations. Children receiving special education services may be referred to OT, or the child may qualify for services under Section 504. The **individual educational program team** (parent, teacher, special educator, OT clinician, etc.) determines a student's need for services (including OT). Children needing assistance with fine motor skills typically require evaluation by an occupational therapist. Likewise, students showing cognitive skill deficits require evaluation by a special educator; speech and language concerns are referred to a speech therapist. The professional members are responsible for evaluating the child and determining whether s/he would benefit from related services. The interdisciplinary team collaborates and reviews the needs of the student to determine his or her eligibility for related services.

EVALUATION

After a referral for OT services is received and parental consent to evaluate is obtained, an evaluation can be initiated. (Some state and Medicaid conditions require a doctor's order as a prerequisite to initiating these services.) Evaluations measure the student's abilities at that particular time. Therefore, it is important to consider the viewpoint of everyone involved with the student, including teachers and parents. Knowledge of the student's strengths and needs may be gained from consultation with the teacher, parent, child, and staff. Standardized tests and clinical observations provide important information. State, local, and school policies may dictate what type of assessment will be used. However, clinicians must consider the child's needs in choosing an assessment. Observation of the child in the classroom, cafeteria, playground, and bathroom provides information about his or her functional skills.[1] Many children perform skills in a quiet one-on-one situation but have difficulty generalizing or modulating them in a busy classroom. Students may also perform better when they are aware that someone is watching or observing. Consultation with the teacher is a key in identifying the specific problems and needs of the student. A teacher questionnaire or referral form is helpful to the team. The OTR is responsible for completing the evaluation (with input from the COTA), interpreting the information, and presenting the report to the IEP team. The skills of the student should be reassessed before different objectives are written for a new IEP. Students are reevaluated as needed or requested by the parents, teachers, or team members. They must be reevaluated at least every 3 years.

ELIGIBILITY

The IEP team determines the student's eligibility once all evaluations are completed. Eligibility for services in public schools is based on **exceptional educational need** (EEN). The IEP team must consider all of the information obtained by means of evaluation in order to determine whether the disability or condition interferes with the student's ability to participate in an educational program and whether related services are required for that student in order to benefit from an educational program.[5,10] The presence of a disability does not necessarily mean that a student cannot participate in the educational program nor does it mean that the student has an EEN.

For example, consider Mary, an 8-year-old girl in the second grade who is diagnosed with cerebral palsy (left hemiplegia). Her parents requested an evaluation through the school district; it in turn conducted an IEP team evaluation and meeting to determine whether she was eligible for OT services. On referral the team members conducted an evaluation. The reports found that Mary has age-appropriate learning and thinking skills (cognition) and communication skills, although she sometimes drools and speaks unclearly. Mary walks independently, moves around the building, and independently performs classroom tasks (e.g., printing, managing materials). Observations from team members found that she interacts well with her teacher and classmates and is an active participant in the classroom. The OT practitioner reports that Mary has mild spasticity in her left upper extremity, decreased control (isolation and precision) of her left upper extremity, and difficulty with bilateral tasks, but she successfully compensates for these factors and can participate in all classroom activities. She plays with others on the playground and handles feeding well. Mary participates in regular gym class. She is independent in toileting.

The IEP team determined that while Mary has a documented disability (cerebral palsy), it does not interfere with her ability to receive an appropriate education. Therefore, an EEN does not exist and OT services are not required for Mary to participate in and benefit from her educational program. If Mary's family thinks she would benefit from OT services in order to address issues related to her muscle tone, range of motion (ROM), fine motor skills, and bilateral coordination skills, the family can seek and secure them in a clinic on an outpatient basis. For a child to be eligible to receive OT services in the public school setting, the services and goals must be educationally relevant.

INDIVIDUAL EDUCATIONAL PROGRAM

For school-age children (3 to 21 years of age) who are receiving special education services, an IEP is developed to outline the goals and objectives for the school year. It is a written plan as well as a *process*. The IEP team consists of the student's parent(s) or caregivers, regular education teacher, special education teacher or provider, a representative of the school district who is knowledgeable about the general curriculum, an individual who can interpret the instructional implications of evaluation results (i.e., the way certain factors may affect the student's ability to learn), and related services personnel. The representative of the school district is frequently given the title of Local Education Agency (LEA) representative and may be the principal. The LEA representative is responsible for making sure that the programs out-

BOX 4-2

Components of an Individual Educational Plan

- Statement of a child's present level of educational performance, including the way the child's disability affects his or her involvement in the general curriculum or age-appropriate activities
- Statement of measurable annual goals, including short-term objectives related to increased involvement and progress in the general curriculum and other (non)educational needs, such as those involving social and extracurricular activities
- Description of special education and related services and supplementary aids and services
- Description of program modifications or support to be used by school personnel to enable the child to attain goals; be involved and progress in general curricular, extracurricular, and nonacademic activities; and be educated and participate in activities with other children, both with and without disabilities
- Explanation of the extent to which the child will not participate in the regular classroom and IEP activities with children who do not have disabilities
- Statement of any individual modifications needed for the child to participate in formal assessments of student achievement (e.g., statewide or districtwide tests)
- Projected date for beginning services and educational modifications; anticipated frequency, location, and duration of services
- Transition services, including linkage with other agencies
- Statement of the way that progress toward annual goals is measured
- Descriptions of methods to regularly inform parents of their child's progress (at least as often as the parents of children without disabilities are informed)

IEP, Individual educational plan.

lined on the IEP are followed through in the educational environment. The person who interprets the evaluation results is often the school psychologist or a clinical psychologist. The student may be present at the meetings. The parents may invite anyone they wish to be present, such as a private therapist or parent advocate. If the family brings a lawyer to the IEP meeting to assist with the process, then the school district may also bring a legal representative.

When developing the IEP, the team considers all evaluation results and the extent of the student's educational needs.[5] Goals, objectives, and methodologies (service and frequency) are developed at the meeting. The IEP is reviewed at least annually or sometimes more frequently if requested or necessary. The format of the IEP varies by state and school district. Box 4-2 contains information that must be included in an IEP. (See the Appendix to Chapter 4 for a sample IEP form.)

Sometimes when a child enters school at age 3, s/he already has a written IFSP. This document is the result of collaboration between the parents and the Birth to Three program professionals and is reviewed every 6 months. IFSPs emphasize the family's goals for the child, whereas an IEP focuses on educational goals that the student works on in school and is reviewed annually (Box 4-3). Both documents require the parents to accept all or a portion of the recommended services. The parents or the school district have the option of going to due process if the team is unable to agree on the program or services recommended for the child. Children receiving special services are given progress notes with each report card.

The progress note (Figure 4-3) details the child's objectives, frequency of performance in selected tasks, and success to date (Figure 4-4). Performance is measured in a variety of contexts, with the goal being integration. Progress notes rely on consultation and collaboration with teachers and staff to ensure that the performance represents actual achievement in the occupation (e.g., education).

CLINICAL *Pearl*

OT objectives embedded in the special education teacher's goals and objectives are reinforced by other team members. As a result, everyone on the team is responsible for the goals and objectives of the IEP.

Tips for Working with Parents

1. *Parents know their children!* Listen to what they have to say and try to address their concerns. They may not know why their child is behaving in a particular manner (professionals may help with this), but they are aware of the behaviors.
2. Parents and caregivers may not be used to the language professionals use in meetings. Present information in layman's terms so that explanations are not needed. For example, say "John has trouble getting around without tripping or bumping into things" instead of "John has dyspraxia." (Note: Even as an OTR attending an Individualized Educational Plan (IEP) meeting for my son, I felt turned off by the use of jargon. The professionals used a lot of jargon but did not understand my son.)
3. Parents attending IEP meetings may be nervous and feel uncomfortable. Help them feel at ease by beginning the meeting asking them what they hope to achieve from the meeting, or ask them what they see as their child's strengths.
4. IEP team meetings frequently highlight the child's weaknesses and present only briefly the child's strengths. Begin your report with the child's strengths; follow it by describing the problem areas, with a plan for how to address these concerns.
5. Try to speak with parents before your evaluation. Ask them what they see at home and how they view the situation. This will help provide a focus for your evaluation and insight into the child.

BOX 4-3

Components of an Individual Family Service Plan

The format of the written plan may differ from program to program, but an IFSP must contain the following information.

- Child's current level of development
- Summaries of evaluation reports
- Family's concerns
- Desired outcomes (goals)
- Early intervention services and support necessary to achieve outcomes
- Frequency of, method for providing, and location of services
- Payment arrangements (if any)
- Transition plan

IFSP, Individual family service plan.

Name Sample

Date:	9/16	10/19	11/17	1/7	2/9	3/17	4/27	5/30
1. Will place 5 out of 9 pieces in an individual inset puzzle with minimal assistance	30% with 1 5% with 2	40% with 2 10% with 2						
2. Will snip with scissors 5 times, placing scissors in hands correctly with minimal assistance	5% with 1 and assistance for placement	25% with 1						
3. Will drink from a cup with consecutive swallows—no spillage.	10% front of shirt wet	15% minimal wet on shirt						
4. Will finger feed. Identify food:	24% chips	30% fries, pears, cheese						

FIGURE 4-3 An example of a data collection sheet for the individual educational plan in the appendix.

6. When discussing the child's performance, be clear about what has been tried in the classroom and how it has or has not worked. This gives the team information on future goals, objectives, and intervention strategies.
7. Parents may become frustrated with a long list of problems. Prioritize the list of problem areas so that the most important ones may be targeted for intervention. You can always address other problems later.
8. Ask the parents what works or doesn't work at home. You may be able to provide them with strategies to help their child, or they may be able to help you with strategies. Children benefit when both the parents and professionals are working on the same page.
9. Provide suggestions and/or strategies for helping the child function within the classroom. Using a previously developed list is acceptable, but make sure you have individualized it to the child. Use his or her

Name **Sample**

Date:	8/9	8/16	8/23	8/30	9/6	9/13
4 out of 9 pieces	1/9	2/9	1/9	2/9	N	2/9
Snip	1 snip	1 snip	1 snip	1 snip	N	1 snip
Scissor correctly	No	No	No	No	N	No
Drink—consecutive swallows	1 swallow	2 swallows	1 swallow	1 swallow	N	2 swallows
Spillage	Top half of shirt	Top half of shirt	Top half of shirt	Top half of shirt	N	Top quarter of shirt
Finger feed	10% chips	30% chips, pears	25% chips, pears, cheese	30% chips, cookies, pears	N	25% chips, pears, cheese

N, No school.

FIGURE 4-4 An example of a data collection sheet for therapy.

name. Remember that any written information sent to others is a reflection of you. You do not want to give the parents the impression that you are too busy to work with their child.

10. Follow up with the parents. Sending letters home with the child, e-mail messages, and brief phone calls all let the parents know you are working with them to help their child. Keep information confidential and protected. For example, there are some things you do not want to e-mail, but letting the parents know that "John had a great day in OT" is always welcomed.

Tips for Working with Teachers

1. Most importantly, remember that the OT practitioner's job in a school setting is to help the child function within the classroom. The teacher is in charge of the classroom. Therefore, the OT practitioner must observe the teacher's style, rules, and classroom expectations before designing the intervention for a specific child.
2. Spend time in the classroom without making suggestions and judging the teacher.
3. Ask the teacher what s/he sees as the problem areas for the child. Ask the teacher how you could help the child function better within the classroom.
4. Prioritize strategies for the teacher. S/he must work with the entire class, so providing them with one or two effective strategies for a child is sufficient. You can always add more later.
5. Provide the teacher with short written strategies, and follow up with him or her as necessary.

6. Respect the teacher's time. Teachers get very few breaks during the day. Discussing a child over lunch may seem like a good solution to the OT practitioner but may add stress to the teacher's day and not allow for a much-needed break. Another solution may be to ask to lead a 1-hour "handwriting" seminar for the entire class every Friday morning. The OT practitioner can work with the entire class, targeting the needs of a small group at the same time. This provides a break for the teacher and helps build rapport while benefiting the entire class.
7. E-mails and short notes are effective means of communication with teachers.
8. Help determine good child-teacher fits. Once a clinician understands the style and expectations of a classroom, they can assist in the placement of children with special needs. For example, some teachers are extremely organized and may work best with children who have difficulty with organization. Other children require flexibility and accommodation.
9. Present yourself to teachers as a resource. For example, providing them with writing kits full of activities to enhance writing skills, fine motor games, visual motor games, or crafts that may be easily implemented into the classroom may be helpful. Clinicians may lead morning exercises or warm-ups to address the sensory needs of the students while modeling activities for teachers.
10. Help teachers out by using OT resources. Establish a relationship between the nearby OT or COTA school. College students are frequently looking for projects that may help teachers and schools. Box 4-4 lists some examples of projects that may assist teachers and OT/COTA students.
11. Provide solutions to teachers concerning children with special needs. Gain their trust through collaboration, which works best by listening, discussion, and follow-through. Team members must be able to critically analyze their work and look for alternative solutions.
12. Use layman's terms when speaking with teachers. It is best to describe the student's behavior rather than use medical or psychological terms to describe it. Speaking about what one observes limits misunderstanding. For example, instead of saying "John is tactually defensive, which is why he has trouble modulating his behavior," say "John does not like to be touched by other children unexpectedly; he finds this type of contact annoying, which is why he may hit other children." Then the OT clinician can provide a solution (e.g., allow John to be in the back of the line. Sometimes he will also want to be in the front of the line. When John is the "line leader," observe carefully and ask him to lead the way from the front. You do not want John to feel left out and never be allowed to be the line leader).

BOX 4-4

Projects That May Assist Teachers and Students in Programs for Occupational Therapy/Certified Occupational Therapy Assistant

Design a fine-motor kit for a classroom of first graders.
Develop games associated with spring.
Make pieces of equipment, toys, or other items needed for the classroom (positioning equipment must be checked out by the clinician).
Develop a finger-puppet show (to improve finger individuation) that follows a book (to encourage reading).
Participate in a health fair at a local school.
Volunteer for story time; find a book about children with special needs.
Volunteer for a field trip or evening workshop.
Develop teacher/parent handouts with strategies for children with organizational problems.
Organize a teacher appreciation day.

Tips for Providing Intervention in the Classroom

1. Develop a good rapport with the teacher before providing intervention in the classroom. Be aware of the teacher's style, rules, routine, and classroom expectations.
2. Discuss with the teacher what you would like to do. Decide on a time that this fits in with other classroom activities. Be open to adjusting your plan to fit in with the teacher's agenda.
3. Working in small groups makes the intervention less obvious and intrusive.
4. Keeping a regular schedule allows the class to feel comfortable with you.
5. Walk into the class at a nondisruptive time (e.g., after the bell rings, when the children are settling down). It is not helpful if you interrupt quiet reading or testing to work with a child.
6. Provide intervention as the child participates in the activities. For example, a child with poor handwriting may complete a worksheet by repeating correct strokes during writing practice. The COTA may help a child with hand movements to a song while standing by providing trunk stabilization so that the child can move his or her arms.

7. Providing intervention in the classroom requires the COTA to adjust the intervention so that the child can be successful at the activities. In this example the teacher chooses the activities; the COTA adapts and grades the activities. This requires COTAs to be flexible and "think on their feet." It would be helpful if the COTA has the child's goals and objectives firmly in his or her mind.
8. Flexibility is easily achieved if the COTA is aware of the child's goals and objectives. If the classroom activity changes, the COTA may select a different goal for the session. Once the COTA is clear about the desired objective, s/he may adapt and modify the activity to address it.

CASE *Study*

Tamara, the COTA, intended to work with Jovan in his first-grade classroom during art class. The objective for the session was for Jovan to hold a crayon with a static tripod grasp and imitate a circle. However, when Tamara entered the classroom, the teacher informed her that the class was canceled; they were now involved in playing "Simon Says" and other inside games because it was raining and the kids were all "wound up." Instead of insisting that Jovan participate in the scheduled art activity, Tamara decided to incorporate Jovan's second goal of improving postural control for writing activities. She quickly changed her intervention to facilitate the trunk and upper arm strengthening required for writing. Tamara asked if she could be the leader of the game. The teacher appreciated the break after a hectic and rainy morning. Tamara led activities for the entire class and provided hands-on help to Jovan as needed. The children performed arm pushups, wheelbarrow walks, crab walks, and sit-ups, among other physical activities. Jovan was proud of himself because he knew how to do the crab walk and got to show the others. Tamara ended the session by asking the children ("Simon says") to sit in their seats, put their heads down, count quietly to 20, and then look up. This quieted down the children. The teacher enjoyed seeing the variation of "Simon Says" activities. Tamara explained that these were great prehandwriting activities and that all the children could benefit from them. Tamara agreed to write them down for the teacher.

1. Depending on the teacher, child, and classroom setting, it may be wise to schedule breaks for intervention in the classroom. The COTA may want to schedule direct service intervention monthly to allow the teacher a break from having someone enter the classroom. This must be included in the IEP.
2. Be responsible for developing a weekly lesson for the entire class. Attend the class at the same time (for consistency) and work from the teacher's lesson plan. For example, if the first-grade class is learning about animals, the COTA could design an entire session on animals. Students could make animal noises and walk like the animal (gross motor), match animal cards with the mother and cub (visual perceptual), pick out animal shapes (fur for a bear, slippery snakeskin) (stereognosis), and make an animal craft (cutting, drawing, coloring) (fine motor).
3. Communicate clearly with the teacher. The COTA could e-mail the teacher to let her know the plan for the following week. It is important to be respectful of the teacher by being prepared and letting her know in advance if you are unable to attend the class. It would be very helpful if all the materials are prepared (along with the lesson plan) in case you are unable to attend.
4. Ask for and accept feedback. Set up a system whereby the teacher can give you feedback. Make changes based on the feedback and follow up with suggestions of your own. Teachers are more likely to listen to you if they feel you are listening to them. Be sure to ask how the children responded to your sessions. Some of these sessions may make the children more attentive for the rest of the day, whereas others may cause the children to become restless.

TRANSITIONS

Children undergo a variety of transitions from infancy to 21 years of age. The students' services and programs change as they enter and leave the Birth to Three program and the public school system. A transition plan includes the steps that should be taken to support the students and their families as they go through these changes so that the transitions can be smooth and successful. Transition planning informs the family about the different services and agencies available.

When a student reaches age 14, transition services such as vocational education and job coaches are discussed with the student and family to help in identifying his or her interests and preferences. Students nearing the age of majority (sometimes at age 17) are informed of their rights under IDEA-R. The family is notified that all rights accorded to parents transfer to the student but that they will continue to receive required parental notices. For the parents to retain their rights, they must be recognized as the student's legal guardians by the courts.

ROLES OF THE REGISTERED OCCUPATIONAL THERAPIST AND CERTIFIED OCCUPATIONAL THERAPY ASSISTANT

OTRs and COTAs have related but distinct roles in the educational setting. A successful partnership between the two ensures effective and efficient use of education and training, encourages creativity, and promotes professional growth and respect.[3] All OT services provided in the educational setting must comply with federal and state regulations. Additionally, professional standards of practice help OTRs and COTAs with **role delineation** in the educational setting. The OT practitioners must work together to provide the best possible service to the child.

OT practitioners may be employed directly by the local educational agency (school district) or contracted through a local hospital, health care agency, or private practice. Those employed by the local educational agency must comply with the supervision and employment practices of the school district's structure. If the OT services are contracted through another agency (e.g., a hospital or health care agency), the practitioners are considered employees of that agency and may be supervised by one of its employees. Supervision guidelines and expectations should be closely coordinated between the employer and the local educational agency. In either situation, all licensing and state regulations regarding caseload and supervision standards must be followed.[3,5]

The OTR is legally responsible for all aspects of the OT process. COTAs are responsible for providing services within their established level of competence. Professional supervision is a partnership that requires communication and mutual responsibility to clarify competencies and responsibilities. The practice standards established by the American Occupational Therapy Association (AOTA) delineate levels of supervision (see Chapter 1). The required level of supervision depends on many factors, such as the COTA's level of experience and service competency, the complexity of the evaluation and therapy methods used, and the current practice guidelines and regulations of the state or local educational agency. Supervision in a school district can often be a challenge because of the large number of schools and the geographic distance. Having the OTR and COTA work together in the same school at the same time allows ongoing supervision of and communication with the COTA. The OTRs are ultimately responsible for service performance.[3] If an OTR is not comfortable with a COTA's performance of a particular task, it should no longer be delegated to the COTA. Likewise, a COTA who is not comfortable performing a certain task is responsible for communicating this concern to the supervising OTR.

Each of the practitioners has a role in screening and evaluation, IEP formation, treatment planning, and intervention. During the evaluation, OTRs determine which data are collected and the tools and methods to be used. COTAs can observe and assist with data collection by making clinical observations and administering and scoring tests within their service competency level. OTRs are responsible for analyzing, interpreting, and reporting information verbally and in writing. During the IEP formation, COTAs assist with developing goals and may attend the IEP meeting (under the direction of an OTR) to report the findings and recommendations. Although COTAs do not interpret the findings or negotiate changes in levels of service or goals, they may suggest changes or reevaluation. COTAs are responsible for communicating observations, ideas, interpretations, and suggestions.

For the intervention phase, COTAs must first demonstrate service competency to the OTR. Then they are responsible for developing intervention activities related to the goals and objectives (after initial direction from an OTR). Therefore, COTAs provide intervention aimed at improving occupations as varied as printing, cutting with scissors, using a keyboard, and performing lunchroom skill activities to managing clothing for toileting or recess. COTAs also collaborate and work with teachers and other school personnel on appropriate positioning of the student and determining which materials or methods can be used in the classroom to increase the student's ability to participate successfully. COTAs are responsible for informing OTRs of changes in the student's environment and providing current data regarding his or her performance.[3]

COTAs may be responsible for collecting data to establish evidence-based intervention. Since the domain of OT practice is occupation, the data must address occupation. Although goals and objectives must be measurable, practitioners must ensure that they are also meaningful to children, families, and educators. See Table 4-2 for a sample of goals and intervention activities. By collecting the data on activities that are valued by educators, families, and children, practitioners support the importance of the profession. Goals and objectives that are too far removed from the actual occupation may be measurable, but if they are not meaningful much time is wasted. For example, consider the following goal: Marcie will cross the street with 75% accuracy. Although this goal is measurable, it is not meaningful and is in fact dangerous. Her mother's comment is "What about the 25% of the time that she does not meet this goal?" Another commonly written goal states the following: "Mike will bring a spoon halfway to his mouth." As this goal is written, Mike does not even get any food during mealtime. A better goal would be as follows: Mike will bring a spoon to his mouth; the first half of the distance will be hand over hand, and he

TABLE 4–2

Sample School-Based Goals and Intervention Activities

GOAL	ACTIVITY
Sam will write four sentences with 80% accuracy (spelling, legibility)	Hand strengthening, warm-up exercises Compensatory techniques, incuding lap top, frequency words available, Benbow Hand program, Adaptive writing tool
Sam will remember to write all his assignments in his daily planner, with verbal reminders from the teacher for 10 school days	Teacher and parent will begin by reminding him. Clinician adds a fun game to the assignment; if Sam remembers it, he gets a reward (i.e., bring in a picture of you and your pet).
Sam will participate in regular gym class, with modifications made as needed	Clinician will consult with gym teacher to provide modifications as necessary. Occupational therapy clinician will consult with gym teacher about games and activities that the whole class may benefit from (e.g., parachute games, relay races, "Simon Says," dancing, etc.).

will complete the second half of the distance 7 out of 10 spoonfuls. COTAs can assist the OTR in developing measurable and meaningful goals by describing the behaviors in the context of the classroom. Once the goals are established the COTA may be responsible for collecting and recording the data regularly.

CLINICAL MODELS VERSUS EDUCATIONAL MODELS

Providing OT services in an educational setting requires a shift in thinking and a change in philosophy from the clinical (medical) model. OT clinicians are traditionally trained under a medical model that views services for children based on dysfunction and its underlying components. In this model therapists evaluate and treat physical problems, while environmental factors that can support or hinder a child's performance are not a primary concern. The focus of a medical model is the remediation of underlying components of dysfunction and removal of pathological processes so that development can continue.[9,10] Federal, state, and local educational agency regulations have established guidelines for the provision of OT services in the school system.[5] Box 4-5 contains questions to assist clinicians in determining whether a student needs OT services and which level of service is recommended. Having an EEN designation and significantly delayed skills does not necessarily mean that a student should receive OT services in school; this is especially true for older students with severe cognitive deficits. Their needs (e.g., working on functional skills such as self-care) can and should be addressed in their educational program. Practitioners in schools may serve more children by working with them in groups. This provides peer support and is a natural part of school. Consulting with the teacher and classroom staff helps resolve many problems and may have an impact on many children. The OT practitioner may become more directly involved if a student's skills deteriorate or the practitioner thinks that a short period of direct service will help the student become more independent.

CLINICAL *Pearl*

Goal writing is much easier if the clinician takes the time to ask the teacher, parent, or child what they hope to get out of the OT sessions. Start out very broadly (e.g., "What would you like to do better?" "What is causing you trouble in school?" "What is interfering with the child's ability to learn?") and ask specific questions (e.g., "What aspects of reading are causing you trouble?" "What about your writing: Is it a problem?" "Do you tire easily?" "Is it messy?" "Do you have trouble holding the pencil?" "What does the child do in class that interrupts others?") until you have a clear visual picture of what the child hopes to accomplish. Make the goals as specific as possible without losing their focus. Write the goals in simple terms so that all team members can understand.

BOX 4-5

Determining the Need for Occupational Therapy in the School

Does the child have an EEN? Because occupational therapy is a related service, the child must have an EEN or qualify under Section 504 of the Rehabilitation Act to be eligible to receive the services provided by the school system.

Does the evaluation indicate the need for occupational therapy services? The evaluation may consist of standardized tests, portfolio reviews, classroom and school environment observations, and consultations with parents and teachers.

Does the child demonstrate a significant delay in motor, sensory or perceptual, psychosocial, or self-help skills compared with the established norms of other children of the same age? A significant delay is one that is >1 SD below the norm and affects school performance.

Is occupational therapy a related service that may be required for the child to benefit from and participate in an educational program? Factors that affect the answer to this question include the child's program, other related services received, and the demands of the classroom, the child's level of function, and the potential for improvement or skill development.

Does the child require the specialized skills of an occupational therapy practitioner, or can tasks and interventions be carried out by other personnel? For example, a teacher may be able to help a child learn eating skills by using adaptive equipment provided by an occupational therapy practitioner.

In the school system, the therapist evaluates the student's performance in the classroom to see if the physical, emotional, or behavioral aspects interfere with his or her ability to perform the tasks required by all students. In the educational environment, a student's abilities are described in functional terms (rather than disability or diagnosis) and the capacity to meet classroom demands. The focus of treatment in an educational model is on developing the skills necessary to function within a particular environment.[5,10]

Although OT practitioners working in schools can bill Medicaid for educationally related services, Medicaid was created to provide medical and health-related services for the financially needy. However, it pays for health services for those who are eligible and is not dependent on where the services are provided. When therapy is provided in the school, it decreases the student's absence from school and is an effective way to provide medical care related to the education of children.

Consider the previous example of Mary, the 8-year-old girl with left-sided hemiplegia. Using a medical model, the COTA working in an outpatient clinic might design activities to address muscle tone, ROM, strength, and isolated muscle control for fine motor skills. Intervention sessions would focus on refining performance skills. Conversely, because Mary was able to perform in the classroom and complete tasks at an age-appropriate level, OT services were not recommended for her in the school setting. Mary's mild motor impairments do not interfere with her educational goals.

Although children with medical conditions or diagnoses may benefit from OT in the school, the practical emphasis is to help children function in the classroom, gym, cafeteria, and playground. Providing services in an LRE often means working in the classroom. OT practitioners provide educationally relevant services, making them a part of the educational team. In recent years, educational agencies and third-party payers have increased their requests for OT clinicians to use outcome-based practices in pediatric settings. Practitioners must quantify documents and publish the outcomes of therapy. Therapists are being asked to not only identify and treat problem areas but also to qualify functional performance and consider factors other than neuromuscular and psychosocial processes, such as the student's potential for improvement, social skills, environmental demands, and family priorities.[9,10]

CLINICAL *Pearl*

OT services provided in the classroom are the most integrated. An informal exchange of ideas and effective intervention strategies naturally evolve among team members when the OT practitioner works with children in their classrooms. This allows for the carryover of strategies and changes that allow children to be successful in school.

LEVELS OF SERVICE

OT services can be delivered through direct service, monitoring, or consultation. The members of the IEP team decide on which service delivery level is appropriate for each child. Therapy emphasizes the child's ability to perform in the school environment rather than in the therapy room.[16] IDEA mandates that children participate in the regular curriculum to the maximum extent possible, so therapy in the classroom is recommended whenever possible. OT plays a supportive role in helping the student participate and benefit from the special education program. This requires continuous collaboration between the teacher or other school staff member and the therapist.

In the classroom, paraprofessionals (such as teacher aides) benefit from training and explanations of how to work with children with special needs. For example, the COTA can teach and model how to perform proper body mechanics while lifting and handling a child that is severely handicapped. In addition, explaining to the staff how to feed, dress, and position students with a variety of diagnoses is essential to carrying out integrated services and creating a safe educational environment.

Direct Service

With direct services, the practitioner works with the student so that he or she can acquire a skill. Direct therapy may be conducted one on one with the child or in a group setting; the time and frequency depend on the needs of the child.

For example, a clinician working with several students in a regular second-grade class could treat the children in the classroom during the regularly scheduled handwriting time. S/he would be present for the handwriting session and work directly with the children designated in the IEP. Before the handwriting session, the COTA may encourage warm-up exercises. The entire class may do these exercises, but the COTA pays attention to the children under the IEP. While the students work on assignments, the COTA may review posture, provide cues for beginning the assignment, help with pencil grip, and provide verbal or tactile feedback, among other strategies. Direct service requires collaboration with the parent or teacher for follow-through and optimum learning. Clinicians who work as partners with teachers show the most success in this type of approach.

Monitoring Service

Clinicians following monitoring services create programs for the child that the teacher, other staff member, or family can follow. The practitioner contacts them frequently so that the program can be updated or altered as necessary. The personnel who follow the program are well trained and need to have a clear understanding of its goals. Clinicians provide simple activities to be followed in a safe manner without the presence of a qualified practitioner. Billing procedures or state regulations may not acknowledge the monitoring service. Under this service, the clinician is responsible for ensuring that the child's goals are met.

Consultation Services

Consultation services are provided when the therapist's expertise is used to help other personnel achieve the child's objectives. Clinicians may contact others only once or on an as-needed basis as set up by the team. Ongoing contact with the teacher or caregiver may be necessary. Consultation services are useful for adapting task materials or the environment, designing strategies to improve posture and positioning, or demonstrating how to handle a situation.

For example, a practitioner may consult with the teacher about a sensory diet for a student in the classroom who needs help organizing sensory input. The clinician would work together with the teacher to create sensory diet suggestions for the child in the classroom. Equipment such as a weighted vest, trampoline, vibrator, and weighted lap pad would be purchased or made for the students' and staff's use as necessary. Sensory diet suggestions could be outlined for the staff to use with the student daily. Table 4-3 is an example of an outline with sensory strategies that could be provided to the teacher. The practitioner would then consult with the staff to set up a daily schedule of sensory diet needs, which could be adjusted as necessary.

DISCONTINUING THERAPY SERVICES

Discharging a child from OT services can be difficult because of the rapport that has been established among the child, family, and practitioner. Children may be discharged from OT when all of the intervention goals and objectives have been accomplished or therapy is not resulting in changes. In cases of plateauing (i.e., the child does not make any progress toward the goal), children may benefit from working with another therapist or an alternative approach. If possible, clinicians should avoid discharging children from therapy when they are undergoing a transition, such as changing schools. Frequently, students are eased out of therapy by decreasing its quantity and going from direct therapy to consultation service to discharge.[7] Children may require consultation on positioning when undergoing physical changes. Any change in service (including frequency) is discussed with the IEP team (including parents). For example, students entering middle school may not have had refined fine motor and self-care skills addressed. Service delivery is dynamic, with flexibility and adaptability to the changing needs of the school and child. Consultation with the teacher may serve the child's needs. If this type of delivery does not work, the practitioner may decide to provide direct service. It is helpful to explain to parents the dynamic nature of services and the IEP process.

CLINICAL *Pearl*

Remember that the teacher is the manager of the classroom. The OT practitioner is a guest, and his or her presence should not disrupt the routine.

TABLE 4-3

Sensory Strategies for Jim

WHAT IT LOOKS LIKE FOR JIM	SENSORY DIET
TACTILE SENSE	
Seeks touch and deep pressure	Provide deep pressure.
Seeks touch by touching objects and people around him	Provide weighted vest or weighted lap pad.
Likes and seeks soft, silky material	Provide silklike sheets or clothing. Place a piece of silk on his seat. Provide a piece of silk to calm Jim.
VESTIBULAR SENSE	
Seems to seek vestibular movement by spinning or rocking	Equipment suggestions: swing, rocking chair, etc. Activity suggestions: "Sit and move" chair cushion.
Gets overstimulated by activities in the environment	Encourage Jim to go to the quiet area in the corner of the room. Rock in the rocking chair.
PROPRIOCEPTIVE SENSE	
Seeks high impact by touching other people	Equipment: weights, joint compression, vibration, etc.
Pushes himself against other people	Provide weighted vest, joint compression, and vibration.
AUDITORY SENSE	
Very sensitive to noise	Work in noiseless environment. Try mufflers or headset to decrease noise. Play quiet ocean sounds in the background. Try rhythmic sounds, like a metronome.
Easily distracted by sound	Keep verbal cues to a minimum and avoid extraneous noise.
VISUAL SENSE	
Easily distracted by objects	Decrease visual distractions.
Gets easily overstimulated by too much visual stimulation	Remove visual distractions from the wall. Work in a cubicle.

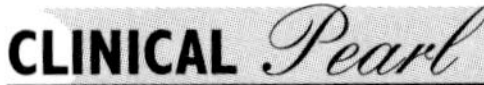

CLINICAL Pearl

Adolescents may need OT consultation to discuss their strengths and weaknesses for vocational activities. Children entering high school may benefit from consultation with an OT practitioner about study habits, strategies to succeed, and issues surrounding physical changes.

SUMMARY

OT clinicians must possess the technical knowledge and skills as well as be knowledgeable about child development, family systems, learning theory, community resources, and current federal and state regulations. Although there are federal regulations that dictate broad policies, OT practitioners must keep abreast of state regulations and local educational agency procedures to ensure compliance in all areas.

Communicating and working as a team is the key to school-based practice. Practitioners must be prepared to discuss OT knowledge in language that educators and families understand. Successfully functioning as part of a team requires the members to value the educational philosophy and listen carefully to the parents and teachers. Practitioners working in schools have the unique opportunity to help children function in the place that they work (school). Incorporating therapy into classroom activities takes skill and negotiation. Practitioners may need to "think outside the box" and provide therapeutic activities in a busy, crowded classroom. OT practitioners are responsible for modeling and teaching skills to others so that the educational staff can provide services to children on a daily basis. Clinicians working in educational settings analyze children in terms of their ability to perform occupations in the school, family, and community rather than in terms of their deficits in performance components. By working with a team of dedicated professionals, clinicians may improve a child's ability to learn, socialize, and function in school.

References

1. American Occupational Therapy Association: *Occupational therapy practice framework: domain and process*, Bethesda, Md, 2002, The Association.
2. American Occupational Therapy Association: *Occupational therapy services for children and youth under IDEA*, Rockville, Md, 1997, The Association.
3. American Occupational Therapy Association: Roles of occupational therapists and occupational therapy assistants in schools, *Am J Occup Ther* 41:798, 1987.
4. American Occupational Therapy Association Pediatric Curriculum Committee: *Guidelines for curriculum content in pediatrics*, Rockville, Md, 1991, The Association.
5. Bober P, Corbett S: *Occupational therapy and physical therapy: a resource and planning guide*, Madison, Wis, 1996, Wisconsin Department of Public Instruction.
6. Carver C: Crossing the thresholds. *OT Practice* 3:18, 1998.
7. Daniel RR v State Board of Education, 874 F, 2d, 1036, 1989.
8. Haley S, Coster W: *Pediatric evaluation of disability inventory*, Boston, 1992, New England Medical Center Hospitals.
9. Kramer P, Hinojosa J: *Frames of reference for pediatric occupational therapy*, ed 2, Baltimore, 1999, Williams & Wilkins.
10. Martin E, Martin R, Terman D: The legislative and litigation history of special education, *Future Child* 6:25, 1996.
11. Public Law 101–336, Americans with Disabilities Act, 1990.
12. Public Law 101–3476, Individuals with Disabilities Education Act, 1990.
13. Public Law 99–3457, The Education of the Handicapped Act, Amendments of 1986.
14. Public Law 105–317, The Individuals with Disabilities Education Act, Amendments of 1997.
15. Swinth Y, Handley-More D: Update on school-based practice, *OT Practice* 8:22, 2003.
16. Swinth Y, Hanft B: School-based practice; moving beyond 1:1 service delivery, *OT Practice* 7:12, 2002.
17. United States Code of Federal Regulations, title 34, subtitle B, chapter III, part 290.
18. United States Code of Federal Regulations, title 34, subtitle B, chapter III, part 300.

Recommended Reading

Hanft B, Place P: *The consulting therapist: a guide for OTs and PTs in schools*, Tucson, 1996, Therapy Skill Builders.

REVIEW *Questions*

1. What are some of the federal laws that have an impact on the provision of OT services in the public school system?
2. Which factors determine whether a child is eligible to receive OT services in a school setting?
3. In what ways do therapy services provided according to an educational model differ from those provided according to a medical model?
4. In what ways do the roles of an occupational therapist and a COTA differ in a school setting?

SUGGESTED *Activities*

1. Visit or volunteer in a public school and observe the various programs and environments that have been developed for students with special needs, such as a learning disabilities resource room and a self-contained classroom.
2. Be politically aware and active. Keep abreast of changes in local, state, and federal laws. Participate in public hearings and contact legislators when laws affecting the provision of therapy services are being debated.
3. Volunteer with an OTR or COTA in the public school system to understand how to integrate therapy services in the regular classroom.

CHAPTER 4 APPENDIX

Individual Educational Program

SCHOOL DISTRICT OF JANESVILLE

Meeting Type _x_ Initial ___ Annual Review ___ Interim ___ Reevaluation
___ Special Review ___ Extended School Year ___ Transition

Name: Sample IEP **Birthdate:** 3/20/01
Social Security number: ____________ **Medicaid number:** ____________
Sex: ___M___ **Grade:** ___-1 (preschool)___

Primary disability: ___Preschool___ **Other disabling conditions:** ___Speech and language___

Date of meeting: Monday, May 17, 2005 **Anticipated annual review:** Tuesday, May 17, 2006
Time of meeting: 7:30 AM **IEP initiation date:** Monday, August 9, 2005
Location of meeting: Janesville Elementary School **IEP ending date:** Tuesday, May 30, 2006

Present Levels of Performance

Area: Cognitive **Method: Brigance** **Date: 5/10/2005**

Findings: Sample follows verbal directions and sometimes chooses to disobey.

Sample has little interest in books, turning several pages at once. Sample enjoys routine songs and has begun to use his own hands to imitate gross arm motions to the music. Sample will touch eight body parts, match color, and sort by color. He picks out a named color for 10 colors.

Area: Fine motor **Method: Peabody Developmental Motor Test (fine motor subtest) Therapist Observation** **Date: 5/10/2005**

Findings: Sample is able to string beads with encouragement to stay on task. He tolerates textures such as lotion and shaving cream for short periods of time. He is able to tear paper into strips after minimum setup and throws beanbags into a target. Sample scribbles spontaneously but is unable to imitate strokes.

Area: Fine motor **Method: Peabody Development Motor Test (gross motor subtest) Therapist Observation** **Date: 5/10/2005**

Findings: Sample ambulates independently in the school and on uneven surfaces. He is able to ascend and descend the stairs with his hand held on or with the support of the railing. Running patterns are very immature, and he requires moderate assistance to play on outdoor playground equipment. Sample becomes hesitant and somewhat anxious or fearful of having his feet off a supporting surface. He continues to be hesitant and reluctant to try new sensorimotor activities, but with reassurance he will participate momentarily. Sample is able to throw and catch a medium-size ball.

CHAPTER 4 APPENDIX—cont'd

Individual Educational Program

Area: Language **Method: Brigance/Therapist Observation** **Date: 5/10/2005**

Findings: Sample says "sss" for "yes." He shakes his head for "no." He waves bye-bye and shows affection with hugs and an "aww" sound. Recently, Sample has been responding to requests to name an object with a one-syllable grunt.

Sample will participate in a group with picture symbol (pic/sym) exchange. He will also use a cheap talk device with eight pictures. He can produce the consonants /m/ and /p/ and the vowels /o/ and /a/. He has attached meaning to them in groups and stories.

Area: Self-help **Method: Brigance/Therapist Observation** **Date: 5/10/2005**

Findings: Sample is able to drink from a sipper cup without assistance but not able to consecutively swallow. He continues to be resistant to the feeding process but has broadened his variety of foods. Recently, he has been using a spoon on his own to feed himself.

Area: Social skills **Method: Brigance** **Date: 5/10/2005**

Findings: Sample watches other children play near him and may attempt to join in. He laughs and dances as he watches others play. Sample searches for hidden objects that he wants. He works with an adult for 10 minutes on activities. Sample begins to put things away at cleanup time when given prompts and gestures.

Strengths: Sample matches and sorts colors. He also picks out 10 named colors. Sample can follow one-step verbal directions. He says "sss" for "yes" and shakes his head for "no."

How does the student's disability affect involvement and progress in the general curriculum?
Not applicable for preschool because there are no other 3 year olds present in the school setting.

How does the student's disability affect his or her participation in appropriate activities?
Sample has delays in language development, which require small-group instruction or teaching of curriculum at a slower pace.

Related Services

(Goals, objectives, and levels of performance are required for all related services other than routine or maintenance types, which require descriptions of the service. However, if an instructional activity is involved, the goals, objectives, and levels of performance are required.)

Service	Description	Minutes	Frequency	Instructional
Speech-language	Group	60	Weekly	Yes
Occupational therapy	Direct individual	30	Weekly	Yes
Physical therapy	Direct individual	30	Weekly	Yes
Transportation	Special education bus	N/A	Daily	No

CHAPTER 4 APPENDIX—cont'd

Individual Educational Program

Special Factors

The IEP team has considered these special factors.

Yes	No	
x		The strengths of the student and the concerns of the parents for enhancing the education of their child.
x		The results of the initial evaluation or most recent evaluation of the student.
x		As appropriate, the result of the child's performance on any general state or district-wide assessment program.
x		In the case of a student whose behavior impedes his or her learning or that of others, the strategies, including positive behavioral interventions, strategies, and supports to address that behavior if appropriate.
x		In the case of a student with limited English proficiency, the language needs of the student as such should relate to the student's IEP.
x		In the case of a student who is blind or visually impaired, provide for instruction in and the use of Braille unless the IEP team determines, after an evaluation of the student's reading and writing skills, needs, and appropriate reading and writing media (including an evaluation of the student's future needs for instruction in and the use of Braille), that this instruction is not appropriate for the student.
x		The communication needs of the student, and in the case of a student who is deaf or hard of hearing, consider the student's language and communication needs, opportunities for direct communication with peers and professional personnel in the student's language and communication mode, academic level, and the full range of needs, including opportunities for direct instruction in the student's language and communication mode.
x		Whether the student requires assistive technology devices and services.
x		If, in considering these factors, the IEP team determines that a student needs a particular device or service (including an intervention, accommodation, or other program modification) in order for the student to receive FAPE, the IEP team must include a statement to that effect in the student's IEP.

LRE Documentation—Preschool Student

How does the nature and severity of this child's disability support placement in a separate (self-contained) class for children with disabilities?

A regular education curriculum is not appropriate at this time because Sample has not met prerequisite skills.

How would this child's presence in a regular preschool class/program substantially and consistently disrupt the performance of his or her classroom peers?

Sample needs individualized instruction to a degree that requires an excessive amount of teacher time, taking time away from the needs of nondisabled students.

What interventions were attempted in the home or preschool environment to facilitate this child's participation in a regular preschool class/program?

Location	Intervention	Begin	End	Results
Special education	Individual assistance	9/05/2005	5/5/2006	Moderately successful, but requires additional time

CHAPTER 4 APPENDIX—cont'd

Individual Educational Program

Assemblies	Individual assistance	9/05/2005	5/10/2006	Moderately successful, but requires shorter time
Cafeteria	Individual assistance	9/05/2005	5/10/2006	Moderately successful, but requires moderate assistance

What opportunities for interacting with nondisabled peers are to be provided for this child?

Activity	**With Whom**	**Where**	**Minutes**	**Frequency**
Assemblies	Nondisabled students	Auditorium	30	As provided
Lunch	Nondisabled students	Cafeteria	30	Daily
Playground	Nondisabled students	Playground	20	Daily

Based on this child's complete IEP and the IEP/staffing committee's consideration of each option listed on the continuum below, the appropriate placement for this child is:

Self-contained; in a separate (self-contained) class established primarily for children with disabilities
The school is at another location: Janesville Elementary School

Physical education will not take place because 3 year olds do not participate in physical education.

Transition services will not be discussed at this time because the child is under the age of 14 and has not reached the age of majority.

Extended School Year (ESY) will be discussed at a future date.

Testing Participation

Based on this student's present level of performance and his or her goals and objectives, the student will not participate in any statewide and/or districtwide testing that other students in his or her grade level are taking at grade −1.

Promotion/Retention

Are alternative promotion/retention standards required?

Yes ***Sample must complete 70% of IEP objectives, with consideration given to chronological age.***

CHAPTER 4 APPENDIX—cont'd

Individual Educational Program

Reporting to Parents

Progress toward annual goals will be reported to parents every 9 weeks through progress reports and will be measured by:

Accomplishment of short-term objectives

Modifications to Regular Education

What supplementary aids and services will be provided to the student, or on behalf of the student, for his or her advancement toward the attainment of the annual goals and participation in academic, nonacademic, and extracurricular activities in the general education curriculum and environment? Describe specific supplementary services/program modifications or support to be provided and indicate the anticipated location(s).

Supplementary Services/Program Modifications or Support

Supplementary Aids

Area: Augmentative communication Location: Special education Min: 30 Frequency: Daily
Aid: Cheap talk
Description: Used to say his name, friends, choose activity

Area: Augmentative communication Location: Special education Min: 30 Frequency: Daily
Description: Picture symbol exchange to choose activity and indicate needs

LRE Recommendations

Minutes/week in special education: 720

Minutes/week in regular education: 0

Individual Educational Program Goals and Objectives for Sample IEP

Assessment area: Cognitive

Goal: Sample will increase his cognitive abilities by completing these short-term objectives.

Location(s)	Person(s) Responsible	Goal Type(s)
Special education	Special education teacher	Academic

CHAPTER 4 APPENDIX—cont'd

Individual Educational Program

Short-Term Objectives	Criteria	Assessment Method	Critical
Sample will identify 16 named body parts by (1) touching or 2) pointing.	80%	Classroom observation	No
Sample will identify 10 named pictures or objects by (1) touching or (2) pointing.	80%	Classroom observation	Yes

Assessment area: Fine motor

Goal: Sample will improve his fine motor skills by accomplishing 80% of the following short-term objectives.

Location(s)	Person(s) Responsible	Goal Type(s)
Special education	Special education teacher Occupational therapist	Academic Related service

Short-Term Objectives	Criteria	Assessment Method	Critical
Sample will put 5 out of 9 pieces in an individual inset puzzle with (1) minimum assistance or (2) independently.	80%	Classroom observation	No
Sample will snip 5 times with regular or adapted scissors, placing the scissors in the hand correctly with (1) minimum assistance or (2) independently.	80%	Classroom observations	No

Assessment area: Gross motor

Goal: Sample will improve his gross motor skills by accomplishing 80% of the following short-term objectives.

Location(s)	Person(s) Responsible	Goal Type(s)
Special education	Special education teacher Physical therapist	Academic Related service

Short-Term Objectives	Criteria	Assessment Method	Critical
Sample will access and play on the playground equipment independently and safely.	0%	Classroom observation	No
Sample will ascend a small set of stairs without the use of a railing or support.	80%	Classroom observations	No

CHAPTER 4 APPENDIX—cont'd

Individual Educational Program

Assessment area: Language

Goal: Sample will improve his language skills by accomplishing 80% of the following short-term objectives.

Location(s)	Person(s) Responsible	Goal Type(s)
Special education	Special education teacher Speech-language pathologist	Academic Related service

Short-Term Objectives	Criteria	Assessment Method	Critical
Sample will communicate a desire to stop an activity by selecting pictures/ symbols representing all done or stop.	80%	Classroom observations	No
Sample will follow unfamiliar one-step directions when given visual and verbal prompts.	80%	Classroom observations	Yes

Assessment area: Self-help

Goal: Sample will improve his self-help skills by accomplishing 80% of the following short-term objectives.

Location(s)	Person(s) Responsible	Goal Type(s)
Special education	Special education teacher Occupational therapist	Academic Related service

Short-Term Objectives	Criteria	Assessment Method	Critical
Sample will drink independently from a cup, demonstrating consecutive swallows and no spillage.	80%	Classroom observations	Yes
Sample will finger-feed himself the food of the adult's choice without overreactions.	80%	Classroom observations	Yes

CHAPTER 4 APPENDIX—cont'd

Individual Educational Program

Assessment area: Social skills

Goal: Sample will improve his social skills by accomplishing 80% of the following short-term objectives.

Location(s)	Person(s) Responsible	Goal Type(s)
Special education	Special education teacher	Academic

Short-Term Objectives	Criteria	Assessment Method	Critical
Sample will participate in simple games such as Ring Around the Rosy during circle time.	80%	Classroom observations	Yes
Sample will share a toy with another child with (1) minimum assistance or (2) independently.	80%	Classroom observations	No

Individual Educational Program

Committee Members

The individuals listed below have attended the IEP/LRE meeting and participated as equal members in the development of this IEP.

By the signature below we agree with the educational and related services to be provided to this student as delineated in this IEP. Our LRE recommendations and this student's placement are based on the completed IEP and the regulations under the Individuals with Disabilities Education Act.

Disability: **Preschool** Placement: **Self-contained**

Attendee	Representing	Signature	Date
Sue Jump	Speech-language pathologist		
Jill Johnson	Physical therapist		
Stephanie Marks	Special education teacher		
Virginia Gray	Occupational therapist		
Rebecca White	Regular education teacher		
Debbie Smith	LEA representative		

CHAPTER 4 APPENDIX—cont'd

Individual Educational Program

______ I have attended the IEP/ LRE meeting and have participated as an equal member of the committee in developing this IEP and determining the least restrictive environment and placement for my child.

______ I have read the IEP/LRE documents or had them read to me and understand their contents.

______ I agree with the educational and related services to be provided to my child as delineated in the IEP.

______ I have received a copy of the IEP/LRE documents.

______ I understand the IEP/LRE process.

Signature of Parent/Level Guardian/Surrogate Parent MM DD YY

FAPE, Free appropriate public education; *IEP*, individual educational program; *LEA*, local education agency; *LRE*, least restrictive environment.

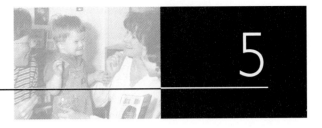

5

Principles of Normal Development

DIANNE KOONTZ LOWMAN
JEAN W. SOLOMON

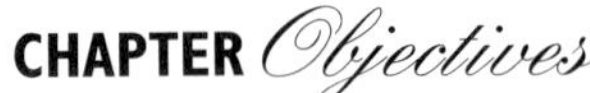

CHAPTER Objectives

After studying this chapter, the reader will be able to accomplish the following:

- Explain the importance of knowing and understanding the characteristics of typical development while working in the pediatric occupational therapy arena
- Discuss the relationship among typical development, areas of performance, and contexts
- Define and briefly describe the periods of development
- Describe the general principles of development
- Apply the general principles of development and justify a developmental sequence of skill acquisition in performance and areas of occupation

KEY TERMS

Normal
Typical
Development
Growth
Context
Periods of development
Principles of development

CHAPTER OUTLINE

Sally is a certified occupational therapy assistant (COTA) who is employed by the local public school system. She has been assigned a new client, a 3-year-old girl named Amy. The supervising registered occupational therapist (OTR) has begun the occupational therapy (OT) evaluation and has requested that Sally schedule a visit to assess the child's self-care and play skills in order to determine whether the child is functioning at the appropriate age level in these areas. Sally realizes that to accurately assess Amy's skills relative to her chronological age, she needs to review normal development definitions and principles.

The OT practitioner must understand the process of typical development. The sequence of acquisition in relation to occupational performance skills and areas is the foundation for OT assessment of and intervention with children who have special needs. The sequence of skill acquisition is predictable in the typically developing child.[1] The OT practitioner's knowledge of normal development guides the order of expectations and choice of activities for children who are not developing typically. In atypical development, delays in performance skills may make it difficult or impossible for a child to perform activities of daily living (ADLs), engage successfully in play activities, or acquire functional work and productive skills. The OT practitioner identifies deficits in the occupational performance skills (e.g., motor and process skills) that interfere with a child's functional independence. The practitioner relies on knowledge of typical development to assist the child in developing useful, functional skills.

GENERAL CONSIDERATIONS

An OT practitioner who is attempting to grasp the basis of normal development must consider general pediatric terms, the predictable sequence of skill acquisition in normal development, the principles of development, and the relationship between development and context. An understanding of the general terms used by pediatric therapists is necessary for effective communication. The pediatric therapist also needs to know the predictable sequence of skill acquisition in a typically developing child. The OT practitioner must understand the relationship between typical development and the occupational performance contexts as delineated in the American Occupational Therapy Association's (AOTA's) Occupational Therapy Practice Framework.[3]

Definitions of Terms

A basic understanding of the generic terms used by OT clinicians who work in pediatrics helps practitioners and other individuals working in the area of pediatrics to communicate effectively. **Normal** is defined as that which occurs habitually or naturally.[2] In this chapter "normal" is used interchangeably with **typical** in the discussions on development. **Development** is the act or process of maturing or acquiring skills ranging from simple to more complex.[2] **Growth** is the maturation of a person.[2] Because the concepts of development and growth are analogous, these terms are used interchangeably in this chapter (Box 5-1).

BOX 5-1

Definition of Typical Development

Typical development is defined as the natural process of acquiring skills ranging from simple to complex.

Predictable Sequence of Skill Acquisition

The normal development of skills in terms of performance and areas of occupation occurs in a predictable sequence.[1,4,5,7] The OT practitioner uses knowledge of typical development while working with children who have special needs to identify the areas in which there are deficits and develop a plan to improve their ADLs, play, and work skills. Although developmental checklists and other tools may help a practitioner identify the presence or absence of certain skills, understanding the process of how and why children are able to develop these skills is more useful in the clinical setting. For example, an OT practitioner could use an observational checklist to determine whether a child can independently finger-feed. A practitioner who has knowledge of normal development and its predictable sequence of events would know that children usually learn to eat with their fingers before learning to eat with a spoon. Therefore, if a child is not yet finger feeding, the practitioner would not introduce spoon feeding (depending on the circumstances). Knowledge and understanding of normal development guide the OT practitioner in the treatment planning process.

Relationship Between Typical Development and Context

OT practitioners need to understand the relationship between typical development and the AOTA's meaning of **context.** Because the events of normal development are sequential and predictable,[1,4,5,7] the chronological age of the child (i.e., how old the child is) has an impact on the child's level of skill development in performance and areas of occupation. Although practitioners obviously cannot change the age of a child, they can offer age-appropriate activities during intervention sessions. Being familiar with age-appropriate activities helps OT practitioners choose tasks for therapy sessions with children. For example, a practitioner may use colored blocks while performing fine motor and sorting activities with a 3-year-old child, but the use of blocks would not be suitable in a session with a 14-year-old adolescent. It would be more appropriate to have the adolescent use objects like coins for fine motor and sorting activities.

Although normal development is predictable and sequential, the rate of skill acquisition varies among children. This variability greatly depends on the contexts (delineated in AOTA's Occupational Therapy Practice Framework) (Box 5-2). These contexts include cultural, physical, social, personal, spiritual, temporal, and virtual factors.[3]

The physical, or nonhuman, aspects of the environment[3] have an impact on the rate of skill acquisition in both performance and areas of occupation. For example, if a child lives in a climate that requires warm clothing, s/he will learn to don and doff a sweater or a coat more quickly than one who lives in a temperate climate. A child who lives in a two-story house will more likely learn to ascend and descend stairs before one who lives in a single-story house.

BOX 5-2

Contexts

CULTURAL CONTEXT
Customs, beliefs/values, standards, and expectations

PHYSICAL CONTEXT
Nonhuman aspects of the environment

SOCIAL CONTEXT
Significant others and the larger social group

PERSONAL CONTEXT
Features of the person such as age, gender, socioeconomic status, and educational level

SPIRITUAL CONTEXT
That which inspires and motivates; the essence of a person

TEMPORAL CONTEXT
Stage of life, time of day, and time of year

VIRTUAL CONTEXT
Computer or airways, simulators, chat rooms, and radio

Adapted from the American Occupational Therapy Association: Occupational therapy practice framework, *Am J Occup Ther* 56:623, 2002.

The social environment, or the availability and anticipation of behaviors by significant others,[3] influences the rate of skill acquisition in performance and areas of occupation. An infant who is breastfed will not acquire the ability to drink from a bottle or cup as quickly as one who is bottle-fed. An infant who is carried frequently may not develop gross motor and mobility skills as quickly as one who is allowed to move around on the floor or in a playpen.

The personal context includes the child's age, gender, socioeconomic status, and educational level.[3] For example, a 2-year-old boy from a rural community will have different goals and enjoy different activities than a 10-year-old girl from an inner city.

The spiritual context consists of that which inspires and motivates the child, including the essence of the person and what gives greater or higher purpose.[3] For young children, the spiritual context includes those things that motivate and are interesting to them. Children who love to sing or draw may find these experiences spiritual. Nature or music may be spiritual for others. Practitioners may need to discuss the views of the parents because they may influence the child's spiritual nature.

The cultural environment, which comprises customs, beliefs, activity patterns, and behavior standards,[3] also influences the rate of skill development in performance and areas of occupation. *Anticipation of behaviors* refers to an individual's expectation of repetition of a daily schedule (e.g., waking up, eating, bathing, and dressing—in that order) or consistency of cause and effect behaviors (e.g., washing the dishes and cleaning the room, causing the mother to be pleased with the child). An adolescent whose parents believe that only adults should be employed may develop work skills later in life than one whose parents believe that summer and after-school jobs are appropriate and should be encouraged. In certain cultures, using eating utensils is not the adult norm. Children in this type of cultural environment may never learn to use a fork or spoon.

It is important for OT practitioners working with children to understand the *temporal context,* which refers to the stage of life, time of year, and length of occupation.[3] Adolescents and toddlers have very different goals and experiences. Toddlers experience the "terrible twos" for a short period of time (it ranges for each child). However, a 5-year-old child should be well past this phase, so the observation of this behavior past the expected duration indicates a cause for concern.

The virtual context includes communication by means of computers and airways.[3] Children use computers, cell phones, and other electronic means to communicate. These virtual environments provide opportunities for children but also must be monitored.

Studying the process of normal development allows practitioners to learn about its predictable sequences and contextual variability. Although this knowledge is important, having the skills to solve problems related to the developmental process is more useful than memorizing the sequences of skill acquisition in performance and areas of occupation. Carefully studying this chapter as well as the next two and participating in the suggested activities give practitioners an excellent basis for using the problem-solving approach in the developmental process. One framework to use when studying development is that based on the generally accepted periods of development. Another framework involves the general principles used by therapists while working in pediatrics.

PERIODS OF DEVELOPMENT

Periods of development are intervals of time during which a child increases in size and acquires specific skills in performance and areas of occupation.[2] Pediatric OT practitioners work with children of varying chronological ages. The following normal developmental periods are used as the basis for comparison in subsequent chapters dealing with normal development (Box 5-3).

Gestation and Birth

Gestation refers to the developmental period of the fetus or unborn child in the mother's uterus. This period begins with conception and ends with birth.[2] The gestational period is also referred to as the *prenatal* (before-birth) *period*.[2] Gestation typically lasts 40 weeks.[2] The birthing process is also known as the *perinatal* (around-birth) *period*. This period varies greatly in duration for a variety of reasons, which are beyond the scope of this book. The perinatal period ends when the infant is able to independently sustain life without placental nutrients from the mother. The *postnatal* (after-birth) *period* is the immediate interval of time following birth. During the postnatal period, the infant is known as a *neonate*, or *new baby*.[2]

BOX 5-3

Periods of Development

GESTATION AND BIRTH
From conception to the moment at which the neonate can survive on its own without placental nutrients

INFANCY
From birth through 18 months of age

EARLY CHILDHOOD
From 18 months through 5 years of age

MIDDLE CHILDHOOD
From 6 years of age until the onset of puberty (12 years of age for females and 14 years of age for males)

ADOLESCENCE
From puberty until the onset of adulthood (usually 21 years of age)

Infancy

Infancy is the period from birth through approximately 18 months of age.[8] It is characterized by significant physical and emotional growth.[8] Normal infants grow considerably in height and weight during the first 18 months of life.[8] They develop sensory and motor skills, and by 18 months of age they are walking, talking, and performing simple self-care tasks such as eating with a spoon, drinking from a cup, and undressing.

Early Childhood

Toddlers and preschool children represent the period of early childhood, which begins at 18 months of age and lasts through 5 years of age.[2,8] During the early-childhood period, children become increasingly independent and establish more of a sense of individuality.

Middle Childhood

Middle childhood begins at 6 years of age and lasts until puberty, which begins at approximately 12 years of age in females and 14 years of age in males.[8] Children in this developmental period spend the majority of their time in educational settings; therefore, the major influence on the child shifts from parents to peers.

Adolescence

Adolescence is the period of physical and psychological development that accompanies the onset of puberty. Puberty is a stage of maturation in which a person becomes physiologically capable of reproduction. This period is marked by hormonal changes and their resulting challenges.[2] Adolescence ends with the onset of adulthood (usually 21 years of age), when individuals begin to function independent of their parents.[2]

OT practitioners use the periods of development as reference points while working with children with special needs. Knowledge of the sequence of development within each period is used as a guide for the OT process. Practitioners need to know the general principles of development in order to understand the reasons children gain skills predictably and sequentially.

PRINCIPLES OF NORMAL DEVELOPMENT

The general **principles of development** are widely accepted in the various pediatric disciplines (Box 5-4). The following principles are tools used by OT practitioners to solve problems during the pediatric OT process.

- **Normal development is sequential and predictable.** The rate (speed) and direction (vertical or horizontal) of development vary among children, but the sequence remains the same.[1,4,5,7] For example, infants who are typically developing acquire head control before trunk control (an example of vertical development). Head and trunk control are necessary for them to sit independently. Infants learn to roll, then sit, then creep, and finally walk. Although most developmental theorists agree that the sequence is the same for all children, recent research in motor control theory demonstrates that motor development does not always follow a set sequence.[1] In either case, each child acquires these skills at a unique rate.
- **Maturation and experience affect a child's development.**[4-6] Maturation and experience influence the rate and direction of normal development. Maturation is the innate (natural) process of growth and development,[2] and experience is the result of interactions with the environment. In addition, current research on motor control introduces the concepts of arousal states and motivation as additional factors that have an impact on motor learning. The child must be aroused in order to be motivated to move and interact with the environment.[1] Although most developmental theorists agree that maturation, experience, arousal state, and motivation have an impact on a child's development, their opinions vary about which one is the more significant.
- **Throughout the course of normal development, changes occur in the biological, psychological, and social systems.**[5] Therefore, development is a dynamic and continuously changing process. Changes in the biological system include those related to the functions and processes of internal structures.[8] Changes in the psychological system affect the emotional and behavioral characteristics of the individual.[8] Changes in the social system include those that affect individuals in their immediate environment and society as a whole.[8] These changes occur in all three systems throughout the course of typical development. A change in one of the systems has an impact on the other two.
- **Development progresses in two directions: vertical and horizontal.**[5] As children progress through the various developmental levels related to the specific performance skills or areas of occupation, they are progressing vertically. For example, in the occupational area of ADLs, children learn to eat with their fingers before they learn to eat with a spoon. As children learn to roll, then crawl, then creep, and finally walk, they are progressing vertically in the gross motor performance skills. In both of the examples, development is occurring in a vertical direction within a specific performance skill or area of occupation. Development that involves different performance skills and areas of occupation is horizontal progression. A child who is simultaneously learning to finger-feed, use a pincer grasp, and creep is progressing horizontally because several different skills in performance and areas of occupation (i.e., ADLs, fine motor skills, and gross motor skills) are involved.
- **Motor development follows three basic rules.**
  1. *Development progresses cephalad to caudad, or head to tail.*[5] For example, a baby is first able to control head and neck movements (beginning at around 2 months), then the arms and hands (grasping begins at about 3 months), then the trunk (most babies sit well by 8 months), and finally the legs and feet (most children walk by 14 to 15 months).
  2. *Development progresses in a proximal to distal direction, which means that children develop control of structures close to their body (such as the shoulder) before they develop those farther away from their body (such as the hand).*[4] For example, a baby can swat at an object by 3 to 4 months but cannot reach straight ahead and grasp an object in the fingers until around 8 months.

BOX 5-4

General Principles of Development

Development is sequential and predictable.
Maturation and experience affect development.
Development involves changes in the biological, psychological, and social systems.
Development occurs in two directions: horizontal and vertical.
Development progresses in order in three basic sequences.
- Cephalad to caudad
- Proximal to distal
- Gross to fine

3. *Development progresses from gross control to fine control, which means that children gain control of large-body movements before they do more refined movements.*[4] For example, children are able to catch a large ball using both arms and their body before they learn to catch a tennis ball with one hand. They use the larger arm muscles to catch a large 8-inch ball and the smaller wrist and hand muscles to catch a tennis ball.

These general principles of development provide a framework for OT practitioners to use while solving developmental problems. The principles can be used to guide the treatment planning process while working with children who have special needs.

SUMMARY

Normal development is sequential and predictable. OT practitioners rely on their knowledge and understanding of typical development while working with children who have special needs. Practitioners must also consider the relationship between normal development and contexts.

The periods and general principles of development help to provide a framework for organizing and understanding information related to typical development. The periods include gestation and birth, infancy, early childhood, middle childhood, and adolescence. The general principles of development, which are widely used in the various pediatric disciplines, help OT practitioners plan evaluations and interventions while working with children who have special needs.

References

1. Alexander R, Boehme R, Cupps B: *Normal development of functional motor skills*, Tucson, 1993, Therapy Skill Builders.
2. *American heritage dictionary of the English language*, ed 4, Boston, 2000, Houghton Mifflin.
3. American Occupational Therapy Association: Occupational therapy practice framework: domain and process, *Am J Occup Ther* 56:609, 2002.
4. Boehme R: *Improving upper body control: an approach to assessment and treatment of tonal dysfunction*, Tucson, 1988, Therapy Skill Builders.
5. Case-Smith J: *Occupational therapy for children*, ed 5, St Louis, 2005, Mosby.
6. Kielhofner G: *Conceptual foundations of occupational therapy*, Philadelphia, 1997, FA Davis.
7. Kramer P, Hinojosa J: *Frames of reference for pediatric occupational therapy*, ed 2, Philadelphia, 1999, Lippincott Williams & Wilkins.
8. Meyer WJ: Infancy, *Microsoft Encarta 98 encyclopedia*, Redmond, Wash, 1997, Microsoft.

Recommended Reading

Bly L: *Motor skills acquisition in the first year: an illustrated guide to normal development*, Tucson, 1994, Therapy Skill Builders.

Green M, Palfrey JS, editors: *Bright futures: guidelines for health supervision of infants, children, and adolescents*, ed 2, Arlington, Va, 2002, National Center for Education in Maternal and Child Health. Retrieved June 30, 2004 from www.brightfutures.org.

Gilfoyle ZM, Grady AP, Moore JC: *Children adapt*, ed 2, Thorofare, NJ, 1990, Slack.

Zero to Three: Brain wonders: helping babies and toddlers grow and develop, Washington, DC, 2004, Zero to Three. Retrieved June 30, 2004 from www.zerotothree.org/brainwonders/.

REVIEW *Questions*

1. Explain the following terms: normal, typical, development, growth.
2. List and describe the periods of development.
3. List and describe the general principles of development.
4. Define context.
5. Describe how contexts have an impact on intervention.

SUGGESTED *Activities*

1. Visit a daycare center or playground to observe children playing. Notice the variety of approaches that are used by different children to accomplish the same task.
2. In small study groups, discuss the general principles of development and then describe these principles in your own words. Give examples of these principles in relation to your own development.
3. In small study groups, describe your cultural background and how it influences your goals and the occupations in which you perform. How would it influence the treatment of a child?
4. Provide examples of how contexts (cultural, physical, personal, social, spiritual, temporal, and virtual) influences development. Discuss the techniques practitioners could use to address each context.

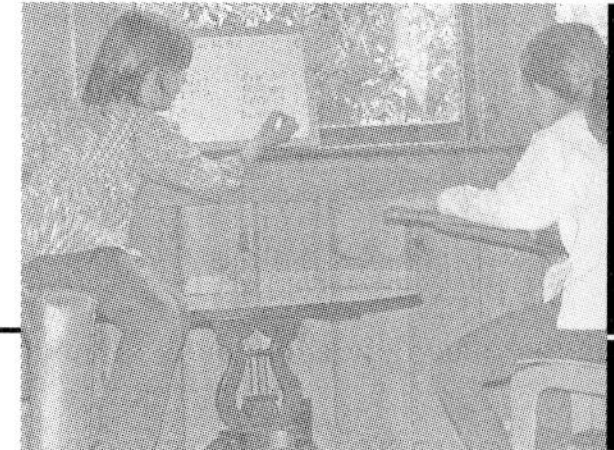

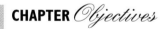

6

Development of Occupational Performance Skills

DIANNE KOONTZ LOWMAN

CHAPTER *Objectives*

After studying this chapter, the reader will be able to accomplish the following:

- Describe significant physiological changes that occur at each stage of development
- Identify the sequences of motor skill development (gross and fine motor)
- Outline the stages of process development (cognitive, defined by Piaget's theory)
- Describe the issues in each phase of communication and interaction development (psychosocial) using the theories of Erikson and Greenspan

KEY TERMS

Performance skills
Motor skills
Gross motor skills
Primitive reflexes
Righting reactions
Equilibrium reactions
Fine motor skills
Process skills
Communication/interaction skills
Psychosocial

CHAPTER OUTLINE

Three generations of family members have gathered for a family reunion. While looking at the grandmother's photograph album, conversation centers around how much the 2-year-old grandson looks like his father and grandfather did at the same age. The family is amazed to see how their bodies, sizes, proportions, and postures look similar, even though their clothing and environments are significantly different!

From birth through adolescence the child progresses through the periods of development. Development that occurs within each period is described in the literature in terms of the physiological, motor, cognitive, language, and psychosocial domains. In the Occupational Therapy Practice Framework, the occupational **performance skills** are **motor skills (gross** and **fine motor)**, **process skills** (cognition), and **communication/interaction skills** (language and psychosocial) (Box 6-1).[2] Deficits in any of these skills may interfere with the child's performance in the areas of self-care, play, education, and social participation. The normal developmental sequences are presented in this chapter to assist practitioners in identifying potential deficits or delays. Sequences may vary, and physical, temporal, social, and cultural aspects of the environment may affect developmental progression.

BOX 6-1

Occupational Performance Skills

MOTOR SKILLS (GROSS AND FINE)
Motor skills are those involved in moving and interacting with objects or the environment and include posture, mobility, coordination, strength, effort, and energy. Examples of motor skills include stabilizing the body and manipulating objects.

PROCESS SKILLS (COGNITION)
Process skills are those used in completing daily tasks and include energy, knowledge, temporal organization, organizing space and objects, and adaptation. Examples of process skills include maintaining attention to a task, choosing appropriate tools and materials for the task, and accommodating the method of task completion in response to a problem.

COMMUNICATION/INTERACTION SKILLS (LANGUAGE AND PSYCHOSOCIAL)
Communication and interaction skills refer to those needed to interact with other people and include physicality, information exchange, and relations. Examples of communication and interaction skills include gesturing to indicate intention, expressing affect, and relating in a manner that establishes rapport with others.

From the American Occupational Therapy Association: Occupational therapy practice framework: domain and process, *Am J Occup Ther* 56:612, 2002.

As children follow a developmental sequence within an individual performance skill, they are also developing in other performance skills. For example, an 18-month-old toddler travels and explores independently, has a precise grasp, is beginning to use tools to solve problems, and demonstrates an understanding of the function of objects in play.

INFANCY

Phillip is an active and happy 1 year old. It is his first birthday party, and he is busy experimenting with his new toys. As family and friends watch, he attempts to sit on his push toy and make it move across the kitchen floor. When his older siblings offer help, he pushes them away because he wants to play alone.

Physiological

The newborn's average weight at birth is 7 lb, 2 oz and the average length between 19 and 22 inches. The appearance of the newborn may be characterized by a covering comprising a layer of fluid called the *vernix caseosa;* a large, bumpy head; a flat, "board" nose; reddish skin; puffy eyes; external breasts; and fine hair called *lanugo* covering the body.[13] At 1 minute after birth the newborn's physiological status is tested using the Apgar scoring system, which rates each of the following five areas on a scale of 0 to 2: color, heart rate, reflex irritability, muscle tone, and respiratory effort. The scores are computed at 1 and 5 minutes after birth. The closer the score to 10, the better the condition of the newborn; scores of 6 or less indicate the need for intervention.[12]

The infant's first 3 months of life are characterized by constant physiological adaptations. Structural changes in the newborn's circulatory system include the expansion of the lungs and increased efficiency of blood flow to the heart. The developing central nervous system participates in the body's regulation of sleep, digestion, and temperature.[10]

Physical growth is dramatic—from birth to 6 months of age, infants experience a more rapid rate of growth than at any other time except gestation.[19] During the first year, infants triple their body weight and increase 10 to 12 inches in height. Their body shape changes, and by 4 months the sizes of their heads and bodies are more proportionate. By 12 months, average infants weigh 21 to 22 lb and are 29 to 30 inches tall. During the second year of life, physical growth slows. By 24 months, an average toddler weighs about 27 lb and is 34 inches tall. The posture of toddlers is characterized by *lordosis* (forward curvature of the spine) and a protruding abdomen, which toddlers retain well into the third year.[33]

At 4 months sleep patterns begin to be regulated, and some infants may sleep through the night. By 8 months the average infant sleeps 12 to 13 hours per day, but the range can vary from 9 to 18 hours per day. By 6 to 7 months the average infant acquires the first tooth, a lower incisor. As a result, saliva production increases, which leads to drooling. At approximately 8 months the upper central incisor teeth begin to surface, at 9 months the upper lateral incisors appear, and at 12 months the first lower molars are seen.[28]

Motor

Brazelton[9] identified six behavioral states observed in the newborn: (1) deep sleep; (2) light sleep; (3) drowsy or semidozing; (4) alert, actively awake; (5) fussy; and (6) crying. The infant's state should be noted when observing the way s/he responds to stimulation.[13]

Sensory skills

Newborns have vision at birth and can see objects best from about 8 inches away, which is the typical distance between the caregiver's face and the infant.[29] By the first month of life an infant shows a preference for patterns and can distinguish between colors. By 3 months visual acuity develops enough to allow distinction between a picture of a face and a real face.[10] By 12 months the infant's visual acuity is about 20/100 to 20/50.[24]

Hearing is well developed in newborns and continues to improve as they grow. They tend to respond strongly to their mother's voice.[25] During the first 2 months, infants respond to sound with random body movements. At 3 months, they move their eyes in the direction of sound.[10] At 6 months, they localize sounds to the left and right.[5] At birth newborns are able to taste sweet, sour, and bitter substances. Between birth and 3 months, infants are able to differentiate between pleasant and noxious odors. They are very sensitive to touch, cold and heat, pain, and pressure; one of the most important stimuli for infants from birth to 3 months is skin contact and warmth.[27] Holding and swaddling the infant provide skin contact and maintain temperature.[13]

Gross motor skills

The newborn's body is characterized by physiological flexion, a position of extremity and trunk flexion.[8] This flexion tends to keep the infant in a compact position and provides a base of stability for random movements to occur. These movements are characterized by a motion called *random burst*, in which everything moves as a unit.[1] The newborn has numerous **primitive reflexes** that are genetically transmitted survival mechanisms. These automatic responses to stimuli help the newborn adapt to the environment. Primitive reflexes are controlled by lower levels of the central nervous system. As higher levels of the central nervous system mature, the higher systems inhibit the expression of the primitive reflexes. As infants learn about the environment, primitive reflexes are integrated into their overall postural mechanism, with the more mature righting and equilibrium responses that dominate their movements.[34] Under stress these reflexes may be partially present, but they are never obligatory in normal development. Some primitive reflexes are present at birth, whereas others emerge later in the infant's development (Table 6-1).

As shown in Table 6-2, infants' **gross motor skills** become gradually more complex as they develop.[1,8,13] They begin to combine basic reflexive movements with higher cognitive and physiological functioning to control these movements in the environment (Box 6-2). Between birth and 2 months, infants can turn their heads from side to side while in both the prone and supine positions. As physiological flexion diminishes, they appear more hypotonic (have less muscular and postural tone) and the movements of each side of their body appear asymmetrical. The asymmetrical tonic neck reflex (ATNR) holds infants' heads to one side. By 4 months, they can raise and rotate their heads to look at their surroundings. In the supine position (on the back), 4-month-old infants begin to bring their hands to their knees and can deliberately roll from the supine position to the side. The increased head and trunk control observed at this age is the result of emerging **righting reactions** and better postural control (see Box 6-2). At 5 months, infants can bring their heads forward without lagging when pulled to a sitting position. By 6 months, they can shift their weight to free extremities to reach for objects while in the prone position (on the stomach). In the supine position, 6-month-old infants can bring their feet to their mouths and are able to sit by themselves for short periods. At 7 to 8 months, they are able to push themselves from a prone to a sitting position, roll over at will, and crawl on their stomachs. Between 6 and 9 months, infants develop upper extremity protective extension reactions that allow them to catch themselves when pushed off balance (Figure 6-1). From 7 to 21 months, they develop **equilibrium reactions** that allow them to maintain their center of gravity over their base of support; these reactions are critical for transitional movements patterns (i.e., movements from one position to another) and ambulation (see Box 6-2; Figure 6-2). At 10 to 11 months, infants are practicing and enjoying creeping. By 12 months, they are learning to shift their weight and step to one side by cruising around furniture. At 13 or 14 months most infants take their first steps, and between 12 and 18 months they spend much of their time practicing motor skills by

TABLE 6-1

Reflexes and Reactions

NAME OF REFLEX OR REACTION	POSITION (P) STIMULUS (S)	POSITIVE RESPONSE	AGE SPAN: AGE OF ONSET OR INTEGRATION	LACK OF INTEGRATION OR ONSET
Rooting	P: Supine S: Light touch on side of face near mouth	Open mouth and turn head in direction of touch.	Birth to 3 mo	Interferes with exploration of objects and head control
Suck/swallow	P: Supine S: Light touch on oral cavity	Close mouth, suck, and swallow.	Birth to 2-5 mo	Interferes with development of coordination of sucking, swallowing, and breathing
Moro's	P: Supine, head at midline S: Drooping head, more than 30 degrees extended	Arms, extend and hands open, then arms flex and hands close; infant usually cries.	Birth to 4-6 mo	Interferes with head control, sitting equilibrium, and protective reactions
Palmar grasp	P: Supine S: Pressure on ulnar surface of palm	Fingers flex.	Birth to 4-6 mo	Interferes with releasing objects
Plantar grasp	P: Supine S: Firm pressure on ball of foot	Toes grasp (flexion).	Birth to 4-9 mo	Interferes with putting on shoes because of toe clawing, gait, and standing and walking problems (e.g., walking on toes)
Neonatal positive support—primary standing	P: Upright S: Being bounced several times on soles of feet (proprioceptive stimulus)	LE extensor tone increases and plantar flexion is present. Some hip and knee flexion or genu recurvatum (hyperextension of the knee) may occur.	Birth to 1-2 mo	Interferes with walking patterns and leads to walking on toes
ATNR	P: Supine, arms and legs extended, head in midposition S: Head turned to one side	Arm and leg on face side extend; arm and leg on skull side flex (or experience increased flexor tone)	Birth to 4-6 mo	Interferes with reaching and grasping, bilateral hand use, and rolling
STNR	P: Quadruped position or over tester's knees S: 1. Flexed head 2. Extended head	1. Arms flex and legs extend (tone increases). 2. Arms extend and legs flex (tone increases).	Birth to 4-6 mo	Interferes with reciprocal creeping (children "bunny hop" or move arms and then legs in quadruped position) and walking
TLR P:	1. Supine, head in midposition, arms and legs extended 2. Prone S: Position (laying on floor); being moved into flexion or extension	1. Extensor tone of neck UE, and LE increases when moved into flexion. 2. Flexor tone of neck UE, and LE increases when moved into extension.	Birth to 4-6 mo	Interferes with turning on side, rolling over, going from laying to sitting position, and creeping In older children, interferes with ability to "hold in supine flexion" or assume a pivot prone position

TABLE 6-1

Reflexes and Reactions—cont'd

NAME OF REFLEX OR REACTION	POSITION (P) STIMULUS (S)	POSITIVE RESPONSE	AGE SPAN: AGE OF ONSET OR INTEGRATION	LACK OF INTEGRATION OR ONSET
Landau	P: Prone, held in space (suspension) supporting thorax S: Suspension (usually), also active or passive dorsiflexion of head	Hips and legs extend; UE extends and abducts. Elbows can flex. (Typically used to determine overall development)	3-4 mo to 12-24 mo	Slows development of prone extension, sitting, and standing Early onset (1 mo); may indicate excessive tone or spasticity
Protective extension UE Parachute, downward Forward, sideways, backward	P: Prone, head in midposition, arms extend above S: Suspension by ankles and pelvis and sudden movement of head toward floor P: Seated S: Child pushed: 1. Forward 2. Left, right 3. Backward		Shoulders flex and elbow and wrist extend (arms extend forward) to protect head Infant catches self in directions pushed: 1. Shoulder flexes and abducts; elbow and wrist extend (arms extend forward). 2. Shoulder abducts, elbow and wrist extend (arms extend to side). 3. Shoulders, elbows, and wrists extend (arms extend backward) to protect head.	Interferes with head protection when center of gravity displaced
Staggering LE Forward, backward, sideways	P: Standing upright S: Displacement of body by pushing on shoulders and upper trunk: 1. Forward 2. Backward 3. Sideways	Infant takes one or more steps in direction of displacement. UEs often also have a protective reaction, with elbow, wrist, and fingers extending: 1. Shoulder flexes. 2. Shoulder abducts and extends. 3. Shoulder abducts.	15-18 mo, continues throughout life	Interferes with ability to catch self when center of gravity displaced, causes trips and falls
Equilibrium—sitting	P: Seated, extremities relaxed S: Hand pulled to one side or shoulder pushed	*Head righting: non-weight-bearing side*—trunk flexes; UE and LE abduct and internally rotate; and elbow, wrist, and fingers extend *Head righting: weight-bearing side*—trunk elongates; UE and LE externally rotate; and elbow, wrist, and fingers abduct and extend.	7-8 mo, continues throughout life	Interferes with ability to sit or maintain balance when reaching for objects or displacing center of gravity

TABLE 6-1

Reflexes and Reactions—cont'd

NAME OF REFLEX OR REACTION	POSITION (P) STIMULUS (S)	POSITIVE RESPONSE	AGE SPAN: AGE OF ONSET OR INTEGRATION	LACK OF INTEGRATION OR ONSET
Standing	P: Standing upright, extremities relaxed S: Body displaced by holding UE and pulling to side	*Head righting: non-weight-bearing side*—trunk flexes; UE and LE abduct and internally rotate; and elbow, wrist, and fingers extend. *Head righting: weight-bearing side*—trunk elongates; UE and LE eternally rotate; and elbow, wrist, and fingers extend and abduct.	12-21 mo, continues throughout life	Interferes with ability to stand and walk and make transitional movements
Equilibrium or tilting—prone, supine	P: Prone or supine on a tilt board, extremities extended S: Board tilted to left or right	*Head righting: non-weight-bearing side*—trunk flexes; UE and LE abduct; and elbow, wrist, hip, and knee externally rotate and extend. *Head righting: weight-bearing side*—UE and LE internally rotate and abduct and elbow, wrist, fingers, knee, and hip extend.	5-6 mo, continues throughout life	Interferes with ability to make transitional movements, sit, and creep

Adapted from Alexander R, Boehme R, Cupps B: *Normal development of functional motor skills*, Tucson, 1993, Therapy Skill Builders; Bly L: *Motor skills acquisition in the first year: an illustrated guide to normal development*, Tucson, 1994, Therapy Skill Builders; Fiorentino MR: *Reflex testing methods for evaluating CNS development*, ed 2, Springfield, Ill, 1981, Charles C Thomas; Simon CJ, Daub MM: Human development across the life span. In Hopkins JL, Smith HD, editors: *Willard and Spackman's occupational therapy*, ed 8, Philadelphia, 1993, Lippincott.

LE, Lower extremity; *UE*, upper extremity; *ATNR*, asymmetrical tonic neck reflex; *STNR*, symmetrical tonic neck reflex; *TLR*, tonic labyrinthine reflex.

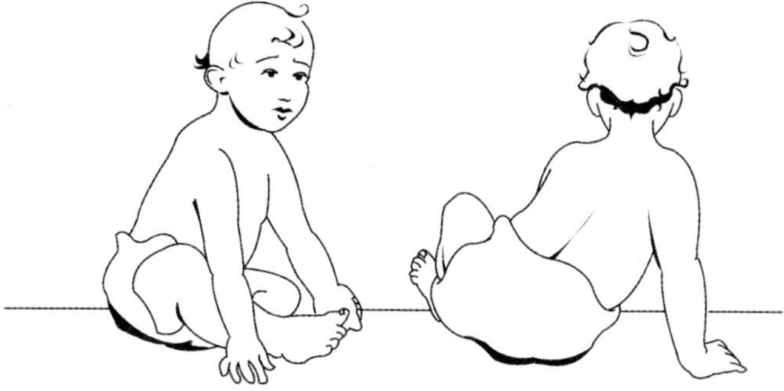

FIGURE 6-1 Equilibrium reactions allow infants to protect themselves by automatically moving forward and sideways after losing balance in a sitting position or from one position to a different one.

TABLE 6-2

Normal Development of Sensorimotor Skills

AGE	GROSS MOTOR COORDINATION	FINE MOTOR COORDINATION
BIRTH OR 37-40 WK OF GESTATION	Is dominated by physiological flexion Moves entire body into extension Turns head side to side (protective response) Keeps head mostly to side while in supine position	Visually regards objects and people Tends to fist and flex hands across chest during feeding Displays strong grasp reflex but has no voluntary grasping abilities Has no voluntary release abilities
1-2 MO	Appears hypertonic as physiological flexion Practices extension and flexion Continues to gain control of head Moves elbows forward toward shoulders while in prone position Has ATNR with head to side while in supine position When held in standing position, bears some weight on legs	Displays diminishing grasp reflex Involuntarily releases after holding them briefly has no voluntary release abilities
3-5 MO	Experiences fading of ATNR and grasp reflex Has more balance between extension and flexion positions Has good head control (centred and upright) Supports self on extended arms while in prone position pops self on forearms Brings hand to feet and feet to mouth while in supine position Props on arms with little support while seated Rolls from supine to prone position Bears some weight on legs when held proximally	Constantly brings hands to mouth Develops tactil awareness in hands Reaches more accurately usually with both hands Palmar grasp Begins transferring objects from hand to hand Does not have control of releasing objects may use mouth to assist
6 MO	Has complete head control Possesses equilibrium reactions Begins assuming quadruped position Rolls from prone to supine position Bounces while standing	Transfers objects from hand to hand while in supine position Shifts weight and reaches with one hand while in prone position Reaches with one hand and supports self with other while seated

Adapted from Alexander R, Boehme R, Cupps B: *Normal development of functional motor skills,* Tucson, 1993, Therapy Skill Builders; Case-Smith J, Shortridge SD: The developmental process: prenatal to adolescence. In Case-Smith J, Allen AS, Pratt PN, editors: *Occupational therapy for children,* ed 3, St Louis, 1996, Mosby; Clark GF: Oral-motor and feeding issues. In Royeen CB, editor: *AOTA self-study series: classroom applications for school-based practice,* Rockville, Md, 1993, American Occupational Therapy Association; Erhardt RP: *Developmental hand dysfunction: theory, assessment, and treatment,* ed 2, Tucson, 1994 Therapy Skill Builders.
ATNR, Asymmetrical tonic neck reflex.

walking, jumping, running, and kicking. Mobility changes infants' perceptions of their environment. A chair is a one-dimensional object in the eyes of a 6 month old; it is only when the infant can finally climb over, under, and around the chair that s/he discovers what a chair really is.[18]

Fine motor skills

Between birth and 3 months, most interactions with the environment are through visual inspection. The grasp reflex allows the infant to have contact with objects placed in the hand. At 4 months s/he demonstrates visually directed reaching skills. At 5 months the infant can use a palmar and an ulnar palmar grasp. The child's fingers are placed on the top surface of an object. The fingers then press the object into the center of the palm toward the little finger (Figure 6-3, A). At 5 to 6 months, transferring objects from one hand to another is a two-step process (the taking hand grabs the objects deposited by the releasing hand before the releasing hand lets go). By 6 months s/he is coordinated enough to reach for an object while in a sitting or prone position. A 6-month-old

TABLE 6-2

Normal Development of Sensorimotor Skills—cont'd

AGE	GROSS MOTOR COORDINATION	FINE MOTOR COORDINATION
6 MO—cont'd		Reaches to be picked up Uses radial palmar grasp begins to use thumb while grasping Shows visual interest in small objects rakes small objects Begins to hold objects in one hand
7-9 MO	Shifts weight and reaches while in quadraped position Creeps Develops extenson flexion and rotation, movements, while increase number of activities that can be accomplished while seated May pull to standing position while holding on to support	Reaches with supination Uses index finger to poke objects Uses inferior scissors grasp to pick up small objects Use radial digital grasp to pick up cube Displays voluntary relases abilities
10-12 MO	Displays good coordination while creeping Pulls to standing position using legs only Cruises holding on to support with one hand Stands independently Begins to walk independently Displays equilibrium reactions while standing	Uses superior pincer grasp with fingertip and thumb Use 3-jaw chuck grasp Displays controlled release into large containers
13-18 MO	Walks along Seldom falls Begins to go up and down stairs	Displays more precise grasping abilities Precisely releases objects into small containers
19-24 MO	Displays equilibrium reactions while walking Runs using a ore narrow base support	Use finger to palm translation of small objects
24-36 MO	Jumps in place*	Uses palm to finger and finger to palm translation of small objects Displays complex rotation of small objects Shifts small objects using palmr stabilization Scribbles Snips with scissors

* From this point on, skills learned during the first 24 months are further refined.

infant uses a radial palmar grasp (in which the object is held between the thumb and the radial side of the palm) (Figure 6-3, *B*) to transfer objects from hand to hand in a one-stage process (with the taking hand and releasing hand executing the transfer simultaneously). Grasping skills change significantly between 7 and 12 months. At 7 months the infant uses a radial digital grasp (in which objects are held between the thumb and fingertips), and the ability to voluntarily release an object begins to emerge. At about 9 months s/he learns to use an inferior pincer grasp (the pad of the thumb is pressed to the pad of the index finger) to pick up a small object. By 10 months the infant can release an object into a container. By 12 months s/he uses a superior pincer grasp (the tip of the thumb is pressed to the tip of the index finger) (Figure 6-4) and consistently puts objects into containers. By 12 months the fine motor skills are developed enough to allow the infant to combine objects and explore their functional uses. These skills facilitate the development of functional and symbolic play skills.[6,13,16]

Interrelatedness of development skills

It is important to note how the interrelatedness of skills affects development. When the newborn is placed in the prone position during periods of alertness, the physiological flexion position raises the pelvis off the surface, transferring much of the infant's weight to the head and shoulders. In addition, this position places the hands beside the cheeks. As the infant turns the head, the mouth and cheeks rub against the surface, providing the sensory

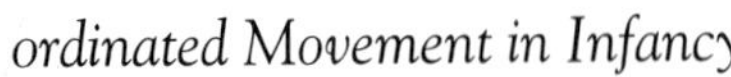

ordinated Movement in Infancy

ɔN → LATERAL FLEXION → ROTATION

XES

are automzatic movemnets that are usually stimulated by sensory factors and performed without conscious e reflexes cause the first involuntarily movements to occur and allow for extension movements to emerge. es are controlled at the lower levels of the central nervous system. As the higher levels (cerebral hemisp mature the expresion of the primitive reflexes is inhibited by these higher levels (i.e., they seem to disappear).

RIGHTING REACTIONS

Righting reactions are postural responses to changes of head and body positions. Righting reaction bring the head and trunk back into an upright position. These reactions involve movements called extension *flexion abdution, adduction* and *lateral flexion.*

EQUILIBRIUM REACTIONS

Equilibrium reactions are automatic, compensatory movements of the body parts that are used to maintain the center of gravity over the base of support when either the center of gravity or the supporting surface is displaced. These complex postural responses combine righting reactions with movements known as *rotational and diagonal patterns.* Essential for volitional movement and mobility, the use of lighting ractions begins at 6 months and continues throughout life.

PROTECTIVE EXTENSION RESPONSES

Protective extension responses are postural reactions that are used to stop a fall or to prevent injuru when equilibrium reactions fail to do so. These responses involve *straightening of the arms or legs* toward a supporting surface. Essential for mobility, the use of protective extension reactions begins between 6 and 9 months and continues throughout life.

Adapted from Alexander R, Boehme R, Cupps B: *Normal development of functional motor skills,* Tucson, 1993, Therapy Skill Builders; Bly L: *Motor skills acquistion i the first year: an illustrated guide to normal development,* Tucson, 1994, Therapy Skills Builders: Florentino MR: *Reflex testing mthods for evaluating CNS development,* ed 2, Springfield, Ill, 1981, Charles C Thomas; Simon CJ, Daub MM: Human development across the life span. In Hopkins JL, Smith HD, editors: *Willard and Spackman's occupational therapy,* ed. 8, Philadelphia, 1993, Lippincott.

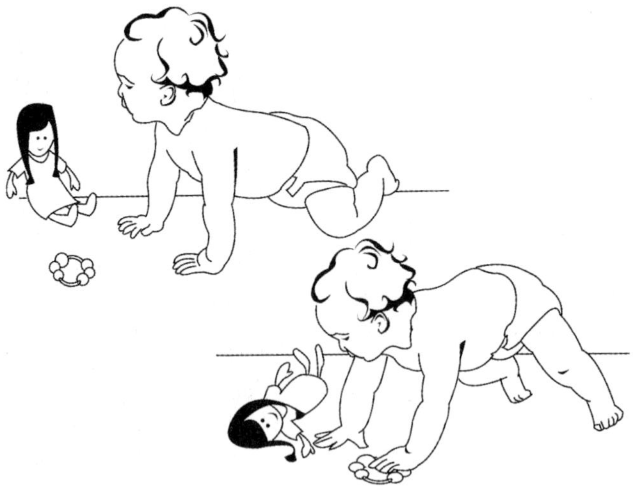

FIGURE 6-2 Infant transition from quadruped (hands and knees) to vaulting position.

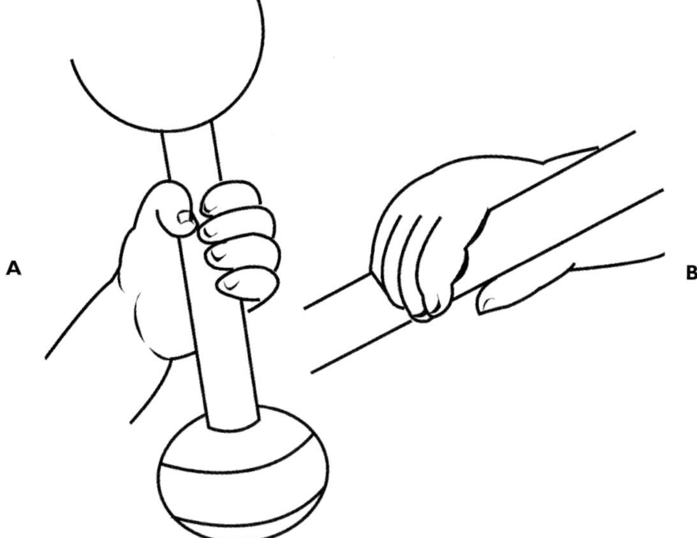

FIGURE 6-3 **A,** When using an ulnar palmar grasp the infant places his or her fingers on the top surface of the object, pressing it into the center of the palm toward the little finger. **B,** When using a radial palmar grasp, the infant holds the object between the thumb and the radial side of the palm.

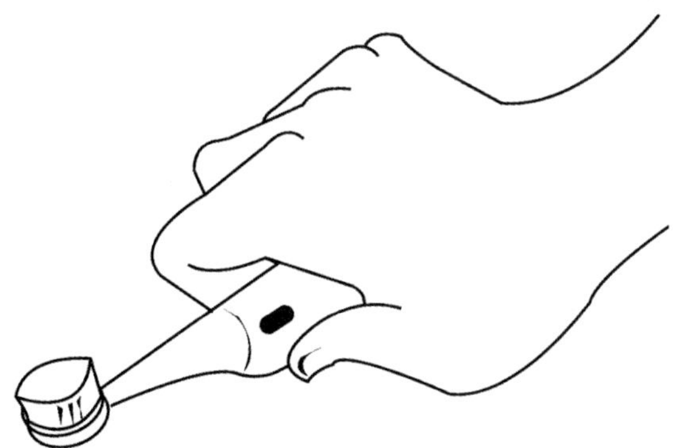

FIGURE 6-4 When using a superior pincer grasp, the infant holds a small object between the tips of the index finger and thumb. The wrist is slightly extended, with the ring and little fingers curled into the palm.

input necessary to elicit the rooting reflex. When s/he turns the head and opens the mouth to root, s/he can suck on the hands.[1] This input to the cheeks also helps develop oral motor skills, such as sucking and chewing. As the infant grows, time in the prone position (or "tummy time") will afford the opportunity for him or her to raise the head and provide deep-pressure input to the ulnar side and the palm of the hands. This input to the hands facilitates the development of the ulnar and palmar grasps. By 6 months, as the infant shifts weight in the prone position, this position provides deep-pressure input to the radial side of the hand, facilitating the radial digital grasp. It is important for the occupational therapy (OT) practitioner to emphasize "tummy time" to facilitate the development of oral motor and fine motor skills.

Process/Cognition

The infant's cognitive development can be described by the use of Piaget's theory. He stated that individuals pass through a series of stages of thought as they progress from infancy to adolescence. These stages are a result of the biological pressure to adapt to the changing environment and organize structures of thinking. According to Piaget, cognitive development is divided into four stages: sensorimotor, preoperational, concrete operational, and formal operational. During the sensorimotor stage the infant develops the ability to organize and coordinate sensations with physical movements and actions. As shown in Table 6-3, the sensorimotor period has six substages.[19,27,30]

During the first stage, known as the *reflexive stage*, behavior is dominated by reflexes such as sucking and the palmar grasp. A rattle placed in an infant's hand is retained by the grasp reflex. Random motor movement causes the infant to accidentally shake the rattle. In the second stage, referred to as *primary circular reactions*, the infant repeats the reflexive movements and patterns simply for pleasure. During this stage s/he may accidentally get the fingers to the mouth and begin to suck on them. The infant then searches for the fingers again but has trouble getting them to the mouth because the coordination to do so has not been mastered. The infant repeats this action until the fingers get to the mouth. In the third stage, called *secondary circular reactions*, the infant begins

TABLE 6-3

Normal Development of Cognitive Skills

AGE	PIAGET'S SENSORIMOTOR PERIOD (BIRTH-2 YR)	COGNITIVE MILESTONES
BIRTH OR 37-40 WK OF GESTATION	**REFLEXIVE STAGE**	Uses entire body during vocalizations Primarily uses abdomen to breathe Becomes quiet in response to a voice Slowly follows moving objects visually (tracks)
1-2 MO	**REFLEXIVE STAGE (1 mo)** Begins displaying primitive reflexes Does not differentiate between self and objects or between sensation and action	Still closely associates all sounds with movement Still primarily uses abdomen to breathe, displays rhythmic breathing patterns while at rest Begins to explore environment by mouthing objects Stops all activity and experiences a change in breathing patterns while focusing on an object or person Has smoother visual tracking skills
3-5 MO	**PRIMARY CIRCULAR REACTIONS (2-4 mo)** Repeats reflexive sensory motor patterns for pleasure	Begins to put hand on bottle and find mouth Experiences transition from watching own hands to mouthing own hands Increases variety of sounds; has less nasal crying Understands conception of object permanence Experiences transition from searching for only dropped objects to searching for partially hidden objects Pats bottle during feeding
6 MO	**SECONDARY CIRCULAR REACTIONS (5-8 mo)** Begins to show true voluntary movement patterns Repeats actions that create pleasurable sensations Has a primitive awareness of cause and effect	Calls out to get attention Repeats own sounds Uses increasingly varied sounds Increasingly dissociates sounds from movement Understands concept of cause and effect repeats certain patterns of actions involving objects or people to achieve a particular result
7-9 MO	**CIRCULAR REACTIONS (2-4 mo)**	Puts objects in containeers Copies movements such as banging objects together Begins to search for objects in containers Responds to word no Explores spatial concepts such as in/out and off/on by experimenting with different movements while playing

Adapted from Case-Smith J, Shortridge SD: The developmental process: prenatal to adolescence. In Case-Smith J, Allen AS, Pratt PN, editors: *Occupational therapy for children,* ed 3, St Louis, 1996, Mosby; Maier HW: *Three theories of child development,* rev ed, New York, 1965, Harper & Row.

to use voluntary movements to repeat actions that accidentally produced a desirable result. At this age an infant who accidentally hits a rattle with the foot while kicking would repeat the same kicking movement to reproduce the sound, thus creating a learned *scheme*, or mental plan, that can be used to reproduce the sound. During the fourth stage, referred to as *coordination of secondary schemata*, several significant changes take place. The infant readily combines previously learned schemes and generalizes them for use in new situations. For example, the infant may visually inspect and touch a toy simultaneously. The major advancement during this period is the emergence of object permanence. The infant searches for an object that has disappeared. In addition, s/he uses existing schemes to obtain a desired object. For example, the infant may pull a string to get an attached toy or object. During the stage called *tertiary circular reactions*, s/he repeatedly attempts a task and modifies the behavior to achieve the desired consequences. The repetition helps the infant understand the concept of cause/effect relationships. Another important hallmark of this stage is the use of tools, such as using a cup to drink from. During the last stage of the sensorimotor period, known as *inventions of new means through mental combinations*, the toddler begins using trial and error to solve problems. For example, s/he learns that pulling on a tablecloth will bring

TABLE 6-3

Normal Development of Cognitive Skills—cont'd

AGE	PIAGET'S SENSORIMOTOR PERIOD (BIRTH-2 YR)	COGNITIVE MILESTONES
10-12 MO	**COORDINATON OF SECONDARY SCHEMATA (9-12 mo)** Begins to participate in object permanence problem-solving activities Begins to be capable of decentralized thought (i.e. realization that objects exist apart from self, in different contexts and when out of sight)	Shows a desire for independence in motor development and skills Follows simple directions Uses objects to reach goal in independent problem-solving activities
13-18 MO	**TERTIARY CIRCULAR REACTIONS (12-18 mo)** Begins to use tools Searches for new schemes	Solve problems by trial and error Uses objects conventionally and begins to group Uses speech to name, refuse, call, greet, protest and express feelings
19-24 MO	**INVENTIONS OF NEW MEANS THROUGH MENTAL COMBINATIONS (18-24 mo)** Begins to show insight begins to purposefully use tools Mental representation is the hallmark of this stage Develops stability to use mental representation (i.e. label and symbolically use mental schemes to present concepts)	Follow two-step directions. Understands object permanence and engages in systematic searching Uses speech as a significant means of communication

Adapted from Case-Smith J, Shortridge SD: The developmental process: prenatal to adolescence. In Case-Smith J, Allen AS, Pratt PN, editors: *Occupational therapy for children*, ed 3, St Louis, 1996, Mosby; Maier HW: *Three theories of child development*, rev ed, New York, 1965, Harper & Row.

down a plate of cookies to the floor. During the last stage the child also uses "pretend" play to create new roles for various objects. For example, stuffed animals that were previously used for teething or banging other objects are considered playmates (see Table 6-3).[19,27,30]

Communication and Interaction/Psychosocial

Language

The development of language is closely related to both cognitive and psychosocial development.[13] Undifferentiated crying characterizes the newborns' "language." By 3 months, their vocalizations are called *cooing* and usually consist of pleasant vowel sounds. At around 4 months they begin to *babble*, or repeat a string of vowel and consonant sounds. From birth to 4 months, infants are "universal linguists"—they are capable of distinguishing among each of the 150 sounds that constitute all human speech. By 6 months, they recognize only the speech sounds of their native language.[23] By the age of 8 months infants develop a sense of the existence of others, recognizing and imitating the actions of caregivers. They repeat sounds, which is known as *lallation* when the repetition is accidental and *echolalia* when the repetition is conscious. By 12 months, infants know between two and eight words and babble short sentences. Their vocabulary increases significantly during the second year. By 24 months, toddlers may have 50 to 200 words in their spoken vocabulary.[13]

Psychosocial

The **psychosocial** development of newborns begins with the earliest emotional connections and interactions with their caregivers. The development of this emotional connection, or feeling of love, between newborns and their caregivers was first examined in the context of attachment, or the development of affectionate ties on the part of the infant to the mother. Ainsworth[3] outlined four stages in the development of infants' attachment to their caregivers.

Initial attachment: At 2 to 3 months, infants exhibit nondiscriminating social responses.

Attachment in the making: By 4 to 6 months, infants begin to discriminate among familiar and unfamiliar persons.

Clear-cut, or active, attachment: By 6 to 7 months, infants attach more to one primary caregiver, seeking proximity to and contact with that person.

Multiple attachments: After 12 months, infants attach to persons other than their primary caregivers.

Another facet of the infant and caregiver relationship is called *bonding*, which is characterized by behaviors such as stroking, kissing, cuddling, and prolonged gazing. These behaviors serve two functions: expressing affection and sustaining an interaction between caregivers and infants. By the time infants are 1 month of age, most parents are attuned to them and are able to interpret their cries and comfort them; in other words, a *goodness of fit*, or a match between infants' temperaments and their environments, exists between their needs and their caregivers' reactions. Caregivers also begin to recognize the early indicators of changes in their infants' temperaments and know ways to calm them or prevent overstimulation.[3,9,27]

Two theories of psychosocial and emotional development in infancy are highlighted in Table 6-4. According to Greenspan,[22] the first stage is called *self-regulation and interest in the world*. During the first few months after birth, the infant is focused on organizing the internal and external worlds, and the job of the primary caregiver(s) is to help him or her regulate these influences. Around the second or third month the infant moves into the *falling in love* stage, in which s/he forms strong a attachment to the primary caregiver(s). S/he responds to the facial expressions and vocalizations of the caregivers with smiles and coos. From 3 to 10 months the infant begins to learn the art of *purposeful communication*. At this stage smiling is purposeful; s/he has learned that smiling causes the adults to smile back. At around 9 or 10 months the infant develops an *organized sense of self* and begins to realize the way behavior is used to get different reactions from others.[22]

EARLY CHILDHOOD

Four-year-old Phillip spends time practicing his fine motor skills. He enjoys drawing pictures and telling long, sometimes exaggerated stories to go with his pictures. When playing with the other children in the neighborhood, Phillip tends to participate with the other boys. The boys tend to play rougher games than the girls.

Physiological

The beginning of the early childhood period is "marked by the development of autonomy, the beginning of expressive language, and sphincter control."[13] The rapid growth of infancy slows as children enter their second and third years. Their limbs begin to grow faster than their heads, making their bodies seem less top-heavy. By 6 years the legs make up almost 45% of the body length, and the children are about seven times their birth weight. The brain of a 5 year old is 75% of its adult weight.[14,33,34] Changes in physiological pathways give the children the sphincter control necessary for toilet training.[13]

The physiological differences between children in the early childhood stage and adults are significant. The

TABLE 6-4

Psychosocial and Emotional Development

PERIOD	AGE (yr)	ERIKSON	GREENSPAN	TYPICAL BEHAVIORS
INFANCY	0–1	**TRUST VERSUS MISTRUST** Has needs gratified Gives to others in return Develops drive and hope	**SELF-REGULATION (0-3 mo)** Calms self Regulates sleep Notices sights and sounds Enjoys touch and movement	Has fussy periods to relieve stress Smiles Imitates gestures Uses special smiles for different people and events May experience joy and anger
			FALLING IN LOVE (2-7 mo) Is wooed by significant others Responds to facial expressions and vocalizations Attachment **PURPOSEFUL COMMUNICATION (3-10 mo)** Displays reciprocal interactions when inflated by adult Initiates interactions	Fears strangers (8 mo) Gives affection Learns about cause and effect Understands concept of object permanence

Courtesy Jayne Shepherd. Adapted from Erikson EH: *Childhood and society*, ed 2, New York, 1963, WW Norton; Greenspan SI: *Playground politics: undersranding the emotional life of your school-aged child*, Reading, Mass, 1993, Addison-Wesley; Greenspan S, Greenspan N: *First feelings: milestones in the emotional development of your baby and child*, New York, 1985, Viking Penguin.

TABLE 6-4

Psychosocial and Emotional Development—cont'd

PERIOD	AGE (yr)	ERIKSON	GREENSPAN	TYPICAL BEHAVIORS
EARLY CHILDHOOD	1-3	**AUTONOMY VERSUS SHAME AND DOUBT** Considers self separate from parents Develops self-control and will power Struggles with a conflict between holding on and letting go	**EMERGENCE OF ORGANISZED SENSE OF SELF (9-18 mo)** Knows ways to get different types of reactions Is focused and organized while playing Initiates complex behaviors Is capable of feeling embarrassment, pride, shame, joy, empathy, anger	**Early** Attaches to transitional object (such as blanket) Imitates others Understands function of objects and means of behaviors May experience joy and anger **Late** Is egocentric Experiences separation anxiety (2 yr)
			CREATING EMOTIONAL IDEAS (18-36 mo) Uses words and gestures Participates in pretend play with others Learns to recover from anger or temper tantrums Starts associating particular functions with certain people	Loves and audience and attention Often says phrases like me do, "it" and "no" Has difficulty sharing Begins to become independent and spend time alone
		INITIATIVE AND IMAGINATION VERSUS GUILT Displays purpose in actions Has a lively imagination Tests reality Imitates parental actions and roles Seeks new experiences that if successful lead to sense of initiative, needs balance between initiative and responsibility for own actions Accepts consequences of actions Makes choices and plans	**EMOTIONAL THINKING (30-48 mo)** Differentiates between real and not real Follows rules Understands relationships among behaviors feelings, and consequences (is capable of feeling guilty) Interacts in socially appropriate ways with adults and peers	Seems optimistic and confident Asks why Is spontaneous Seeks other playmates Fears monsters, spiders, etc, has bad dreams (4-5 yr) Plays with imaginary playmates Tells exaggerated stories

Courtesy Jayne Shepherd. Adapted from Erikson EH: *Childhood and society*, ed 2, New York, 1963, WW Norton; Greenspan SI: *Playground politics: undersranding the emotional life of your school-aged child*, Reading, Mass, 1993, Addison-Wesley; Greenspan S, Greenspan N: *First feelings: milestones in the emotional development of your baby and child*, New York, 1985, Viking Penguin.

eustachian tube is shorter and positioned more horizontally than that of adults, making children more susceptible to middle ear infections. The digestive tract is not fully mature and the shape of the stomach is straight, resulting in frequent upset stomachs. Because of the immaturity of the retina, young children are farsighted.[13]

Motor

All of the basic components of motor development, such as vision, touch, gross motor skills, and fine motor skills, exist physiologically during the second and third years. These components are developed as the skills are refined through interactions with the environment. Balance and strength increase during the early childhood period. At

TABLE 6-4

Psychosocial and Emotional Development—cont'd

PERIOD	AGE (yr)	ERIKSON	GREENSPAN	TYPICAL BEHAVIORS
MIDDLE CHILDHOOD	1-3	**INDUSTRY VERSUS INFERIORITY** Sees work as pleasurable Develops sense of responsibility and competence Learns work habits Learns to use tools Likes recognition for accomplishments Is sensitive to performance in comparison with others Tries new activities Becomes scholastically and socially competent	**THE WORLD IS MY OYSTER (5-7 yr)** Carries out self-care and self-regulatory functions with minimum assitance Enjoys relationship with parents Takes simultaneous interest in wants and needs of parents, peers and "me first" Forms relationships with peers Struggles to assert own will with peers Better handled not getting own way Better understands reasons for reality limits **THE WORLD IS OTHER KIDS (8-10 yr)** Cares about role in peer group Has best friends and regular friends Maintains nurturing relationship with parents Continues to enjoy fantasy Follows rules Orders emotions and groups them into categories Experiences competition without becoming aggressive or compliant	**Early (5-7)** Acts assertive and bossy: acts like a "know-it-all" Is critical of self Experiences night-terrors Shares and takes turns May experience joy and anger **Late (9-11)** Desires privacy Acts with impulsivity and more control Looks up to and focuses on being like a certain person a "hero" ("hero worship") Becomes more competitive Expects perfection from others (1 yr)
ADOLESCENCE		**SELF-IDENTITY VERSUS ROLE CONFUSION** Has a temporal perspective Experiments with roles (parents friends, various groups) Enters sexual relationship Shares self with others Develops ideological commitments	**THE WORLD IS INSIDE ME (11-12 yr)** Has a developing internal sense of right and wrong Enjoys one or a few intimate friends Takes interest in adults as role models Uses rules flexibly by understanding context Takes interest in opposite sex Has feelings of privacy about own body Has concerns about body and personality related to puberty	Acts as if *right now* is most important thing in life Accepts and adjusts to changing body Plays to imaginary audience Believes in personal fable (of infallibility) and characterized by the phrase "It won't happen to me" Begins working Achieves emotional independence

Courtesy Jayne Shepherd. Adapted from Erikson EH: *Childhood and society*, ed 2, New York, 1963, WW Norton; Greenspan SI: *Playground politics: undersranding the emotional life of your school-aged child*, Reading, Mass, 1993, Addison-Wesley; Greenspan S, Greenspan N: *First feelings: milestones in the emotional development of your baby and child*, New York, 1985, Viking Penguin.

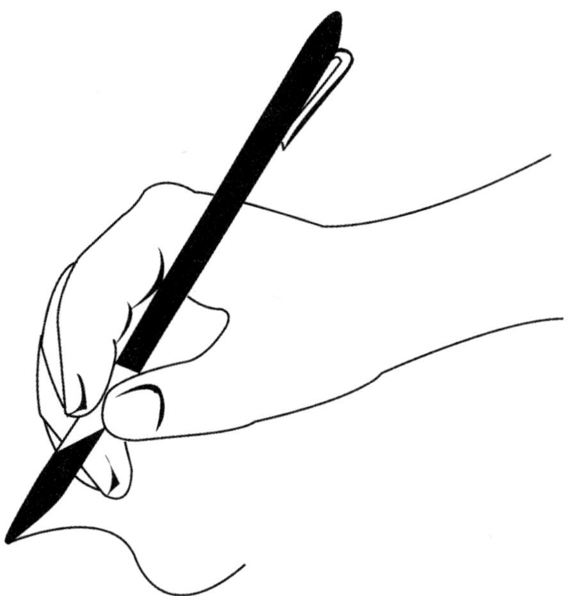

FIGURE 6-5 When using a dynamic tripod grasp, the child holds a pencil with the thumb and index and middle fingers. The fingers move while other joints of the arm remain stable.

2 years of age toddlers walk with an increased stride length, and by 4 years their walking pattern more closely resembles that of an adult. The ability to run develops at around 3 to 4 years; by 5 or 6 years a mature running pattern develops. Two-year-old children can climb stairs without holding on to a support; by 3½ years, children are able to walk up and down the stairs without holding on and with alternating feet.[13]

Like gross motor skills, the coordination and precision of hand and finger movements are refined with maturation and practice, especially when children enter preschool and school. At 2 years, one of the major accomplishments of children is learning to draw. The first type of grasp they learn is a palmar one; however, during the second year, they develop the ability to hold a pencil in their hand rather than fist. As thumb, finger, and hand precision improve enough to allow children to use a tripod grasp, their drawings progress from scribbles to deliberate lines and shapes. A mature, dynamic tripod grasp develops by 5 years (Figure 6-5). Three-year-old children are able to snip paper with scissors, and more mature skills with scissors develop at around 5 to 6 years.[11,13]

Process/Cognition

Piaget's second phase of development, the *preoperational period*, occurs between the ages of 2 and 7 years; 2 to 4 years olds are in the preconceptual substage of preoperational thought. The beginning of symbolic thought and strong egocentrism and the emergence of animism characterize this substage. The ability to use *symbolism* means that the child is able to mentally consider objects that are not present. *Egocentrism* is the inability of individuals to realize that others have thoughts and feelings that may not be the same as their own. *Animism* is the mental act of giving inanimate objects lifelike qualities; this characteristic develops at around age 3.[34] Children between the ages of 5 and 7 are in a substage of preoperational thought called *intuitive thought*.

Communication and Interaction/Psychosocial

Language

During this phase, cognitive and language development is characterized by the use of symbolism. At this time children begin to engage in symbolic, or pretend, play and tend to think more logically. They are able to use words and gestures to represent real objects or events.[13] Their vocabulary expands rapidly, increasing from a repertoire of 200 words at 2 years to 1500 words at 3 years. Two year olds label items and ask simple questions, whereas 3 year olds can express their thoughts and feelings in simple sentences. By age 4 children can narrate long stories, which are sometimes exaggerated. Five- or 6-year-old children are able to enunciate clearly and use their advanced language skills as a tool for learning. For example, they commonly ask questions such as "What is this for?," "How does this work?," and "What does it mean?"[11]

Psychosocial

According to Erikson, the 2- to 4-year-old period of early childhood is referred to as the stage of *autonomy versus shame and doubt*. During this stage a need to be autonomous dominates children's psychosocial development; they are determined to make their own decisions and be independent. Central to this stage is the period known as the *terrible two's*, in which 2 year olds try to prove their independence. According to Erikson's theories, children begin to doubt themselves and feel ashamed if they are not given adequate opportunities for self-regulation.[10,13,17] Those between the ages of 4 and 6 are in the stage Erikson calls *initiative and imagination versus guilt*. Children show initiative in activities in which their behavior produces successful, effective results and meets with parental approval. On the other hand, guilt results when children assume a sense of responsibility for their own behavior. By imitating others, they learn to take responsibility for their own actions and develop a sense of purpose. Gender role development is also during this stage.[11,13,36]

The early childhood years comprise two of Greenspan's stages, which are called *creating emotional ideas* and *emotional thinking*. In the stage of creating emotional ideas,

2 year olds express them by using words and gestures, engaging in pretend play, and starting to associate certain functions with certain people. In the stage of emotional thinking, 3 and 4 year olds are able to differentiate between what is and is not real, follow rules, and understand the relationship between behaviors and feelings.[22]

MIDDLE CHILDHOOD

Ten-year-old Phillip is very concerned about being accepted in his peer group—he insists on wearing the same tennis shoes as the other boys. He and his friends spend hours playing seemingly endless baseball games. They follow the rules but don't really keep score.

Physiological

Between the early childhood years and the growth spurt of adolescence, the growth rate slows down. Although wide variations in growth occur in both sexes during the middle childhood years, girls and boys typically grow an average of 2 to 3 inches per year, with their legs becoming longer and trunks slimmer.[34] Girls typically grow taller than boys during this period. Facial features become more distinct and unique, partly because baby teeth have been replaced by permanent teeth. The digestive system matures, so children retain food in the digestive system longer; they eat less frequently but have increased appetites and eat in greater quantities.[13] By the age of 10, head and brain growth is 95% complete. Hearing acuity increases, and changes in the location of the eustachian tube decrease the risk of middle ear infections.[12,34]

Motor

Because the rate of physical development slows down during middle childhood, children have the opportunity to refine their gross motor skills and become generally more adept at handling their bodies. Children tend to focus on the refinement of previously learned skills. Hours of repetition leads to mastery of these skills, which creates higher self-esteem and greater acceptance from peers.[7] Increased muscle strength and endurance allow children to become more physical; their favorite activities often include running, climbing, throwing, riding a bicycle, swimming, and skating.[34] Refined fine motor skills allow children to improve their performance of tasks such as sewing, using garden tools, and writing. The task of writing is a combination of refined grasping skills and coordinated movements that result in smooth writing strokes and smaller letters. By the age of 10 years, most children have converted from writing in printed letters to writing in cursive letters.[13]

Process/Cognition

The middle childhood years include the Piaget stage of *concrete operations*, which includes children from 7 to 11 years. This stage marks the beginning of the ability to think abstractly, or to mentally manipulate actions. For example, children are able to envision what might happen if they throw a rock across the room, but they do not actually have to throw the rock to see what is going to happen. Other characteristics of the concrete operational period include the following[34]:

- Children are less self-centered.
- Children can recognize that others may have viewpoints that differ from their own.
- Children can identify similarities and differences among objects.
- Children can use simple logic to arrive at a conclusion.
- Children can simultaneously consider many aspects of a situation rather than just one.
- Children realize that a substance's quantity does not change when its form does.
- Children can order objects by size, indicating an understanding of the relationships among objects.
- Children can imagine objects or pieces as parts of a whole.

Using Piaget's ideas as a basis, Kohlberg formulated schemes of moral development. During the early elementary years (between the ages of 4 and 10), children are in what he calls the *preconventional level* of moral development. They make moral judgments based solely on the basis of anticipated punishment or reward (i.e., a "right," or "good," action is one that feels good and is rewarded, and a "wrong," or "bad," action is one that results in punishment[34]). Between 10 and 13 years, children enter a stage called the *morality of conventional role conformity*. They are eager to please others and therefore tend to internalize rules (by applying them to themselves) and judge their actions according to set standards. Ten and 11 year olds are concerned with meeting the expectations and following the rules of their peer group. This stage is characterized by conforming, following the "Golden Rule" ("Do unto others as you would have them do unto you"), and showing respect for authority and rules.[31]

Communication and Interaction/Psychosocial

Language

During middle childhood the vocabulary of children expands, partly as a result of their focus on reading. Puns and figures of speech become meaningful, and children's jokes are based on the dual meaning of words, slang, curse words, colloquialisms, and secret languages.[19] Communication among children during the middle childhood years has been described as *socialized communication*—conversations center around school activities, personal experiences, families and pets, sports, clothes, movies, television, comics, and "taboo" subjects such as sex, cursing, and drinking.[31]

Psychosocial

When children begin attending elementary school, their families are no longer the sole source of security and relationships. During this period, significant social relationships are developed outside the family in the neighborhood and school. A feeling of belonging is very important to children in the middle childhood years, so they become increasingly concerned about their status among peers. They seem to have their own personal societies, separate from the adult world, that include rituals, heroes, and peer groups.[7,13,31] Peer groups usually comprise children of the same sex. Girls and boys tend to engage in their own activities, with little communication between each other. During this period, children experience more pressure to conform than during any other period of development. Children struggle to simultaneously participate in group activities while balancing the group's identity with their own and establishing their roles within the group.[19]

The middle childhood years include the stage Erikson named *industry versus inferiority*. He believed that children must learn new skills to survive in their culture; if unsuccessful, they develop a sense of inferiority.[19] During this stage the source of children's feelings of security switch from the family to the peer group as they try to master the activities of their friends. Greenspan[21] described the 8- to 10-year-old developmental stage as *the world is other kids*. Children develop a mental picture of themselves that is based on interactions with friends, family members, and teachers. The stage called *the world inside me* is representative of an 11 year old's definition of self, which is based on personal characteristics rather than the peer group's perceptions. At this age, children are able to empathize and understand the feelings of others. They realize that relationships require constant mutual adjustments, so they are able to disagree with a friend but still maintain the friendship.[21]

ADOLESCENCE

Fifteen-year-old Phillip wants to get a job working in the music store at the mall. He thinks he would be good at the job because of his extensive knowledge of popular groups and musicians. An additional benefit is that all his friends hang out at the mall.

Physiological

Adolescence is a period characterized by many dramatic physiological changes, some of which are related to the adolescent growth spurt and some to the onset of puberty. Preadolescence, characterized by little physical growth, is followed by a period of rapid growth, indicating the onset of puberty.[40] The growth spurt is triggered by neural and hormonal signals to the hypothalamus, resulting in the increased production of and sensitivity to certain hormones. The onset of puberty in boys occurs between 10½ and 16 years, with the average age being 12½ years. The onset in girls occurs between 9½ and 15 years, with the average age being 10½ years. Although boys begin their growth spurt later than girls, it tends to be greater, with boys growing 8.3 inches and girls 7.7 inches.[15,26,40]

The onset of puberty is usually associated with the first signs of sexual development. The first visible sign of puberty in girls is breast growth, which begins at around age 10½. The average age for menarche is 12.8.[33] The onset of puberty in boys is signified by enlargement of the testes, which occurs between the ages of 10 and 13½ years.[15] These ages are ranges; the age of the onset of puberty is *quite* variable.

Those boys who mature earlier than others are described more positively by peers, teachers, and themselves. They tend to be the most popular, are better at sports, and begin dating more easily than those who mature later. Boys who mature later are described as less attractive, more childish, and less masculine.[15,32,37] For girls the scenario is reversed. Those who mature the earliest sometimes have a poor body image and low self-esteem. They tend to confide in older adolescents and share their experiences. Girls who mature later develop at the same age as their male peers and are likely to develop a better self-concept than those who mature earlier.[15,32,37] These differences in the rates of development greatly affect adolescents' self-concept and self-esteem. To help ease the transition, adults can educate adolescents about the following:

- Health and preparation for puberty
- Nutrition
- Issues such as smoking prevention, automobile safety, and contraception
- Developing autonomy and independence[39]

Motor

The development of gross motor skills in adolescents is directly related to the physical changes that are occurring. Increased muscle mass provides increased dynamic strength, as evidenced by better running, jumping, and throwing skills.[4] Because boys have a greater percentage of muscle mass than girls, their strength is greater.[7] In addition, motor coordination stops improving in girls at the age of 15 but keeps improving in boys beyond this age. Fine motor abilities also tend to differ between the sexes. Girls show greater rates of improvement in hand-eye coordination, but overall they still do not perform as well as boys.[4,36,40]

Process/Cognition

The development of *formal operational thought* is the hallmark of adolescence.[13] Adolescents have the ability to think about possibilities as well as realities. They can formulate hypotheses about the outcome of a certain situation, and after imagining all the possible results they can test each hypothesis to determine which one is true.[15] This process is called *hypothetical deductive reasoning*.

Adolescents develop their moral thought in the period known as the *conventional level* of Kohlberg's stages. During this stage, adolescents approach moral problems in a social context; they want to please others by being good members of society. Adolescents follow the standards of others, conform to social conventions, support the status quo, and generally try to please others and obey the law.[32]

Communication and Interaction/Psychosocial

Language

In high school, adolescents manipulate language; for example, they use codes, slang, and sarcasm. The use of slang during adolescence is important for establishing group membership and being accepted by peers. They also have the cognitive ability to use language for more than simple communication. For example, they can participate in debates or class discussions and argue for a position that they do not agree with; this abstract use of language is not understood by children at younger ages.[7]

Egocentrism

Adolescents tend to believe that if something is of great concern to them, then it is also of great concern to others. Because they believe that others have the thoughts similar to their own, they tend to be self-conscious, or *egocentric*. This egocentrism manifests itself in adolescents as an *imaginary audience*, or a perception that everyone is watching them. Another way egocentrism manifests itself is through the *personal fable*, or the idea that they are special, have completely unique experiences, and are not subject to the natural rules governing the rest of the world. Egocentrism is the cause of much of the self-destructive behavior shown by adolescents who think that they are magically protected from harm.[32]

Identity

Erikson referred to the adolescent stage of development as *identify versus identity confusion*. The main goal during this stage is for adolescents to find or understand their identity. They work to form a new sense of self by combining past experiences with future expectations. This process allows adolescents to understand themselves in terms of who they have been and who they hope to become.[17]

The establishment of an occupational identity is one part of the establishment of ego identity. A number of theories about occupational development exist. Ginzberg[20] outlined three periods that apply to this stage: a fantasy period, a tentative period, and a realistic period. Two of Super's[38] stages also apply to adolescents: the growth stage and the exploration stage. Adolescents explore various occupations, identify with workers in a specific occupation, discover which occupations they enjoy, and develop basic habits of work and an identity as a worker.

Peers

Peer groups support adolescents as they experience the transition from childhood to adulthood.[13] Involvement in peer groups provides opportunities for them to accomplish the following.

- Share responsibilities for their own affairs
- Experiment with new ways of handling new situations
- Learn from each other's mistakes
- Try out new roles[26]

Early adolescence (ages 12 to 14 years) is the time when children are most concerned with conforming to the values and practices of their peer group. Older adolescents are less likely to conform to a group and more likely to rely on their own independent thinking and judgment.[26]

Parents

Even though adolescents spend more time with friends, the parents still have considerable effects on them. Although adolescents seek the advice of peers on matters such as social activities, dress, and hobbies, they seek the advice of their parents on issues such as occupations, college, and money.[35]

SUMMARY

From birth through adolescence, infants and children progress through a series of stages of development. The sequences of physiological, sensorimotor, cognitive and language, and psychosocial development outlined in this chapter are typical; however, it should be noted that each individual child progresses through these sequences at a different rate. The OT practitioner should consider any physical, social, and cultural factors in the environment that may affect a client's developmental sequence.

Acknowledgment

I would like to thank the occupational therapy students at Virginia Commonwealth University's Department of

Occupational Therapy for researching the material in this chapter and field testing the review questions and suggested activities.

References

1. Alexander R, Boehme R, Cupps B: *Normal development of functional motor skills*, Tucson, 1993, Therapy Skill Builders.
2. American Occupational Therapy Association: Occupational therapy practice framework: domain and process, *Am J Occup Ther* 56:609-639, 2002.
3. Ainsworth M: Attachment retrospect and prospect. In Parkes CM, Stevenson-Hind M, editors: *The place of attachment in human behavior,* New York, 1982, Basic Books.
4. Ausubel DP: *Theories and problems of adolescent development*, ed 3, 2002, Writers Club Press, Universe.com.
5. Bax M, Hart H, Jenkins SM: *Child development and child health: the preschool years*, Oxford, 1990, Blackwell Scientific.
6. Benbow M: *Neurokinesthetic approach to hand function and handwriting*, Albuquerque, 1995, Clinician's View.
7. Berger KS: *The developing person through childhood and adolescence*, ed 5, New York, 1999, Worth Publishers.
8. Bly L: *Motor skills acquisition in the first year: an illustrated guide to normal development*, Tucson, 1994, Therapy Skill Builders.
9. Brazelton TB: *Neonatal behavioral assessment scale*, ed 2, Philadelphia, 1984, Lippincott.
10. Caplan T, Caplan F: *The first twelve months of life*, New York, 1995, Bantam Books.
11. Caplan T, Caplan F: *The early childhood years: the 2 to 6 year old*, New York, 1984, Bantam Books.
12. Case-Smith J, Rogers J: School-based occupational therapy. In Case-Smith J, editor: *Occupational therapy for children*, ed 5, St Louis, 2005, Mosby.
13. Case-Smith J, Shortridge SD: The developmental process: prenatal to adolescence. In Case-Smith J, editor: *Occupational therapy for children*, ed 4, St Louis, 2001, Mosby.
14. Dacey JS, Travers JF: *Human development across the lifespan*, ed 6, New York, 2001, McGraw-Hill.
15. Dusek JB: *Adolescent development and behavior*, ed 3, Englewood Cliffs, NJ, 1995, Prentice Hall.
16. Erhardt RP: *Developmental hand dysfunction: theory, assessment, and treatment*, ed 2, Tucson, 1994, Therapy Skill Builders.
17. Erikson EH: *Childhood and society*, ed 2, New York, 1963, WW Norton.
18. Fraiberg SH: *The magic years: understanding and handling the problems of early childhood*, New York, 1959, Scribner.
19. Freiberg K: *Human development,99/00* (annual editions), Guilford, Conn 1998, McGraw Hill/Dushin.
20. Ginzberg E: Toward a theory of occupational choice: a restatement, *Voc Guide Quart* 20:169, 1972.
21. Greenspan S: *Playground politics: Understanding the emotional life of your school-aged child*, Reading, Mass, 1993, Addison-Wesley.
22. Greenspan S, Greenspan N: *First feelings: milestones in the emotional development of your baby and child*, New York, 1994, Viking Penguin.
23. Grunwald L: The amazing minds of infants. In Junn EN, Boyatzis CJ, editors: *Annual editions: child growth and development*, Guilford, Conn, 1995, Dushkin.
24. Haywood KM: *Life span motor development*, Champaign, Ill, 1986, Human Kinetics.
25. Hetherington EM, Parke RD: *Child psychology: A contemporary viewpoint*, New York, 1993, McGraw-Hill.
26. Kimmel DC, Weiner IB: *Adolescence: a developmental transition*, New York, 1995, John Wiley & Sons.
27. Lamb ME, Bornstein M, Teti DM: *Development in infancy: an introduction*, ed 4, Mahwah, NJ, 2002, Lawrence Erlbaum Associates, Publishers.
28. Leach P: *Your baby and child*, New York, 1994, Knopf.
29. Lief NR, Fahs ME, Thomas RM: *The first three years of life*, New York, 1991, Smithmark.
30. Maier HW: *Three theories of child development*, rev ed, New York, 1965, Harper & Row.
31. Minuchin P: *The middle years of childhood*, Pacific Grove, Calif, 1977, Brooks/Cole.
32. Papaplia DE, Olds SW: *Human development*, ed 2, New York, 1992, McGraw-Hill.
33. Payne VG, Isaacs LD: *Human motor development: a lifespan approach*, ed 2, London, 1991, Mayfield.
34. Santrock JW: *Life span development*, ed 9, New York, 1995, McGraw-Hill Humanities.
35. Sigelman CK, Rider, EA, Van De Veer DA: *Life span human development*, ed 4, Pacific Grove, Calif, 2003, Brooks/Cole.
36. Simon CJ, Daub MM: Human development across the life span. In Hopkins JL, Smith HD, editors: *Willard and Spackman's occupational therapy*, ed 8, Philadelphia, 1993, Lippincott.
37. Steinberg L: *Adolescence*, ed 6, New York, 2001, McGraw-Hill.
38. Super DE: *The psychology of careers*, New York, 1957, Harper & Row.
39. Vaughan VC, Litt IF: *Child and adolescent development: clinical implications*, Philadelphia, 1990, WB Saunders.
40. Watson RI, Lindgren HC: *Psychology of the child and the adolescent*, ed 4, New York, 1979, Macmillan.

Recommended Reading

Bee HL, Boyd, DR: *The developing child*, ed 10, Needham Heights, Mass, 2003, Allyn & Bacon.

Berk LE: *Infants, children, and adolescents*, ed 4, Boston, Mass, 2001, Allyn & Bacon.

Dixon SD, Stein MT: *Encounters with children: pediatric behavior and development*, ed 3, St. Louis, 2000, Mosby.

Santrock J: *Life-span development*, ed 9, New York, 2003, McGraw-Hill Humanities.

Sigelman CK, Rider EA, Van De Veer DA: *Life-span human development*, ed 4, Pacific Grove, Calif, 2003, Brooks/Cole.

REVIEW *Questions*

1. What are primitive reflexes, righting reactions, equilibrium reactions, and protective extension?
2. Briefly describe the gross and fine motor skills of children at the following ages: 1 month, 6 months, 12 months, and 18 months.
3. What are four sequences of Piaget's stages of cognitive development? Give an example of a behavior that might be observed during each stage of cognitive development.
4. Why is Greenspan's stage for 2 to 7 month olds called *falling in love*? Why is Greenspan's stage for 5 to 7 year olds called *the world is my oyster*?
5. What are Erikson's five stages of development? Briefly describe each.

SUGGESTED *Activities*

1. Visit a nursery or child-care center that serves infants and toddlers. What postural reactions do you observe? Which can you elicit while playing with the infants?
2. Go to a nearby playground and watch normal children at play. Using the American Occupational Therapy Association's Occupational Therapy Practice Framework[2] as a guide, record your observations. Develop a chart like the following one to summarize development throughout childhood.

	NEW-BORN	1 YEAR	4 YEARS	10 YEARS	15 YEARS
Physiological development					
Motor skills: gross					
Motor skills: fine					
Process/ cognition					
Communication and interaction/ psychosocial					

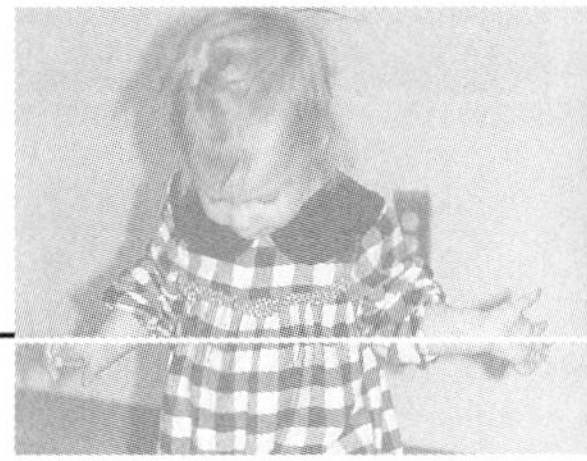

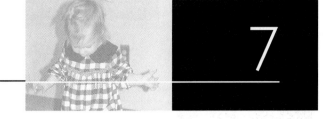

7

Development of Areas of Occupation

DIANNE KOONTZ LOWMAN
JANE CLIFFORD O'BRIEN
JEAN W. SOLOMON

CHAPTER *Objectives*

After studying this chapter, the reader will be able to accomplish the following:

- Describe the developmental sequence of oral motor control
- Identify the sequences of feeding and eating, dressing and undressing, and grooming and hygiene development
- Identify the types of food and utensils that are appropriate for infants and young children of different ages
- Identify the variables affecting a child's development of self-care skills
- Describe age-appropriate home management activities
- Discuss care of others as it relates to humans and animals or pets
- Describe developmentally appropriate activities considered as work or productive in the context of the Occupational Therapy Practice Framework
- Explain the difference between formal and informal educational activities
- Identify age-appropriate vocational activities
- Define *play* and *leisure skills*
- Describe the progression of play skills
- Explain the relevance of play to occupational therapy practice
- Identify occupational therapy professionals who have made significant contributions to the study of play

KEY TERMS

Area of occupation
Activities of daily living
Eating
Feeding
Oral motor development
Dressing and undressing
Personal hygiene and grooming skills
Oral hygiene
Bathing and showering
Toilet hygiene
Instrumental activities of daily living
Readiness skills
Home management activities
Community mobility
Care of others
Educational activities
Work
Vocational activities
Play
Leisure activities
Social participation

CHAPTER OUTLINE

Occupational therapy (OT) practitioners focus on improving a child's ability to perform daily living, education, work, play and leisure, and social activities. These activities occur in cultural, physical, social, personal, and temporal contexts. The OT practitioner evaluates a child's ability to perform in these areas by examining the performance skills of each area. Knowledge of each **area of occupation** is therefore important to pediatric OT practice. This chapter provides a description of the areas of occupation within the framework of normal development.

Activities of Daily Living

DEFINITION AND RATIONALE

Activities of daily living (ADLs) constitute one of the areas of occupation described in the American Occupational Therapy Association's (AOTA's) "Occupational Therapy Practice Framework."[2] The ADLs listed in Box 7-1 are the most basic tasks that children learn as they grow and mature.[35] Basic self-care skills include feeding and eating, dressing and undressing, and grooming and hygiene.[2] Because eating is a critical daily living skill essential to the child's survival, growth, health, and well-being, it falls within the OT practitioner's domain of concern.[3] A child with sufficient **eating** skills is able to actively bring food to the mouth without assistance. A child who requires **feeding** must receive assistance in the activity of eating.[3] Oral motor control relates to the child's ability to use the lips, cheeks, jaw, tongue, and palate.[37] **Oral motor development** refers to feeding, sound play, and oral exploration.[29] Feeding is an oral motor skill, but some oral motor skills, such as oral motor awareness and exploration, do not involve food at all.[14]

BOX 7-1

Activities of Daily Living

Bathing and showering
Bowel and bladder management
Toileting hygiene
Dressing and undressing
Eating and feeding
Functional mobility
Personal device care
Personal hygiene and grooming
Communicative device use
Community mobility
Health management/medication routine
Meal preparation and cleanup

From the American Occupational Therapy Association: Occupational therapy practice framework: domain and process, *Am J Occup Ther* 56:609, 2002.

The normal development of oral motor skills related to eating and feeding involves sucking from a nipple, coordinating the suck-swallow-breathe sequence, drinking from a cup, and munching and chewing solid foods.[12,25,26] The maturation of these skills is closely tied to the physical maturation of the infant.

FEEDING AND EATING SKILLS

Oral Motor Development

The infant's oral mechanisms differ anatomically from those of the adult; the oral cavity of the infant appears to be filled by the tongue. The small oral cavity, coupled with sucking fat pads that stabilize the infant's cheeks, allows the infant to compress and suck on a nipple placed in the mouth. The limited mobility of the tongue results in the back and forth movement of the tongue known as *suckling*.[25,29,30] As the size ratios in the mouth change with the infant's growth, a more mature oral motor pattern emerges. By 4 to 6 months of age the area inside the infant's mouth increases as the jaw grows and the sucking fat pads decrease. These changes allow increased movement of the infant's cheeks and lips. A "true sucking" pattern develops, as the infant's tongue can move up and down as well as forward and backward. Increased control of the jaw, lips, cheeks, and tongue allows the infant to move food and liquid toward the back of the mouth and prepares the infant to accept and control strained baby food.[29,31]

Full-term infants are born with reflexes that allow them to locate the source of food, suck, and then swallow. The following describes these reflexes in relation to oral motor development.[31]

- *Rooting reflex:* When the infant's cheeks or lips are stroked, s/he turns toward the stimulus. This reflex allows the infant to search for food and is maintained for a longer period in breast-fed infants.
- *Suck-swallow reflex:* When the infant's lips are touched, his or her mouth opens and sucking movements begin.
- *Gag reflex:* The gag reflex protects the infant from swallowing anything that may block the airway.[29] At birth the gag reflex is highly sensitive and elicited by stimulation to the back three fourths of the tongue. This reflex gradually moves to the back one fourth of the tongue as the infant matures and engages in oral play.
- *Phasic bite-release reflex:* When the infant's gums are stimulated, s/he responds with a rhythmic up and down movement of the jaw. This reflex forms the basis for munching and chewing.

TABLE 7-1

Normal Development of Sensorimotor, Oral-Motor, and Feeding Skills

AGE	SENSORIMOTOR SKILLS	ORAL-MOTOR SKILLS	FEEDING SKILLS
BIRTH/ 37-40 WK GESTATION	Is dominated by physiological flexion Moves total body into extension or flexion Turns head side to side in prone position (a protective response) Keeps head mostly on side in supine position Tends to keep hands fisted and flexed across chest during feeding Has strong grasp reflex	Possesses strong gag reflex Possesses rooting reflex Possesses autonomic phasic bite-release pattern Sucks and suckles when hand or object comes into contact with mouth Shows minimal drooling in supine position and increased drooling in other positions	Begins bottle or breast feeding with total sucking pattern Uses mixture of suckling and sucking on bottle (dependent on head position) Possesses incomplete lip closure Is unable to release nipple
1-2 MO	Appears hypotonic as physiological flexion diminishes Practices extension and flexion Continues to gain control of head Moves elbows forward toward shoulders in prone position Possesses ATNR, with head to side in supine position Experiences weakening grasp reflex Does not possess voluntary release skills	Continues to show strong gag reflex Continues to show rooting reflex Continues to show automatic phasic bite-release pattern Continues to suck and suckle when hand or object comes in contact with mouth Drools more as jaw and tongue move in wider excursions	May lose coordination of sucking-swallowing-breathing pattern with increased head movements Opens mouth and waits for food Possesses better lip closure Uses active lip movement when sucking
3-5 MO	Experiences diminishing ATNR and grasp reflex Possesses more balance between extension and flexion Has good head control (centered and upright) Brings hands to mouth constantly Supports on extended arms and props on forearms in prone position Brings hand to feet and feet to mouth in supine position Props on arms, with little support in sitting position Develops tactile awareness in hands Reaches more accurately, usually with both hands Begins transfer of objects from hand to hand Does not possess controlled release skills; may use mouth to assist	Experiences diminished rooting reflex and autonomic phasic bite-release pattern Experiences diminished strong gag reflex at 5 months Drools less in positions with greater postural stability Uses mouth to explore objects Begins to show new oral movements in association with increased head and body control	Anticipates feeding; recognizes bottle and readies mouth for nipple Demonstrates voluntary control of mouth during bottle drinking or breast feeding Loses liquid from lip corners Is able to receive solid food from a spoon at 5 months Uses suckling during spoon feeding; gags on new textures Shows tongue reversal after spoon is removed; ejects food involuntarily

Adapted from Alexander R, Boehme R, Cupps B: *Normal development of functional motor skills,* Tucson, 1993, Therapy Skill Builders; Bly L: *Motor skills acquisition in the first year: an illustrated guide to normal development,* Tucson, 1994, Therapy Skill Builders; Case-Smith J, Humphrey R: Feeding and oral motor skills. In Case-Smith J, Allen AS, Pratt PN, editors: *Occupational therapy for children,* ed 2, St Louis, 1995, Mosby; Clark GF: Oral-motor and feeding issues. In Royeen CB, editor: *AOTA self-study series: classroom applications for school-based practice,* Rockville, Md, 1993, American Occupational Therapy Association; Glass RP, Wolf LS: Feeding and oral-motor skills. In Case-Smith J, editor: *Pediatric occupational therapy and early intervention,* Boston, 1993, Andover Medical; Lowman DK, Murphy SM: *The educator's guide to feeding children with disabilities,* Baltimore, 1999, Paul H Brookes; Lowman DK, Lane SJ: Children with feeding and nutritional problems. In Porr S, Rainville, EB, editors: *Pediatric therapy: a systems approach,* Philadelphia, 1999, FA Davis; Morris SE, Klein MD: *Pre-feeding skills: a comprehensive resource for feeding development,* Tucson, 1987, Therapy Skill Builders.
ATNR, Asymmetrical tonic neck reflex.

TABLE 7-1

Normal Development of Sensorimotor, Oral-Motor, and Feeding Skills—cont'd

AGE	SENSORIMOTOR SKILLS	ORAL-MOTOR SKILLS	FEEDING SKILLS
6 MO	Has total head control Shifts weight and reaches with one hand in prone position Begins shifting weight in quadruped position Transfers objects from hand to hand in supine position Reaches with one hand while supporting with other in sitting position Reaches to be picked up Begins to use thumb in grasp Begins to hold objects in one hand Shows visual interest in small things	No longer has rooting reflex or autonomic phasic bite-release pattern Experiences decrease in strength of gag reflex Maintains lip closure longer in supine, prone, and sitting positions Drools when babbling, reaching, and teething; drools less during feeding	Sucks from bottle or breast with no liquid loss and long sequences of coordinated sucking-swallowing-breathing Suckles liquid from a cup, with liquid loss Coughs and chokes when drinking too much liquid from cup Moves upper lip down to scrape food from spoon and uses suckling with some sucking to move food back Gags on new textures Opens mouth when spoon approaches Uses phasic up-and-down jaw movements, suckling, or sucking when presented with solids Moves tongue laterally when solids placed on side-biting surfaces Begins finger feeding Plays with spoon
7-9 MO	Shifts weight and reaches in quadruped position Creeps Develops extension, flexion, and rotation; expands movement options in sitting position May pull to stand and hold on to support Reaches with supination Uses index finger to poke Develops voluntary release skills	Experiences diminished gag reflex; becomes more similar to an adult protective gag reflex Uses facial expressions to convey likes and dislikes Uses mouth in combination with visual examination and hand manipulation to investigate new objects Bites on fingers and objects to reduce teething discomfort Produces more coordinated jaw, tongue, and lip movements in supine, prone, sitting, and standing positions; rarely drools except when teething	Suckles liquid in cup; loses liquid when cup is removed Takes fewer sucks and suckles before pulling away from cup to breathe Independently holds bottle Feeds self cracker using fingers Holds jaw closed on soft solids to break off pieces Uses variable up-and-down movement while chewing; moves tongue laterally and jaw diagonally when solids placed on biting surfaces Assists with cup and spoon feeding

Adapted from Alexander R, Boehme R, Cupps B: *Normal development of functional motor skills,* Tucson, 1993, Therapy Skill Builders; Bly L: *Motor skills acquisition in the first year: an illustrated guide to normal development,* Tucson, 1994, Therapy Skill Builders; Case-Smith J, Humphrey R: Feeding and oral motor skills. In Case-Smith J, Allen AS, Pratt PN, editors: *Occupational therapy for children,* ed 2, St Louis, 1995, Mosby; Clark GF: Oral-motor and feeding issues. In Royeen CB, editor: *AOTA self-study series: classroom applications for school-based practice,* Rockville, Md, 1993, American Occupational Therapy Association; Glass RP, Wolf LS: Feeding and oral-motor skills. In Case-Smith J, editor: *Pediatric occupational therapy and early intervention,* Boston, 1993, Andover Medical; Lowman DK, Murphy SM: *The educator's guide to feeding children with disabilities,* Baltimore, 1999, Paul H Brookes; Lowman DK, Lane SJ: Children with feeding and nutritional problems. In Porr S, Rainville EB, editors: *Pediatric therapy: a systems approach,* Philadelphia, 1999, FA Davis; Morris SE, Klein MD: *Pre-feeding skills: a comprehensive resource for feeding development,* Tucson, 1987, Therapy Skill Builders.

TABLE 7-1

Normal Development of Sensorimotor, Oral-Motor, and Feeding Skills—cont'd

AGE	SENSORIMOTOR SKILLS	ORAL-MOTOR SKILLS	FEEDING SKILLS
10-12 MO	Creeps with good coordination Cruises holding on to support with one hand Stands independently Learns to walk independently Uses superior pincer grasp with fingertip and thumb Smoothly releases large objects	Produces more coordinated jaw, tongue, and lip movements when sitting, standing, and creeping on hands and knees; rarely drools except when teething	Easily closes lips on spoon; uses upper and lower lips to remove food from spoon Uses controlled, sustained biting motion on soft cookies or crackers Chews with mixture of up-and-down and diagonal rotary movements Feeds self independently using fingers Likes to feed self but needs assistance with using spoon; inverts spoon before putting in mouth
13-18 MO	Walks alone Learns to go up and down stairs Has more precise grasp and release	Moves upper and lower lips By 15-18 months has excellent coordination of sucking, swallowing, and breathing	Uses an up-and-down sucking pattern to obtain liquid from a cup Shows well-coordinated rotary chewing movements by 18 months Has well controlled and sustained biting movements Practices self-feeding; becomes neater Holds cup and puts cup down without spilling liquid
19-24 MO	Demonstrates equilibrium reactions while standing and walking Runs with more narrow base of support	Uses up-and-down tongue movements and tip elevation Develops internal jaw stabilization Swallows with easy lip closure	Efficiently drinks from cup Has well graded and sustained bite
24-36 MO	Jumps in place* Pedals tricycle* Scribbles* Snips with scissors*	Uses tongue humping rather than tongue protrusion to initiate swallowing	Possesses circular rotary jaw movements* Closes lips while chewing* Holds cup in one hand* Handles spoon more accurately* Uses fingers to fill spoon* Begins to drink from straws*

* From this point on, skills learned during the first 24 months are further refined.

- *Grasp reflex*: When a finger is pressed into the infant's palm, s/he grasps the finger. As the infant sucks the grasp tightens, indicating a connection between sucking and the grasp reflex. Most of these early reflexive patterns begin to change or disappear between 4 and 6 months of age, when the cortex develops.[29,31]

Infancy

Oral skills develop concurrently and are closely related to the overall development of sensorimotor skills. Table 7-1 presents a brief overview of normal sensorimotor, oral motor, and feeding development during the first 3 years of life. Feeding initially requires that the adult provide head support and head-trunk alignment to allow the infant to coordinate the suck-swallow-breathe sequence. The infant's first suckling pattern predominates for the first 3 to 4 months of life.[12] Beginning at 4 months a "true sucking" pattern—an up and down tongue movement—develops as head and jaw stability appears.

At 6 months the infant has complete head control and more jaw stability, allowing for better control of tongue movements. This stability allows the infant to effectively suck from a bottle and remove soft food from a spoon.[25] At 4 to 5 months the infant demonstrates a reflexive phasic bite-release pattern when presented with a soft cracker. With practice, the rhythm progresses into a munching pattern involving an up and down jaw movement. The munching pattern is effective with baby food or other dissolvable foods.[12,25] By 7 to 8 months, some diagonal jaw movements are added to the munching pattern. Infants use their fingers to eat soft crackers and cookies.[12,25]

At around 12 months, infants enjoy and prefer eating with their fingers. Rotary chewing movements and a well graded bite are observed. At this time, many infants experience the transition from a bottle to a cup. While learning to drink from a cup, the infant's jaw initially continues to move in the up and down sucking pattern. In addition, the infant bites the rim of the cup to stabilize the jaw. By 15 months the infant demonstrates some diagonal rotary movements of the tongue and jaw while chewing food. Between 15 and 18 months the infant begins to independently eat with a spoon.[12]

Early Childhood

By 24 months of age the foundation has been established for all adult eating patterns.[28] At age 2 children eat independently, consuming most meats and raw vegetables (Figure 7-1). Circular rotary chewing develops between the second and third year of life and allows toddlers to eat almost all adult foods.[25,31]

By 24 months, children can hold a spoon and bring it to the mouth with the wrist supinated into the palm-up position.[29] At 30 to 36 months, children experiment with forks to stab at food. A variety of spoons are available for children learning to use utensils.[22] The size of the spoon's bowl should match the size of the child's mouth. Children learning to use spoons typically use ones with shallow bowls; they must work harder to eat food from spoons with deeper bowls. Child-size spoons and forks are easier for children to hold and manipulate, and bowls and plates with raised edges are also easier for children to scoop against.[22,29]

By 24 months, toddlers can also efficiently drink from cups. Children may begin drinking through straws between 2 and 3 years of age, especially if they have been exposed early to the use of straws. Given the variety of silly long, short, and decorated straws available, children are happy to independently use their own straws.[22] By

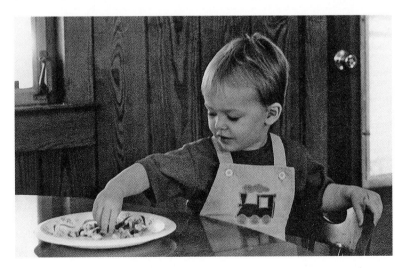

FIGURE 7-1 At age 2 children are able to sit up at the table, feed themselves, and eat almost all adult foods.

30 to 36 months, children try to serve themselves liquids and family-style servings of food.[29]

DRESSING AND UNDRESSING SKILLS

Dressing and undressing are also essential, basic self-care skills learned in infancy and early childhood.[2] Dressing includes selecting clothing and accessories appropriate for the weather and occasion, putting clothes on sequentially, and fastening and adjusting clothing and shoes.[2] Young children develop independent dressing skills at various ages according to the family's cultural expectations for self-dressing and the types of clothing worn, opportunities for practice, and the child's motivation for independence.[10] Dressing skills require coordinated movements of almost every body part.[32] The development of independ-

TABLE 7-2

Developmental Sequence for Self-Care Skills

AGE (yr)	DRESSING AND UNDRESSING SKILLS	GROOMING AND HYGIENE
1	Cooperates in dressing (e.g., holds foot up for shoe or sock, holds arm out for sleeve) Pushes arms through sleeves and legs through pants	Cooperates during hand washing and drying Has regular bowel movements
1½	Takes off loose clothing (such as mittens, hat, socks, and shoes) Partially pulls shirt over head Unties shoes or takes off hat as an act of undressing Unfastens clothing zippers with large pull tabs Puts on hat	Allows teeth to be brushed Pays attention to acts of eliminating Indicates discomfort from soiled points Begins to sit on potty when placed there and supervised (for a short time)
2	Removes unfastened coat Purposefully removes shoes (if laces are untied) Helps pull down pants Finds armholes in over-the-head shirt	Attempts to brush teeth in imitation of adults Washes own hands with assistance Shows interest in washing self in bathtub Urinates regularly
2½	Removes pull-down pants or shorts with elastic waist Removes simple clothing (such as open shirt or jacket) Assists in putting on socks Puts on front-button-type coat or shirt Unbuttons large buttons	Dries hands Wipes nose if given a tissue and prompted to do so Has daytime control of bowel and bladder; experiences occasional accidents Usually indicates need to go to toilet; rarely has bowel accidents
3	Puts on over-the-head shirt with some assistance Puts on shoes without fastening (may be on wrong feet) Puts on socks with some difficulty positioning heel Independently pulls down pants or shorts Zips and unzips coat zipper without separating or inserting zipper Needs assistance to remove over-the-head shirt Buttons large front buttons	Washes own hands Uses toothbrush with assistance Gets drink from fountain or faucet with no assistance Uses toilet independently but needs help wiping after bowel movements

Adapted from Case-Smith J: Self-care strategies for children with developmental deficits. In Christiansen C, editor: *Ways of living: self-care strategies for special needs,* Bethesda, Md, 1994, AOTA; Coley IL: *Pediatric assessment of self-care activities,* St Louis, 1978, Mosby; Cook RE, Tessier A, Klein MD: *Adapting early childhood curricula for children in inclusive settings,* Columbus, Ohio, 1996, Merrill; Johnson-Martin NM: *The Carolina curriculum for preschoolers with special needs,* ed 2, Baltimore, 2004, Paul H Brookes; Johnson-Martin NM: *The Carolina curriculum for infants and toddlers with special needs,* ed 3, Baltimore, 1990, Paul H Brookes; Klein MD: *Pre-dressing skills: skill starters for self-help development, revised.* Tucson, 1983, Communication Skill Builders; Orelove, FP, Sobsey, D: *Educating children with multiple disabilities: a transdisciplinary approach,* ed 3, Baltimore, 1996, Paul H Brookes; Shepherd J, Procter SA, Coley IL: Self-care and adaptations for independent living. In Case-Smith J, Allen JA, Pratt PN, editors: *Occupational therapy for children,* ed 2, St Louis, 1996, Mosby.

TABLE 7-2

Developmental Sequence for Self-Care Skills—cont'd

AGE (yr)	DRESSING AND UNDRESSING SKILLS	GROOMING AND HYGIENE
3½	Usually finds front of clothing Snaps or hooks clothing in front Unzips front zipper on coat or jacket, separating zipper Puts on mittens Buttons series of three or four buttons Unbuckles belt or shoe Puts on boots Dresses with supervision (needs help with front and back)	Pours well from small pitcher Spreads soft butter with knife Seldom has toileting accidents; may need help with difficult clothing
4	Removes pullover garment independently Buckles belt or shoe Zips coat zipper, inserting zipper Puts on pull-down pants or shorts Puts on socks, with appropriate heel placement Puts on shoes, with assistance in tying laces Consistently knows front and back of clothing	Washes and dries hands and face without assistance Brushes teeth with supervision Washes and dries self after bath with supervision Cares for self at toilet (may need help with wiping after bowel movement)
4½	Puts belt in loops	Runs brush or comb through hair Tears toilet tissue and flushes toilet after use
5	Puts on pullover shirt correctly each time Ties and unties knots Laces shoes Dresses unsupervised	Scrubs fingernails with brush with coaching Brushes and combs hair with supervision Cuts soft food with knife Blows nose independently when prompted Wipes self after bowel movements
5½	Closes back zipper	Performs toileting activities, including flushing toilet, independently
6	Ties bow knot Ties hood strings Buttons back buttons Snaps back snaps Selects clothing that is appropriate for weather conditions and specific activities	Brushes and rinses teeth independently

ent dressing skills typically occurs at age 4 to 5 years.[10,20,36] Table 7-2 lists the general sequence of dressing and undressing skills.

Infancy

During the first year of development, the infant is established in the daily routine and begins to cooperate in dressing activities.[16] S/he learns to remove loose-fitting clothing such as hats, mittens, and socks. By age 1 the infant has achieved many of the motor skills needed for the development of dressing skills. They can separate movements so that the arms or legs can move separate from the trunk, have begun to stabilize with one hand the action of the other, and can adjust their posture during reaching.[21] Infants have the necessary control to push arms and legs through sleeves and pants or play at pulling off a hat.[21]

Early Childhood

By age 2, refined balance and equilibrium reactions provide children with the necessary motor skills to raise their arms to pull shirts over their heads. They can move their hands behind them to attempt to put their arms into the sleeves of a button-front shirt. By 3 years, children are more aware of details and can find arm and leg holes

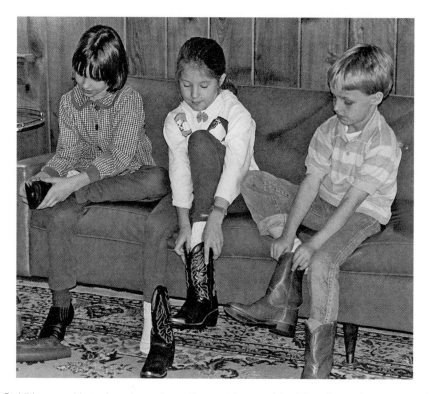

FIGURE 7-2 By age 5, children are able to dress themselves without adult supervision. They show adequate strength, balance, equilibrium, and fine motor coordination.

easily. By 4 years they recognize correct and incorrect sides; as fine motor skills progress they can also use buckles, zippers, and laces. By 5 years all skills of balance, equilibrium, and fine motor coordination are refined enough to allow children to dress themselves unsupervised.[16,21] Figure 7-2 shows children putting on their boots before going outdoors.

PERSONAL HYGIENE AND GROOMING

Grooming and hygiene are important self-care skills that tend to develop after eating and dressing skills. (See Table 7-2 for the general sequence of personal hygiene and grooming.) The cultural expectations and social routines of the family determine when independence in grooming and hygiene is achieved.[36] Face washing, hand washing, and hair care are typical **personal hygiene and grooming skills** learned in early childhood. The infant cooperates in hand washing. By age 2, children can wash the hands but need assistance turning on water and getting soap. By age 4, children wash the hands and face unsupervised. With supervision and coaching, 5 year olds can scrub fingernails with a brush and comb hair.[16]

In early childhood, **oral hygiene** involves brushing teeth.[2] Before age 2, infants allow their parents to brush their teeth. Two year olds imitate parents who are brushing their teeth. Children continue to brush their own teeth with supervision until the age of 5 or 6 years.[36] At that time, refinement of skill in the use of tools enables children to independently complete all steps of caring for their teeth, including preparing, brushing, and rinsing them.[12]

BATHING AND SHOWERING

Bathing and showering involves soaping, rinsing, and drying the body. At around age 2, children begin to show interest in bathing by assisting in washing while in the bathtub. Because bathing is a pleasurable activity for most children and parents, learning to wash themselves begins in the context of play.[12] Typically, most children are able to wash and dry themselves with supervision by age 4. It is not until age 8 that most children can independently prepare the bath or shower water, wash, and dry themselves.[36]

TOILET HYGIENE

Toilet hygiene involves clothing management, maintaining toileting position, transferring to and from toileting, and cleaning the body. Physiologically, voluntary control of urination does not usually occur until between 2 and 3 years of age. Independent toileting is a developmental milestone with wide variation among children.

During infancy, regularity in bowel movement and urination gradually develops. The infant may also indicate when diapers are wet or soiled and even sit on the toilet when placed. Toilet training is not typically introduced until the child remains dry for 1 or more hours at a time, shows signs of a full bladder or need to toilet, and is at least 2½ years old.[32] Daytime bowel and bladder control is usually attained between 2½ and 3 years of age, although the child may still need assistance with difficult clothing or fasteners.[16] Nighttime bladder control may not be attained until age 5 or 6. During the day, 5 year olds can anticipate immediate toilet needs and completely care for themselves while toileting, including wiping and flushing the toilet.[16]

Instrumental Activities of Daily Living

Instrumental activities of daily living (IADL) are the complex activities of daily living needed to function independently in the home, school, or community.[2] During childhood, children learn home management tasks that help them participate in family routines and community mobility skills in order to be active outside the home. As they get older, they are given the responsibility of caring for others.[36]

READINESS SKILLS

Readiness skills are necessary for successful participation in home management, community mobility, and care of others' activities. Specific readiness skills are related to particular tasks. Activity analysis (breaking an activity into steps) can determine the readiness skills needed to perform a specific task. For example, making a bed requires the coordination of the two sides of the body, sequencing skills, and a pad-to-pad pinch. Setting the dinner table requires sequencing, balance, and dexterity while carrying and placing plates and silverware. The different readiness skills necessary to care for others can be illustrated by comparing the requirements for caring for a pet with babysitting a sibling. These two tasks obviously require different abilities.

HOME MANAGEMENT ACTIVITIES

Home management activities are tasks that are necessary to obtain and maintain personal and household possessions.[2] Temporal and environmental performance contexts significantly influence a child's or adolescent's participation in home management tasks. Children's ages and physical, social, and cultural environments determine their roles in this domain. Children and adolescents may have chores that they are expected to complete on a regular schedule. Examples of chores include making the bed, setting the dinner table, and cutting the grass. Some children and adolescents have the incentive of a monetary allowance to complete the assigned chores, whereas others do not have a monetary incentive but are still expected to assist in the maintenance of their households.

COMMUNITY MOBILITY

Mobility in the community outside the home is critical to the child's development. During the preschool years **community mobility** may mean accompanying parents, while during adolescence it may be driving to run errands. Environmental factors that have an impact on mobility might be crowds, street crossings, public transportation, and architectural barriers.[36] Family and cultural expectations also determine the age and independence of community mobility skills.

CARE OF OTHERS

The **care of others** refers to the physical upkeep and nurturing of pets or other human beings.[2] As with household management, the care of others is also significantly influenced by performance contexts. In large families, older siblings may be required to assist their parents in the care of younger siblings. A child living on a farm may assist with feeding and caring for the farm animals. A child living in an urban area may walk the family dog several times a day in the park.

SUMMARY

The ADLs of feeding and eating, dressing and undressing, personal hygiene and grooming, and toilet hygiene are the most basic tasks learned by children as they grow and mature. The IADLs of home management, community mobility, and caring for others are critical to the child's development and ability to be active outside the home. The specific age at which young children develop independent ADL and IADL skills varies according to the family's cultural expectations, opportunities for practice, and the child's motivation for independence. OT practitioners are in an excellent position to teach parents and teachers ways to facilitate the development of self-care skills in children.

Education

READINESS SKILLS

Readiness skills are those performance abilities that are necessary to effectively engage in educational and vocational activities. *Readiness* is a stage of preparedness for "what comes next."[17,36] Different readiness skills are necessary for different tasks. Readiness skills must be considered within the temporal and environmental contexts of the Occupational Therapy Practice Framework. The chronological age of the child or adolescent is directly related to the necessary readiness skills. For example, different readiness skills are expected of a kindergarten student and a high school student. Social, cultural, and physical environments also influence expectations of readiness.

The readiness skills necessary for successful participation in formal educational activities vary according to performance contexts. This section discusses educational readiness skills for children enrolled in preschool programs, kindergarten, and elementary school.

Preschool Readiness Skills

Children entering preschool programs need certain readiness skills, which include independence in toileting with a minimum of assistance from fasteners, independence in self-feeding, and cooperative play behavior. Children attending a preschool program are also expected to understand rules and schedules. They need to exhibit the beginning of behavioral and emotional maturity (i.e., controlling tempers and mood swings).

Kindergarten Readiness Skills

The child attending kindergarten is expected to have the readiness skills of a typical preschooler with additional preacademic and academic skills. S/he must be able to sit quietly while listening to a story and should have adequate fine motor skills for coloring and manipulating small objects.[11,17] S/he must possess gross motor skills such as running, hopping, and jumping and is expected to recognize letters and numbers.

Elementary School Readiness Skills

Children attending elementary school are expected to have greater independence and skill in the occupational performance areas than those of younger children. Independence in the bathroom and cafeteria is necessary. In addition to independence in eating, children in elementary school are expected to carry their lunch trays and assist in cleaning the table at the end of a meal. They must remain in their classroom chairs for extended periods of time. The ability to remain "on task" and attend to work while seated is termed *in-seat behavior*.

Expectations of reading, writing, spelling, and math skills increase with grade level. The child attending elementary school should have adequate perceptual and motor skills to participate in games and organized sports.

Middle Childhood and Adolescent Readiness Skills

Educational readiness skills for middle childhood and adolescence build on the competencies gained during the preceding periods. Appropriate social skills and manners are expected, and increased skill in creative thinking, problem solving, and the development of ideas is re-

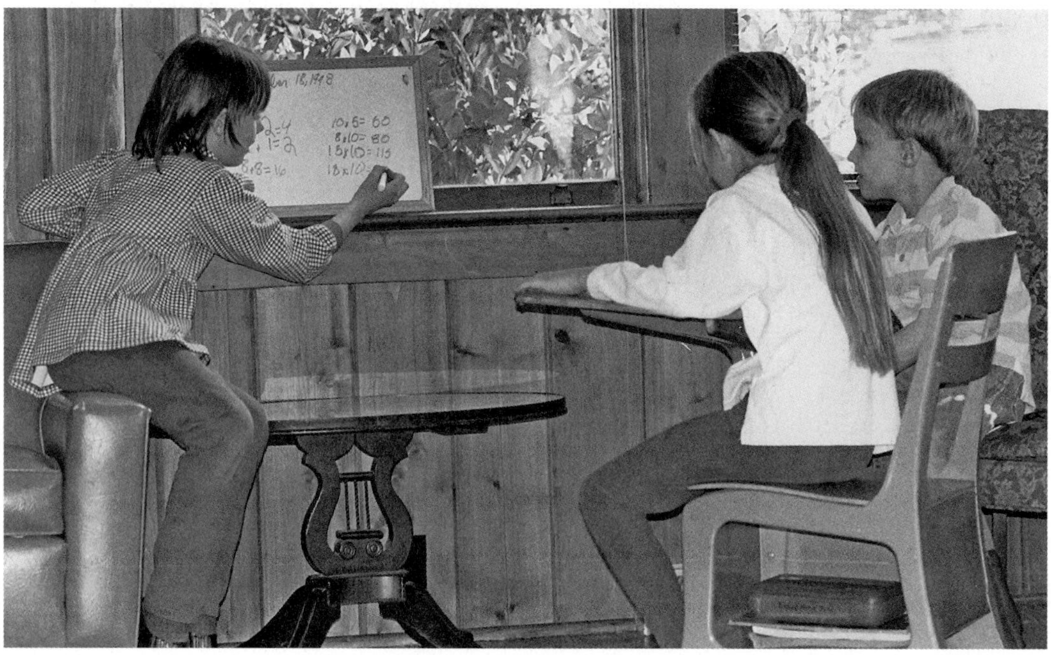

FIGURE 7-3 Children enjoy "playing school," a typical informal educational activity. Notice the students attending to the "teacher."

quired. Expressive writing is learned during this period. During middle childhood, children and adolescents also begin to seek independence. They question authority figures but must learn to work with them effectively in educational settings.

EDUCATIONAL ACTIVITIES

Educational activities are the opportunities that facilitate learning for children and adolescents.[36] These activities can be formal or informal. Formal educational activities are structured and may be mandated by public law for specific age groups. These activities are provided in settings such as preschool programs, daycare, public schools, and Sunday school classes. Informal educational activities are less structured and occur in a variety of settings. Examples of these activities, in which younger children engage, include playing school with an older sibling and playing a shopping game with peers. Figure 7-3 shows children engaged in "playing school," a typical informal educational activity. Adolescents frequently study together, creating opportunities for informal learning.

Work/Vocational Activities

In preparation for entering the world of **work** as adults, adolescents engage in a variety of **vocational activities**. These activities are work related and typically have a monetary incentive or salary. Like educational activities, vocational activities can be formal or informal. An example of a formal vocational activity is having a job. Public laws determine the age at which a person may hold a job. Informal vocational activities include neighborhood lemonade stands and cutting a neighbor's grass for a fee. Figure 7-4 shows a child "selling" cookies to a friend. Like home management and the care of others, vocational activities in which a child or adolescent might participate are significantly influenced by performance contexts for that individual.

Readiness skills for formal and informal vocational activities are as varied as and depend greatly on performance contexts. To successfully engage in formal vocational activities, skills such as promptness, appropriate dress, and effective communication with peers and supervisors are important. Activity analysis is beneficial when considering appropriate formal and informal vocational activities.

SUMMARY

Education and work are two of the areas of occupation described in the Occupational Therapy Practice Framework. Readiness skills also develop during childhood and can differ according to each child's age and the task being performed. Although all children and adolescents participate in educational tasks, great variability exists in the ways they participate in home management activities, the care of others, and vocational activities.

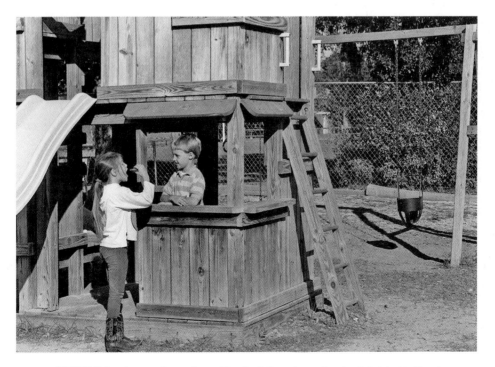

FIGURE 7-4 A young boy sells cookies, (an informal vocational activity) to his friend.

Play/Leisure Activities

Play is the occupation of childhood. Through play children learn cognitive, social-emotional, motor, and language skills.[4,5,15,33,35] In adulthood play often takes the form of **leisure activities,** which are not associated with time-consuming duties and responsibilities.[2] During play and leisure activities people refine skills, relax, reflect, and engage in creativity.

Children must have certain skills to engage in play. OT practitioners evaluate the play of children to determine ways to facilitate play and enable children to play at their highest potential. In this way, OT practitioners assist children in gaining skills for adulthood.

DEFINITION OF PLAY

Scholars have struggled for centuries to define *play*.* Play has been viewed as (1) a method to release surplus energy, (2) a link in the evolutionary change from animal to human being (recapitulationtheory), (3) a method to practice survival skills, and (4) an attitude or mood.[27,32] More recent theories have asserted that play provides the stimulation needed to satisfy a physiological need for optimum arousal.[33]

Theorists describe play in terms of the development of cognitive, emotional, social, language, and motor skills.[4,5,15,33,35] These theorists propose that play develops as children learn necessary skills. For example, Piaget proposed that children's play developed from sensorimotor (practice) play to symbolic play to games with rules as the child acquires cognitive skills.[35] Table 7-3 describes Piaget's stages of play. McCune-Nicolich proposed that children engage in more make-believe play as their language skills develop.[35] See Table 7-4 for a description of the progression of symbolic or make-believe play. Figure 7-5 shows an 18-month-old toddler playing "dress-up" with her mother's shoes. Early theorists such as Erikson and Freud believed that children work out emotional conflicts during play.[35] Psychoanalysts also theorized that they could use play to evaluate these conflicts.

Developmental theorists describe the changes in play in terms of motor skill progression.[5,23,33] In doing so, they divide play into the categories of functional (sensorimotor), constructive (manipulative), dramatic ("pretend"), and formal (rule governed).[33] Parham identified the social aspects of play as progressing from solitary to parallel to group play.[33] Figure 7-6 shows two children engaged in cooperative play.

Play encompasses a variety of skills and occupies much of the child's day. Thus, OT practitioners have a firm understanding of its complexities. Occupational Therapy Practice Framework defines *play* or *leisure activities* as "...any spontaneous or organized activity that provides enjoyment, entertainment, amusement, or diversion."[2]

OT practitioners view play as a performance area in addition to ADLs and work and productive activities. As such, OT practitioners work with children to facilitate and remediate play skills. The following OT theorists have made significant contributions to the study of play in OT practice.

*References 6, 7, 13, 15, 18, 19, 33-35.

TABLE 7-3

Piaget's Stages of Play

AGE (YEARS)	STAGE
0-2	**Sensorimotor:** Practices games, exploratory behaviors, reflexive behaviors, repetition
2-6	**Symbolic:** Uses imaginary objects, pretend play
6-10	**Games with rules:** Participates in team sports, activities with flexible rules, goals

TABLE 7-4

Symbolic Play

AGE (MONTHS)	PLAY CHARACTERISTICS
12	Play directed towards self Imitation of patty-cake and other movements Simple pretend play directed toward self (eating, sleeping) Imitation of familiar actions
18-24	Role-playing with objects (such as feeding a doll) Use of nonrealistic objects in pretend
24-36	Engagement in multistep scenarios (such as giving doll a bath, dressing the doll, and putting the doll to bed)
36-48	Use of language in play Advance plans and development of stories Acting out sequences with miniatures
48	Imaginary play Role-playing entire scenarios Creation of stories with "pretend" characters

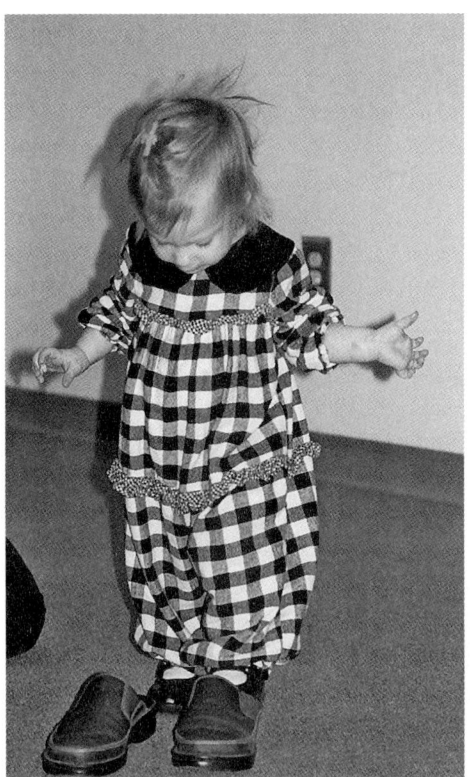

FIGURE 7-5 A toddler enjoys playing "dress-up" with her mother's shoes, a typical activity for an 18 month old.

OCCUPATIONAL THERAPY THEORISTS AND THEIR CONTRIBUTIONS TO PLAY

Reilly

Mary Reilly, a noted occupational therapist and researcher, described play as a progression through three stages: exploratory behaviors, competency, and achievement.[34] *Exploratory behaviors* are intrinsically motivated and are engaged in for their own sake.[34] Infants engage in exploratory behaviors that focus on sensory experiences.[34] The second stage of development, *competency*, occurs when children search for challenges, novelty, and experimentation. In this stage they often want to do everything alone and "their way."[34] It is often present in early and middle childhood. The *achievement* stage of play emphasizes performance standards (such as winning) and competition. Children at this stage of development take more risks in their play.

Takata

Occupational therapist Nancy Takata developed the *Play History* to provide OT practitioners with a format for obtaining information about a child's play.[34] The interview format helps describe a child's play skills. OT practitioners with a solid knowledge of typical play patterns can use this information to design treatment.

Knox

The *Knox Preschool Play Scale* (PPS) was constructed by occupational therapist Susan Knox and is based on the

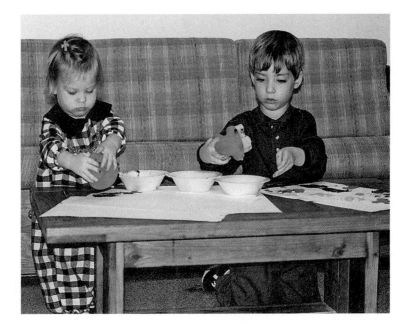

FIGURE 7-6 Children share their paints as they create pictures. They are absorbed in the play process.

work of Piagetian cognitive stages and Parham's social stages.[33] The Knox PPS divides play into four domains: space management, material management, imitation, and participation. The scale provides age equivalents for each domain and an overall play age. This scale is easy to administer and provides information on the motor skill requirements for play.

Bundy

Professor and occupational therapist Anita Bundy designed the *Test of Playfulness* (ToP) to objectively measure playfulness.[7,8] Bundy found that a child's attitude about and approach to activities (i.e., playfulness) provide valuable information for OT practitioners. Some children who do not possess the skills for play may still be playful. Others have the skills but do not appear to be having fun.

The ToP examines the context in which children perform play activities.[7,8] For example, two 4-year-old boys playing "Godzilla" may engage in rough and tumble "fighting." Because the context of the fighting is play, the children are not being mean spirited or hurtful. They are clearly playing and not fighting.

PLAY SKILL ACQUISITION

Children acquire play skills as they mature and develop. Play affords opportunities for them to develop. For example, a child needs balance and coordination to ride a bike. At the same time, riding the bike improves the child's balance and coordination. A variety of play opportunities are important for development. Table 7-5 provides an outline of toys and play activities suitable for different age groups.

Infancy

Infants explore the environment and learn through their senses.[5,24] They enjoy visual, tactile, auditory, and movement sensations.[6] Toys with bells and noise encourage infants to explore the environment.[23] Play should focus on enhancing their capabilities while furnishing new opportunities for exploration. OT practitioners and caregivers must allow them to repeat activities until they have mastered them.[5,34] Infant play encourages body awareness. They typically explore their hands and feet spontaneously. Playing games such as patty-cake helps them understand that their bodies are fun, as does face-to-face play with an adult.[4,5,14] Peek-a-boo is a favorite game at this age. Enjoyable toys encourage mobility, elicit actions, increase motor skills, and facilitate natural creativity.

Parents and caregivers establish bonds with infants by playing comfortably with them. Adults must respond to their cues. Those that indicate stress include crying, hiccups, gaze aversion, yawning, finger splaying, and tantrums.[6,27] If infants cry or show signs of stress, they should be comforted and the type of play changed. OT practitioners should remember that play is fun.

TABLE 7-5

Toys and Play Activities for Various Ages

AGE (YEARS)	TOYS AND ACTIVITIES
0-1	**Manipulative, sensory:** rattles, musical sounds, bells, swings, soft toys, boxes, pots and pans, wooden spoons, books
1-2	**Movement, manipulative, sensory:** push-pull toys, balls, pop-beads, pop-up toys, toy phones, musical books, noisy toys, ride-on toys, trucks, cause and effect toys
2-4	**Pretend play, movement, manipulative, sensory:** dolls, trucks, action figures, playdough, markers, water play, balls, blocks, Legos, books, dress-up toys, hats, shoes, clothes, tricycles
4-6	**Pretend play, craft activities, movement:** swings, gyms, bicycles, scooters, ball games, beads, painting, play dough, arts and crafts, dolls, cooking, group games (for example, follow-the-leader, tag, red rover)
6-8	**Pretend play, craft activities, movement:** gymnastic play, jumping rope, coordinated games (for example, keep-away with ball), arts and crafts, wood kits, model airplanes, painting, drawing, skating, bike riding, swimming
8-10	**Movement, group games, manipulative:** basketball, baseball, soccer, bike riding, skateboarding, tennis, swimming, volleyball, arts and crafts requiring more skill, cooking, collecting
10 and up	**Movement, games that challenge, skilled manipulative resulting in products:** competitive sports, strenuous activities, sewing, knitting, woodworking, bowling, walking, going to the beach, flying kites, boating, camping, reading

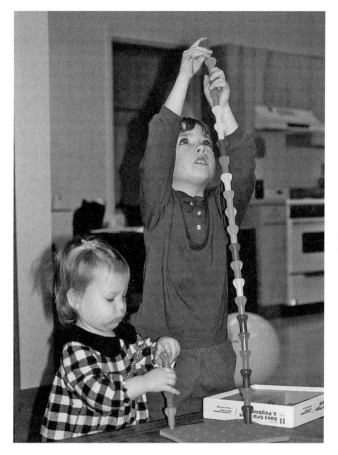

FIGURE 7-7 Children challenge their motor, social, and cognitive skills during play. They must use their fine motor skills to build a tower.

Early Childhood

Continued exploration and the development of friendships accentuate childhood play.[6,24] Play provides children with opportunities to learn negotiation, problem-solving, and communication skills. Figure 7-7 shows children challenging their skills in play. It also develops and refines motor skills.[6,15,24] Adults should be cautious about intervening too quickly during play. Children need opportunities to work out differences among themselves.

Children enjoy manipulative play, imitation, games, and social play with other children of the same sex.[6] They enjoy dramatic and rough and tumble play.[6,35] Role-playing scenarios that facilitate dramatic play stimulates a child's imagination, creativity, and problem-solving abilities.

Middle Childhood

Middle childhood is a time of the refinement of skills, such as speed, dexterity, strength, and endurance. Children become more competent in play activities. They enjoy games with rules and competition. Childhood is a time for them to experiment with many play activities. Some of these activities are easy, whereas others are difficult. Children should be encouraged to play, have fun, and realize that everyone has different talents. This is all part of growing up and finding their identities.

Adolescence

Adolescents are in search of independence.[6,24] Parents need to facilitate socially appropriate play and leisure activities. Adolescents enjoy activities in which they can participate with peers.[6,24] They may wish to participate in school or community clubs. Practitioners and parents need to listen carefully to adolescents to help them discover their goals and talents. At this stage of development, play is beneficial in the establishment of independence.

DEVELOPMENTAL RELEVANCE OF PLAY AND LEISURE

Play is important in each stage of development. It provides children with opportunities to develop motor, social-emotional, cognitive, and language skills. (The Appendix ["Play Analysis Guide"] at the end of this chapter provides a guide to the observation of play.) Play also allows children to interact with others, challenge themselves, and learn their strengths and weaknesses; therefore, play contributes to the quality of life. Play and leisure remain important throughout a person's life. People engage in play and leisure activities because they enjoy them and are intrinsically motivated to participate in them.[9]

SUMMARY

Play and leisure activities are crucial components of child development for the acquisition of skills children will use in adulthood. These activities provide the foundation for problem solving, skill development, social interaction, and negotiating.

OT practitioners can be key players in teaching parents, teachers, and peers the ways to play and be playful with children who have special needs. OT practitioners also have the skills required to assist children and their families in developing play skills so that the children may reach their potential.

Social Participation

Social participation activities are associated with the organized patterns of behavior expected of a child interacting with others within a given social system, such as the family, peer group, or community.[2] Children with delays or disabilities are members of a family system. Interventions that have an impact on one member of the family system do so on all members of that system. Therefore, it is important for OT practitioners to understand the family system. Refer to Chapter 2 for a detailed description of the patterns associated with the family system. Likewise, peers can positively or negatively influence a child's willingness to perform a task.[36] For example, if they ridicule an adaptive device, it will not be used. Consideration of the child's social routines and cultural and physical contexts is critical in determining the appropriate intervention techniques.

Chapter Summary

OT practitioners should have a firm knowledge of the areas of occupation of daily living, education, work, play and leisure, and social participation to effectively work with children and their families. OT practitioners use their knowledge of performance contexts in which the activity occurs because these contexts can influence the activity and the success of the child. Finally, the ability to analyze each of the areas of occupation through activity analysis is essential to effectively work with children and adolescents.

References

1. *American Heritage Dictionary*, ed 4, Boston, 2000, Houghton Mifflin.
2. American Occupational Therapy Association: Occupational therapy practice framework: domain and process, *Am J Occup Ther* 56:609, 2002.
3. Avery-Smith W: Eating dysfunction positions paper, *Am J Occup Ther* 50:846, 1996.
4. Axline VM: Play therapy procedures and results. In Schaefer C, editor: *The therapeutic use of play*, New York, 1976, Jason Aronson.
5. Bantz DL, Siktberg L: Teaching families to evaluate age-appropriate toys, *J Pediatr Health Care* 7:111, 1993.
6. Berger KS: *The developing person through the lifespan*, ed 5, New York, 1999, Worth.
7. Bundy AC: Assessment of play and leisure: delineation of the problem, *Am J Occup Ther* 47:217, 1993.
8. Bundy AC: Play and playfulness: what to look for. In Parham LD, Fazio LS, editors: *Play in occupational therapy for children*, St Louis, 1997, Mosby.
9. Bundy AC: Play theory and sensory integration. In Fisher AG, Murray EA, Bundy AC, editors: *Sensory integration: theory and practice*, Philadelphia, 1991, FA Davis.
10. Case-Smith J: Self-care strategies for children with developmental deficits. In Christiansen C, Matuska K, editors: *Ways of living: self-care strategies for special needs*, ed 3, Bethesda, Md, 2004, American Occupational Therapy Association.
11. Case-Smith J, editor: *Occupational therapy for children*, ed 4, St Louis, 2001, Mosby.
12. Case-Smith J, Humphrey R: Feeding intervention. In Case-Smith J, editor: *Occupational therapy for children*, ed 4, St Louis, 2001, Mosby.
13. Cass JE: *The significance of children's play*, London, 1971, Batsford.
14. Clark GF: Oral-motor and feeding issues. In Royeen CB, editor: AOTA *self-study series: classroom applications for school-based practice*, Rockville, Md, 1993, American Occupational Therapy Association.
15. Cohen D: *The development of play*, New York, 1987, New York University Press.
16. Coley IL: *Pediatric assessment of self-care activities*, St Louis, 1978, Mosby.
17. ERIC Clearinghouse on Elementary and Early Childhood Education, University of Illinois at Urbana-Champaign, Children's Research Center. http://www.npin.org/respar/tests/learning/kinrea.htm/.
18. Florey L: Development through play. In Schaefer C, editor: *The therapeutic use of play*, New York, 1976, Jason Aronson.
19. Greenstein DB: It's child's play. In Galvin J, Sherer M, editors: *Evaluating, selecting, and using appropriate assistive technology*, Gaithersburg, Md, 1996, Aspen.
20. Johnson-Martin NM: *The Carolina curriculum for infants and toddlers with special needs*, ed 3, Baltimore, 2004, Paul H Brookes.
21. Klein MD: *Pre-dressing skills: Skill starters for self-help development*, rev ed, Tucson, 1983, Communication Skill Builders.

22. Klein MD, Delaney TA: *Feeding and nutrition for the child with special needs: handouts for parents*, Tucson, 1994, Therapy Skill Builders.
23. Linder TW, editor: *Transdisciplinary play based assessment*, rev ed, Baltimore, 1993, Paul H Brookes.
24. Llorens LA: *Application of a developmental theory for health and rehabilitation*, Rockville, Md, 1976, American Occupational Therapy Association.
25. Lowman DK, Lane SJ: Children with feeding and nutritional problems. In Porr S, Rainville EB, editors: *Pediatric therapy: a systems approach*, Philadelphia, 1999, FA Davis.
26. Lowman DK, Murphy SM: *The educator's guide to feeding children with disabilities*, Baltimore, 1999, Paul H Brookes.
27. Marfo K, editor: *Parent-child interaction and developmental disabilities*, New York, 1988, Praeger.
28. Millar S: The psychology of play, New York, 1974, Aronson.
29. Morris SE, Klein MD: *Pre-feeding skills: A comprehensive resource for mealtime development*, ed 2, Tucson, 2000, Therapy Skill Builders.
30. Murphy SM, Caretto C: Anatomy of the oral and respiratory structures made easy. In Lowman DK, Murphy SM, editors: *The educator's guide to feeding children with disabilities*, Baltimore, 1999, Paul H Brookes.
31. Murphy SM, Caretto C: Oral-motor considerations for feeding. In Lowman DK, Murphy SM, editors: *The educator's guide to feeding children with disabilities*, Baltimore, 1999, Paul H Brookes.
32. Orelove FP, Sobsey D, Silberman, R: *Educating children with multiple disabilities: a collaborative approach*, ed 4, Baltimore, 2004, Paul H Brookes.
33. Parham LD, Primeau L: Play and occupational therapy. In Parham LD, Fazio LS, editors: *Play in occupational therapy for children*, St Louis, 1997, Mosby.
34. Reilly M, editor: *Play as exploratory learning: Studies in curiosity behavior*, Beverly Hills, 1974, Sage.
35. Rubin K, Fein GG, Vandenberg B: Play. In Mussen PH, editor: *Handbook of child psychology*, ed 4, New York, 1983, Wiley.
36. Shepherd J: Self-care and adaptations for independent living. In Case-Smith J, editor: *Occupational therapy for children*, ed 4, St Louis, 2001, Mosby.
37. Wolf LS, Glass RP: *Feeding and swallowing disorders in infancy: assessment and management*, Tucson, 1992, Therapy Skill Builders.

REVIEW *Questions*

1. Describe the developmental sequence of oral motor control, feeding, and eating skills.
2. Which foods and utensils are appropriate for children at various ages?
3. List the developmental sequences of dressing and undressing, toilet hygiene, grooming, bathing and showering, and oral hygiene.
4. Provide examples describing the progression of play skills.
5. Which terms describe play?
6. Describe the contributions of Reilly, Takata, Knox, and Bundy to the study of play in occupational therapy.
7. What is the difference between formal and informal work and productive activities? Give an example of each.
8. List the readiness skills expected for a child entering kindergarten. Why are these skills important?

SUGGESTED *Activities*

1. In a small group, list and discuss examples of how different cultural expectations might affect the development of self-care skills.
2. Visit a local child-care center.
   a. Observe preschool children of different ages eating lunch. What similarities and differences do you notice?
   b. Note all the different ways you see children putting on their coats.
   c. Visit the 2-year-old class. How many children are in diapers? How many are toilet trained?
3. Participate in play with an infant, child, and adolescent. Describe the way their play differed.
4. Watch a child playing for 15 minutes. Describe the way Reilly, Knox, Takata, and Bundy would describe the child's play.
5. Describe your favorite play activities as a child, adolescent, and adult. Record the setting, materials, group members, and feelings. Share your activities with classmates. How are the activities the same? Different?
6. In a small group, discuss your recollection of your formal education. In what ways do your stories differ and at what age?
7. Make a log of home management, the care of others, and vocational activities that you remember engaging in as a child and adolescent. Compare logs with classmates.

CHAPTER 7 APPENDIX

Play Analysis Guide

NAME OF CHILD: **DATE OF EVALUATION:**

DATE OF BIRTH:

CHILD'S AGE:

I. **Describe the physical setting.**
   Who was present?

II. **Describe the activities performed by the child.**
   A. *Gross Motor*
      Balance:
      Coordination:
      Motor Planning:
      Sequencing:
      Endurance:
      Mobility:
      Quality of Movement:
      Overall Skill:
   B. *Fine Motor*
      Manipulation of Objects:
      Grip:
      Strength:
      Overall Effectiveness:
   C. *Social*
      Participation:
      Negotiating:
      Peer Interactions:
      Sharing:
   D. *Imitative*
      Creativity:
      Novelty:
      Use of Toys:
   E. *Language*
      Expression:
      Communication:
      Imagination:
   F. *Attitude*
      Approach:
      Affect:
      Spontaneity:
      Teasing:
      Mischief:

III. **Describe the adult supervision. Did it facilitate or inhibit play?**

IV. **Other**

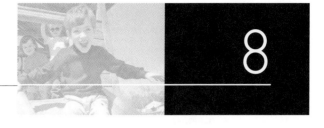

8

Adolescent Development: The Journey to Adulthood

KERRYELLEN G. VROMAN

CHAPTER *Objectives*

After studying this chapter, the reader will be able to accomplish the following:

- Describe the physical, cognitive, and psychosocial development of adolescents
- Recognize the interrelationship between health and adolescent development
- Identify the role and responsibilities of the occupational therapy assistant in facilitating the adolescent client's healthy transition to young adulthood
- Recognize that adolescent developmental issues affect the choice of therapeutic activities, interventions, and strategies used with adolescent clients

KEY TERMS

Self-esteem
Self-concept
Body image
Self-efficacy
Cognition
Identity
Leisure

CHAPTER OUTLINE

"Of all the stages of life, adolescence is the most difficult to describe. Any generalization about teenagers immediately calls forth an opposite one. Teenagers are maddeningly self-centered and yet capable of impressive acts of altruism. Their attention wanders like a butterfly, and yet they can spend hours concentrating on seemingly pointless involvements. They are lazy and rude, and yet when you least expect it they can be loving and helpful."[13]

Most accounts of adolescent development, such as the quote above, seek to capture the intense physical, emotional, and social changes that characterize this turbulent stage of human development. Evoking the full spectrum of emotions, adolescents experience moments of joy, overwhelming loneliness, laughter and fun, seemingly unbearable emotional pain, anger, frustration, and embarrassment contrasted with moments of supreme confidence and perceived immortality. They experience the closeness of peer friendships; the pleasure of discovering intimacy; and an intense passion for music, sports, or other interests, which for a week, a month, or a year become all-absorbing.

Physical maturation and psychosocial development determine adolescents' capacities to think, relate, and act as a future adult. These developments affect their choices of occupations and the quality of their occupational performance. We can understand adolescent development as a maturational process that can be observed in the common age-related tasks and challenges that adolescents undertake. These developmental tasks include achieving independence from parents; assuming the norms and lifestyles of peer groups; accepting the physical and sexual development of one's body; and establishing a sexual, personal, moral, and occupational identity. If they are successfully achieved, these tasks promote well-being, whereas failure results in ongoing life difficulties.[25]

This chapter describes adolescent development in order to provide an understanding of the developmental transition from childhood to adulthood. While knowledge of the clients' physical, cognitive, and psychosocial presentations is integral to *all* effective occupational therapy (OT) interventions, this information is essential when working with adolescents. Evaluation and intervention for adolescents always includes consideration of their developmental levels and needs. As in other chapters, case studies are used to demonstrate how developmental issues influence OT services, and the practice guidelines offered help the reader apply the developmental information to his or her OT practice. However, to effectively use the information provided in this chapter, the certified occupational therapy assistant (COTA) needs to combine all aspects of development to see it as a dynamic and integrated process of growth. Furthermore, the reader must apply this template of information to his or her unique work setting or socioeconomic and culturally diverse group of adolescents (Box 8-1).

BOX 8-1

Quick Facts: American Teenagers

- 19.9 million teens are between the ages of 10 and 14 and 19.8 million are between the ages of 15 and 19 (US Census Bureau, 2000).
- The adolescent population is becoming increasingly racially and ethnically diverse. Whites comprise 62.9% of the adolescent population; 15% are Hispanic; 14.5% are Black, non-Hispanic; 3.6% are Asian/Pacific Islander, and 1% is American Indian/Alaskan Native (US Census Bureau, 2000).
- More than half of all adolescents live in suburban areas; the highest percentage of adolescents aged 10 to 19 live in the South (35.6%), followed by the Midwest, West, and East at 23.5%, 22.7%, and 18.1%, respectively.
- Two thirds of adolescents between the ages of 12 and 17 live with both parents (2002 data).
- One third of high school students are working.
- One in 6 youths under the age of 18 lives below the federally determined poverty level. Black and Hispanic adolescents are more likely to experience poverty.

Data from Fact Sheet on Demographics: Adolescents, *American Adolescents: Are They Healthy?* ed 3, National Adolescent Health Information Center.

PHYSICAL MATURATION AND MOTOR DEVELOPMENT

The designated age of adolescence varies, but it is the stage of life between 12 and 18 years, or the years of high school, that is the most commonly associated with physical maturation and puberty. For most teens the significant biological changes of puberty include dramatic increases in height and weight and changes in body proportions, especially in the last 4 years of adolescence.[12] The stimulus for the physical growth and physiological maturation of reproductive systems is a complex interaction of hormones. The pituitary gland is responsible for initiating the release of growth and sex-related hormones from the thyroid, adrenal glands, and ovaries and testes at this stage of development.

There is rapid physical growth, which varies in intensity, onset, and duration due to natural individual differences in the general population. In this growth phase, which lasts about 4 years, adolescents gain approximately 50% of their adult weight and 20% of their adult height. The onset of the adolescent growth spurt can be as early as 9 years and may continue in some adolescents to around age 17. In the US, the average peak of growth for girls occurs at around age 11 and for boys age 13.

Bones increase in length, width, and strength as well as change in composition. For example, the calcification of bones makes them denser and stronger than the more cartilaginous bone composition of childhood. In addition, the growth of the skeletal system is not even. The head, hands, and feet reach their adult size the earliest. The body's musculature also experiences an increase in strength and size along with the growth of the bones. Skeletal growth and muscle development result in an overall increase in strength and endurance for physical activities. This increase in strength is greatest at about 12 months after the adolescent's height and weight have reached his or her peak and is associated with an overall improvement in motor performance, including better coordination and endurance. Because of the gain in muscle mass and the increase in heart and lung function that is typically greater for boys, a sex difference in strength and gross motor performance is developed and maintained throughout adulthood.[12] Motor performance peaks for males in late adolescence at around 17 to 18 years of age.[10] Girls will typically show an increase in motor performance that includes enhancements in speed, accuracy, and endurance earlier, at around the age of 14. However, the changes in girls' motor performance is highly variable and influenced by a complex interaction of physical and social factors such as their musculoskeletal development and menses as well as their interest, motivation, participation, and attitude toward physical activities.[10]

The rapid physical growth in adolescence is accompanied by the maturation of the reproductive system and the development of primary sex characteristics. Physical growth brings about changes in the sex organs that are directly involved in reproduction (e.g., menarche in girls and the growth of the penis and testicles in boys). On average, menarche first occurs in American girls at around age 12.[38] However, the onset of menarche is influenced by race, socioeconomic status, heredity, and nutrition. In boys, the development of primary sex characteristics such as penis growth and spermarche (first ejaculations) generally occurs between the ages of 12 and 13. The development of secondary sex characteristics also occurs at this stage (e.g., adolescent boys develop facial hair and a lower voice, girls develop breasts, and both sexes develop pubic hair). The age of sexual development in healthy adolescents varies as much as 3 years from the average age.[6,38]

Implications of Physical Growth and Sexual Maturation

Amy, 14, is an attractive 5-foot, 3-inch girl of average weight. To her friends, family, and teachers she is a successful adolescent. She achieves good grades, plays in the high school orchestra, and is a member of the dance team. However, in the past 6 months she has become increasingly self-conscious, especially about her developing body and the lack of a boyfriend. Amy started dieting and quickly lost weight. However, despite her dramatic weight loss, Amy still believes she is overweight and needs to diet. She has withdrawn from her friends and increased her workout exercise routine. Her mother became concerned when she found Amy purging after eating and hiding food. The psychiatrist diagnosed Amy's condition as anorexia nervosa, a disorder characterized by a distorted self-image.

For some adolescents, physical development is accepted with pride. For others these changes cause confusion, anxiety, or emotional turmoil. With changes in physical stature, physical appearance becomes an important concern in the lives of adolescents. How they view their physical and sexual development contributes significantly to their global **self-esteem.**[45] Part of adolescence involves integrating these physical and physiological changes into a **self-concept** that includes a positive attitude toward the body, referred to as **body image.** Body image affects our emotions, thoughts, and behaviors and influences both our public and intimate relationships.[43] Supporting adolescents in learning about their bodies and understanding that their feelings and thoughts about their bodies are shared by many of their peers can significantly reduce the anxiety associated with physical and sexual development.

Perceptions and attitudes that influence body image are socially constructed. There is a collective social peer view of what is normal and desirable (Box 8-2). For example, an individual's body image is influenced by social and cultural images of the "ideal masculine and feminine" bodies. Ethnic and social groups affect how a teen develops a positive body image. However, a more powerful influence on adolescents' appraisal of their bodies is the pervasive influence of the media (e.g., advertisements, teen magazines, music videos, and the fashion industry). The media markets a physical appearance that bears little relationship to the ethnic or physical appearance of the diverse population of American teens. Therefore, it is not surprising that many adolescents struggle with their actual physical image and are critical of their bodily appearance.[9] A negative body image is associated with low self-esteem as well as mental health problems such as anxiety, depression, and body image disorders. It is estimated that between 40% and 70% of girls, especially in early adolescence, are dissatisfied with two or more aspects of their bodily appearance.[21] Eavesdropping on the conversations of teenage girls would be likely to reveal such utterances as "*Do you think my backside is too big in these jeans?*" or "*I'm too fat...I need to lose weight.*" Studies show that body dissatisfaction is universal and that most girls,

BOX 8-2

Normal Development of Body Image

The practitioner may observe the following behaviors in the early and middle years of adolescence. These behaviors are typical of an adolescent concerned with developing a positive body image.

Early adolescents

- Are preoccupied with self, evaluating their own attractiveness.
- Make comparisons between their body/appearance and that of other teens.
- Have an interest in as well as anxiety about their personal sexual development.

Middle adolescents

- Have achieved pubertal changes and are developing an acceptance of their bodies.
- Are less preoccupied with their physical changes. Their interest now is their appearance, grooming, and "trying to be attractive."
- Eating and other body image–related disorders become established.

Adapted from Radizik M, Sherer S, Neinstein L: Psychosocial development in the normal adolescent. In Neinstein LS, editor: *Adolescent health: a practical guide*, Philadelphia, 2002, Lippincott, Williams & Wilkins.

regardless of ethnicity, express a desire to be thin.[33] Boys experience similar challenges regarding their internalized perception of how they "should" be in relation to peer pressure and images of masculinity. A boy dissatisfied with his body is likely to want to gain weight and develop muscle mass in the upper body (i.e., shoulders, arms, and chest).[55]

In addition to adjusting to the physical changes and developing a healthy body image, identity also involves self-evaluation as it relates to physical abilities and competency in physical activities such as sports. Similarly, physical appearance becomes an expression of individuality (e.g., body piercing and tattoos), and there is the development of sexual identity, which involves exploring one's sexuality and intimacy with others.

Family, friends, and the availability of information will influence the adjustment to the physical and physiological changes of the body. Physical maturation and the associated increase in physical skills have social status among adolescents. An adolescent finds security and social confidence in fitting within the "norm" for physical development. Those adolescents who achieve the "desired standard" of physical appearance and/or level of physical performance (e.g., high school sports teams with high visibility, such as football) receive validation and approval from their peers and adults. This social status reinforces positive self-esteem as well as **self-efficacy** in motor skills.

Sexual maturity also has social implications. Early and late sexual maturity pose both psychological challenges to and advantages for adolescents. For example, those who outwardly appear sexually mature seem older than their actual age and as a result experience demands and expectations that they are not psychologically able to handle. Early-maturing teens can experience pressure from peers and adults, are more concerned with being liked, and are more likely to be governed by rules and routines. The advantages of increased size and enhanced physical performance associated with early maturing promote self-confidence. Studies consistently show that during adolescence early-maturing boys are more popular, described as better adjusted, and reportedly more successful in heterosexual relationships.[55] Early maturity poses challenges for girls. They often demonstrate lower self-esteem and a poor self-concept associated with body image, and they engage in more risky behaviors (e.g., unprotected sex). They also experience more psychological difficulties (e.g., eating disorders and depression) than their more slowly developing girlfriends.

COGNITIVE DEVELOPMENT

Cognition is concerned with the mental processes of construction, acquisition, and the use of knowledge as well as perception, memory, and the use of symbolism and language.[41] The quality of thinking changes in adolescence, which Piaget referred to as the development of logical thinking or formal operations.[26,55] Adolescents' ability to think becomes more creative, complex, and efficient (speed and adeptness). It is also more thorough, organized, and systematic than it was in late childhood.[12] Adolescents' ability to problem-solve and reason becomes increasingly sophisticated, and they develop the capacity to think abstractly (i.e., they do not require concrete examples). For example, the adolescent develops the ability to use hypothetical-deductive reasoning. This type of reasoning involves thinking about possibilities without requiring actual examples. In this process of reasoning, a person identifies and explores many imagined possible outcomes to determine the most likely one for a particular situation or problem as well as the relationship between present actions and future consequences. Hypothetical-deductive reasoning is essential for problem solving and the process of arguing. Preadolescents consider possibilities as generalizations of actual, real events, whereas the adolescent understands that the actual world is one of the possibilities.[41]

It is teens' cognitive abilities that enable them to achieve independence in thought and action.[11] For the first time in their lives, adolescents develop a perspective of time and become interested in the future. Thus, cognitive development not only contributes to school performance (i.e., educational achievement) but is central to the development of occupational skills and the personal, social, moral, and political values that denote membership in adult society. This development of moral and social reasoning enables adolescents to deal with concepts such as integrity, justice, truth, and self-identity.[41]

One important cognitive development is that adolescents learn to understand the consequences of their actions and the values influencing their decision making. With abstract thinking abilities and a concern for the future comes a capacity for making choices about behavior that considers the consequences. The American Occupational Therapy Association's (AOTA's) Occupational Therapy Practice Framework defines self-regulation as the ability to control and monitor one's behavior and emotions appropriately relative to the situation and social cues.[1] Impulsive, ill-conceived behaviors with little regard for the future or without an assessment of the consequences are more typical of a junior high or early high school student than the late adolescent. However, adolescents with cognitive impairments will have long-term difficulties moderating their behavior, comprehending the consequences of their actions, or recognizing the subtleties of social cues. They will make impulsive decisions without considering future consequences. These types of behavioral difficulty are common in adolescents with head injuries. Box 8-3 lists some strategies for working with adolescents who have cognitive difficulties resulting from such cognitive conditions as head injuries and mild mental retardation.

BOX 8-3

Strategies for Working with Adolescents with Cognitive Impairments

- Identify how each teen learns best. Ask the teen, family, or teachers.
- Identify strengths and build from existing skills.
- Offer a selection of choices (*Which of these three things would you like to do?*) rather than an open-ended choice (*What would you like to do?*).
- Select activities that match the teen's abilities, needs, and interests. Offer activities that are age related but within the performance level of the teen (e.g., themes that deal with developmental needs such as relationships, appearance, grooming, and self-identity).
- Break down activities into simple steps that are achievable but provide a challenge.
- Keep instructions simple:
  Present only one instruction or step at a time.
  Increase instructions only if the client consistently follows current directions.
  Present directions systematically.
  Use many methods of instruction (e.g., verbal instructions, demonstrations, visual cues such as pictures, step-by-step diagrams, and the hand-over-hand technique).
- Develop and learn a new skill in a familiar setting before using the skill in novel settings (e.g., the community).
- Give specific feedback with concrete examples. State the correct or incorrect skill or behavior demonstrated. "*Good*" is an example of encouragement; it does not give clear feedback on performance.
- Be consistent and use repetition.
- Do not introduce variety without a reason. Change can mean new cognitive demands for the teen and increase the stress of learning. Flexibility and behavioral and cognitive adaptations are difficult for adolescents with cognitive impairments.

PSYCHOSOCIAL DEVELOPMENT

Achieving a stable, positive self-identity is regarded as a critical yet complex psychosocial task of adolescence, involving the adolescent in a process of self-reflection and self-understanding.[24] This process defines an adolescent's future values, beliefs, and perceptions of himself or herself as a self-determining and valued member of society. It is an egocentric process of being self-absorbed and preoccupied with oneself, one's body and appearance, one's interests, and one's friends. An interest in family activities lessens and the importance of peer relationships increases.[44] It is the beginning of emotional separation and independence from parents.

Psychosocial development has three characteristic phases. Table 8-1 outlines common behaviors in each of these phases. Phase 1, early adolescence, occurs during the middle school years between the ages of 10 and 13. Phase 2, middle adolescence, occurs during the high school years between the ages of 14 and 17. Phase 3, late adolescence, between the ages of 17 and 21, typically the first years of work or college.[2,44] The middle years of adolescence constitute the most intense period of psychosocial development. In this phase, peers replace parents as the primary influence in the adolescent's life. Conformity with peer groups is desirable, and the opinions of friends and peers matter the most.

Late adolescence is a period of consolidation. By this last phase, adolescents are ideally developing into responsible young adults who are able to make decisions, have a stable and consistent value system, and can successfully take on adult roles such as a worker and a contributing member of the community. A stable, positive sense of self and awareness of their own abilities enable late adolescents and young adults to establish healthy relationships.

However, difficulties or failure to navigate the psychological and social developmental tasks of adolescence

TABLE 8-1

Summary of the Typical Characteristics of Psychosocial Development

PHASE	CHARACTERISTICS
Early adolescence	Engrossed with self (e.g., interested in personal appearance) Separate from parents emotionally (e.g., reduce participation in family activities); teens display less overt affection to parents Decrease in compliance with parents' rules or limits as well as challenge other authority figures (e.g., teachers, coaches) Questioning of adults' opinions (e.g., critical of and challenge their parents' opinions, advice, and expectations); begin to see parents as having faults Have changeable moods and behavior Mostly have same-sex friendships, with strong feelings toward these peers Demonstrate abstract thinking Idealistic fantasizing about careers; think about possible future self and role(s) Privacy is important (e.g., they have own bedroom with door closed, writing diaries, private telephone conversations) Interested in experiences related to personal sexual development and explore sexual feelings (e.g., masturbation) Self-conscious, displays modesty, blushing, awkwardness about self and body Ability to self-regulate emotional expression and behavior is limited (e.g., do not think beyond immediate wants or needs and are therefore susceptible to peer pressure) Experiment with drugs (cigarettes, alcohol, and marijuana)
Middle adolescence	Continue to move toward psychological and social independence from parents Increase involvement in peer group culture, displayed in adopting peer value system, codes of behavior, style of dress, and appearance, which demonstrates in an overt way individualism and separation from family Involvement in formal and informal peer group activities such as sports teams, clubs, and gangs Acceptance of developing body and sexual expression and experimentation (e.g., dating, sexual activity with partner) Explore and reflect on the expressions of their feelings and those of other people Increase their realism in career/vocational aspirations Increased creative and intellectual ability as well as interest in intellectual activities and capacity to do work (e.g., mentally and emotionally) Underscoring the risk-taking behaviors are feelings of omnipotence (sense of being powerful) and immortality; risky behaviors include reckless driving, unprotected sex, high alcohol consumption, and drug use Experiment with drugs (cigarettes, alcohol, marijuana, and other illicit drugs)
Late adolescence	Sense of who they are becomes more stable (e.g., interests and consistency in opinions, values, and beliefs) Strengthen relationships with parents (e.g., parental advice and assistance valued) Increase their independence in decision making and ability to express ideas and opinions Have increased interest in the future and consider the consequences of current actions and decisions regarding the future; this behavior leads to delayed gratification, setting personal limits, ability to monitor own behavior, and reach compromises Earlier angst with puberty, physical appearance, and attractiveness largely resolved Peer influence diminished, with increased confidence in personal values and sense of self Show a preference for one-to-one relationships and start to select an intimate partner Become realistic in vocational choice or employment, establishing worker role and financial independence Value system (e.g., regarding morality, belief, religious affiliation, and sexuality) defined and increasingly stable

Data from Radizik M, Sherer S, Neinstein LS: Psychosocial development in normal adolescent. In Neinstein LS, editor: *Adolescent health care: a practical guide*, ed 4, Philadelphia, 2002, Lippincott, Williams & Wilkins; American Academy of Child and Adolescent Psychiatry website: http://www.aacap.org/publications. Retrieved 9/7/2004.

can have adverse and far-reaching health and social outcomes. In addition to mental and behavioral problems that are associated with adolescence, such as eating disorders, dropping out of school, suicide, depression, and substance abuse (e.g., drug, solvent, and alcohol abuse), and behavioral problems such as oppositional defiance disorder, there are lifelong health and social consequences. Effective interventions are vital at this developmental stage.

Identity Formation: "Who Am I?"

Identity formation is a lifelong process. From birth, a child works toward achieving a sense of himself or herself as a separate entity. Throughout life, a person's sense of self continues to evolve. However, adolescent psychosocial development is about the quest to define this self-identity.[12] Self-identity has two elements, an individualistic component (*"Who am I?"*) and a contextual component (*"Where and how do I fit in my world?"*), which is concerned with a broad understanding of one's relationship to the world.[30] A person experiences his or her sense of identity as a solid, core feeling from which s/he can interact with the world.[34] To other people, a person's identity appears as his or her values, beliefs, interests, and commitments to a job and career as well as a social role such as daughter or parent.[34]

Erik Erikson was the first developmental theorist to propose the process of acquiring a sense of identity (identity formation) as a central task of adolescent psychosocial development. His perspective on adolescent identity formation as a process of crisis resolution (i.e., a period of exploration and experimentation) and a process of commitment (i.e., an invested set of values, beliefs, interests, and occupations) has continued to dictate how identity formation is viewed in current research and clinical practice. This view of identity is that of a complex process comprising spiritual and religious beliefs; intellectual, social, and political interests; and a vocational or career path that provides a work identity. It includes relationships and gender orientation (i.e., awareness and acceptance of one's female or male identity, not just one's biological sex), culture and ethnicity, and perceptions of one's personality traits (e.g., introverted, extroverted, open, conscientious).

Daydreams and fantasies about real and imagined selves energize and motivate adolescents. In the process of developing an identity, adolescents actively attempt to try to make sense of their world and find meaning in what happens to them. To achieve this they explore different roles, express a variety of opinions and preferences, make choices, and interpret their experiences. They try different activities and lifestyles before settling on any particular viewpoint, set of values, or life goals. This process involves adolescents in self-reflection and introspection (internalized thinking about the self and making social comparisons between themselves and peers as well as evaluating how they are possibly viewed by family, friends, etc.). They set goals, take action, and resolve conflicts and problems.[30] All of these behaviors help teens identify what makes them an individual (Figure 8-1).

Adolescents' behaviors, thoughts, and emotions can seem contradictory, typically between the ages of 13 and 15. For example, a teen might have body piercing, regu-

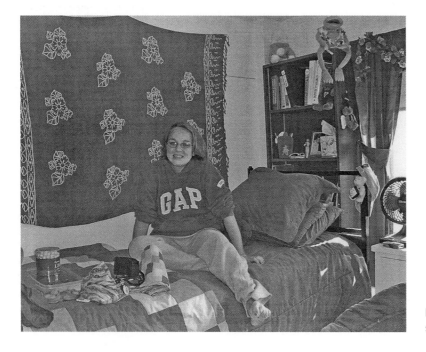

FIGURE 8-1 A teenager's use of personal space reflects her evolving identity.

larly break parental rules, and attend school erratically while at the same time responsibly hold a job, dress appropriately for the work setting, and be a reliable employee. Similarly, adolescents will choose healthy behaviors such as being vegetarians or participating in sports but will also experiment with alcohol, tobacco, and other unhealthy substances. They will explore different belief systems, argue passionately against their parent's political views, or express disinterest in relationships with the opposite sex but the following day hang out exclusively with a girlfriend or boyfriend. As a teen was heard to retort to a parent's comment, "I don't have to be responsible, I am an adolescent." Society has permissive tolerance toward adolescents that permits this period of experimentation and exploration. The expected outcome is one in which young adults have defined themselves as individuals and whose thinking, emotions, and behaviors are congruent with each other and with the social norms and values of their community.

Some developmental theorists claim that describing identity as a series of states implies that there is an end state of identity formation rather than a complex and ongoing process of negotiation, adaptation, and decision making. However, the descriptive identity states proposed by the developmental theorist Marcia are commonly used and helpful in explaining the characteristics of an adolescent's identity development.[34] Identifying this state of developmental identity is of assistance in the planning of OT interventions that are appropriate to psychosocial needs and will further encourage exploration and resolution of identity issues.

Marcia[34] suggested that adolescents experience states of identity diffusion and moratorium or prematurely enter a state of identity foreclosure. Successfully working through a process of identity formation leads to a state of identity achievement.

Identity diffusion, common in early adolescence, is the least defined sense of personal identity. Adolescents have little or no interest in exploring their options. They have not made any commitments to choices, interests, or values. The question "who am I" is not a significant issue in this state of identity formation. Those who continue to experience identity diffusion well into their middle and late adolescent years have difficulty meeting the psychosocial demands of adolescent development. They may demonstrate impulsivity, disorganized thinking, and immature moral reasoning.[12] Identity diffusion is associated with lower self-esteem, a negative attitude, and dissatisfaction with one's life, parents' lifestyle, and school.[12] In a state of identity diffusion, adolescents seldom anticipate and think about their future. They are observed to have difficulties meeting the day-to-day demands of life such as completing schoolwork and participating in sports or extracurricular activities.[6] Because they have not explored their interests or considered their strengths in relation to work, they sometimes have problems finding employment.

Moratorium, common in early and middle adolescence, is the active state of exploring and developing an identity. The difference between moratorium and diffusion is that in a state of identity diffusion the adolescent avoids or ignores the task of exploring his or her identity, whereas in a state of moratorium finding an identity is a project that s/he vigorously pursues. It is a time of openly exploring alternatives, striving for autonomy and a sense of individuality. A late-stage adolescent experiencing a state of identity moratorium is likely to still be undecided about his or her major course of study and plans. The uncertainty of the moratorium status, especially a prolonged moratorium, can increase anxiety, self-consciousness, impulsiveness, and depression.[12]

Some adolescents avoid experiencing an identity crisis and do not engage in the process of self-exploration and experimentation. This state is described as foreclosure and involves premature decision making and commitment to identity. Adolescents demonstrating identity foreclosure commonly accept their parents' values and beliefs and follow family expectations regarding career choices without considering other possibilities. Foreclosing prematurely on identity is associated with approval-seeking behaviors and a high respect for authority. Such adolescents are more conforming and less autonomous than their peers and prefer a structured environment.[12] These adolescents are less self-reflective, less intimate in personal relationships, and less open to new experiences than their peers.[12] However, foreclosure makes them less anxious than many of their peers, who struggle with developing their identities over the period of adolescence.

Identity achievement, common for adolescents in their final years of high school or in college or those in the work force, represents healthy psychosocial development. Adolescents who have resolved their identity issues are able to change and adapt in response to personal and social demands and do so without undue anxiety. A relatively stable sense of self as a competent individual gives the adolescent self-esteem and confidence in his or her abilities.

Identity achievement typically follows a state of moratorium. It is a commitment to the interests, values, gender orientation, political views, career or job, and moral stance that have been reached after exploring the possibilities. Adolescents and young adults who reach identity achievement are more autonomous and independent. They are also less self-absorbed and self-conscious and are less vulnerable to peer pressure than those who have not reached this state. They are open and creative in their thinking.[12] In addition, a sense of identity gives a person a greater capacity for intimacy, self-regulation, and mature moral reasoning. Identity achievement results in congruency between a person's identity and his or her self-expression and behaviors[45] (Box 8-4).

Adolescents who are unable to develop a stable and distinct sense of self as a competent self-directed individual have difficulties. In late adolescence, the inability to achieve one's identity is associated with a lack of self-confidence and lower self-esteem. As adults they have problems with work and establishing and maintaining intimate relationships and are challenged by the countless other responsibilities of adult life, such as parenting and being a contributing member of the community.

Promoting psychosocial development is implicit in adolescent OT services. A person's roles have behavioral expectations and are closely associated with identity and social status. For example, being an OT assistant is associated with your occupational identity, and other people attribute certain qualities to you because you work in a health care profession. They expect you to behave in a particular way, such as being patient and caring. Adolescents who require OT services often lack access to roles and activities that have social status or promote self-esteem. They may also have roles that are not viewed positively or as being socially desirable. One example is the role defined by the term *disabled* or *special needs*. Therefore, within the structure of therapy, COTAs can have a significant influence in helping adolescents define and shape their beliefs and self-perceptions.

BOX 8-4

Behavioral Indicators of Self-Esteem

Positive Self-Esteem
- Expresses opinions
- Mixes with other teens (e.g., interacts with social group of teens)
- Initiates friendly interactions with others
- Makes eye contact easily when speaking
- Faces others when speaking with them
- Observes comfortable, socially determined space between self and others
- Speaks fluently in first language without pauses or visible discomfort
- Participates in group activities
- Works collaboratively with others
- Will give directions or instructions to others
- Will volunteer for tasks and activities

Negative Self-Esteem
- Avoids eye contact
- Overly confident, for example, brags about achievements or skills
- Verbally self-critical, makes self-deprecating comments; makes fun of self as a form of humor
- Speaks loudly or dogmatically to avoid response of others
- Submissive, overly agreeable to others' requests or demands
- Reluctant to give opinions or views, especially if it will draw attention to himself or herself
- Monitoring behaviors, for example, hypervigilant of surroundings and other people
- Makes excuses for performance, seldom evaluates personal performance as satisfactory
- Engages in putting others down, name calling, gossiping, and at worst bullying

Adapted from Santrock JW: *Adolescence*, New York, 2003, McGraw-Hill.

As OT practitioners, we can observe adolescents' identity exploration in the activities they choose as well as the roles they have and express a desire to have in the future. As they perform in their roles, a COTA gains information about how teens see themselves in the present and the future. The COTA's task in promoting psychosocial development is to offer within therapy a broad range of activities and experiences that will assist in the development of skills leading to successful performance in the adolescent's chosen activities and roles and will offer a social environment in which self-identity can be explored. Choice, variety, and opportunities for self-directed exploration through participation in age-related activities develop identity. OT sessions are facilitating self-identity as they develop and explore work and leisure activities or promote the acquisition of social and life skills. OT services focus on facilitating an adolescent's independence in activities of daily living (ADLs) and instrumental activities of daily living (IADLs). For the adolescent this also promotes a sense of independence, which is an important aspect of psychosocial development. However, his or her identity as an autonomous, self-determining person does not always require actual physical independence. Autonomy may take many forms, such as an adolescent with a physical disability assuming responsibility for instructing his or her own attendant caregiver or determining the pattern and organization of his or her own daily routine. Independence is an individual interpretation, a personal perception of autonomy.

OCCUPATIONAL PERFORMANCE IN ADOLESCENCE

The Occupational Therapy Practice Framework identifies ADLs, IADLs, education, work, leisure, and social participation as the performance areas of occupation.[1] Here we focus on three areas—work, leisure, and social participation—which are particularly significant in healthy adolescent development. These areas of occupation offer opportunities for learning new skills, promoting self-expression, and contributing to identity development. For example, adolescents are likely to take on the values associated with the type of work and leisure and social activities in which they participate.[17] Through their participation in meaningful occupations, adolescents explore activities that reflect their curiosity, values, interests, and needs. Competence in occupational performance, especially in social, sports, work, and academic activities, plays a significant role in the process by providing peer acceptance, social status, and enhancement of self-esteem.

Work

Work includes paid employment and volunteer activities. Paid employment is the norm for American adolescents over the age of 16. Studies examining work patterns of American teenagers report that approximately 70% of them work while in school.[4] In addition to paid employment, the 2000 edition of *America's Children: Key National Indicators of Well-Being* reported that 55% of high school students also participated in volunteer activities.

In addition to their academic experiences, work contributes to an adolescent's interests and values.[29] In the work setting adolescents interact with adults on a more equal level, have opportunities to assume responsibilities, learn work behaviors and values, and develop knowledge of possible preferences for adult occupations. Working also develops life and social skills such as managing money, organizing time, developing a routine, working collaboratively with other people, and communicating with social groups outside family and school. The disposable income earned gives adolescents discretionary spending and a sense of economic independence. However, other adolescents assume responsibility for helping to support their families.

OT programs for adolescents typically focus on strategies such as the acquisition of work skills to assist them in the transition from school to work. However, work skills and behaviors represent only one aspect of the transition from school. Another significant aspect of identity development involves acquiring an occupational identity. This involves combining interests, values, and abilities in the pursuit of a realistic choice of a job or career path. In the successful transition to work, a choice of occupation that integrates personal identity is as important as matching one's skills and job requirements. Therefore, OT programs that address the transition to work need to start early in adolescence with developing an occupational identity in conjunction with specific skill-based training.

Occupational identity begins in early adolescence. With the development of abstract thinking and the capacity to think about the future, adolescents start to fantasize about their future occupations. These daydreams are initially idealistic and combine aspirations and dreams about the possible adult self. By middle adolescence these job/vocational idealizations become more realistic, and by late adolescence there is a realism based on interests, values, and the match between one's performance abilities and actual job demands. When adolescents attend tertiary colleges and universities, the transition to work is delayed and occupational identity deferred. Work is the end product of an adolescent's life coming together.[22] When it happens, full-time work is a societal indicator of adulthood. The student role of the child and adolescent is replaced by the worker role, along with financial independence.

Leisure and Play

Similar to work and education, **leisure** is an area of occupational performance in which adolescents can explore and try out new behaviors and roles, establish likes and dislikes, socialize, and express themselves within the peer group. American adolescents spend more than half of their waking hours in free time and leisure activities, and how they use this time is important to their development.[31] In an OT study exploring how teens view leisure, they stated that for them leisure represented enjoyment, freedom of choice, and "time out."[44] Leisure (i.e., discretionary) activities give adolescents opportunities to assess their strengths, values, interests, and positions in the social context in a way that is different from their experiences in the more structured school and work setting.[52]

Some leisure activities provide constructive use of time spent out of school. Participation in organized leisure activities (e.g., extracurricular activities) promotes the development of physical, intellectual, and social skills.[18] Structured leisure activities that are part of extracurricular school programs (e.g., sports teams, school band or orchestra, drama club, and cheerleading) or community-based activities such as scouts, music, and dance classes involve challenge and are goal directed but are also fun. They offer choices that promote healthy development and the acquisition of skills that encourage higher academic performance and occupational achievement.[7] Additional positive benefits include an increased likelihood of attending college (e.g., lower-achieving and lower socioeconomic male students who play sports are more likely to finish high school), better interpersonal skills, and greater community involvement as well as lower alcohol and drug use and antisocial behavior.[18,23,35]

Physical leisure activities have additional lifestyle advantages, as patterns of activity in adolescence are predictive of adult physical activity levels.[50] Furthermore, the increase in obesity and chronic health conditions among American adolescents and young adults has made the patterns and levels of physical activity in adolescence

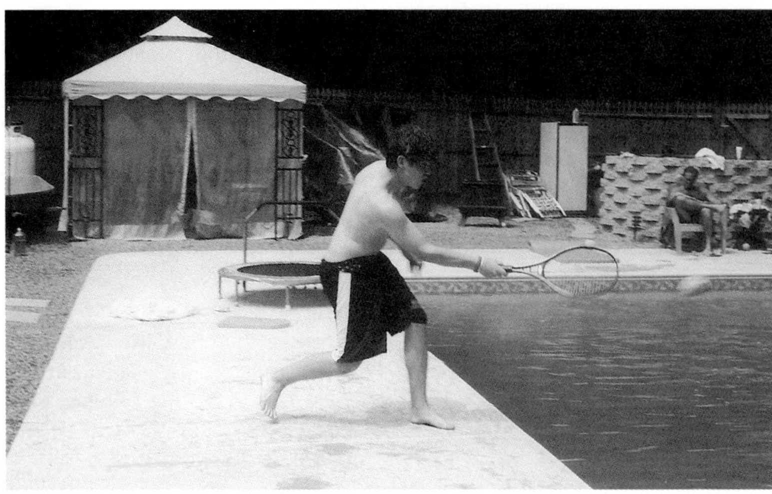

FIGURE 8-2 Teenagers participating in physical activity with their friends. (Courtesy Chloe Troia.)

increasingly important.[27] Many high school, college, and community programs promote participation in physical activity during the adolescent years as a public health objective. However, there is an overall decline in this participation, including sports activities, during adolescence. While studies have identified that many factors (parents, teachers [school], peers) influence an adolescent's physical activity level, one of the strongest influences is that of his or her friends.[50] Adolescent boys are more likely to participate in and have a positive attitude toward physical activities than girls because of the relationship between masculine identities and sports activities, competition, and achievement (Figure 8-2).[50]

Adolescents spend much of their unstructured time watching television and playing computer games. These passive and less social leisure activities do not have the same positive benefits, and poor choices of leisure activities can have adverse consequences. The main criticism of passive activities is that they contribute to boredom, which is associated with a greater risk of dropping out of school, drug use, and antisocial/delinquent activities.[51]

Leisure activities represent a valuable therapeutic area of OT practice in which occupational performance skills can be developed. In developing leisure and related skills such as those determining social behavior, therapy may enable adolescents to be more successful in extracurricular activities and participate in the social peer group activities in their schools and communities. As previously mentioned, it is developmentally beneficial that adolescents join extracurricular activities. Choosing activities in therapy sessions that are popular and will transfer easily beyond the context of therapy builds self-efficacy and autonomy. A long-term goal of therapy is to always facilitate a positive life trajectory by improving performance and preparing teens to assume roles in the school, community, and family contexts.

Social Participation

Social participation, defined as the patterns of behavior and activities expected of an individual, is a significant area of occupational performance. In adolescence, social roles and relationships are explored and developed by engaging in a spectrum of social activities.[42] Peer-focused social interactions and relationships formed in school and leisure activities provide social status and develop adolescents' social identity separate from that associated with their families. This change represents moving from family members as the primary source of support to a reliance on friends, peers, and adults who are not family members for emotional and social support.[5,11]

Social integration (i.e., a sense of belonging, acceptance, and having friends) plays a significant role in adolescent development and emotional adjustment.[53,54] Common in adolescence are cliques, which are small, cohesive groups of teens that have a somewhat flexible membership, meet personal needs, and share activities and communication. Participation in cliques provides a normative reference for comparison with peers and significantly influences adolescents' developing social attitudes and behaviors as well as academic adjustment.[5] The transition from junior high to high school can be made easier by membership in supportive and peer-recognized cliques. Initially in early and middle adolescence, the membership of cliques develops spontaneously around common interests, school activities, even neighborhood affiliations. These groups offer a broad range of activities and enjoyment. In junior high the cliques are usually constituted of the same sex, but by middle to late adolescence these groups expand to include the opposite sex. In late adolescence the clique weakens and is replaced by loose associations among couples.[11] The lack of participation in peer groups and social exclusion from

BOX 8-5

Quick Facts: Health of American Teenagers

- Between 16% and 22% of American adolescents are obese or overweight.
- Approximately 50% of high school students are sexually active; by graduation, two thirds of them will have had sex.
- The teenage pregnancy rate is dropping. Between 1991 and 1998 the birth age for teens 15 to 19 years of age declined by 18%.
- The three leading causes of death among American teens aged 15 to 19 are (1) accidents, (2) homicide, and (3) suicide.
- 25% of female and 15% of male high school students stated that they had attempted or seriously considered suicide.
- Typically, the initial drug use for girls is cigarettes and for boys alcohol. It is not restricted to urban areas. Rural teens have equal access. American adolescents reporting daily cigarette use for the past 30 days were 4.5 % of 8th graders, 8.9 % of 10th graders, and 15.8% of 12th graders. This represents a decrease compared with levels reported in previous Monitoring the Future Study (MFS) surveys.
- The percentage of 8th and 10th graders reporting the use of illicit drugs declined in 2003 to the lowest level since 1993 and 1997. 48.8% of high school seniors reported past or current use of marijuana. The use of ecstasy is more prevalent than cocaine. Other illicit drugs that have increased in use by teenagers are anabolic steroids and heroin. In 2003, seniors reported that Vicodin was the second most common drug used after marijuana (MFS survey).
- Alcohol is the most widely used substance by adolescents: 18.6% of 8th graders, 35.2% of 10th graders, and 48% of 12th graders drank alcohol in the previous month (MFS, 2000).

Compiled from *Monitoring the Future Study (2001-2004)*, a continuing study of American youth, http://www.nida.nih.gov/Infofacts/HSYouthtrens. html; Neinstein LS: *Adolescent healthcare: a practical guide*, ed 4, Philadelphia, 2002, Lippincott, Williams & Wilkins; *Profile of American's youth*, http://www.acf.hhs.gov/fysb/youthinfo/profile.html. Retrieved January 2005.

cliques come with a cost. There is a sense of rejection, a lack of opportunity to participate in activities, social isolation, and a lack of social status. An adolescent who does not find his or her niche in a clique is more likely to be depressed and lonely and have psychological problems.[11] Exclusion from cliques and the resulting lack of choices are suggested as possible reasons for joining less constructive peer groups such as gangs or those groups who engage in illegal and/or antisocial activities (Box 8-5).

Friendships, which are different from peer groups or clique relationships, are also important in adolescent development. They are more emotionally intense, involve openness and honesty, and are less concerned with social acceptance.[12] Adolescent girls generally have more friends than boys. Their friendships are interdependent and reflect a preference for intimacy, whereas boys' friendships are congenial relationships established around shared interests such as sports, music, or other common activities.

Teens' friendships evolve over time and reflect their cognitive and psychosocial development.[11] Initially, adolescent friendships are between individuals of the same sex that develop around sharing activities and possessions and a closeness of mutual understanding. In middle adolescence, friendships are based around shared loyalty and an exchange of ideas. During these years, there are an emotional intensity and shared confidence that heighten the vulnerability associated with friendships.[12] However, by the latter years of adolescence the nature of friendships evolves to incorporate elements of both autonomy and interdependence, so the dependence on friends and sharing of all activities are no longer essential features of the relationships. Furthermore, the development of meaningful, intimate relationships in late adolescence shifts the primary focus away from friendships (Figure 8-3).

The social participation and closeness achieved in adolescent friendships provide intimacy and social and emotional adjustments that contribute to interpersonal skills and self-knowledge. Adolescents talk to their friends and share concerns and fears, especially as the emotional separation from parents creates a time when they are apt to claim that "parents don't understand." Friendships facilitate the development of self-identity; consequently, adolescents who have close friendships have better self-esteem and social skills than peers who lack them. Furthermore, having friends is associated with less anxiety and depression in adolescence.[12]

Although we talk at length about peer relationships being a central feature of an adolescent's life, the stability and security provided by parents and/or significant adults are essential to navigating this transition from childhood to adulthood. There is physical and emotional separation from parents as well as questioning the parents' values and beliefs, but contrary to popular opinion, major conflicts between parents and adolescents are not a normal part of the adolescent-parent relationship.[32] Those conflicts that do exist are more common in early adolescence and decrease with age. In addition to the relationship with parents, relationships with adults who are not family members are required for healthy adolescent development. Involvement in nonacademic extracurricular and leisure activities is consistently linked with positive, healthy adolescent development. These structured out-

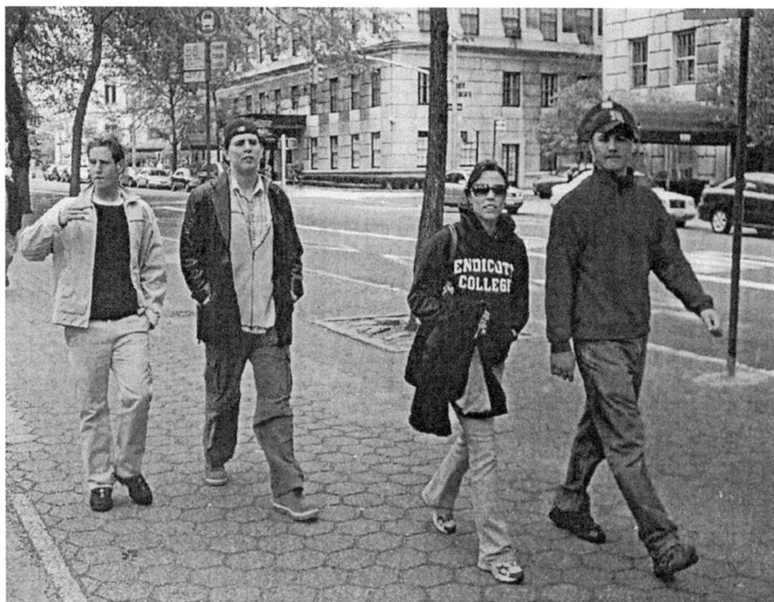

FIGURE 8-3 Taking the city by storm! Teens enjoy spending time together.

of-school activities provide the venue for relationships with nonfamilial adults. Positive experiences with coaches, adult leaders, and teachers who give attention to adolescents in these activities facilitate problem solving, provide social support, increase self-esteem, and promote skill acquisition and competency.[18]

CONTEXT OF ADOLESCENT DEVELOPMENT

Salient contexts are those aspects of the environment that influence an adolescent's occupational performance, such as the social contexts of friends, team members, other students, parents, siblings, extended family, coaches, and teachers. The relationship between adolescents and their environment is reciprocal; it has an impact on what they do and how they do it.[28] The physical context, such as the adolescent's school and community, provides opportunities and resources, imposes expectations, and creates barriers. Both the social and physical contexts of the adolescent are shaped by the culture.[28] Culture represents the beliefs, perceptions, values, and norms of the group and society that an adolescent belongs to, such as the family's ethnic group as well as the prevailing American culture. An important aspect of context is that society ascribes socially constructed characteristics to roles. These characteristics are universally understood within a particular cohort (i.e., a group of people with similar attributes, such as age and cultural affiliation) and place demands and constraints on those individuals who have these roles. For example, adolescent roles such as hockey player, cheerleader, geek, nerd, and jock each have a set of common behaviors and expectations as well as either a positive or negative status.

Understanding an adolescent's social and cultural contexts is vital for practitioners who work with the diverse population of American teens. [47] The culturally competent practitioner working in diverse cultural settings needs to be cognizant of the norms and expectations of the ethnic and sociocultural backgrounds that shape adolescents' self-perceptions and the development of a constructive self-esteem.[48] These factors will influence their choices of activities and interests, the expectations of their family, and the values they develop. Likewise, the adolescent's social peer context will shape "adaptive social and emotional development."[5]

It cannot be assumed that all adolescent activities have the same influence. Context determines the importance and value of particular adolescent activities.[23] For example, successful participation in school sports activities in poorer communities is linked to the status of a "good student," whereas in higher socioeconomic communities, where academic achievement is valued highly, other types of extracurricular activities are associated with the good student and are positively reinforced.[23]

Context can have adverse consequences on an adolescent's development. Low socioeconomic status and family disorganization increase the likelihood that a child or adolescent will exhibit deviant and high-risk behaviors leading to adverse outcomes.[36] This is because these environments limit adolescents' (often from minorities) access to information and resources and opportunities to develop self-esteem, personal mastery, and complex cognitive development.[36] Therefore, experiences in school, therapy, and extracurricular activities have an increased role in meeting their needs and ameliorating the effects of their social and home environments.

TABLE 8-2

Contextual Factors That Contribute to Healthy Adolescent Development

CONTEXTUAL FACTOR	CHARACTERISTICS
Support	Family support including positive parent-adolescent communication Parental involvement in school activities and schoolwork Constructive relationships with other adults Caring neighborhood and school environment
Empowerment	Community values the youth Adolescents are given useful and valued roles in the community Community involves adolescents in community service activities and values their contributions Safe home and community environments
Boundaries and expectations of adolescents	Family boundaries that include rules and consequences School and neighborhood boundaries that include rules, consequences, and community monitoring of behavior Adult role models Positive peer influences High expectations—family, friends, and school expect adolescent to do well

From the Search Institute, 2004, http://www.search-institute.org.

The complex influence of context is a factor in any intervention program for teens. All of its aspects should be considered in planning and implementing therapy. Using a context that facilitates development, such as peer partnerships, participation in extracurricular activities, and mentoring by caring adults, promotes healthy adolescent development and discourages the self-limiting effect of involvement in unhealthy groups. For example, the context of client-centered therapy facilitates development by providing choices, opportunities for decision making, and autonomy, which in turn provide a sense of personal control. Similarly, a therapeutic milieu offers the adolescent opportunities for self-directed exploration in a safe, stable, supportive environment and provides acceptance and positive regard. Table 8-2 lists some of the contextual characteristics that support and foster adolescent self-development and acquisition of skills.

NAVIGATING ADOLESCENCE WITH A DISABILITY

It is estimated that between 23% and 35% of American adolescents have chronic health conditions or special health care needs.[19,39] These adolescents experience the same development as others, but because of their special needs or dependence on parents they have fewer opportunities to develop a sense of their own abilities. The successful transition from school to work is similar to the transition of non-disabled adolescents. Adolescents with disabilities experience and resolve the psychosocial issues of adjusting to the physical changes of puberty, psychological independence from parents or caregivers, social relationships with the same and opposite sexes, and the process of establishing a sense of identity. Undertaking these developmental tasks is the prerequisite of choosing a job, being out of school, and working.[14,22] Parents who have been the primary support and caregivers for their adolescents and in particular had to advocate vigorously for their needs when they were children can be challenged by the task of "letting go" so that the adolescent can develop and become an autonomous individual.

Adolescents with disabilities have fewer opportunities to engage in typical adolescent experiences, make their own choices, engage in social relationships, and/or explore the world of ideas, values, and cultures different from those of their families.[8,49] Exploration and experimentation are needed to provide these teens with experiences of success and failure, both of which are required if they are to develop a sense of the boundaries of their competence.[54] Adolescents with disabilities face additional challenges, including their negative self-perceptions and lower expectations of themselves. They also face barriers such as a lack of resources, problems related to mobility and environmental access, discrimination, and the stigma of disability (Figure 8-4).[16]

Adolescents with physical disabilities report experiencing more loneliness and feeling more isolated than their non-disabled peers, and even those teens who have good social relationships in school have less contact with friends outside the school setting than their non-disabled peers.[20] They have difficulty with inclusion in peer and structured extracurricular activities and struggle with social acceptance from peers in and out of the school setting.[16,49] Factors affecting the social acceptance of teens with physical disabilities include role marginalization (where they are perceived as lacking a clear role and unable to undertake the tasks of many typical life roles), lower social achievement, and limited contact with peers.[37] The limited peer interaction is due not only to a lack of opportunity but also because they do not have the skills necessary to engage in typical adolescent activities. For example, in early and middle adolescence, play and

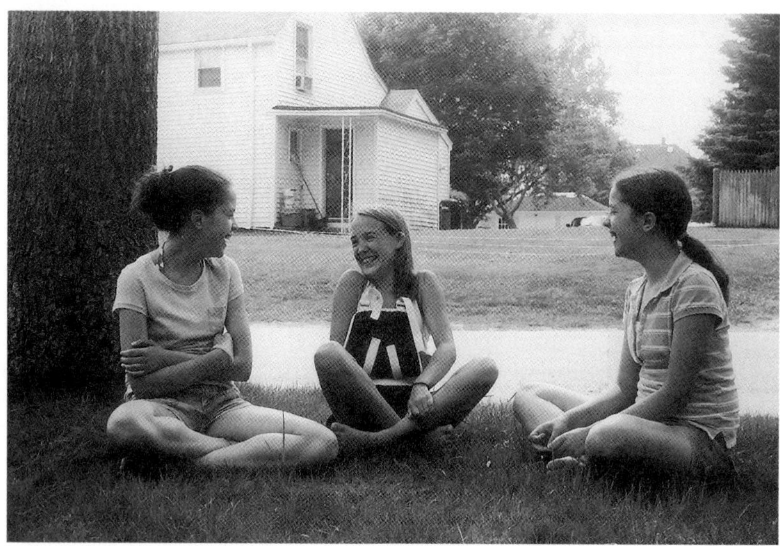

FIGURE 8-4 Adolescents with special needs value "hanging out" with friends. (Courtesy Chloe Troia.)

leisure activities are often physical and consequently exclude adolescents with disabilities.[3] In addition, non-disabled adolescents consider their peers with physical disabilities as less socially attractive and report that they are less likely to interact with them socially.[20] However, academic achievement can promote better social acceptance for adolescents with disabilities.[37]

How teens with disabilities view themselves also creates barriers to their social acceptance and integration. Doubt and McColl[16] shared this account of one student's attempt to be included.

> I approached the [hockey team] about being a statistician because I really wanted to get involved in the team. This is probably the closest without playing...that I could.... plus I'm doing work for them too, so I am useful and that's a good way to get involved...and it really gives me a chance to be one of the guys finally. A secondary guy but one of the guys nonetheless (p. 149).

Adolescents strive for conformity and to identify with their peers. Yet for a teen with a disability this is extremely difficult because social status among adolescents is often attributed to areas such as excelling in sports. Similarly, body image includes comparison with an ideal that is unrealistic for many adolescents, but it is particularly challenging for those with obvious physical disabilities. To "fit in" with non-disabled teens, adolescents with disabilities will attempt to mask their disabilities or make fun of them or use self-exclusion. These strategies are often aimed at making non-disabled peers more comfortable with disability.

Adolescents with physical disabilities struggle with the paradox of striving to achieve the typical adolescent emotional and psychological independence and an identity as an autonomous individual while remaining physically dependent on their parents or caregivers. In contrast, at-risk teens and/or those with emotional disturbances can have pseudoindependence (i.e., a false sense of independence). Because of their difficult personal, social, and economic circumstances, these adolescents find themselves prematurely independent of a stable care-giving environment, although developmentally they still need the support and nurturing of a home and parents. These adolescents struggle with the normal developmental processes while dealing with issues such as violence, poverty, school failure, and discrimination.[53]

OCCUPATIONAL THERAPY PRACTITIONER'S ROLE AND RESPONSIBILITIES

Working with adolescents is both rewarding and frustrating. Flexibility, a sense of humor, and the capacity to first see adolescents' strengths before identifying their weaknesses are assets for COTAs who choose to work with them. Equally important is a COTA's ability to integrate the adolescent's developmental needs into the therapy process and interventions. This requires a comprehensive understanding of the biological factors and cognitive, psychological and social development as well as the influence of the social context (school, family, friends) in adolescence. When working in health care and education it is easy to develop a distorted view of adolescents, since many of them who receive services have difficulties such as substance abuse, mental health disorders, academic difficulties, delinquency, and truancy. However, we need to be aware that most teens successfully navigate adolescence.[46]

Tom is a 15-year-old African-American youth with Down syndrome. Psychological test scores achieved by Tom place him in the mildly retarded group under the guidelines of the fourth edition of the Diagnostic and Statistical Manual (DSM-IV). Until high school, Tom participated well in mainstream school activities, with some accommodations. As the cognitive demands of education have increased during high school, he spends most of his day in a special class setting. The prioritized goals of Tom's recent Individualized Educational Program (IEP) facilitate his transition from high school to the community and work.

Adolescents with special needs such as Tom require significant assistance to achieve developmental milestones such as independence, understanding the physical changes they are experiencing, forming friendships, and the transition from an educational setting to the community and a work environment. The Individuals with Disabilities Education Act (IDEA) of 1997 recognized the need to facilitate the transition from high school for students like Tom when it introduced an amendment requiring the Individualized Transition Plan (ITP) for adolescents with special needs from the age of 14 years.

The COTA's work involves helping students such as Tom learn the life and social skills required for independence in the community. In working with adolescents with cognitive impairments, the COTA needs to understand the functional level and types of difficulty for each person and how these disabilities affect the ability to do everyday skills. For example, in Tom's case his cognition influences how he understands information and is able to learn, how much information he can handle at one time, and the complexity of instructions he can follow. An adolescent's cognitive ability determines how well s/he will remember and recall information, and it will determine the strategies the COTA might use for teaching new skills. The challenge for the COTA is to optimize each adolescent's ability to function within the constraints of his or her disability. Therefore, the skilled practitioner develops expectations that include just the "right" amount of challenge. With tasks targeted appropriately to an adolescent's level, it is also essential to modify the demands of the environment to help him or her function effectively. An example would be providing a visual list of the sequence of activities to ensure safety in the kitchen or improving accessibility to assist with mobility.

The role of the OT practitioner in the school system is often one of consultation or periodic review and monitoring. The transition from high school is an opportune time to advocate OT reassessment and collaborative interdisciplinary program planning in life and prevocational skills. OT practitioners must work collaboratively with students, their families, and teachers to establish each student's strengths and weaknesses so that they can assist them with the development of the basic lifeskills and emotional resources that they will need in the future.

All adolescents with special needs are eligible for OT services.

- Under the 1975 Public Law 94-142, Education of All Handicapped Children's Act, OT practitioners may evaluate, treat, and recommend services for children and adolescents from the ages of 3 to 21.
- In 1997 Public Law 105-17, Individuals with Disabilities Education Act, required that the ITP be included in the IEP of every adolescent, with special education before the student reaches age 14.
- By age 16 a statement of the needed transition services as well as goals, objectives, and activities should be included in a student's IEP.
- An amendment to the IDEA (PL105-17) expanded the scope of alternative education programs from only at-risk students to include all those with disabilities and behaviors that need to be addressed outside the mainstream educational system.

Mainstream and alternative high schools have identified the areas of need for OT as transition from school to work and services for adolescents with cognitive deficits; sensory impairments; and physical, communicative, and behavioral disabilities.[15,49] Students with special needs and those attending alternative schools show decreased participation in leisure activities and hobbies, poor time management, and poor coping skills such as self-regulation of anger

CLINICAL *Pearl*

Adolescents with disabilities have the challenge of achieving a sense of identity that constructively integrates their differences into a coherent and healthy self-concept. Referring to adolescents with special needs as "disabled teens" or using similar labels is not acceptable in the client-centered context of OT. Self-conscious and acutely aware of themselves, adolescents want to be "like everyone else," namely other teenagers in their social group. This social acceptance is highly valued. The OT practitioner's role is to actively assist adolescents with disabilities in developing an identity that does not make their disabilities the central or defining characteristic of their identities. For example, labeling Jane "the cerebral palsy student" or Doug "disruptive" encourages adolescents with health issues or disabilities to shape their identities around the disabilities and limitations rather than focus on the abilities and strengths that make them feel more like other adolescents. Identifying abilities as part of self-identity promotes self-efficacy and self-esteem.

and stress as well as unhealthy lifestyle behaviors.[15] Although there is support for OT services in high schools, there is a lack of OT practitioners working in this setting.[15,49] The COTA working in the school system or a health care setting has an important role in helping adolescents participate fully in the social and academic opportunities provided by the school and community.

SUMMARY

Even though growing up and making the transition from a child to young adult in today's society is challenging and characterized by change and adjustment, most American teens successfully make this journey and become healthy young adults. Fundamental to an adolescent's growth and well-being is the formation of social relationships and the development of a sense of competency through participation in all areas of occupational performance. OT practitioners have the expertise and responsibility to promote the healthy development of the adolescent in the school system as well as health care setting. However, it will be only through the active recruitment of OT practitioners that specialize in the high school setting that adequate OT services will be provided to meet the unique needs of adolescents with special needs or disabilities.[40,49]

References

1. American Occupational Therapy Association: *Occupational therapy practice framework: domain and process*, Bethesda, Md, 2002, The Association.
2. Arnett JJ: Emerging adulthood: a theory of development from the late teens through the twenties, *Am Psychol* 55:469, 2000.
3. Arnold P, Chapman M: Self-esteem, aspirations and expectations of adolescents with physical disability, *Devt Med Child Neurol* 34:97, 1992.
4. Bachman JG, Schulenberg J: How part-time work intensity relates to drug use, behavior, time use and satisfaction among school seniors: are these consequences or merely correlates? *Dev Psychol* 29:220, 1993.
5. Bagwell CL, Coie JD, Terry RA, Lockman JE: Peer clique participation and social status in preadolescence, *Merrill-Palmer Quart* 46:280, 2000.
6. Berger KS, Thompson RA: *The developing person through the life span*, ed 4, New York, 1998, Worth.
7. Broh BA: Linking extracurricular programming to academic achievement: who benefits and why? *Sociol Educ* 75:69, 2002.
8. Brollier C, Shepherd J, Markey KF: Transition from school to community living, *Am J Occup Ther* 48:346, 1994.
9. Cash TF, Putzinsky T: *Body image*, New York, 2002, Guilford.
10. Cech DJ, Martin S: *Functional movement development across the life span*, ed 2, Philadelphia, 2002, WB Saunders.
11. Coleman JC, Hendry L: *The nature of adolescence*, ed 2, New York, 1990, Routledge.
12. Conger JJ, Galambos NL: *Adolescence and youth: psychological development in a changing world*, ed 5, New York, 1997, Longman.
13. Csikszentmihayli M, Larson R: *Being adolescent: conflict and growth in the teenage years*, New York, 1984, Basic Books, p xiii.
14. Davis SE: Developmental tasks and transitions of adolescents with chronic illness and disabilities, *Rehabil Counseling Bull* 29:69, 1985.
15. Dirette D, Kolak L: Occupational performance needs of adolescents in alternative education programs, *Am J Occup Ther* 58:337, 2004.
16. Doubt L, McColl MA: A secondary guy: physically disabled teenagers in secondary schools, *Can J Occup Ther* 70:139, 2003.
17. Eccles JS, Barber BL: Student council, volunteering, basketball, or marching band: what kind of extracurricular involvement matters? *J Adolesc Res* 14:10, 1999.
18. Eccles JS, Barber BL, Stone M, et al: Extracurricular activities and adolescent development, *J Soc Issues* 59:865, 2003.
19. Foundation for Accountability: *A portrait of adolescents in America 2001: a report from the Robert Wood Johnson Foundation national strategic indicator surveys*, Portland, 2001, The Foundation for Accountability.
20. Frederickson N, Turner J: Utilizing the classroom peer group to address children's social needs: an evaluation of the circle of friends intervention approach, *J Special Educ* 36:234, 2002.
21. Gilligan C, Lyons NP, Hanmer TJ: *Making connections: the relational worlds of adolescent girls at Emma Willard school*, Cambridge, 1990, Harvard University Press.
22. Goldberg RT: Towards an understanding of the rehabilitation of the disabled adolescent, *Rehab Lit* 42:66, 1981.
23. Guest A, Schneider B: Adolescents' extracurricular participation in context: the mediating effects of schools, communities, and identity, *Sociol Educ* 76:89, 2003.
24. Harter S: *The construction of self*, New York, 1999, Guilford.
25. Hooker K: Developmental tasks. In Lerner RM, Petersen AC, Brooks-Gunn T, editors: *Encyclopedia of adolescence*, vol 1, London, 1991, Garland Publishing.
26. Keating DP: Cognition, adolescents. In Lerner RM, Petersen AC, Brooks-Gunn T, editors: *Encyclopedia of adolescence*, vol. 1, p 987, London, 1991, Garland Publishing.
27. Kemper HCG: The importance of physical activity in childhood and adolescence. In Haynan L, Mahon MM, Turner JR, editors: *Health behavior in childhood and adolescence*, p 105, New York, 2002, Springer Publishing.
28. Kielhofner G: *Model of human occupation*, ed 3, Baltimore, 2002, Lippincott Williams & Wilkins.
29. Kirkpatrick JM: Social origins, adolescents' experiences and work value trajectories during the transition to adulthood, *Soc Forces* 80:32, 2002.
30. Kunnen ES, Bosma HA, VanGeert PLC: A dynamic systems approach to identity formation: theoretical background and methodological possibilities. In Nurmi JE, editor: *Navigating through adolescence: European perspectives*, p 251, New York, 2001, Routledge Falmer.

31. Larson R, Verma S: How children and adolescents spend time across the world: work, play and developmental opportunities, *Psychol Bull* 125:701, 1999.
32. Laursen B, Coy KC, Collins WA: Reconsidering changes in parent-child conflict across adolescence: a meta-analysis, *Child Dev* 69:817, 1998.
33. Levine MP, Smolak L: Body image development in adolescence. In Cash TF, Putzinsky T, editors: *Body image*, p 74, New York, 2002, Guilford.
34. Marcia JE: Identity and self-development. In Lerner RM, Petersen AC, Brooks-Gunn T, editors: *Encyclopedia of adolescence*, vol 1, p 529, London, 1991, Garland Publishing.
35. Marsh HW, Kleitman S: Extracurricular school activities: the good, the bad and the nonlinear, *Harvard Educ Rev* 72:465, 2002.
36. Mechanic D: Adolescents at risk: new directions, *J Adolesc Health* 12:638, 1991.
37 Mpofu E: Enhancing social acceptance of early adolescents with physical disabilities: effect of role salience, peer interaction, and academic support interventions, *Internat J Disabil Dev Educ* 50:435, 2003.
38. Neinstein LS, Kaufman FR: Normal physical growth and development. In Neistein LS, editor: *Adolescent health care: a practical guide*, ed 4, p 3, Philadelphia, 2002, Lippincott Williams & Wilkins.
39. Newacheck PW, Halfon N: Prevalence and impact of disabling chronic conditions in childhood, *Am J Public Health* 88:610, 1998.
40. Orentlicher ML, Michaels CA: Some thoughts on the role of occupational therapy in the transition from school to adult life: Part II, *School Sys Special Interest Sect Quart* 7:1, 2000.
41. Overton WF, Byrnes JP: Cognitive development. In Lerner RM, Petersen AC, Brooks-Gunn T, editors: *Encyclopedia of adolescence*, vol 1, p 151, London, 1991, Garland Publishing.
42. Passmore A, French D: The nature of leisure in adolescence: a focus group, *Br J Occup Ther* 66:419, 2003.
43. Putzinsky T, Cash TF: Understanding body images: historical and contemporary perspectives. In Cash TF, Putzinsky T, editors: *Body image*, New York, 2002, Guilford.
44. Radzik M, Sherer S, Neinstein LS: Psychosocial development in normal adolescents. In Neinstein LS, editor: *Adolescent health: a practical guide*, ed 4, p 52, Philadelphia, 2002, Lippincott Williams & Wilkins.
45. Santrock JW: *Adolescence*, ed 9, New York, 2003, McGraw-Hill Higher Education.
46. Scales PC, Leffert N: *Developmental assets: a synthesis of the scientific research on adolescent development*, ed 2, Minneapolis, 2004, Search Institute.
47. Schwartz SJ, Montgomery MJ: Similarities or differences in identity development? The impact of acculturation and gender on identity process and outcome, *J Youth Adolesc* 31:359, 2002.
48. Spencer MB, Dupree D, Hartman T: A phenomenological variant of ecological systems theory (PVEST): a self-organization perspective of content, *Dev Psychopathol* 9:817, 1997.
49. Stewart DA, Law MC, Rosenbaum P, Willms DG: A qualitative study of the transition to adulthood for youth with physical disabilities, *Phys Occup Ther Pediatr* 21:3, 2001.
50. Vilhjalmsson R, Krisjansdottir G: Gender difference in physical activity in older children and adolescents: the central role of organised sport, *Soc Sci Med* 56:363, 2003.
51. Widmer MA, Ellis GD, Trunnell ER: Measurement of ethical behavior in leisure among high and low risk adolescents, *Adolescence* 31:397, 1996.
52. Wynn JR: High school after school: creating pathways to the future for adolescents, *New Directions Youth Dev* 97:59, 2003.
53. Youngblood J, Spencer MB: Integrating normative identity process and academic support requirements for special needs adolescents: the application of an identity focused cultural ecological (ICE) perspective, *Appl Dev Sci* 6:95, 2002.
54. Zajicek-Faber ML: Promoting good health in adolescents with disabilities, *Health Social Work* 23:203, 1998.
55. Zastrow CH, Kirst-Ashman KK: *Understanding human behavior*, ed 6, Belmont, Calif, 2004, Brooks/Cole-Thomson Learning.

REVIEW *Questions*

1. What are the physical and cognitive changes of adolescence?
2. How is body image viewed in adolescence?
3. What are some of the psychosocial issues for each stage: early, middle, and late adolescence?
4. What are some behavioral indicators of positive and negative self-esteem?
5. What are the characteristics of play/leisure and social participation in adolescence?
6. What are some of the issues that children with special needs may face in adolescence?

SUGGESTED *Activities*

1. Interview a teen to learn about interests, hobbies, concerns, and occupations that are important to him or her.
2. Read some teen magazines and in class discuss how the themes and images might influence an adolescent reader.
3. Have students present to each other on current teen trends, such as music, dress, styles, and social behaviors. Discuss cultural differences.
4. Develop a list of activities that teens enjoy that could easily be incorporated into occupational therapy intervention.
5. Spend time with a teenager alone for a few hours, in a group, and at home. How does he or she show individuality? How does his or her behavior change with context? How does he or she "fit in" each setting?
6. View the "Breakfast Club" and delineate the roles of adolescence. How is this film typical of adolescent development?
7. Compare and contrast adolescent or teen culture in America with another culture.

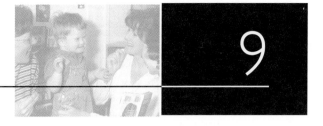

9

General Intervention Considerations

JEAN W. SOLOMON
JANE CLIFFORD O'BRIEN

CHAPTER *Objectives*

After studying this chapter, the reader will be able to accomplish the following:

- Explain the way in which assessment relates to program planning and intervention
- Differentiate among long-term goals, short-term objectives, and mini objectives
- Apply activity analysis to intervention
- Apply the knowledge of activity adaptation to a given case
- Be aware of the importance of culture and family-centered intervention
- Discuss discharge planning
- Understand a top-down approach to intervention
- Identify and describe the tools of practice

KEY TERMS

Referral
Screening
Evaluation
Intervention plan
Activity analysis
Task-focused activity analysis
Child- and family-focused activity analyses
Legitimate tools
Activity synthesis
Activity configuration
RUMBA criteria
Top-down approach
Occupational Therapy Intervention Process Model (OTIPM)

CHAPTER OUTLINE

This chapter discusses specific treatment considerations that arise during the occupational therapy (OT) process. This process begins with the referral, screening, and evaluation; continues with the intervention plan, goal setting, and treatment implementation; and then moves on to reevaluation and discharge planning.

The roles of the registered occupational therapist (OTR) and certified occupational therapy assistant (COTA) in the OT process differ. The OTR is responsible for selection of the assessments used during the evaluation, interpretation of the results, and development of the intervention plan. The COTA may gather evaluative data under the supervision of the OTR using an approved structured format but is not responsible for the interpretation of the assessment results; s/he may contribute knowledge of the client gained during the assessment process.

REFERRAL, SCREENING, AND EVALUATION

The referral, screening, and evaluation aspects of the OT process are concomitantly referred to as the *evaluation period*. During this period the OT practitioner meets the child, family, or other referral source (e.g., teacher, early interventionist) to collect information that will assist in setting goals and developing an activity configuration for the child.

Referral

Children are usually introduced to OT by means of a **referral.** The specific need for a referral depends on the individual state licensure law or regulations within the area of practice. It is the responsibility of the OT practitioner to know the laws and regulations that govern his or her area of practice. Some states require a referral before an OT practitioner can see a client. Other states require a referral only for the intervention process. A physician or a nurse practitioner generally gives the referral, depending on the state's laws; it is called a *physician's referral* or *doctor's orders*.

According to the *Standards of Practice for Occupational Therapy* published by the American Occupational Therapy Association (AOTA) in 1998,[1] only the OTR may accept a referral for assessment. COTAs, if given a referral, are responsible for forwarding it to a supervising OTR and educating "current and potential referral sources about the scope of occupational therapy services and the process of initiating occupational therapy referrals."[1] COTAs may acknowledge requests for services from any source. However, they do not accept and begin working on cases at their own professional discretion without the supervision and collaboration of the OT.

Screening

Clients may come to OT through **screening.** Both OTRs and COTAs can conduct such screenings. For example, a COTA may be hired to screen children in a well-baby clinic or an incoming kindergarten class to determine the need for additional evaluation before entering school. Once the COTA has identified the need for a more complete evaluation, the OTR determines the specific evaluation or format to be used. The data gathered by the COTA is interpreted by the OTR. A COTA "may contribute to this process under the supervision of a registered occupational therapist."[1]

Evaluation

The **evaluation** is a critical part of the OT process. The OTR is responsible for determining the type and scope of the evaluation. An evaluation includes assessments of an individual's areas of performance (e.g., activities of daily living [ADLs], instrumental ADLs [IADLs], work, education, play/leisure, social participation), client factors (e.g., neuromusculoskeletal, specific and global mental functions, body system), performance skills, performance patterns, contexts, and activity demands.[2] According to the AOTA's *Occupational Therapy Roles*, an entry-level COTA "assists with data collection and evaluation under the supervision of the occupational therapist."[3] An intermediate- or advanced-level COTA "administers standardized tests under the supervision of an occupational therapist after service competency has been established."[3] Although the COTA may participate in the evaluation process, the OTR is responsible for interpreting the results and developing the intervention plan.

Levels of performance

The evaluation provides the OT practitioner with a picture of the child's occupational needs, including strengths and weaknesses. This occupational profile consists of a description of the level of performance at which the child functions. A child's level of function may differ in relation to task, pattern, and context. For example, a child may feed himself or herself independently at home after setup but be unable to do so at school in the time period provided while sitting at the table with the loud noises and confusion of the lunch room.

Functional independence

Functional independence refers to the completion of age-appropriate activities with or without the use of assistive devices and without human assistance (e.g., eating independently with an offset spoon).

Assisted performance

Assisted performance refers to a child's participation in a specific age-appropriate task with some assistance from the caregiver (e.g., putting on a shirt and receiving assistance with buttoning).

Dependent performance

Dependent performance occurs when a child is unable to perform an age-appropriate task. A caregiver is required to perform the task for the child (e.g., holding a cup for a child with cerebral palsy who is unable to drink from one).

INTERVENTION PLANNING, GOAL SETTING, AND TREATMENT IMPLEMENTATION

Intervention Planning

The OTR develops the **intervention plan** after the evaluation is complete. It includes parental concerns, the client's strengths and weaknesses, a statement of the client's rehabilitation potential, long-term goals, and short-term objectives. The plan describes the type of media (i.e., specific types of materials) and modalities (i.e., intervention tools) that will be used and the frequency and duration of treatment. The plans for reevaluation and discharge as well as the level of personnel providing the intervention are also included.[1]

The intervention plan is based on a selected frame of reference (see Chapter 1). The frame of reference provides guidelines and intervention strategies. The COTA utilizes knowledge of the selected frame of reference and activity analysis and the selection, gradation, and adaptation of activities to carry out the intervention plan.

Legitimate tools

Legitimate tools are the instruments or tools that a profession uses to bring about change. Legitimate tools change over time based on the growing knowledge of the profession, technological advances, and the needs and values of both the profession and society.[12] OT practitioners use occupations, purposeful activities, activity analysis, activity synthesis, and therapeutic use of self as tools to help children.

Occupation

The goal of OT is to help children participate in their desired occupations. Their occupations include social participation, self-care tasks (e.g., feeding, dressing, bathing), academics, and play. Intervention is designed to help them participate to the fullest in these occupations. Therefore, OT practitioners analyze occupations to determine why the child is not performing and use the tools of practice to assist them. Intervention is then designed to remediate or rehabilitate the underlying skills that are causing difficulties, compensate for problem areas, or adapt the requirements of the skills so that the child may be successful at performing in a different way.

OT practitioners strive to provide occupation-based intervention.[2,8] This intervention involves participation in the actual occupation with which the child struggles. For example, intervention to improve a child's ability to play with others may consist of inviting a child to the treatment session and facilitating play with others.

Purposeful activities

Purposeful activities are defined as goal-directed behaviors or tasks that constitute occupations.[9] An activity is purposeful if the individual is a voluntary, active participant and the activity is directed toward a goal that the individual considers meaningful. OT practitioners use purposeful activity to evaluate, facilitate, restore, or maintain individuals' abilities to function in their daily occupations.

Purposeful activity provides opportunities for individuals to achieve mastery, while successful performance promotes feelings of personal competence. Those involved in purposeful activities focus on the goals rather than the processes required for achievement of those goals. Purposeful activity occurs within the context of personal, cultural, physical, and other environmental conditions and requires a variety of client factors (e.g., neuromusculoskeletal, global, and specific mental functions and systems).[2] Purposeful activities are specific to the individual; therefore, the OT practitioner grades or adapts a chosen activity for the individual.[9]

Activity analysis

Activity analysis refers to the process of analyzing an activity to determine how and when it should be used with a particular client.[3] It is the identification of the components or client factors involved in performing an activity.[3] Several methods are used to analyze activity, two of which are discussed in this chapter.

The first method is **task-focused activity analysis.** This method of analyzing activity identifies the physical, social, and mental factors involved in a specific task. The OT practitioner uses an activity analysis to describe the materials needed for the activity, the sequential steps of the activity, and safety concerns.[4] Task-focused activity analysis identifies the most and least important performance components needed to complete the activity. The physical, personal, social, and cultural conditions and influences are described. Using this analysis, the OT practitioner identifies how the activity may be graded and adapted for the client.

Task-focused activity analysis is used to understand the activity in terms of skills and personal and cultural meanings to help the OT practitioner understand how

TASK-FOCUSED ACTIVITY ANALYSIS

CHILD'S NAME: ***Kellie Penalta*** DATE: ***12/30/05***

ACTIVITY DESCRIPTION: ***Closing Velcro tabs on shoes***

SUPPLIES/EQUIPMENT: ***Socks, shoes, chair***

STEPS OF ACTIVITY:
1) ***Prepare work area with chair, socks and shoes.***
2) ***Position child on chair.***
3) ***Put socks and shoes on.***
4) ***Demonstrate how to close tabs.***
5) ***Allow the child to practice closing tabs with hand-over-hand assistance.***
6) ***Allow child to begin practicing closing tabs.***

LIST THE MOST IMPORTANT PERFORMANCE COMPONENTS REQUIRED FOR THIS ACTIVITY:

Sensorimotor	Cognitive	Psychosocial/Psychological
1) Sensory awareness	***1) Level of arousal***	***1) Values***
2) Tactile	***2) Attention span***	***2) Interests***
3) Proprioception	***3) Sequencing***	***3) Role performance***
4) Kinesthesia	***4) Learning***	***4) Self-expression***
5) Fine coordination / dexterity	***5) Concept formation***	***5) Coping skills***

LIST THE LEAST IMPORTANT PERFORMANCE COMPONENTS REQUIRED FOR THIS ACTIVITY:

Sensorimotor	Cognitive	Psychosocial/Psychological
1) Oral-motor control	***1) Orientation***	***1) Self-concept***
2) Reflexes	***2) Recognition***	***2) Social conduct***
3) Pain response	***3) Categorization***	***3) Interpersonal skills***
4) Olfactory	***4) Spatial operations***	***4) Time management skills***
5) Gustatory	***5) Problem-solving skills***	***5) Self-control***

ENVIRONMENTAL CONTEXTS:

1. Physical	2. Social	3. Cultural
Activity can be done in the child's room or another room in the home. Area should be well lighted. Child can sit on chair or floor.	***Practitioner and child will work together until task is learned. Mother will practice with child.***	***In own culture, people are expected to wear shoes.***

Gradation	Adaptation	Safety Hazards
Method of instruction can vary to accommodate child's learning needs. Task can be taught using hand-over-hand method.	***D rings can be placed on tip of tabs to facilitate grasping the tabs.***	***None***

FIGURE 9-1 Task-focused activity analysis form for Kellie Penalta.

CHILD-AND FAMILY-FOCUSED ACTIVITY ANALYSIS

DATE: *12/30/05*

CHILD'S NAME: *Kellie Penalta* AGE: *2 years, 7 months*

DIAGNOSIS: *Pervasive Development Disorder-Austism*

SETTING: *Home Based* FREQUENCY OF OT: *5 times per week*

DURATION: *1 hour per session*

Strengths	Limitations
Strong family support system *Enjoys proprioceptive activities* *Enjoys vestibular activities*	*Decreased eye contact* *Delays in fine motor skills* *Delays in gross motor skills* *Delay with self-care skills*

OBJECTIVE: ***Kellie will be able to engage in at least three activities without tantrums within 6 months***

Planned Activities	Materials	Supplies and Equipment
1) Hair brushing ***2) Vestibular activities*** ***3) Dressing activities***		***1) Hair brush*** ***2) Therapy ball*** ***3) Clothing, shoes***
Position of Child and Practitioner	**Performance Results**	**Recommendations**
1) Child sits on floor in front of therapist.	***1) Child had difficulty tolerating hairbrushing.***	***1) Continue with deep pressure hairbrushing with corn brush. Allow child to initiate hairbrushing activity.***
2) Child initially sits on a 9-inch ball. Practitioner is positioned behind child and supports child at hips.	***2) Child was able to tolerate sitting on ball. She was able to carry out a task while sitting on a ball.***	***2) Introduce a 12-inch ball during next session.***
3) Child sits on floor in front of practitioners, Practitioner also sits on floor.	***3) Child was receptive and able to follow directions. Hand-over-hand assistance was required.***	***3) Mother should practice activity with child everyday. Discrete trial teaching will be used during therapy sessions.***

FIGURE 9-2 Child- and family-focused activity analysis form for Kellie Penalta.

the activity can be used therapeutically. This type of analysis enables him or her to quickly identify the demand of an activity (Figure 9-1).[6] The second method comprises both **child- and family-focused activity analyses** (Figure 9-2). The OT practitioner analyzes the actual intervention and identifies the child's and family's strengths and weaknesses. S/he then identifies the objectives and plans activities that are specifically designed to meet those objectives. The practitioner describes the types of materials, supplies, and equipment that will be needed; identifies the position of the child and the OT practitioner during intervention; and documents the expected results or recommendations. Several activities may meet the plan.

There is a degree of overlap between the two types of activity analysis. Although each one emphasizes distinct aspects of activity, both require that the practitioner understand the needs of the child, a variety of theoretical approaches, and the context of intervention.

Activity synthesis

Activity synthesis includes adapting, grading, and reconfiguring activities and is considered a legitimate tool used in OT practice.

Adaptation refers to the process of changing specific steps during an activity so that the client is able to engage in it. An activity is adapted by modifying or changing the sequence of its steps, the way in which the materials are presented, or the way in which the child is positioned or by presenting the activity in such a way that the child is expected to perform only certain aspects of it. Activities can also be adapted by changing the characteristics of the materials that are used, such as their size, shape, texture, or weight.[12] For example, for a child who is fearful of movement and needs to improve or develop righting reactions, the practitioner could place him or her on a therapy ball to elicit righting reactions. However, because of the child's fear of movement, the practitioner could begin the intervention with a smaller ball that allows his or her feet to stay on the ground and provides slow, controlled movements. The practitioner can make the activity easier or more difficult to find the right challenge for the child.

Grading refers to the process of arranging the steps of an activity in a sequential series to change or progress, allowing for gradual improvement by increasing the demand for a higher level of performance as the child's abilities increase. The OT practitioner determines the type and extent of grading based on clinical reasoning. By participating in activities that are graded for his or her needs, a client's level of performance changes. Once the practitioner has adapted and graded an activity, it is presented in its "real" form, thus synthesizing the analysis, adaptation, and grading into the activity itself.[11] For example, as a child is learning self-feeding, finger feeding is acceptable. The activity is then adapted by the introduction of a utensil. It would be acceptable initially for the child to hold the utensil and attempt to use it to scoop or spear food. The practitioner ultimately expects the child to grasp the utensil, spear the food, and bring it to the mouth, thus synthesizing the activity of self-feeding into the child's repertoire of abilities. The goal of adapting and grading activities is participation in occupations in the given context.

Activity configuration

Activity configuration is the process of selecting specific activities to use during the intervention process based on a child's age, interests, and abilities. For example, a long-term goal may be for the child to be able to feed independently. One short-term objective may be for the child to be able to scoop with a spoon. A session objective may be for the child to learn how to control the grasp and release of a spoon.

Therapeutic use of self

Therapeutic use of self refers to the ability of the OT practitioner to communicate with the child and the child's family or caregivers while being aware of his or her own personal feelings. OT practitioners use their individual characteristics to relate to families, interact with children, and help them perform occupations. As such, those practitioners who are aware of their own strengths and weaknesses may show insight into how one's use of self has an impact on intervention so that they may help children and their families more effectively.

In a therapeutic relationship the practitioner helps the child and family without any expectation of the help being reciprocated. [10] S/he develops and maintains a good relationship with the child and family.[5] Therefore, OT practitioners must possess a basic knowledge of family dynamics, cultural and ethnic concepts in the provision of services, and family systems. As Suzanne Peloquin said, "...concern for the patient as a person remains essential to effective practice."[13]

OT practitioners recognize that a child is treated with consideration of the context, including the family, culture, and environment. His or her role is to create an atmosphere of freedom and an appropriate challenge within the structure of the intervention. The intervention should not be so simple that the child becomes bored or so difficult that s/he feels inadequate. The practitioner prepares a setting to meet the child's needs by guiding him or her toward mastery of the skill.[13]

OT practitioners work with the family to guide them as they care for the child. Because families experience emotional turmoil caused by dealing with a child with special needs, they may not be able to participate in the therapeutic process. Clinicians must work with parents where they are and not place unreal expectations or judgments on when the parents should "get through" things. Working on goals that are important to a family at a particular time is an effective way to help them. Parents will understand their children as they work with the OT practitioner to meet the agreed-upon goals.

Tyrone is an 18-month-old child with developmental delays; he is unable to walk, speaks very little, and does not manipulate toys. His mother has three other children (ages 9, 7, and 3), lives alone, and receives public assistance. The

OT practitioner provides the mother with an extensive home program, which she refuses to do. The practitioner documents the fact that the mother is noncompliant and in denial over her son's diagnosis.

In this scenario, the OT practitioner has failed to examine the context and therefore has too quickly judged Tyrone's mother. She may be overwhelmed with this new diagnosis and the demands of caring for three young children by herself on limited income. She may not be following through with the home program because she has no time or energy to do it. The OT practitioner has not targeted the goals that support the mother and family.

Consider the same case, in which the OT practitioner provided the mother with techniques to include the other children in playing with Tyrone to improve his abilities. This would allow the mother some free time and involve all the children in activity. The OT practitioner may even provide games that they could all do together as "family time" (e.g., "Simon Says" or finger plays). The OTR may work more closely with the mother in determining how Tyrone's developmental delays are having an impact on the family. After identifying that feeding Tyrone is problematic, the OT practitioner may target feeding issues. Targeting the issues of concern to parents is the best way to involve them in the intervention process. OT practitioners who target parental concerns seldom find parents who are in "denial."

CLINICAL *Pearl*

Examining situations from all angles provides insight that may help OT practitioners working with children.

CLINICAL *Pearl*

The parents may not understand the entirety of the diagnosis, but they generally understand their child. They can learn about their child's strengths and weaknesses during the intervention process. OT practitioners can help the parents understand their child by involving them in goal setting.

CLINICAL *Pearl*

Parents want the best from their children. OT practitioners help them care for their children and play a role in empowering parents.

CLINICAL *Pearl*

Making eye contact, getting to the child's level, and pointing out his or her strengths to the parents help practitioners gain trust from the child and family. These abilities are considered part of the therapeutic use of self.

One way to help parents understand their child is through *modeling* behaviors. Parents report that they learn more easily by observing the practitioner work with the child. Being able to observe and ask questions helps them develop skills and routines to care for their child.[6,9] OT practitioners model handling techniques, management, and attitudes toward the child. Clinicians also model patience, understanding, and acceptance, which in turn help parents show the same. Practitioners learn from parents by listening and opening lines of communication; this therapeutic relationship empowers parents. While the OT practitioner comes into contact with many children with special needs, the parents may find this new experience overwhelming. Therefore, a clinician who models understanding, caring, and acceptance of their child may teach them the same, which has an impact on the child and family in ways that cannot be measured. This is the essence of the therapeutic use of self.

The therapeutic use of self requires that OT practitioners be aware of their body language; read parents' verbal and nonverbal cues; and interact in a caring, nonjudgmental manner. Making eye contact, nodding one's head, and making facial expressions to communicate are all aspects of the therapeutic use of self that clinicians must understand and use effectively.

Multicultural implications

Maria is a 2-year-old girl diagnosed with spastic quadriplegia. She is from the Dominican Republic. Her parents have recently immigrated to the United States. Maria is evaluated at the early intervention center by the OTR, physical therapist, and speech therapist. The team decides that Maria needs all the services. The OTR meets with the parents to decide on the goals for the sessions. The social worker, who speaks Spanish, is present. Using a family-centered approach (per the early intervention laws), the OT practitioner asks the parents what their concerns are and what they would like to work on in therapy sessions. The parents are hesitant to respond throughout the whole meeting. The OT practitioner feels that the parents are not interested in receiving services for their daughter. The OT practitioner and social worker meet after the meeting to discuss the events.

This case study illustrates the need to understand cultural expectations. The OT practitioner does not understand why the parents do not quickly express their desires for Maria. The practitioner interprets this as a lack of caring and disinterest in the child's progress.

The social worker explains to the OT practitioner that while many American parents feel empowered to discuss their concerns and advocate for their child, parents from the Dominican Republic look to the professional to tell them what to do. Maria's parents have not yet been socialized to the American system. They are not disinterested but rather somewhat confused as to why a medical health care professional (e.g., the OT practitioner) would ask them what they wanted. They view health care professionals as the experts and as such will follow through with any requirements made by the team.

Once the OT practitioner understands this cultural difference, s/he holds the next meeting in a different way, is more directive, and provides the parents with the team's recommendations. However, the team acknowledges that Maria will require services when she enters school, and as such they will have to help socialize the parents to advocate for their child with professionals. However, the OT practitioner may first have to be more direct than what might be necessary with parents socialized to the American system.

Cultural values have an impact on all areas of family life. OT practitioners need to understand the cultural context in which the child belongs in order to meet the child's and family's needs. Although the OT practitioner may not have direct understanding of each culture, sensitivity and open communication may bridge the gap. Disregard for cultural concerns may interfere with establishing rapport; as a result, the practitioner may find that the child or caregiver is not invested in the intervention. When this happens, the lack of compliance and satisfaction generally makes the therapy process ineffective.

Goal Setting

The COTA collaborates with the OTR and family on the development of the long-term goals and short-term objectives for any child they are treating. Through this collaborative process, the OTR, COTA, and family agree on the needs of the child as well as the appropriate priorities for intervention. This makes the intervention process more efficient and effective and leads to a better understanding of the child. Based on the evaluation and discussion of needs, realistic goals for the child can be established.

Long-term goals

Long-term goals are statements that describe the occupational goals the client should achieve after intervention. These goals should be measurable, observable, and clear and written in behavioral terms. Goals need to be very specific and address the problems that have been identified. A practitioner can use the mnemonic device referred to as the **RUMBA criteria** to evaluate the goal statements they write (Box 9-1).[7]

BOX 9-1

RUMBA Criteria

R (RELEVANT)
A relevant goal reflects the client's current life situation and future possibilities. Everyone involved in the client's care (client, therapist, family, and members of other disciplines) should agree on the goal.

U (UNDERSTANDABLE)
An understandable goal is stated in clear language. Jargon and very specialized or difficult words should be avoided.

M (MEASURABLE)
A measurable goal contains criteria for success.

B (BEHAVIORAL)
A behavioral goal focuses on the behavior or skill that the client must eventually demonstrate.

A (ACHIEVABLE)
An achievable goal describes a behavior or skill that the client should be able to accomplish in a reasonable period of time.

Adapted from Early MB: *Mental health concepts and techniques for the occupational therapy assistant,* ed 2, New York, 1993, Raven Press.

Short-term objectives

Short-term objectives are the steps the client needs to achieve to meet the long-term goal. They are statements that describe the skills that should be mastered in a relatively short period. For example, consider a client whose long-term goal is independent dressing. The short-term objectives may include developing a pincer grasp for buttoning, learning to button, and the developing sequencing skills for dressing.

Treatment Implementation

Treatment implementation (intervention) involves working within the system through which the child is receiving therapy, working with the family, and working directly with the child. Working with the child involves planning each session, developing and analyzing activities, and then grading and adapting those activities as necessary. This process is geared toward reaching the short-term objectives first and then the long-term goals.

Intervention includes the methods used to work toward meeting the goals, the media or activities used during the intervention, and documentation of the child's progress or lack of progress.

Session objectives (mini objectives)

Mini objectives are the goals the practitioner has set for a specific intervention session. They are planned before the session in collaboration with the child and parents. Sometimes mini objectives will last for several sessions because it may take more than one intervention to meet them.

Once the mini objectives are identified, the OT practitioner analyzes the activities that will facilitate meeting the objective.

Frames of reference

The OTR and COTA collaborate during the development of the intervention plan.[3] The OTR develops the plan based on a frame of reference. The COTA, with knowledge of the frame of reference, carries out the plan.

A frame of reference provides the conceptual framework for organizing practical material, outlining the theoretical concepts of a particular approach, providing guidelines for assessing functional capacities of the client, and providing a method for conceptualizing and initiating intervention. Various frames of reference are used in OT. (See Chapter 1 and other textbooks for more details.)

REEVALUATION AND DISCHARGE PLANNING

Reevaluation

Although the OTR determines whether a reevaluation is indicated, the COTA is responsible for reporting any change in the child's condition to the supervisor. Therefore, if the COTA observes changes, they must be brought to the attention of the OTR, and the COTA should suggest a reevaluation. The COTA participates in the reevaluation in collaboration with and under the supervision of the OTR.[3]

Discharge Planning

In pediatric OT the discharge planning and date may be mandated by specific laws that govern the type of system in which the child receives OT services. Regardless of the system, the discontinuation process is the responsibility of the OTR. The COTA collaborates in the discontinuation process under the supervision of the OTR by reporting on the child's progress and making suggestions regarding future needs.

Services are typically discontinued once the child has met the predetermined goals and achieved maximum benefit from OT or the parents or child determine that the child no longer wants to receive OT. Services may be discontinued when the child moves or enters another system. The COTA may recommend discontinuation of services to the OTR when any of the mentioned conditions exist. Discontinuation plans should include a plan for follow-up when indicated. Figure 9-3 provides a summary of the OT process from the referral to the follow-up plan.

While many systems do not allow for children to be discharged and readmitted, this may in fact be the best method. For example, a child may need to receive OT services one time in junior high school due to changes in body or advanced requirements.

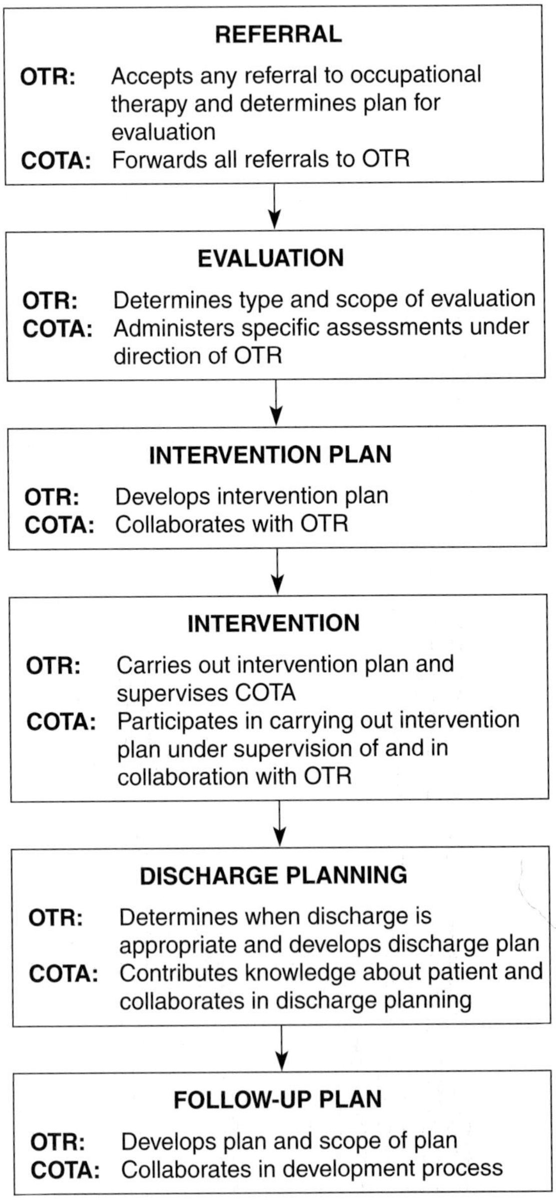

REFERRAL

OTR: Accepts any referral to occupational therapy and determines plan for evaluation

COTA: Forwards all referrals to OTR

↓

EVALUATION

OTR: Determines type and scope of evaluation

COTA: Administers specific assessments under direction of OTR

↓

INTERVENTION PLAN

OTR: Develops intervention plan

COTA: Collaborates with OTR

↓

INTERVENTION

OTR: Carries out intervention plan and supervises COTA

COTA: Participates in carrying out intervention plan under supervision of and in collaboration with OTR

↓

DISCHARGE PLANNING

OTR: Determines when discharge is appropriate and develops discharge plan

COTA: Contributes knowledge about patient and collaborates in discharge planning

↓

FOLLOW-UP PLAN

OTR: Develops plan and scope of plan

COTA: Collaborates in development process

FIGURE 9-3 Responsibilities of registered occupational therapist (OTR) and certified occupational therapy assistant (COTA) in occupational therapy intervention process.

OCCUPATION-CENTERED TOP-DOWN APPROACH

Since OT practitioners are interested in helping children engage in their occupations, evaluation and intervention focusing on occupations are recommended. Fisher proposed a model for OT evaluation and intervention using a client-centered, occupation-based, **top-down approach** called the **Occupational Therapy Intervention Process Model (OTIPM)**.[8]

The following is a case study illustrating how this may look in practice. The focus of this evaluation and intervention plan is on the child's occupations.[8] Later in the process, the OT practitioner will determine the specific client factors or components interfering with performance. However, the goals for intervention can be developed based on overall performance. As highlighted in this case study, OT practitioners are encouraged to address the concerns of the parents, caregivers, and teachers when designing intervention, which focuses on occupational performance. OT practitioners are encouraged to read Fisher's work for more information.[8]

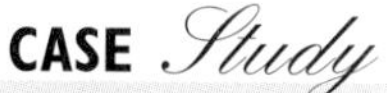

CASE *Study*

Hannah is a 2-year, 7-month-old girl with a diagnosis of pervasive developmental disorder. She was referred to an early intervention program for evaluation by the pediatrician.

Parental Concerns

Her parents expressed concern that Hannah does not talk as clearly as her cousin and never has; becomes agitated very easily and screams, especially during bath time; and does not play with her cousins and sisters. Furthermore, her mother is concerned about the lack of variety in her diet. Hannah's parents are concerned that she is not developing like her sisters (ages 5 and 1), and they are unsure of how to manage her behaviors. Her mother is "worried about Hannah's lack of interest in her mother, father, or siblings."

Areas of Performance

Activities of daily living

- *Feeding.* Hannah is currently able to drink from a bottle but does not like to drink from a cup. She is very particular about the food she eats and likes only very soft, almost liquid types of food. Her food preferences currently include Cheerios with milk, pasta soup, and bland mashed potatoes. Hannah sometimes eats very ripe bananas.
- *Dressing.* Hannah does not yet dress or undress independently. Her mother reports that she likes to wear only long-sleeved shirts and leggings and refuses to walk around barefoot. Hannah is able to remove her socks. She is able to remove mittens, hats, and coats after they are unzipped. She is unable to remove slip-on shoes or unlace or unbuckle other shoes. She is unable to put on or take off pants, skirts, or shirts.
- *Bathing.* Hannah often hides and becomes tearful when her mother announces that it is bath time. She cries, has tantrums, and hits others when placed in the tub. She hates having her face washed; however, her mother reports that sometimes Hannah will rub her face with a washcloth on her own.
- *Toileting.* Hannah does not indicate when she is wet or soiled and shows no discomfort.
- *Sleep.* Hannah sleeps through the night. She goes to bed around 9:00 PM and wakes up around 7:00 AM. She takes a 2-hour nap during the day.

Play

Hannah does not interact with others while playing but plays quietly alone. She enjoys balls and will stare at them for long periods of time. Hannah sometimes enjoys going to the playground, especially when there are few or no other children around. She goes up and down the slide, sometimes as often as 30 times in an hour. She is terrified of the swing and refuses to go in the sandbox. Hannah enjoys roughhousing with her father.

Social Participation

Her mother reports that Hannah prefers to sit in front of the television watching children's programs and does not play with toys. She does not respond to her name when called despite having had a normal audiological examination. Hannah's eye contact is limited; she does not look at her mother when requesting things. She does not verbalize her needs but instead takes her mother's hand to guide her to whatever she wants. Hannah does not initiate conversation with her sisters or parents.

Habits/Routines

Hannah stays at home with her mother and younger sister; her older sister attends morning kindergarten. She lives in a two-story house in the country. Hannah has a playground, with a swing, sandbox, and yard. She has a variety of toys. Hannah eats breakfast around 8:00 AM, lunch at noon, and dinner at 6:00 PM. She takes a 2-hour nap after lunch. Hannah bathes once a week, although her mother would like her to do it more often. The family enjoys taking hikes and spending time together. The children go to gymnastics classes once a week. Hannah frequently does not participate in classes.

Each Sunday the family gets together at the grandmother's house for dinner and socializing. There are many children playing. Hannah has difficulty and frequently goes to a quiet room in the house. The family leaves early on many occasions when she has tantrums.

Assessment

Hannah's family has established routines in which she is able to participate. She shows some difficulties at family gatherings but has also demonstrated the ability to adapt (e.g., finding a quiet space). Hannah is able to indicate her wants by pulling on her mother's hand, which indicates that she has motivations and desires.

Hannah is demonstrating delays in all areas of self-care, play, and social participation. She shows signs of sensory modulation difficulties that interfere with these occupations.

Plan

Hannah will attend an early intervention program three mornings a week, which will include OT services to work on improving her ability to play with others, dress and feed herself, and get along with family members.

BOX 9-2

Goals and Objectives

1. Hannah will be able to dress herself with verbal prompting within 6 months.
   - Hannah will be able to button a shirt with demonstrative prompts 3 out of 4 times.
   - Hannah will be able to unbutton a shirt independently 3 out of 4 times.
   - Hannah will show improved bilateral coordination by putting together five pop beads independently 4 out of 6 times.
2. Hannah will play with her sisters for 15 minutes, sharing toys at least twice during the session.
   - Hannah will engage in parallel play with her sister and cousin (both 5 years old) for 5 minutes without interfering in the play.
   - Hannah will play pass with a ball with her sister (5 years old) for 5 minutes without becoming upset.
   - Hannah will dance with her sisters for 3 minutes as part of family game night.
3. Hannah will seek her mother's help at least five times a day.
   - Hannah will indicate her desires to her mother by pointing to the objects she wants 3 out of 5 times.
   - Hannah will hold her mother's hand to be lead to the objects she wants.
   - Hannah will make eye contact with her mother twice while playing peek a boo.

Abbreviated Intervention Plan

The goals and objectives were designed to meet parental concerns (Box 9-2). The first goal of dressing will help Hannah's parents see that she can participate in daily tasks and may empower them to set other goals. The other goals and objectives center around parental concerns that Hannah does not play with others and shows a lack of interest in her mother, father, and siblings. Since play is so important in a child's life, the OT practitioner decided to start there. Furthermore, her mother repeatedly expressed concern that Hannah was not interested in the family. Therefore, helping the child become part of the family will benefit everyone.

Because Hannah already gets her mother's attention to show her what she wants, the OT practitioner built upon this skill. This will help the parent and child feel successful early on and thereby build a trusting relationship between parent and child in order to meet other goals. Furthermore, the mother is concerned with Hannah's lack of interest in the family, and this goal will reinforce the connections between her and the other family members. Children with a diagnosis of pervasive developmental disorder may not express themselves in the same manner as typically developing children. Therefore, grabbing her mother's hand and expressing her desires by means of pointing at pictures close to her mother may be Hannah's way of staying close to her. This may cause her mother to feel needed and thus connected to her. Once Hannah is accustomed to pointing to pictures, the OT practitioner may give the pictures to the father, sisters, and teachers.

Once the family has seen some progress and Hannah's behaviors are under more control, the OT sessions may focus on the underlying components, such as improving fine motor skills. For example, once Hannah is able to play with her sisters at home with a large ball, the practitioner may recommend coloring activities or other activities that are more challenging for her. The OT practitioner feels that targeting the family issues has the greatest impact on the child's performance. The goal of the sessions is not that Hannah becomes "normal"; instead, the goal is for her to fit in with the family so that the other family members can begin to understand her and make the necessary accommodations.

Frames of Reference

A sensory integration frame of reference will be used to help Hannah modulate sensory information. The OT practitioner will work with the family to determine her sensory needs. S/he can then provide home strategies for the parents that will help manage Hannah's behaviors more easily.

A developmental frame of reference will also be used to help Hannah participate in everyday play activities at home. The OT practitioner will provide the other family members with simple, easily implemented goals to help them relate to and understand Hannah. Hannah will learn how to play better through practice and rewards (e.g., sensory or verbal).

Intervention strategies

Intervention strategies are tailored to meet the child's and family's needs and thus require creativity, analysis, and reflection on how the activities are meeting the goals. Since children change, intervention strategies must also change.

Hannah's OT sessions may focus on sensory modulation activities, including brushing programs and tactile exploration (e.g., playing with sand, water, or rice). Many children with pervasive developmental disorder benefit from a sensory integration approach that includes child-directed experiences on suspended equipment, requiring adaptive responses. See Chapter 21 for more treatment suggestions.

The OT practitioner will carefully adapt activities while reading the child's cues so that the child can succeed. Occasionally including the parents and siblings in the sessions helps model how to promote positive behaviors and may provide the parents with strategies to use at home. Because the goal of the sessions is to improve play skills, intervention will resemble play and may even include small play groups with other children. The OT practitioner will give the child a reward for positive behaviors (e.g., sharing), which could be a sticker, positive verbal praise, or an extra turn on the swing.

To help the child ask for assistance from her mother, the clinician sets up a picture board with the activities of the day and teaches the child how to point to the next activity. Hannah will eventually learn to pick out the activities by pointing. This same strategy can be implemented at home by placing pictures on the refrigerator, from which she may choose. The clinician may decide to give the mother an apron with the pictures attached to it so that Hannah has to go to her. Each intervention session includes a variety of play activities, strategies for parents, and successful performances from Hannah. The OT practitioner pays close attention to Hannah and her family's needs.

SUMMARY

OT services are provided to children from birth to 21 years of age. Before engaging in pediatric practice, the practitioner must be familiar with the profession's tools; the OT intervention process; and federal, state, and local laws in order to effectively design OT services. Practitioners in pediatrics work not only with the child but also with the family or caregiver. Specialized training in intervention techniques, family dynamics, and cultural considerations are beneficial. OT practitioners help children participate in everyday occupations. Therefore, a top-down approach focusing on occupations as the means and ends and emphasizing client-centered care is recommended.[8]

References

1. American Occupational Therapy Association: *Standards of practice for occupational therapy*, Bethesda, Md, 1998, The Association.
2. American Occupational Therapy Association: *Occupational Therapy Practice Framework: domain and process*, Bethesda, Md, 2002, The Association.
3. American Occupational Therapy Association: *Occupational therapy roles*, Bethesda, Md, 1994, The Association.
4. Blesedell-Crepeau E: Activity analysis: a way of thinking about occupational performance. In Neistadt ME, Crepeau EB, editors: *Willard and Spackman's Occupational Therapy*, ed 10, Philadelphia, 2003, Lippincott.
5. Case-Smith J: *Pediatric occupational therapy and early intervention*, ed 2, Boston, 1998, Butterworth-Heinemann.
6. Crowe T, Vanheit B, Berghmansk K, Mann P: Role perceptions of mothers with young children: the impact of a child's disability, *Am J Occup Ther* 49:221, 1997.
7. Early MB: *Mental health concepts and techniques for the occupational therapy assistant*, ed 3, Philadelphia, 1999, Lippincott.
8. Fisher A: *OTIPM: A model for implementing top-down, client-centered, and occupation-based assessment, intervention, and documentation*, Durham, NH, January 12-14, 2005, University of New Hampshire.
9. Hinojosa J, Sabari J, Pedretti LW: Purposeful activities, *Am J Occup Ther* 47:1081, 1993.
10. Humphry R, Link S: Preparation of occupational therapists to work in early intervention programs, *Am J Occup Ther* 44:28, 1990.
11. Kramer P, Hinojosa J: Activity synthesis. In Hinojosa J, Blount M: *The texture of life: purposeful activities*, Bethesda, Md, 2004, American Occupational Therapy Association.
12. Luebben A, Hinojosa J, Kramer P: Legitimate tools of pediatric occupational therapy. In Kramer P, Hinojosa J: *Frames of reference in pediatric occupational therapy*, ed 2, Baltimore, Md, 1999, Williams & Wilkins.
13. Peloquin S: The patient-therapist relationship in occupational therapy: understanding visions and images, *Am J Occup Ther* 44:13, 1990.

Recommended Reading

Carver C: Crossing thresholds, *OT Practice* 3:18, 1998.
Case-Smith J: Pediatric assessment, *OT Practice* 2:24, 1997.
Esdaile S: A play focused intervention involving mothers of preschoolers, *Am J Occup Ther* 50:113, 1996.
Fisher A, Murray E, Bundy A: *Sensory integration—theory and practice*, ed 2, Philadelphia, 2002, FA Davis.
Haack L, Haldy M: Making it easy—adapting home and school environments, *OT Practice* 1:22, 1996.

Harris S, Weiss M: *Right from the start—behavioral intervention for young children with autism*, Bethesda, Md, 1998, Woodbine House.

Kranowitz C: *The out-of-sync child*, New York, 1998, Perigee.

Larson E: The story of Maricela and Miguel: a narrative analysis of dimensions of adaptation, *Am J Occup Ther* 50:286, 1996.

Maurice C: *Behavioral intervention for young children with autism*, Austin, Tex, 1996, Pro-ed.

Siegel B: *The world of the autistic child*, New York, 1996, Oxford University Press.

Stancliff B: Autism: defining the OT's role in treating this confusing disorder, *OT Practice* 1:18, 1996.

Stancliff B: Understanding the "whoops" children, *OT Practice* 3:18, 1998.

REVIEW *Questions*

1. In what way does assessment of a child guide the OT practitioner in the processes of program planning and treatment implementation?
2. Define and differentiate among long-term goals, short-term objectives, and mini objectives.
3. What are the components of an activity analysis?
4. In what ways are activity analysis and adaptation used by the OT practitioner during program planning and treatment implementation?
5. What are the levels of performance?
6. Provide an example of using a top-down approach to OT intervention.

SUGGESTED *Activities*

1. Using the task-focused activity analysis form as a guide, analyze the specific daily routines that you personally perform, such as brushing your teeth, getting dressed, and preparing lunch.
2. Visit a daycare center or observe a neighbor's child performing specific tasks. Analyze what you observe using the task-focused activity analysis.
3. Choose an activity in which you typically engage and experiment by changing your position and the materials used for the activity. For example, eat a bowl of ice cream while sitting at the table and then do the same thing on your stomach in front of the television. Try different sizes of bowls and spoons. Write down how the change in your position or in the bowl and spoon made a difference in your performance.
4. Identify *at least* one long-term personal goal. Write short-term objectives about the way you plan on reaching your goal(s). Consider what methods you will use in attaining the objectives and ultimately your goal(s). The goal(s) should be attainable within 12 months. Use the RUMBA criteria when writing your goal(s).
5. Ask parents what they would like for their children in the near future. Write these as measurable goals. Describe the trends you observed and what you have learned that may help you in practice.

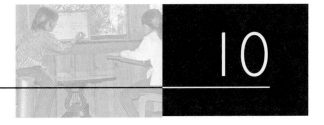

10

Introduction to Pediatric Health Conditions*

JEAN W. SOLOMON
JANE CLIFFORD O'BRIEN

CHAPTER *Objectives*

After studying this chapter, the reader will be able to accomplish the following:

- Describe the signs and symptoms of pediatric cardiopulmonary, musculoskeletal, and neuromuscular disorders
- Describe general intervention considerations for these conditions
- Describe the signs and symptoms of developmental disorders
- Describe general intervention considerations for developmental disorders
- Describe the signs and symptoms of genetic and chromosomal disorders, giving specific examples
- Describe the signs and symptoms of neoplastic disorders
- Describe the types of burns
- Describe the various ways to classify burns
- Describe/define obesity
- Describe general intervention considerations in the treatment and prevention of obesity
- Identify the role of team members in the intervention of pediatric conditions

*The section on developmental coordination disorder (DCD) was written as part of a doctoral dissertation. Special thanks go to Harriet Williams, PhD; Anita Bundy, ScD; Jim Lyons, PhD; and Bruce McClenaghan, PhD, for their assistance. The authors would like to acknowledge the children who participated in the study from Waterboro Elementary School; Saint Mary's School; Occupational Therapy Associates in Watertown, Mass; and the University of New England Community Occupational Therapy Clinic.

KEY TERMS

Cardiac disorders
Soft tissue injury
Contusion
Crush wound
Dislocation
Sprain
Fracture
Traumatic brain injury
Developmental disorder
Pervasive developmental disorder
Autism
Rett syndrome
Asperger syndrome
Attention deficit hyperactivity disorder
Developmental coordination disorder
Cri du chat syndrome
Fragile X syndrome
Prader-Willi syndrome
Leukemia
Burns
Obesity

CHAPTER OUTLINE

This chapter provides basic information about diseases that affect the mental and/or physical well-being of infants, children, and adolescents. Pediatric health conditions are categorized in a variety of ways, including congenital or acquired, acute or chronic, discrete or pervasive, and body system(s) affected.

The chapter is organized considering all of the categories. Congenital conditions are those diseases present at birth. Acquired conditions are those diseases or disorders that develop after birth and can be associated with trauma or accidents. Acute conditions are those diseases that have a rapid onset and last a relatively short time. Whereas the signs and symptoms of chronic conditions may gradually become apparent and last longer than 6 weeks, discrete conditions affect specific body functions and structures. Pervasive disorders are more diffuse, affecting numerous body functions and structures.

The body system diseases presented are divided into cardiopulmonary, musculoskeletal, and neuromuscular conditions. Potential pediatric team members are discussed throughout the chapter; a description of the team members is provided in Box 10-1. Specific examples of pediatric health conditions not otherwise discussed in this text are presented as examples for this chapter.

CARDIOPULMONARY SYSTEM

The cardiopulmonary system consists of the cardiac (heart and vessels) and respiratory (trachea, lungs, and diaphragm) systems, which are located in the thoracic area of the human body. The following health conditions affect the cardiac and respiratory body structures and consequently one's ability to participate fully in life's roles and occupations.

BOX 10-1

Potential Team Members

- Behavior specialist
- Cardiologist
- Cardiac surgeon
- Emergency medical technician
- Geneticist
- Neonatologist
- Neurologist
- Neuropsychologist
- Neurosurgeon
- Nurse
- Occupational therapist
- Occupational therapy assistant
- Orthopedist
- Orthopedic surgeon
- Orthotist
- Physical therapist
- Physical therapy assistant
- Prosthetist
- Psychologist
- Pulmonologist
- Respiratory therapist

The occupational therapy (OT) clinic receives a referral from a physician to evaluate and treat the feeding ability of a 7-month-old child on the pediatric cardiac unit. The child has undergone surgery to repair a heart defect. The registered occupational therapist (OTR) and certified occupational therapy assistant (COTA), who will be working together, study **cardiac disorders** so that they can be informed before evaluating the child. The following section provides an overview of cardiac disorders.

Cardiac Disorders

Cardiac disorders are conditions that involve the heart and/or vessels (Figure 10-1).

Congenital heart diseases and dysrhythmias are examples of pediatric cardiac health conditions. The referral of children who have cardiac disorders to the pediatric OT practitioner is typically based on secondary deficits associated with the child's primary diagnosis. Oral-motor and feeding issues or sensory processing problems may prompt a referral to a pediatric occupational therapist (Box 10-2).

Congenital heart disease

Most pediatric health conditions that involve the heart or major vessels are congenital. Cardiac health conditions can be serious and sometimes life threatening. The cause of most congenital cardiac health conditions is unknown. However, certain cardiac health conditions are associated with specific syndromes, especially with chromosomal disorders. Examples of congenital heart disorders include

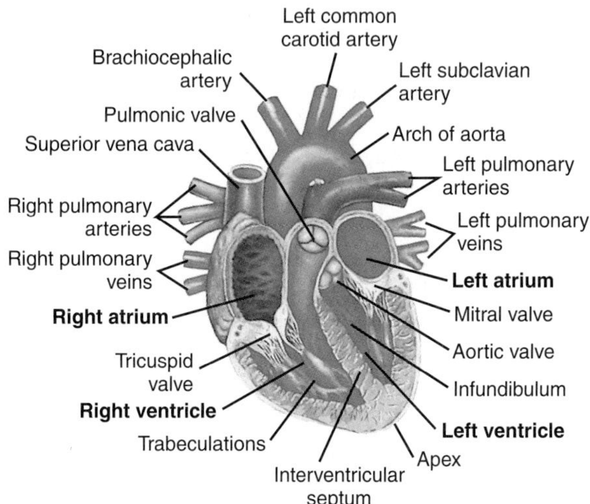

FIGURE 10-1 Frontal section of the heart. (From Canobbio MM: *Cardiovascular disorders*, St Louis, 1990, Mosby.)

BOX 10-2

Cardiopulmonary Disorders: General Signs and Symptoms

Decreased tolerance for exercise
Increased occurrence of respiratory infections
Shortness of breath
Decreased endurance
Small physical size for age
Cyanosis (bluish discoloration of skin and mucous membranes)
Poor distal circulation
Failure to thrive
Persistent cough or wheezing
Pain or discomfort in joints and muscles

atrial septal defects (ASDs), ventricular septal defects (VSDs), and tetralogy of Fallot (TOF).

Atrial septal defects

ASDs are abnormal openings between the atria of the heart. The severity of the signs and symptoms of an ASD is dependent on the size and location of the hole (Figure 10-2, *A*). Typically, the right side of the heart receives deoxygenated blood from the body structures to send to the lungs for oxygenation. When an ASD is present, there are increased amounts of oxygenated blood in the right side of the heart. The primary symptom of an ASD is a heart murmur. Unless the ASD is severe and life threatening, the preferred medical intervention is surgical repair during middle childhood.[3]

Ventricular septal defects

VSDs are the most common of the congenital heart diseases. The defect is an opening in the septum that separates the left and right ventricles of the heart (Figure 10-2, *B*). The opening permits oxygenated blood to flow into the right ventricle and then into the pulmonary artery and lungs. A small VSD will be asymptomatic and close spontaneously. A large VSD will require surgical repair during early childhood. Symptoms associated with a large VSD include irritability, poor weight gain, recurrent infections, and congestive heart failure.

Tetralogy of Fallot

The congenital heart disease known as TOF consists of four distinct defects observed in the heart and its associ-

CLINICAL *Pearl*

Older children who know that they have an ASD are likely to avoid exercise and activity because of fear and decreased endurance.

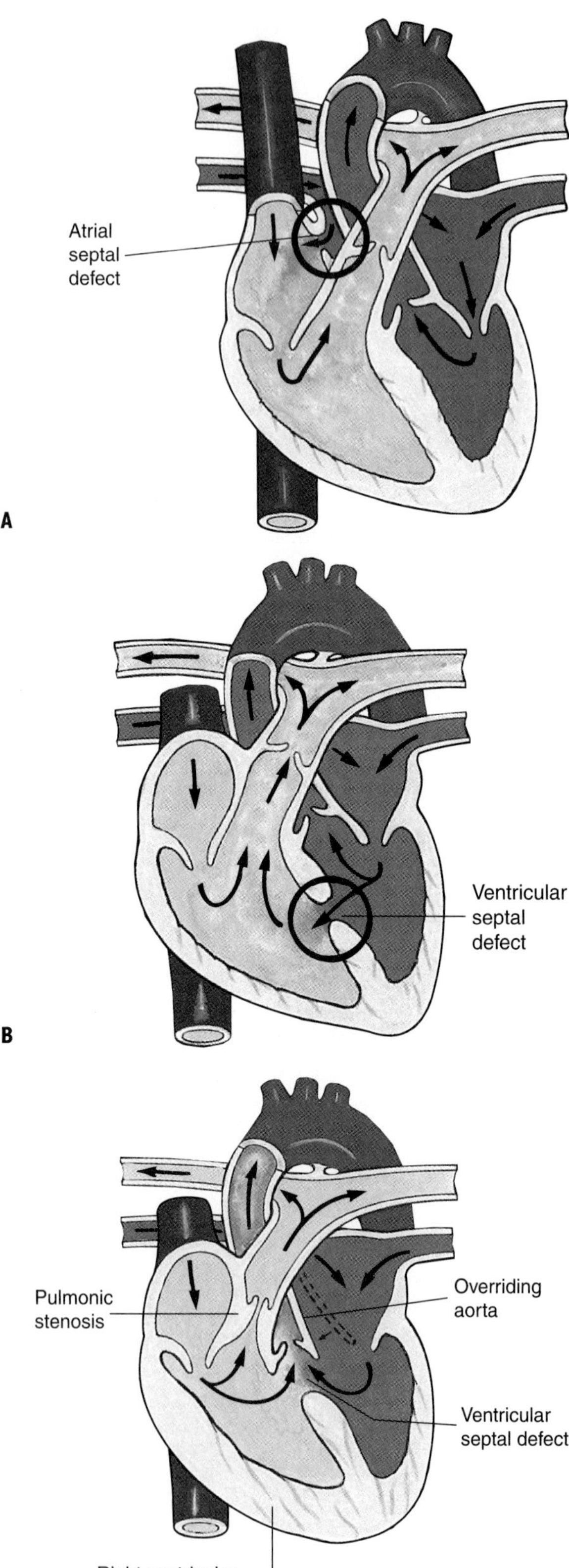

FIGURE 10-2 **A,** Atrial septal defect. **B,** Ventricular septal defect. **C,** Abnormally large right ventricle. (From Hockenberry MJ: *Wong's essentials of pediatric nursing*, ed 7, St Louis, 2005, Mosby.)

ated blood vessels. A VSD is present. There is misplacement of the aorta and narrowing of the pulmonary artery. The right ventricle is abnormally large (Figure 10-2, C). Collectively, these defects lead to decreased blood flow to the lungs. Symptoms of TOF include cyanosis (body structures turn blue), failure to thrive (difficulty with feeding and weight gain), and a heart murmur. Medical intervention involves surgical repair during the first year of life.[3]

Dysrhythmias

A normal heart has recurrent expansion and compression of the chest that maintains proper circulation of the blood and respiration, which together are known as cardiac rhythm. Dysrhythmias are irregular cardiac rhythms. Examples of dysrhythmias include bradydysrhythmia (an abnormally slow heartbeat) and tachydysrhythmia (an abnormally fast heartbeat).

Children with cardiac disorders may experience difficulty with strength (due to the lack of practice), endurance (due to a cardiac disorder), and/or pain or discomfort in the joints and muscles (due to the lack of use or decreased oxygen). These difficulties may result in impaired functioning in the areas of occupation, including difficulty with feeding, playing, education, social participation, play, and self-care (Table 10-1). OT intervention with infants, children, and adolescents who have cardiac disorders focuses on helping them gain strength and endurance for and tolerance to activity so that they may participate in these occupations. Because children with cardiac disorders may experience failure to thrive (secondary to poor endurance and/or inadequate oral-motor strength), intervention begins with providing compensatory techniques during feeding so that the child may be more successful. This may include adaptive nipples, holding the infant's cheeks to help him or her hold on to the bottle, and providing frequent breaks during feeding. OT practitioners may also focus therapy on improving the infant's ability to play for longer periods. Older children may benefit from compensatory techniques to conserve strength and endurance at home or school or during play. Those with cardiac disorders benefit from building endurance through short activity periods with frequent breaks and moving toward longer activity periods with fewer breaks. OT practitioners must be aware of signs of fatigue (e.g., bluish coloring, coughing, wheezing, shortness of breath).

Pulmonary Disorders

Pulmonary disorders are conditions that involve the lungs and one's ability to breathe. Examples of pediatric

TABLE 10-1

Cardiopulmonary Disorders: General Intervention Considerations

CONSIDERATION	DEFINITION AND EXAMPLE(S)
Breathing exercises	Exercises that promote optimum respiration rate by exerting the muscles involved in breathing, including the diaphragm and the oblique muscles
Relaxation techniques	Techniques such as controlled breathing to promote decreased heart rate, lower metabolism, and decreased respiration rate. Additional relaxation methods include visualization of pleasant experiences, yoga, exercises, and biofeedback.
Energy conservation techniques	Principles and methods that promote using the least amount of energy and movement to perform activities. Sitting rather than standing while making a sandwich is one example of an energy conservation technique.
Balance/pacing of activities	Principles and methods that promote equal consideration between work and rest.
Balanced diet	Eating and drinking food with nutritional value to promote physical health and well-being.
Avoidance of internal and environmental "triggers"	Attempting to lower exposure to internal (e.g., stress, lack of rest) and external (e.g., pollen, smoke, dust) stimuli that initiate a negative cardiopulmonary response
Strength and endurance activities	Techniques to increase the participation time in activities through increased repetition and decreased breaks
Emotional/psychosocial issues	Address child's self-concept, perception of their abilities, interests, etc. Help children gain an appreciation of their strengths

CLINICAL *Pearl*

Infants with cardiac disorders may not be able to hold a regular rattle. Pet shops have small, lightweight rattles that they can successfully hold. Practitioners may start with these rattles until the child builds up strength and endurance.

CLINICAL *Pearl*

Children who fail to thrive may benefit from high-calorie foods and drinks. Consultation with a dietitian or nutritionist is helpful in determining the appropriate food for infants and children.

pulmonary diseases include asthma and cystic fibrosis (CF). Children with these diagnoses are referred for OT when they experience problems that interfere with activities of daily living (ADLs), instrumental activities of daily living (IADLs), education, play, and social participation.

Asthma

Asthma is a chronic respiratory condition that is characterized by sudden, recurring attacks of labored breathing, chest constriction, and coughing. It is a reactive disease of the small-airway structures in the lungs. Environmental and internal stimuli can trigger an attack in a child or adolescent who has asthma. Examples of environmental triggers include changes in atmospheric pressure, cold air, and cigarette smoke. Examples of internal triggers are exercise and stress. During an asthma attack, the muscular walls of the airway structures undergo spasm and excessive amounts of mucous are secreted. These occurrences result in laborious breathing. Asthmatic children have described feeling as if they were drowning in their own saliva and unable to catch their breath. Most children and adolescents anticipate oncoming attacks and are able to prevent a trip to the emergency room or doctor by following previously prescribed intervention procedures. Medical intervention often involves inhalant and/or drug therapy.[6]

Cystic fibrosis

CF occurs primarily in Caucasians and is diagnosed during infancy or early childhood. It is an inherited (genetic) disease that affects exocrine (externally excreting) glands. The pancreas, respiratory system, and sweat glands are the organs most affected. The secretions from these glands are abnormally clammy or sticky. Symptoms of CF include frequent greasy stools, failure to thrive (problems in feeding and weight gain), frequent colds, and pneumonia with a chronic cough or wheezing. Chronic obstructive pulmonary disease (COPD) is the most serious complication of CF. Symptoms of COPD include wheezing, infections, and recurrent pneumothorax (partial collapse of a lobe of the lung).

Medical intervention for this pediatric health condition includes antibiotics for infections, inhalant therapy, and supplemental oxygen. Physical therapy may be required to assist with postural drainage and in turn decrease the excessive buildup of sticky mucous in the lungs.

CLINICAL *Pearl*

Children who have CF may benefit from swimming. Care should be taken to provide relaxing swim sessions while still challenging the child. Consultation with the physician and physical therapist is beneficial.

CLINICAL *Pearl*

As part of health management and maintenance, clinicians may help children and adolescents establish a routine for having an inhaler available as needed.

Hematologic Disorders

Hematologic disorders are conditions of the blood. Human blood is a fluid that consists of plasma, blood cells, and platelets. The purpose of blood is to carry nutrients and oxygen to the tissues of the body and to carry waste materials away from the tissues. Anemia is a pathological deficiency in the oxygen-carrying component of the blood, thus depriving body tissue of the necessary nutrients and oxygen. Anemia also leads to a buildup of waste products in human tissue.

Sickle cell anemia is one type that occurs in the black people of Africa or those of African descent. The red blood cells of an affected person are crescent shaped. It is characterized by exacerbation (flare-ups) and remission (lack of symptoms). During exacerbation the person who has sickle cell anemia may experience pain in the joints, fever, leg ulcers, and jaundice (Figure 10-3).

Depending on the severity of the disease, secondary complications might arise, including a hemorrhage or cerebrovascular accident (CVA). Discussions of CVA and other potential secondary complications of sickle cell anemia are beyond the scope of this text.

Children and adolescents who have sickle cell anemia may be referred for OT because of an inability to

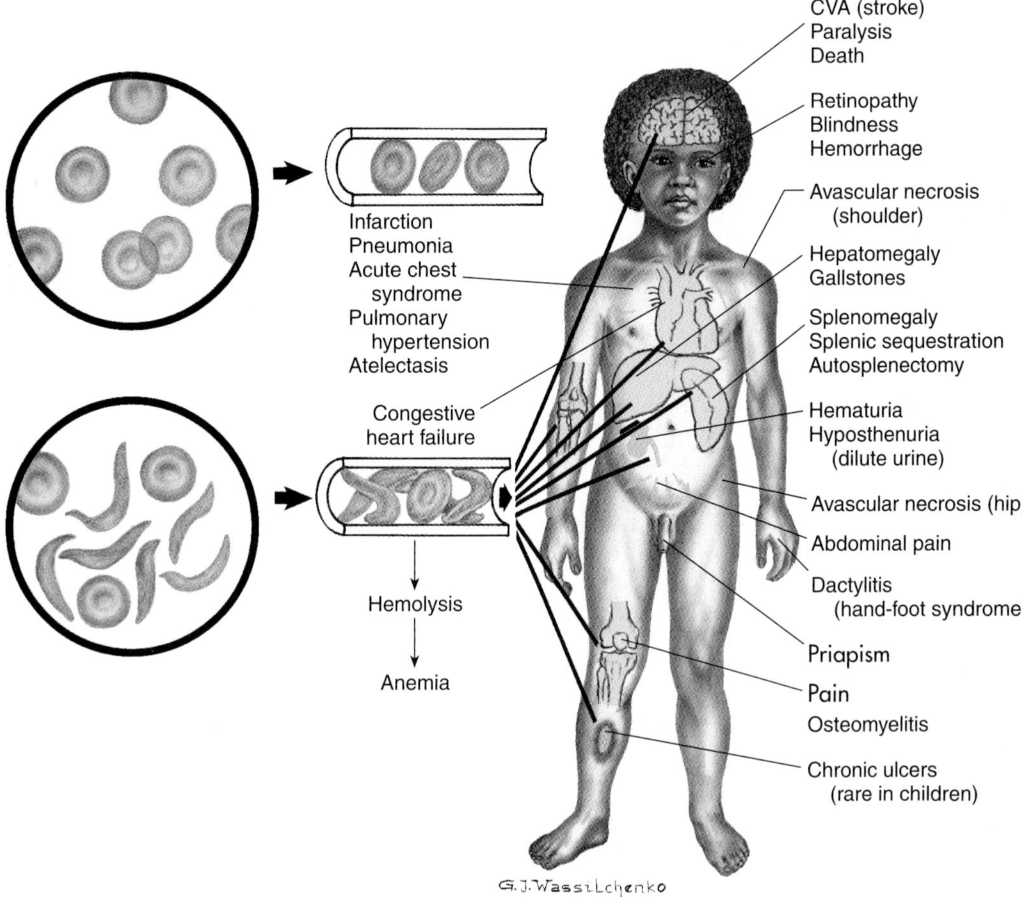

FIGURE 10-3 Sickle cell anemia. (From Hockenberry MJ: *Wong's essentials of pediatric nursing*, ed 7, St Louis, 2005, Mosby.)

function in ADLs, IADLs, education, play, and social participation resulting from pain in the joints. They may require assistance in organizing schoolwork because of missed school days resulting from exacerbation of the disease. Children and adolescents may benefit from energy conservation techniques to handle the flare-ups more efficiently. OT practitioners may provide adaptive positioning, night splints, and other assistive technology services and devices to help the child or adolescent through the flare-up periods. They may also benefit from support groups in order to cope with the impact of the disease on daily functioning.

CLINICAL *Pearl*

Practitioners working in school systems may solicit adolescent children with sickle cell anemia to lead support groups for the younger children. This helps the adolescent "give back" in a volunteer role that benefits all participants in the group.

MUSCULOSKELETAL SYSTEM

The musculoskeletal system comprises the skeletal and muscular systems. The skeletal system consists of bones, joints, cartilage, and ligaments. The muscular system consists of muscles and the fascia covering them. Tendons, which are bands of tough, inelastic fibrous tissue, connect muscles to bones. Muscles are activated by the nervous system and move bone(s) to create movement at a joint. Musculoskeletal disorders can be congenital (present at birth) or acquired. The discussion of musculoskeletal disorders is organized with consideration of whether the pediatric health condition is congenital or acquired.

Congenital Anomalies and Disorders

Congenital anomalies and disorders of the musculoskeletal system include osteogenesis imperfecta (brittle bones), achondroplasia (dwarfism), arthrogryposis multiplex congenita, and congenital hip dislocation (dysplasia of the hip at birth). Additional information on osteogenesis imperfecta and arthrogryposis can be found in Chapter 15.

Achondroplasia

Achondroplasia, or dwarfism, is a pathological condition of arrested or stunted growth. It is a disorder of the growth cartilage. The onset of this pediatric health condition is during fetal development. Typical physical features include a large, protruding forehead and short, thick arms and legs on a relatively normal trunk. Occasionally, medical intervention might include orthopedic surgery.

Congenital dysplasia of the hip

The causes of congenital dysplasia, or dislocation of the hip, can be genetic or environmental. Instability of one or both of the hip joints may be inherited. Sudden passive stretching of an unstable hip or prolonged time in a position that makes the hip vulnerable may cause a dislocation.[9,23]

Medical intervention at an early age is critical to prevent permanent physical or body structure damage. Surgical intervention may be necessary. However, less invasive procedures, such as bracing and casting, may promote proper hip alignment and stability. For additional information regarding orthotics and prosthetics, see Chapter 23.

Acquired Musculoskeletal Disorders

Acquired musculoskeletal disorders are conditions that are not present at birth and involve injury or trauma to the skeletal and/or muscular systems. A general discussion of soft tissue injuries and fractures follows. Soft tissue injuries and fractures can be considered orthopedic conditions that require the attention of an orthopedist, a medical doctor who specializes in diseases of the musculoskeletal system.

Soft tissue injury

A **soft tissue injury** is damage to muscle, nerves, skin, and/or connective tissue. Children and adolescents are subject to soft tissue injuries because of their active lifestyles. Types of soft tissue injury include contusions, crush injuries, dislocations, and sprains.

A **contusion** is an injury that does not disrupt the integrity of the skin and is characterized by swelling, discoloration, and pain. Children and adolescents experience bumps and bruises throughout their developing years. In the absence of any secondary or complicating health conditions, contusions heal with time and do not require medical or therapeutic intervention.

A **crush wound** or injury is a break in the external surface of the bone caused by severe force applied against tissues (e.g., a finger caught in a door). This type of injury may require medical and OT intervention if alignment and immobility are necessary for the injury to heal. Crush injuries that could have benefited from medical attention but did not receive it may result in permanent deformity and pain of the joint(s) involved. The permanent misalignment of a body structure may have functional implications in later life.

A **dislocation** is the displacement of a bone from its normal position, especially from its normal articulation at a joint. Dislocations of the shoulder and hip joints are frequently seen in infants and young children. The shoulder and hip joints are particularly vulnerable because both are freely movable. The shallowness of the shoulder joint increases the likelihood of dislocation occurring at this body structure.

A **sprain** is a traumatic injury to tendons, muscle, or ligaments around a joint and is characterized by pain, swelling, and discoloration. In children and adolescents, a sprain can occur when they lose their balance and consequently use a protective response that makes the wrist and ankle the most vulnerable joints for injury. Sprains are most frequently seen in the ankles and wrists. Most do not require emergency medical attention or therapeutic intervention.

CLINICAL *Pearl*

Immediately apply ice to a soft tissue injury for a minimum of 20 minutes or until the area is numb. The application of ice will reduce swelling at the involved site and relieve pain.

Fractures

Fractures are breaks, ruptures, or cracks in bone or cartilage. They may be defined in a variety of ways. They may be closed or open. A closed fracture is one in which there are no open wounds from the penetration of the skin. An open fracture involves an open wound, with complications being more common. Fractures are frequent in children and adolescents. They require immediate realignment as the first medical intervention. Next, immobilization is necessary to allow the bone(s) to heal. Immobilization may require casts, splints, pins, or other external fixations.

BOX 10-3

Musculoskeletal Disorders: Signs and Symptoms

Misalignment of joints
Swelling
Pain
Warmth to touch
Immobility
Discoloration (redness, blueness, whiteness)

TABLE 10-2

Musculoskeletal Disorders: General Intervention Considerations

CONSIDERATION	DEFINITION AND EXAMPLE(S)
Promote proper joint alignment	Through statics (nonmovement) and dynamics (movement), facilitates the typical alignment of muscles and joints. (Note: In the absence of soft tissue contracture and/or bony deformities)
Apply modalities such as ice or moist heat	Placing a moist heat pack or ice pack on the inflamed area
Immobilize with a cast or splint	Keeping the involved area in proper alignment
Instruct in proper positioning to reduce edema or swelling	Elevating the involved/inflamed area to increase flow of body fluids back to the trunk
Compensation	Helps child engage in occupations through changing the ways or techniques used to participate
Modification/adaptation	Helps child participate in occupations by changing how the activities are performed.
Emotional/psychosocial	Addresses emotional/psychosocial issues associated with disorders. Children may need to work on developing a positive self-concept, body awareness, and sense of control.
Social participation	Promotes social participation in children

Children with musculoskeletal disorders may exhibit difficulty performing ADLs, IADLs, education, play, or social participation because of improper joint alignment (Box 10-3). For example, children with achondroplasia often have difficulty grasping and manipulating objects due to short but large hands. They benefit from practice, modification, and adaptation (Table 10-2). They may need work space modifications (e.g., shorter chair). Furthermore, their physical stature may interfere with play. Clinicians can help children engage in play more easily and consequently enhance social participation. Practitioners may design splints to help with the alignment of joints. Clinicians frequently consult with orthopedists to provide information on the functional outcome of the splint or procedure.

NEUROMUSCULAR DISORDERS

The neuromuscular system includes the nervous system and the muscles of the human body. The nervous system can be subdivided into the peripheral and central nervous systems. The central nervous system (CNS) includes the brain and spinal cord. The peripheral nervous system (PNS) consists of the nerves that originate from the spinal cord and innervate the muscles of the neck, trunk, arms, and legs. An example of a pediatric health condition that affects the CNS is a traumatic brain injury. Discussions of other neuromuscular disorders can be found in subsequent chapters.

Traumatic Brain Injury

A traumatic brain injury (TBI) is a serious injury to the brain. It is also known as a closed head injury (CHI) or head injury (HI). Trauma is the leading cause of health disorders and deaths in the pediatric population.[9,21] This type of brain injury results from damage to the CNS as a result of forces coming into contact with the skull. Damage to the nerve tissue occurs both during and after the immediate trauma.[9] Medical intervention depends on the severity of the head trauma and the presenting signs and symptoms.

Children and adolescents with TBIs are referred for OT because of an inability to function in the areas of occupation (ADLs, IADLs, education, work, play, and social participation) (Box 10-4). The trauma to the brain typically results in motor, cognitive, and emotional changes. Motor deficits may include abnormal muscle

BOX 10-4

Neuromuscular Disorders: Signs and Symptoms of Traumatic Brain Injury

Loss of consciousness
Lethargy
Vomiting
Irritability
Motor: loss of balance, abnormal muscle tone, weakness
Processing, memory loss
Communication/interaction impairments: slurred and/or slowed speech, word-finding problems
Severe headache
Confusion

Data from Case-Smith J: *Occupational therapy for children*, ed 5, St Louis, 2005, Mosby.

TABLE 10-3

Neuromuscular Disorders: General Intervention Considerations (Traumatic Brain Injury)

CONSIDERATION	DEFINITION AND EXAMPLE(S)
Preparatory activities	Prepare the child for activities by making him or her more ready to interact with the environment. "Normalize" sensory awareness/response and muscle tone. Child participates in sensory games, rubbing arms with different textures, and awareness activities.
Enabling activities	Build up skills needed for engagement in occupations (e.g., arm strength, visual attention, memory). Examples include weight-bearing and -shifting activities and development of arm strength through repetitive activities (e.g., weight training, lifting plates, picking up laundry).
Purposeful activities and occupations	Facilitate performing the actual occupation or activity in an environment closest to the natural one. Examples include unbuttoning shirt in preparation for PM shower and preparing lunch at the clinic.

tone (changes in the resting state of a muscle typically resulting in increased muscle tone), hemiplegia (involvement of the arm and leg on one side of the body), and quadriplegia (involvement of both arms and legs) (Table 10-3). As the swelling of brain begins to heal, some of the deficits may improve. Children and adolescents may need to relearn motor patterns. They may require splinting of the extremities to maintain and improve the range of motion (ROM). OT practitioners work to retrain the movements of children and adolescents who have sustained TBIs. OT practitioners address cognitive changes such as loss of memory, word-finding problems, and poor abstract thought and reasoning. Children and adolescents may experience perceptual deficits that include being unaware of their surroundings, poor sequencing, and timing skills. The emotional changes may include lability (moods ranging from happy to tearful or angry), inappropriateness (e.g., cursing, touching, disrobing), and personality changes. Children and adolescents who have had a TBI may demonstrate a "flat" affect, showing little or no emotion. The stages of recovery may include periods of aggressiveness and irritability.

OT practitioners working with children and adolescents who have had a TBI work closely with their parents and a team of professionals (speech and language pathologists, physical therapists, a rehabilitation specialist, a physiatrist, nurses, psychologists, and teachers). The OT practitioner is a key player on this team and has the responsibility of addressing the child's ability to function in everyday occupations.

CLINICAL *Pearl*

Muscle tone in a child or adolescent who has sustained a traumatic brain injury is different than that of a child who has cerebral palsy. The abnormally high tone is more resistant to handling and inhibitory techniques.

CLINICAL *Pearl*

Cotreatment (combining OT and physical therapy services into one session) is an effective intervention strategy while working with larger children. Incorporating the child's total body structure (i.e., the trunk, arms, and legs) into the therapy session is more successful with two practitioners involved.

DEVELOPMENTAL DISORDERS

A **developmental disorder** is a mental and/or physical disability that arises before adulthood and lasts throughout a person's life. **Pervasive developmental disorders** (PDDs) constitute a group of pediatric health conditions affecting a variety of body functions and structures with a wide range of severity. Autism is the most well known of the PDDs. Other examples include Rett syndrome, Asperger syndrome, attention deficit hyperactivity disorder (ADHD), and **developmental coordination disorder** (DCD) (Box 10-5).

BOX 10-5

Developmental Disorders: Signs and Symptoms

- Delays in motor, processing, and communication/interaction skills
- Impaired body functions
- Limited repertoire of behavior
- Stereotypical behaviors present
- Decreased attention to purposeful activities and occupations
- Children not reaching milestones
- Infants showing decreased exploration and interest in environment

Autism

Autism is characterized by severe and complex impairments in reciprocal social interaction, communication skills, and the presence of stereotypical behavior, interests, and activities.[2]

The Centers for Disease Control[10] estimates that four times as many boys as girls are diagnosed as having autism. Children who are autistic come from all racial, ethnic, intellectual, and socioeconomic backgrounds.[9] Autism affects a child's ability to participate in occupations at home and in the community. The behavioral characteristics of autism that are critical to its diagnosis are presented here.[2]

- Disturbances in social interaction that affect the child's ability to meaningfully interact with people and inanimate objects
- Disturbances in communication that may be mild to severe, with mild being minor disarticulation and severe being the absence of meaningful speech
- Disturbances of behavior reflective of intolerance by resistance to change, stereotypical behavior, and bizarre attachments to objects
- Disturbances of sensory and perceptual processing and associated impairments; problems of sensory and perceptual processing that may be either registration (acknowledge/orient to sensation) or modulation (control over input)

Children with autism present with a variety of symptoms that range in severity for each individual child. While therapy for each child varies, certain considerations may benefit those with autism (Box 10-6). Children with autism require a structured environment with clear expectations. Behavior management programs using positive reinforcers (such as the use of stickers) work well. OT practitioners working with children who have autism must be able to read verbal and nonverbal cues quickly. Since these children have difficulty expressing themselves verbally, they may experience frustration when the clinician does not "listen" to them. This may cause them to escalate poor or acting-out behavior.

Children who have autism experience difficulty processing sensory information and thus benefit from a sensory integration approach (see Chapter 21). OT practitioners will need to carefully monitor the child's reaction to activities; it may be difficult for the child to pick the activities. Therefore, asking an autistic child to choose between two activities helps facilitate decision making.

Communication with children who have autism may include simple signs, verbal expressions, demonstrations, pictures, and communication systems. OT practitioners will need to consult with the speech/language therapists, teachers, parents, and other professionals to determine the most effective way(s) to communicate.

BOX 10-6

General Intervention Techniques for Children with Autism

Provide structure and consistency.
Keep the same routine.
Read child's nonverbal and verbal cues.
Communicate through signs, pictures, communication boards, and/or singing.
Work with child at his or her level.
Follow the child's cues.
Redirect when child begins self-stimulation.
Listen to parent(s) for child's preferences.
Provide a quiet setting.
Allow child to play with other children.
Use positive behavioral reinforcers.
Use sensory integration techniques.

- Tactile
- Vestibular
- Proprioceptive
- Olfactory
- Gustatory (Children with autism may enjoy very spicy or sour tastes instead of bland tastes.)

Provide child with choices (may have to start with only two).
Allow child time to respond.
Keep talking to a minimum—use simple directions.
Use behavioral management techniques.
Realize children will have "off days" (may have to change the plan).
Realize practitioners will have "off days"—spend some time thinking about what could have been done differently.
Listen to the parents!
Work on occupation-centered goals so that therapy is meaningful to the child and family.

OT practitioners work with autistic children to improve their ability to participate in ADLs, IADLs, education, work, play, and social participation. Since children with autism typically experience deficits in all of these areas, the clinician must prioritize and identify meaningful goals. These goals are the most effectively developed by collaborating with the parents and/or teacher. For example, holding a spoon during mealtime is easily understood as addressing feeding goals. It is harder for parents and/or teachers to understand how grasping a cube will help with feeding.

Rett Syndrome

Rett syndrome is a progressive neurological disorder occurring exclusively in females. The infant and toddler seem to be developing normally until 6 to 18 months of age, at which time regression in all skills is observed.

Microencephaly, seizures, abnormal muscle tone, mental retardation, and stereotypical patterns of behavior (especially hand wriggling) emerge. Adolescents who have Rett syndrome are generally nonambulatory and do not have functional hand use.

Asperger Syndrome

Asperger syndrome (previously considered a type of autism) is characterized by deficits in social interaction without a significant delay in communication skills. Children who have Asperger syndrome exhibit restrictive, repetitive patterns of behavior, interest, and activity. However, those with this syndrome tend to have age-appropriate cognitive and self-help skills.

Attention Deficit Hyperactivity Disorder

ADHD is the most common neurobehavioral disorder. It occurs in males three times more often than in females. Children who have ADHD have difficulty with attention, hyperactivity, distractibility, and impulsivity. Other features include sleep disorders, emotional lability, poor self-esteem, and poor frustration tolerance.[9]

Children with this disorder benefit from organization and structure. Clinicians and psychologists can provide parents with strategies and/or techniques to help their children with behavior problems. OT practitioners can provide sensory strategies that help these children relax and concentrate. Physical activity may help them modulate their behaviors and pay attention more effectively in class. In fact, some schools encourage walking programs before the start of classes.

Developmental Coordination Disorder

DCD encompasses a wide range of characteristics, the essential feature of which is that the children's motor coordination is markedly below their chronological age and intellectual ability and significantly interferes with ADLs.[2] The diagnosis of DCD cannot be the result of physical, sensory, or neurological impairments.[11,15,17] In addition, children are diagnosed with DCD only if the criteria for PDDs are not met.[2] If mental retardation is present, the motor difficulties must be in excess of those usually associated with the level of severity of mental retardation.

Children with DCD have difficulty forming letters quickly and precisely; this is often manifested in an inability to keep up with classmates and complete assignments efficiently.[15,22] For example, a child may be able to complete only one simple sentence in the time allotted, while other children are able to complete full paragraphs. The extra energy and time that children with DCD spend on the mechanics of writing often interfere with their ability to manage other classroom tasks. They take longer and are less efficient in carrying out everyday self-care tasks, which include such things as brushing the teeth and getting dressed. Tasks that other children accomplish easily (e.g., fastening clothing, tying shoes, or organizing homework) may be problematic for a child who has DCD.[19] These children also often exhibit low self-esteem, show frustration, and begin to expect failure.[13] Feelings of low self-esteem develop as early as 6 years of age,[24] a time when children experience difficulty keeping up with their peers and struggle with sports and play activities. The feelings associated with low perception of physical competence and inadequacy in performing tasks that other children take for granted can and often do result in emotional problems.[18,22,24,26]

Many professionals suggest that they will outgrow these coordination deficits, but evidence indicates that children who have DCD continue to have difficulty in adolescence and adulthood.[20,25] Losse et al[20] followed a group of children for 10 years and reported significant differences in verbal IQ, performance IQ, and academic performance between children with DCD and their peers. Those who had DCD experienced more behavioral problems, had more difficulty with handwriting in art design and technology, demonstrated trouble with home economics, and exhibited lower performance in practical science lessons.

The motor deficits exhibited by children with DCD are many and varied. Among other things, they exhibit poor balance, postural control, and coordination and are more variable in their motor responses.[16,28] Timing and sequencing deficits and slower movement times have also been reported for children who have DCD.[14,28] These children tend to rely more on visual than proprioceptive information, fail to anticipate or use perceptual information, and do not use appropriate rehearsal strategies.[12,27] This in turn impairs quality of movement, especially in situations in which the child has to react to a changing environment.

CLINICAL *Pearl*

Children who have sensory processing deficits may experience the signs and symptoms of ADHD. OT practitioners can provide sensory strategies and intervention that may help children modulate their attention and function within the home and classroom. Diet may also cause ADHD behaviors (although this has not been proven; ask any parent). Overstimulating or anxious environments may cause children to exhibit the behaviors of ADHD. Those experiencing emotional trauma may exhibit the signs of ADHD.

TABLE 10-4

Developmental Disorders: General Intervention Considerations

CONSIDERATION	DEFINITION AND EXAMPLE(S)
Behavior management programs	Programs to promote appropriate daily actions by identifying target behaviors, establishing positive reinforcers, and implementing a behavioral plan and follow-up with data collection
Structured environment	Sets up clear routines with consistency to allow child to understand and practice daily occupations
Total communication approach	Uses a variety of systems to relate to child, such as a communication board, sign language, verbal language, pointing/gesturing, and facilitative communication
Sensory integration intervention	Uses suspended equipment to provide a controlled sensory input so that the child can make an adaptive response. SI theory postulates that this will help with CNS development.
Practice occupations	Repeat skills and occupations such as using backward or forward chaining. Children learn through repetition.
Teach and repeat	Simplify occupations to allow child to participate and increase ability to reach milestones
Education	Teaches child how to perform occupations Educates parents, teachers, and others about child's condition and techniques to support child's occupations
Promote interests	Provides novelty to promote interests and exploration
Emotional/psychosocial issues	Address child's self-concept, self-awareness, and body awareness by providing opportunities for exploration and success

CNS, Central nervous system; *SI,* sensory integration.

According to sensory integration theory, the primary basis for the poor motor performance of children with DCD lies in the central processing of information related to the planning, selecting, and timing of movement. These children have been shown to have difficulty processing tactile, vestibular, and proprioceptive information.[4,5,8]

The treatment of children with DCD may follow a motor control (see Chapter 20) or sensory integration (see Chapter 21) approach (Table 10-4).

BOX 10-7

Genetic and Chromosomal Disorders: Signs and Symptoms

- Microencephaly
- Impaired cognitive development
- Unusual or excessive eating habits/patterns
- Small body structure
- Congenital anomalies
- Facial features characteristic of syndrome
- Simian crease in hands (characteristic of Down syndrome)
- Failure to thrive
- Developmental delays

GENETIC AND CHROMOSOMAL DISORDERS

Genetic and chromosomal disorders are inherited pediatric health conditions secondary to a change in the genetic makeup of the fetus. Because there are so many genes (23 pairs of chromosomes per cell multiplied by 250 to 2000 genes per chromosome), genetic disorders occur. Examples of genetic and chromosomal disorders include Cri du chat, fragile X, and Prader-Willi syndromes. Additional genetic and chromosomal disorders are discussed in subsequent chapters (Box 10-7).

Cri du Chat Syndrome

Cri du chat syndrome (cry of the cat) is a rare genetic condition caused by the absence of part of chromosome 5. The baby and young child with this genetic disorder have a weak, mewing cry. Classic body features documented in children who have cri du chat syndrome include microencephaly; widely spaced, down-slanting eyes; cardiopulmonary abnormalities; and failure to thrive.[7]

Fragile X Syndrome

Fragile X syndrome is a prevalent genetic health disorder. Boys are affected more often than girls. Body functions

CLINICAL *Pearl*

During my clinical practice, I worked with two children who had the medical diagnosis of cri du chat syndrome. Both of them tended to have low muscle tone, feeding issues, behavioral problems, and significant cognitive limitations.

such as brain development and body structures such as the skull, joints, and feet are affected. Classic structural features include elongated faces, prominent jaws and foreheads, hypermobile or lax joints, and flat feet. Children who have fragile X syndrome may be mentally retarded.

Prader-Willi Syndrome

Prader-Willi syndrome is a genetic health disorder that involves chromosome 15. Children and adolescents who have Prader-Willi syndrome exhibit varying degrees of mental retardation, overeating habits, and self-mutilating behaviors such as picking sores until they bleed or biting their fists until large calluses develop.

OT practitioners working with children with genetic or chromosomal disorders address the occupational performance of children (Table 10-5). For example, children with fragile X syndrome may have intellectual disabilities and thus will require assistance to develop ADL skills. These requirements include adaptation to be independent, structure to engage in leisure activities, and training to participate in work. Children and adolescents with Prader-Willi syndrome require intervention for social participation because picking sores and overeating are not socially acceptable behaviors. OT practitioners may provide the families of these children with strategies to help their children function to their maximum potential.

NEOPLASTIC DISORDERS

A neoplasm is an abnormal new growth of tissue (a tumor). It may be localized (in one place) or invasive (in multiple tissues and organs). It may be benign (not immediately life threatening) or malignant (possibly cause death). Tumors are named for location, type of cellular makeup, or the person who first identified it.[3]

Leukemia

Leukemia comprises a group of pediatric health conditions involving various acute and chronic tumor dis-

CLINICAL *Pearl*

To avoid excessive weight gain and obesity in children and adolescents who have Prader-Willi syndrome, a strict diet and eating schedule must be established and maintained.

TABLE 10-5

Genetic and Chromosomal Disorders: General Intervention Considerations

CONSIDERATION	DEFINITION AND EXAMPLE(S)
Failure to thrive	Many genetic disorders have associated feeding difficulties. These may be due to motor, cognitive, or structural functions. The OT practitioner should evaluate and treat them through training, compensation, adaptive technology, or remediation.
Developmental delays	Many genetic disorders have associated delays in motor, social, language, and self-care skills. OT practitioners can help children learn the skills needed for their occupations through intervention.
Cognitive delays	Lower cognitive abilities are frequently a part of genetic disorders. Children may learn skills at a slower rate and may show difficulty in problem solving and with abstract thought and reasoning. Practicing occupations in a variety of contexts helps children generalize skills.
Congenital anomalies	Children with genetic disorders may exhibit certain physical features (short stature, flat hand arches) which interfere with motor skills. OT practitioners can help them compensate or adapt to perform occupations.
Psychosocial/emotional issues	Children with genetic disorders also experience a range of emotional and psychological issues. OT practitioners can help them cope with everyday situations, deal with periods of stress, adapt to life changes, and work with their strengths.
Social participation/ behaviors	OT practitioners work with children, families, and communities to help the children engage in occupations. Children with all levels of ability benefit from social participation. OT practitioners can assist them in fitting into groups by helping them develop socially appropriate behaviors.

OT, Occupational therapy.

BOX 10-8

Neoplastic Disorders: General Signs and Symptoms

Loss of weight
Night sweats
Chronic fatigue
Recurrent headaches
Vomiting
Changes in behavior
Pain
Lumps
Misalignment of bones or joints
Evident growths on bone

orders of the bone marrow. A child or adolescent who has leukemia may experience an abnormal increase in white blood cells; enlargement of the lymph nodes, liver, and spleen; and impaired blood clotting. These body function deficits can cause pain, fatigue, weight loss, recurrent infection, excessive bruising, and/or hemorrhaging (Box 10-8). Medical intervention may include antibiotics, chemotherapy, and blood transfusion. Referral to an occupational therapist is made because of secondary disorders and/or complications.

Tumors of the Central Nervous System

Tumors of the CNS (i.e., those located in the brain and/or spinal cord) are the most common ones of solid tissue in children and adolescents.[9] The causes of CNS tumors are unknown. Medical intervention varies with the differential diagnosis.

Bone Cancer and Tumors

Primary (first to develop) bone tumors are rare during childhood, with the incidence peaking during adolescence. Most bone cancer results from metastasizing or spreading to bone from the primary tumor(s) located in a different body structure. Medical intervention may include surgery and radiotherapy.

Children with neoplastic disorders may require OT intervention to catch up in school after missing many days due to surgery or other medical interventions (Table 10-6). Children may experience physical symptoms and require OT intervention on compensatory strategies. OT practitioners may address the emotional needs of children and their families by instituting play therapy.

OTHER PEDIATRIC HEALTH CONDITIONS

Two significant pediatric health conditions not discussed anywhere else in the text are burns and obesity. OT practitioners working with children must understand the signs, symptoms, and intervention considerations corresponding to these health conditions.

Burns

Burns account for a large number of children and adolescents who must undergo prolonged, painful hospitalization.

TABLE 10-6

Neoplastic Conditions: General Intervention Considerations

CONSIDERATION	DEFINITION AND EXAMPLE(S)
Energy conservation	Children may benefit from learning ways to perform occupations with less physical stress. For example, sitting down while getting ready for school conserves energy.
Compensation techniques	Children may experience physical symptoms and require strategies to perform everyday tasks (e.g., using the left hand instead of the right for eating).
Psychosocial/emotional issues	Children may miss school and feel "left out." They may experience the full range of emotions and stress of a life-threatening illness. Families may be in turmoil over the illness. Children may feel alone and require intervention to help them deal with the illness so that they may engage in their occupations.
Adaptive equipment	Adaptive equipment may be recommended to assist children in their occupations. For example, young children may benefit from a bath seat to make positioning during bath time easier for the caregiver.
Engagement in occupations	Children may feel "left out" of regular activities and require participation in occupations to regain a sense of being. OT practitioners help children return to school, home, and play activities through education, assistive technology, and compensation techniques.

OT, Occupational therapy.

They are caused by accidents involving the use of thermal, electrical, chemical, and radioactive agents.

A thermal burn is caused by hot objects or flames, such as heat from an open fire, an iron, stove, or the tip of a cigarette. An electrical burn results from skin or other body tissue coming into contact with electricity, such as lightning or a direct electrical current coming from an outlet or plug. A chemical burn is caused by a chemical substance such as acid or some other poison (i.e., something or some substance that is destructive or fatal). A radioactive burn is caused by rays or waves of radiation that come into contact with body tissue.

Thermal burns are the most common of the four types.[9] There are specific criteria that determine the severity of a burn and the prognosis for recovery. The percentage of body area burned is assessed according to the total body surface area (TBSA) by the rule of nines in children older than 10. In the rule of nines, 9% is assigned to the head and both arms, 18% to each leg, 18% to both the anterior (front) and posterior (back) of the trunk, and 1% to the perineum. The formula is modified for infants and young children because of their proportionately larger head size. (See Figure 10-4 for the percentage of distribution per area of the body.)

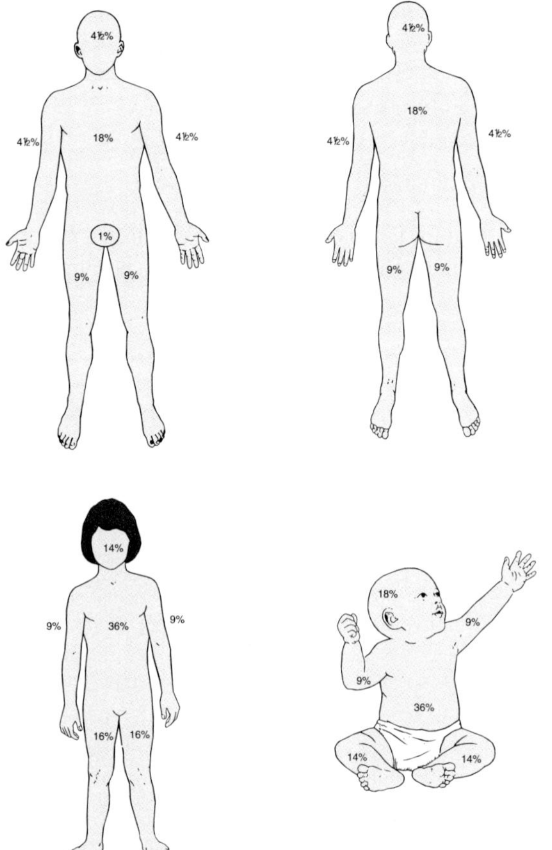

FIGURE 10-4 Percentage of distribution per area of the body. (From *Mosby's medical, nursing, and allied health dictionary,* ed 6, St Louis, 2002, Mosby.)

The American Burn Association[1] also classifies burns as minor, moderate, and severe. In minor burns, less than 10% of the TBSA is covered with a partial-thickness burn; these burns are adequately treated on an outpatient basis. A moderate burn is considered 10% to 20% of the TBSA covered with a partial-thickness burn; it requires hospitalization. A major burn is considered any full-thickness burn or greater than 20% of the TBSA covered with a partial-thickness burn.[1,9]

The depth of a burn is assessed according to the number of layers of tissue involved in the injury (Figure 10-5). Superficial or first-degree burns damage tissue minimally and heal without scarring. Second-degree burns are partial thickness burns and involve the epidermis and portions of the dermis. Although second-degree burns will heal, the process can be painful and scarring may be a result. Deep-thickness burns can be third- or fourth-degree (involving muscle) burns and require emergency and ongoing medical intervention. During the acute medical management of a child or adolescent who has been seriously burned, the prevention of secondary infections, wound débridement (cleaning), and wound closure are critical. During the rehabilitative phase of intervention, team members work closely to accomplish the outcomes of healing of the body structures involved, correction of cosmetic damage, reduction and management of scar tissue, restoration of function, and integration back into the child's or adolescent's natural environment (Table 10-7).

Clinicians working with child and adolescent burn victims begin by working on providing splints to keep the limb immobile for healing and later to facilitate function. OT practitioners work closely with physical therapists on débridement and pain management techniques. OT practitioners can help children and adolescents with burns compensate for physical limitations, or they may help them gain physical skills again. Facilitating play/leisure activities helps children and adolescents release emotions and return to childhood occupations. OT practitioners may address their psychological concerns through play, self-concept activities, and discussion. Practitioners help children and adolescents learn, through participating in everyday occupations, how they may function despite the burns.

Obesity

Obesity is excessively increased body weight caused by an accumulation of adipose tissue or fat. A child's age, sex, and height must be considered relative to his or her body weight. Although childhood obesity is associated with certain pediatric health conditions, the leading causes of this condition are changeable. The three primary

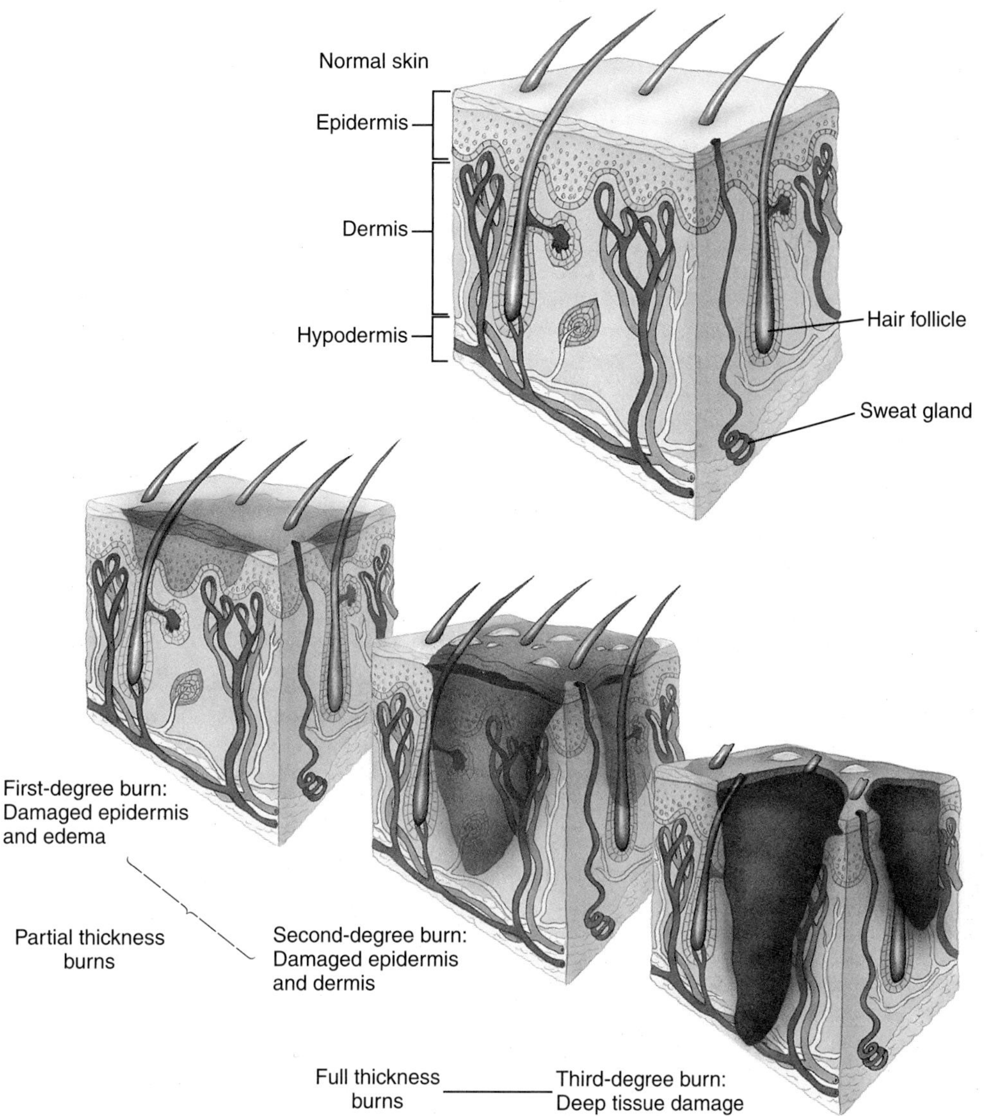

FIGURE 10-5 Classification of burns. (From Thibodeau GA, Patton KT: *Anatomy and physiology*, ed 5, St Louis, 2003, Mosby.)

TABLE 10-7

Burns: General Intervention Considerations

CONSIDERATION	DEFINITION AND EXAMPLE(S)
Positioning and splinting	Splint in functional position to initially aid in healing and later splint to increase function
ROM	Passive and active ROM techniques are used to promote functional range.
Engagement in occupations	Provides remediation, adaptation, and modification so that child may participate in occupations
Social participation	Helps child return to social situations
Scar tissue management	Splinting, desensitization techniques, and pressure garments are used to decrease scarring.
Edema management	Retrograde massage, gentle ranging, and elevation may help manage edema.
Self-concept	Participation in occupations enables child to develop positive self-concept.
Psychological/emotional issues	Provide a range of activities to help child work through emotional issues associated with burns. Children who have burns may experience difficulty with body image.

ROM, Range of motion.

BOX 10-9

Childhood Obesity and Associated Juvenile Diabetes: Signs and Symptoms

Frequent urination
Profuse sweating
Weight loss or gain
Excessive, uncontrolled eating
Recurrent infections
Excessive sugar in blood or urine
Shortness of breath
Poor endurance
Painful hips and knee joints

$$BMI = \frac{\text{Weight (kg)}}{\text{Height (m}^2\text{)}}$$

Body mass index assessment	
19-25	Appropriate weight (19-34 years)
21-27	Appropriate weight (>34 years)
27.5-30	Mild obesity
30-40	Moderate obesity
>40	Morbid obesity

FIGURE 10-6 Calculation of body mass index. (From Thompson JM, Wilson SF: *Health assessment for nursing practice*, St Louis, 1996, Mosby.)

causes of obesity are excessive eating, inadequate exercise, and an eating disorder. Complications of obesity might include heart disease, painful hip and knee joints, juvenile diabetes (Box 10-9), and shortness of breath. Body mass index (BMI) is a formula used to assess obesity. It is calculated by dividing a person's body weight by the square of a person's height (Figure 10-6). Intervention strategies implemented by the team should include a reasonable weight loss program that fosters a proper diet and the proper amount and type of exercise. Family involvement during the intervention phase is critical to the success of a weight loss program (Table 10-8).

OT practitioners can be instrumental in improving the health status of obese children. They are able to adapt and analyze the demands of activities, and in so doing they may design activities appropriate for the age and fitness level of children and their families. Any program designed to help an obese child must work with the family. The OT practitioner may lead a nutrition group (with the nutritionist as the consultant) and exercise program. The exercise program may vary as much as the individual characteristics of children and their families. For example, the OT practitioner may suggest that each night the family dance to their favorite tunes, play "Simon Says" outside, walk around the block, or play outside for 1 hour. Simple nutrition programs with easy check-off sheets for the child and family may be designed.

IMPLICATIONS FOR THE PEDIATRIC OCCUPATIONAL THERAPY PRACTITIONER

The pediatric OT practitioner uses knowledge of pediatric health conditions as a guide to the assessment and

TABLE 10-8

Obesity: General Intervention Considerations

CONSIDERATION	DEFINITION AND EXAMPLE(S)
Education	OT practitioners will consult with dietitian or nutritionist and parents/caregivers to identify the child's current diet. The OT practitioner may reinforce proper diet and exercise through education of child and family.
Physical activity	Participation in activities such as biking, walking, dancing, and swimming
Self-control	Strategies to help child gain control of behaviors may include decreasing TV/video time and increasing active physical activity time.
Self-esteem	Children with obesity frequently experience low self-esteem. OT practitioners can help children develop positive self-esteem through successful participation in activities.
Emotional/psychological issues	OT practitioners may consult with other health care team professionals to best meet the emotional/psychological needs of the child. The role of the OT practitioner is to help the child feel successful through engagement in activities.
Behavior management	Identifies behaviors, develops a plan, and implements the plan, with positive reinforcers and follow-up. Intervention for children with obesity centers on increasing physical activity and controlling diet.

OT, Occupational therapy.

CLINICAL *Pearl*

Obesity interferes with a child's ability to perform everyday occupations. The following list presents ideas that OT practitioners may use to promote healthy lifestyles in children.

- Organize a school walk each morning for OT month. Provide stickers or prizes as incentives.
- Lead a 30-minute after-school "moving along" program where children dance, walk, run, exercise, and have a relay race, among other things. This is easily adapted to all ages.
- Organize a "turn off the TV week" at school. Offer a worksheet of alternative activities (requiring movement) to families.
- Lead an after-school self-concept and physical activity group. Children who are physically active feel better about themselves.
- Organize a fun run in your school or community.
- Meet with the nutritionist, staff, and administrators in the school to discuss the nutritional value of the school lunch program.

intervention process. The practitioner's knowledge in the area of typical development also has an impact on the OT assessment and intervention process. Although attention has been given to potential medical intervention, the pediatric OT practitioner is the most concerned with the child's or adolescent's successful engagement in the occupations and performance of ADLs, IADLs, education, work, play/leisure, and social participation. Specific OT intervention(s) will be based on the evaluation of a client's independence in the areas of occupation and performance skills.

SUMMARY

This chapter has presented an introduction to pediatric health conditions. The information has been organized into categories that include body system(s) affected, acute or chronic, congenital or acquired, and discrete or pervasive. The final section of this chapter discusses burn injuries and obesity in children and adolescents. At the end of each section, general signs and symptoms and general intervention considerations are presented. These considerations on intervention are presented in the tables.

References

1. American Burn Association, 2001.
2. American Psychiatric Association: *Diagnostic and statistical manual of mental disorders* (DSM IV), ed 4, text revision, Washington, DC, 2000, American Psychiatric Association.
3. Anderson DM, Keith J, Novale PD, et al: *Mosby's medical, nursing, and allied health dictionary*, ed 6, St Louis, 2002, Mosby.
4. Ayres AJ: *Sensory integration and learning disorders*, Los Angeles, 1972, Western Psychological Services.
5. Ayres AJ, Mailloux ZK, Wendler CL: Developmental dyspraxia: is it a unitary function? *Occup J Res* 7:93, 1987.
6. Barnhart SL, Czervinche MP: *Perinatal and pediatric respiratory care*, Philadelphia, 1995, Saunders.
7. Batshaw M, editor: *Children with disabilities*, ed 5, Baltimore, 2002, Paul H. Brookes Publishers.
8. Bundy A, Lanc S, Murray E: *Sensory integration: theory and practice*, ed 2, Philadelphia, 2002, FA Davis.
9. Case-Smith J: *Occupational therapy for children*, ed 5, St Louis, 2005, Mosby.
10. Centers for Disease Control and Prevention, 2001, www.cdc.gov/nip/vacsafe/concerns/autism/autism-factshtm.
11. Cermak SA, Gubbay SS, Larkin D: What is developmental coordination disorder? In Cermak SA, editor: *Developmental coordination disorder*, p 2, Albany, 2002, Delmar Thomson Learning.
12. Dewey D, Wilson B: Developmental coordination disorder: what is it? *Phys Occup Ther Pediatr* 20:5, 2001.
13. Fox AM, Lent B: Clumsy children: primer on developmental coordination disorder, *Can Fam Phys* 42:1965, 1996.
14. Geuze RH, Kalverboer AF: Tapping a rhythm: a problem of timing for children who are clumsy and dyslexic, *Adapt Phys Act Q*, 11:203, 1994.
15. Gubbay SS: Clumsiness. In Frederiks JAM, editor: *Handbook of clinical neurology: neurobehavioral disorders*, vol 2, pp. 159-167, Amsterdam, 1985, Elsevier.
16. Gubbay SS: *The clumsy child: a study in developmental apraxia and agnostic ataxia*, London, 1975, Saunders.
17. Hall D: Clumsy children, *Br Med J* 296:375, 1988.
18. Henderson SE, Hall D: Concomitants of clumsiness in young school children, *Dev Med Child Neurol* 24:448, 1982.
19. Klein S, Magill-Evans J: Perceptions of competence and peer acceptance in young children with motor and learning difficulties, *Phys Occup Ther Pediatr* 18:39, 1998.
20. Losse A, Henderson SE, Elliman D, et al: Clumsiness in children—do they grow out of it? A 10-year follow-up study, *Dev Med Child Neurol* 33:55, 1991.
21. Michaud LF, Semel-Concepcion J, Dahaime AC, et al: Traumatic brain injury. In Batshaw M, editor: *Children with disabilities*, ed 5, p 525, Baltimore, 2002, Paul H Brookes Publishers.
22. Missiuna C, Polatjko HJ: Developmental dyspraxia by any other name, *Am J Occup Ther* 49:619, 1995.
23. Salter RB, Dudos JP: The first fifteen years' experience with innominate osteotomy in the treatment of developmental hip dysplasia and subluxation of the hip, *Clin Orthop* 98:72, 1974.
24. Schoemaker MM, Kalverboer AF: Social and affective problems of children who are clumsy: how early do they begin? *Adapt Phys Act Q* 11:130, 1994.
25. Sellars JS: Clumsiness: review of causes, treatment, and outlook, *Phys Occup Ther Pediatr* 15:39, 1995.
26. Shaw L, Levin MD, Belfer M: Developmental double jeopardy: a study of clumsiness and self-esteem in child-

ren with learning problems, *Dev Behav Pediatr* 3:191, 1982.
27. Smyth TR, Glencross DJ: Information processing deficits in clumsy children, *Austr J Occup Ther* 47:919, 1986.
28. Williams HG, Woolacott MH, Ivry R: Timing and motor control in clumsy children, *J Motor Behav* 24:165, 1992.

REVIEW *Questions*

1. What are three types of pediatric health conditions?
2. Name one specific disorder for each type of pediatric health condition identified in the first question.
3. What are the four types of burns? Define each and identify which is the most common.
4. How are burns classified?
5. What is the impact of obesity on a child's occupations?
6. How can obesity be prevented? Brainstorm some strategies you could use in your practice to help children with obesity.
7. Describe intervention strategies for children with specific conditions.

SUGGESTED *Activities*

1. Interview an OT practitioner who works in a pediatric medical system.
2. Interview a firefighter to consider the different types of fires and burns and client factors in the persons s/he has rescued.
3. Research lunch menus in local elementary, middle, and high schools. Compare and contrast, considering food groups and nutritional value.
4. Interview a dietitian who works with children and adolescents who are obese.
5. Analyze your lifestyle, considering diet, exercise, and the balance between work and rest.
6. Interview a family member of a child who has a diagnosis presented in this chapter.
7. Develop a handout for siblings on a particular diagnosis.
8. Using the tables as your guide, develop activities specific to each type of medical condition.

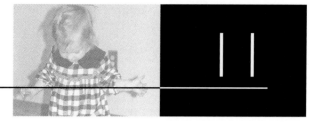

11

Intellectual Disabilities

DIANA BAL

JANE CLIFFORD O'BRIEN

CHAPTER *Objectives*

After studying this chapter, the reader will be able to accomplish the following:

- Identify possible causes of intellectual disabilities
- Explain the difference in the levels of severity of intellectual disabilities
- Identify functional consequences for each level of intellectual disabilities
- Identify the amount of support needed for each level of intellectual disabilities
- Explain the roles of the registered occupational therapist and certified occupational therapy assistant in assessments of and interventions with children who have intellectual disabilities

KEY TERMS

Intellectual disability
Intelligence quotient
Teratogen
Mild mental retardation
Moderate mental retardation
Severe mental retardation
Profound mental retardation
Global mental functions
Specific mental functions

CHAPTER OUTLINE

A child with an intellectual disability has below-average cognitive functioning that causes developmental delays and impairments in multiple areas of occupation, including social participation, education, skills required for activities of daily living (ADLs) and instrumental activities of daily living (IADLs), and play/leisure. The child may also have associated physical disabilities interfering with performance skills. Infants as well as school-age children who have intellectual disabilities benefit from occupational therapy (OT) intervention to promote performance in all areas of occupation. Adults with intellectual disabilities may benefit from OT intervention to adapt to body and life changes.

DEFINITION

The term **intellectual disability** is now used to describe children previously referred to as having mental retardation. Labels such as developmental delay, mental disability, and cognitive delay are all used to describe mental retardation and intellectual disability. The terms *developmental disability*, *mental retardation*, and *intellectual disability* will be used in this chapter to describe these children. Mental retardation is a developmental disorder characterized by significantly below-average intellectual functioning as well as deficits in two or more skill areas (e.g., ADLs, communication, social participation, education, play/leisure, homemaking skills, and skills required to attain and maintain independence).[1] There must be evidence of mental retardation before the child is 18 years of age. Physi-cians consider five assumptions when diagnosing mental retardation.[2]

Limitations in present functioning must be considered within the context of community environments typical of the individual's age, peers, and culture.

Valid assessment considers cultural and linguistic diversity as well as differences in communicative, sensory, motor, and behavioral factors.

Within an individual, limitations and strengths often coexist.

An important purpose for describing limitations is to develop a profile of supports.

With appropriate personal supports over a sustained period, the life functioning of the person with mental retardation generally improves.

MEASUREMENT AND CLASSIFICATION

One of the initial signs of intellectual disability is a significant delay in motor and cognitive development. Although the learning speed of children who are developmentally disabled may be slower than it is for those who are not, all children are capable of learning. It is important to look at how the limitations interfere with functional skills in occupations. The amount of material these children are capable of learning depends on the severity of their intellectual delays. The level of severity is determined by using several factors, including the results of intelligence testing, adaptive functioning, and mental age.[1]

Intelligence Testing

Intelligence is determined by using standardized tests that measure the underlying abilities of the child. These tests help indicate how the child may perform in school and society as well as what types of support services may be required. Intelligence tests are scored on a scale of 0 to 145, with the average score 100 and a standard deviation of 15 points. Therefore, scores between 85 and 115 are considered within normal limits (average **intelligence quotient** [IQ]). Children who score between 70 and 84 fall within the borderline mental retardation range, 55 to 69 represents mild mental retardation; 40 to 54 classifies children as moderate mental retardation, 25 to 39 is considered severe mental retardation, and children with scores lower than 25 are labeled as having profound mental retardation (Table 11-1).[4]

IQ tests such as the revised Wechsler Intelligence Scale (WISC-R), Stanford-Binet Intelligence Scale, McCarthy Scales of Children's Ability, and Bayley Scales of Infant Development are administered by a qualified psychologist. The tests include motor and verbal sections. Administering IQ tests to children with severe disabilities can be challenging, and changes in how the test is administered interfere with standardization and the consequent results. Therefore, clinicians must view the results cautiously. Since infant and child IQ tests require motor responses, those who are physically unable to perform certain motor tasks may receive lower scores.

TABLE 11-1

Categories of Mental Retardation Based on Intelligence Quotient Scores

IQ RANGE	MENTAL RETARDATION CATEGORY
55 to 69	Mild
40 to 54	Moderate
25 to 39	Severe
Less than 25	Profound

IQ, Intelligence quotient.

Adaptive Functioning

Along with cognitive delays, children labeled with mental retardation must demonstrate deficits in at least one area of adaptive functioning, which includes all of the skills required for performance in ADLs, IADLs (e.g., dressing, grooming, and hygiene), social participation, education, and communication.[1,2] A child's functioning is compared with the typical developmental level for the child's chronological age. Functional skills are evaluated in many different settings, with the caregiver or teacher providing input. The *Vineland Adaptive Behavior Scale* uses parental input to evaluate adaptive behavior in terms of communication, daily living, socialization, and motor skills. The *School Functional Assessment* uses input from the teacher to assess the child's ability to perform the occupational tasks necessary in the school setting. The *Support Intensity Scale (SIS)* is an assessment designed to measure the pattern and level of support required for an adult with mental retardation to lead a normal, independent life.[11] The *SIS* measures the amount of support required in the medical, behavioral, and life activity areas. Fifty-seven activities are evaluated according to the frequency, time of day, and type of support required. This is beneficial when developing support plans and can assist with resource allocation and financial planning.[9]

Mental Age

Mental age refers to the age at which the child is actually functioning, whereas chronological age refers to the child's actual age. For example, a 5-year-old child who performs tasks that a typical 3 year old performs would have a mental age of 3. Mental age is based on and determined by performance on standardized tests. These tests allow the child's performance to be equitably compared with the chronological age standard.

ETIOLOGY AND INCIDENCE

The incidence of mental retardation is reported as 3 out of every 100 people in the country.[2] The causes of intellectual disability range from birth defects to genetic disorders to complications during birth to problems in infancy. In some cases the cause is unknown. Children who have intellectual disabilities may also have physical and psychological disabilities. These deficits can include visual impairments, hearing loss, muscle tone problems, seizures, and sensory disorders (see Chapters 15 and 21). Physicians categorize the causes of intellectual disability based on when they occur; prenatal causes occur before birth, perinatal causes occur at birth, and postnatal causes occur from birth to 3 years of age.

CLINICAL *Pearl*

It is possible to estimate IQ in younger children by dividing mental age by chronological age and multiplying by 100. For example,

36 months (mental age) ÷ 72 months (chronological age) × 100 = 50.

The child in this example has an IQ of 50. (Note: This is considered an estimate.)

Prenatal Causes

Genetic

Each human cell contains 23 pairs of chromosomes. Genes on these chromosomes contain deoxyribonucleic acid (DNA), the material that contains the unique physical and genetic plans for each individual. The store of DNA information on each of the genes is called the *genetic code*. The first 22 pairs are called *autosomes* and the twenty-third pair the *sex chromosomes*. During reproduction 23 chromosomes come from the mother and 23 from the father, resulting in a cell with 46 chromosomes.

When too many or too few chromosomes are present (e.g., 47 instead of 46) or an abnormal gene exists, the developing fetus is negatively affected. Genetic disorders may be inherited or caused by errors in cell division. Two examples of genetic conditions associated with mental retardation are Down syndrome and fragile X syndrome. Down syndrome is called *trisomy 21* because individuals with this condition have three copies of chromosome 21 instead of a pair. Individuals with fragile X syndrome have an abnormal, or "fragile," X chromosome that contains a weak area.

Acquired

A **teratogen** is any physical or chemical substance that may cause physical or developmental complications in the fetus.[5] Teratogens can include prescription medications, alcohol, or illegal drugs consumed by the mother; maternal infections; and other toxins. The effects of teratogens on the fetus range from congenital anomalies (defects) to intellectual disabilities. The type of agent, amount of exposure, and point at which exposure occurs during embryonic and fetal development play important roles in the outcome. Exposure to teratogens during the first 12 weeks of pregnancy can be the most dangerous because it is during this time that the fetal brain, spinal cord, most internal organs, and limbs develop.

Perinatal Causes

Anoxia or hypoxia at birth

Anoxia is a total lack of oxygen in a specific area of the body; *hypoxia* is a decreased amount of oxygen.[10] Mental retardation can result when either condition affects the brain. The severity of brain dysfunction depends on (1) the location and size of the area deprived of oxygen, (2) the amount of time the area is without oxygen, and (3) the metabolic changes that take place in the body as a result of cell death in that area.

Anoxia or hypoxia can occur during labor because of a small birth canal, which can result in bleeding around the baby's brain, compression of the umbilical cord, tearing of the placenta (placenta previa), or breech birth (i.e., the child is born with the buttocks first instead of head first).

Prematurity

Infants born before completion of the thirty-seventh week of gestation are considered premature.[10] Numerous factors may cause prematurity, such as poor nutrition, lack of prenatal care, toxemia, multiple fetuses, a weak cervix, numerous previous births, and adolescent mothers.[7] Although prematurity does not necessarily mean that a disability will develop, some complications caused by prematurity may result in mental retardation. For example, prematurity can cause *respiratory distress syndrome (RDS)*, a condition in which the premature infant's lungs are not yet producing *surfactant*, a chemical on the surface of the lungs that helps keep them from collapsing. Another complication of prematurity is *apnea*, a condition in which the infant stops breathing; apnea can last from seconds to minutes. Prematurity can also cause *hydrocephalus*, a condition in which the cerebrospinal fluid accumulates in the brain and can cause the head to grow disproportionately large (Figure 11-1). The extent of the infant's prematurity and associated complications affects the severity of the impairment (if any develops). Premature brain development puts infants at risk for brain hemorrhages (bleeding). The increased amount of blood in the brain causes hypoxia (decrease oxygen) and possible ischemia (cell death), resulting in motor and cognitive disabilities. The extent of the disability depends on the size of the hemorrhage.

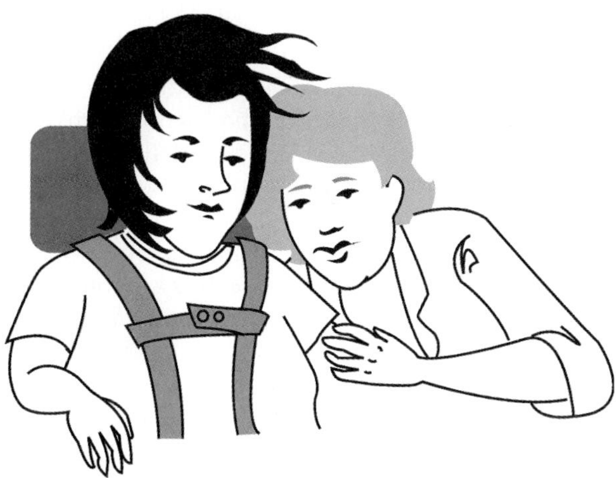

FIGURE 11-1 Adult with disproportionately sized head caused by unshunted hydrocephalus.

Postnatal Causes

Infections

Infections can cause brain damage and resulting disabilities in infants and children. *Viral meningitis* is a condition in which a virus attacks the protective covering around the brain and spinal cord, known as the *meninges*.[7] Several different viruses cause meningitis, including chickenpox. In small children and infants meningitis may cause permanent brain damage that leads to intellectual disability, the severity of which depends on the extent of brain damage. Inflammation of the brain, known as *encephalitis*, may be caused by complications from chickenpox, rabies, measles, influenza, and other diseases.[10] The severity of any resulting disability varies depending on the area and amount of the brain that have been damaged.

Trauma

Any traumatic injury to the brain has the potential to cause brain damage and subsequent intellectual and motor impairments. Automobile accidents represent the most common cause of brain injuries, especially those cases in which the child is not restrained by a seat belt.[6] Falls, bicycle accidents, pedestrian-automobile accidents, near-drowning, and physical abuse also cause brain injuries that lead to mental retardation.

Toxins or pollutants

Toxins are poisonous substances that cause particular problems when ingested.[10] Because infants and small children often place objects and substances in their mouths, certain common household substances can pose serious and life-threatening problems. For example, older homes often have lead-based paint on the walls. Inhaling, licking, or eating paint chips can cause lead poisoning, resulting in developmental problems. Once diagnosed the lead poisoning can be treated, but residual permanent damage may exist. Other common household toxins include mercury from thermometers and cleaning agents.

CLINICAL *Pearl*

While working with children who have multiple disabilities (Figure 11-2), do not underestimate their abilities; they will surprise you. Rachel is severely physically handicapped, requiring full support for her body; however, she showed great success in using an augmented communication system.

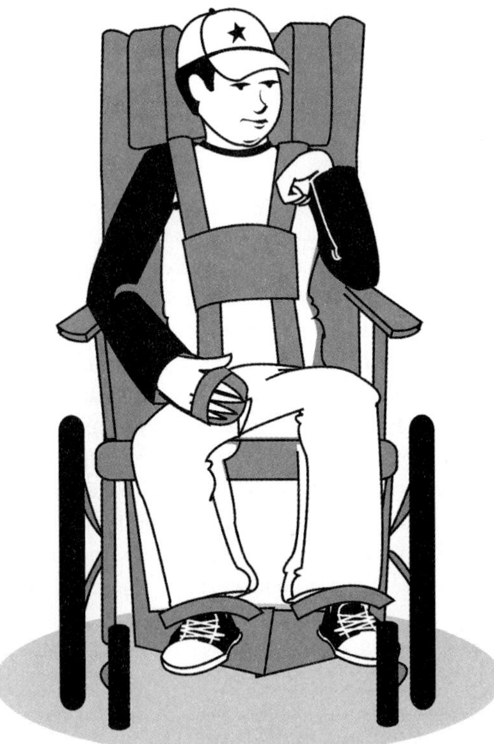

FIGURE 11-2 Adolescent with multiple disabilities and mental retardation.

PERFORMANCE IN AREAS OF OCCUPATION

The capacity of a child with an intellectual disability to perform in the areas of occupation varies greatly depending on the severity of mental retardation and the presence of additional deficits. The following presentation is a general description of expected capabilities based on the categories of intellectual disability.

CLINICAL *Pearl*

The parents or primary caregivers of children who are developmentally delayed have valuable information concerning the children's abilities and the activities that they enjoy. This information will assist practitioners in developing interventions for the child and family.

Mild Intellectual Disability

Carrie is 9 years old and is in the second grade. When she was born her parents realized that she was "floppy" (an indicator of low muscle tone) and weak. Since she could not sustain a sucking pattern, a gastrostomy tube (g-tube) was placed in her stomach at 1 month. The tube was removed when Carrie was 2 years old, and she currently eats a regular diet with Ensure supplements. At school she receives resource help in reading and math from a special education teacher for 1 hour in the morning and 1 hour in the afternoon. Carrie follows the classroom routine and moves around the school independently. She has difficulty with directions and right/left discrimination. Carrie reads sight words and books at a first-grade level. Handwriting is a challenge for her because of directional difficulties, but she is able to copy print from a model. Each day her teacher has her sign in to practice writing her full name quickly in a designated area. Carrie's Individual Educational Plan (IEP) includes adaptations of preferential seating, decreased workload, having tests read to her, the use of a word processor, and extra time for completion of work as needed. For writing assignments she uses the computer/word processor with Co:Writer and Write:OutLoud programs, which read the words on the screen and provide a list of words from which she can select. Carrie is independent in self-care tasks. She learned to tie her shoes last year and needs extra time to get dressed in the morning, so her mother encourages her to bathe and select her clothing the night before. In the future, she would like to be a teacher's aide and help take care of children.

Carrie has ***mild mental retardation.***

Individuals with mild intellectual disability have IQs of 55 to 69, and they usually require support in special circumstances. Children in this category may not seem significantly different from others until they attempt to attain higher levels of cognitive skill and perform tasks that require significant abstract thinking. These individuals usually master academic skills from the third to the seventh grade; however, it takes them longer than average students to attain them. Academic skills include the following:

- Reading at the fourth- or fifth-grade level
- Writing simple letters or lists, such as a grocery list
- Performing simple mathematical functions such as multiplication and division
- Using the computer and Internet to perform simple research or communicate with others

As adults their social, vocational, and self-help skills are usually sufficient to allow them to partially or completely support themselves financially through employ-

CLINICAL *Pearl*

Adolescents or adults who are mildly mentally disabled may show impaired judgment in those areas concerning safety and sexuality. Therapy sessions may address these problem areas through education at the child's cognitive and emotional levels.

ment. Therefore, they can live independently or in a minimally supervised setting in the community.

Moderate Intellectual Disability

Kelly is 7 years old and is enrolled in a self-contained classroom for children who have moderate mental disabilities. He is nonverbal but indicates his needs by pointing to pictures on a simple communication board. He gets upset when he is touched, is wearing certain fabrics, or feels confined by others. Kelly requires minimum to moderate assistance to put on clothing, especially to get them correctly oriented. He requires moderate assistance to fasten them because of alignment and the multistep process. He feeds himself with a spoon but is a very picky eater. Sorting items by color and scribbling on paper are Kelly's favorite activities.

A registered occupational therapist (OTR) recommended that Kelly participate in a classroom and home program to decrease his hypersensitivity. After consultation with the certified occupational therapy assistant (COTA) concerning an intervention plan, the COTA provides direct therapy and consults with the staff and family to promote sensory modulation and oral desensitization. After 3 months the staff and family have a better understanding of what upsets Kelly. He has begun eating a variety of foods at school and home.

Kelly has ***moderate mental retardation.***

Individuals with moderate intellectual disability have IQs of 40 to 54 and need support regularly. They are likely to have deficits in academic, communicative, and social skills. With special education, individuals who have moderate intellectual disabilities are usually able to attain the skills of a first- or second-grade student, which include the following:

- Writing name cursively
- Reading simple texts and emergency words
- Remembering home phone number
- Understanding written numbers and quantities (e.g., being able to select three apples from a pile of apples)
- Understanding basic concepts of money

CLINICAL *Pearl*

The OT practitioner can have a significant impact on the success of an adult who has moderate mental disabilities and is living in a group home or supervised setting. For example, the OT practitioner can train staff in techniques to facilitate routines. The client can use adaptive equipment to be more independent in self-feeding, personal hygiene, and leisure occupations. Therapists can also consult with the work supervisors of individuals with mental disabilities on strategies to ensure success at work.

Children and adolescents with moderate mental retardation require supervision but are able to follow simple sequential-step verbal directions. They may learn repetitive actions such as making a sandwich for lunch. They may be able to participate in simple leisure activities. Children and adolescents with moderate intellectual disabilities can communicate desires and preferences and thus should be provided with opportunities to make choices. Adolescents and adults may require supervision to complete ADLs and IADLs. These individuals can do some meaningful work in sheltered workshops or community-supported employment settings. Numerous adults with moderate mental disabilities live successfully in supervised living arrangements. OT practitioners can provide support and strategies to caregivers on how to address behaviors and physical routines.

Severe Intellectual Disability

Thomas is a 9-year-old boy who attends the self-contained class at his local elementary school. He is short with low muscle tone, and he appears flabby and chubby. He is able to walk, loves to eat, and has mastered feeding himself independently with a spoon but needs prompting to open his milk containers. Thomas is on a toileting schedule at home and school. He counts to two, recognizes colors, and responds to his name. In class, he scribbles on paper but tends to color the table or another student's paper if an adult is not prompting him. He has learned how to put small items into a container but will throw the objects if not monitored. His favorite thing to do is bang objects on the table, and he rocks forward and backward or removes his shirt when he has nothing to do. His language is very limited, but he is able to point to items he wants and use some picture symbols to indicate basic needs (e.g., food, bathroom, favorite toy, computer). He needs adult supervision and someone to hold his hand while changing rooms at school because he will go in any direction.

Thomas has ***severe mental retardation.***

Individuals with severe mental retardation have an IQ between 25 and 39 and therefore require support in all areas of occupational performance on a regular basis. Functional independence depends greatly on their associated physical limitations. Habitual basic self-care skills such as feeding and hygiene tasks may be learned because of the repetitive nature of these activities. Children with severe mental retardation have difficulty with generalizing skills and perform best with routine and consistency. For example, a child might be able to unzip his or her book bag but not the zipper on an unfamiliar jacket. Desires and needs can be communicated verbally or nonverbally by using communication boards or other technologies. As adolescents and adults, those with severe mental retardation may be successful in supervised prevocational training activities. They require extensive supervision and support to live independently. It is unlikely that these individuals will achieve any particular academic grade level in school because tasks such as reading and writing are extremely difficult for them. In special education, an individual with severe mental disabilities can do the following:

- Recognize his or her photograph
- Perform self-care skills that are routinely done (e.g., feed oneself with a spoon, pull pants up/down)
- Learn how to follow simple classroom rules that are done consistently (hang up backpack when entering classroom)

Children and adolescents with severe mental retardation frequently have physical disabilities, including cerebral palsy, seizure disorder, visual impairment, hearing loss, and communication disorder. OT practitioners must evaluate and address the physical demands of activities along with the global and specific mental function demands. Family members who are caring for the child may require education on handling techniques and behavioral management. Practitioners work with the other family members to help them understand the disabled family member so that they may interact, socialize, and enjoy each other.

Profound Intellectual Disability

Danielle is a frail little girl. She is unable to sit or stand because she has poor head and trunk control. She depends on others for all self-care needs, including eating, toileting, and dressing. She eats a mashed-diet texture because of inadequate tongue lateralization secondary to a tongue thrust. Danielle drools because of poor lip control resulting from her limited head control. Although she has wonderful eye contact and visual regard for her environment, she is unable to move her body on command or follow simple requests. Danielle responds to every auditory cue around her. She is very alert to everything in her environment but is also very easily distracted.

Danielle has ***profound mental retardation.***

An IQ of less than 25 classifies individuals as having profound intellectual disability. Because of the numerous physical disabilities that may accompany profound intellectual disabilities, these individuals often have difficulty making developmental progress and require constant support in all areas of occupation.

Depending on the extent of their physical limitations, individuals with profound mental retardation may learn to communicate and perform basic or routine self-care activities such as hygiene and grooming tasks. Extensive assistance is required for all other ADL skills, and continuous support is needed in living arrangements. Maintenance of the physical skills required for everyday occupations assists in preserving the overall health of the child. Practitioners working with children who have profound mental retardation concentrate on the basic skills required for occupations. For example, the goals of therapy may include such tasks as the following:

- Smile on approach
- Indicate food preference
- Feed oneself with a spoon
- Make visual contact
- Allow caregiver to bathe them
- Allow caregiver to touch them
- Cooperate with dressing or self-care

CLINICAL *Pearl*

Nonverbal children with severe mental disabilities can point to pictures mounted on a place mat to indicate their wants and needs during mealtime. For example, they can point to a picture of a cup to let caregivers know that they want more milk.

CLINICAL *Pearl*

Children who have profound mental disabilities have preferences for certain people, toys, and food and typically have a sense of humor. The OT practitioner must respect their preferences and try to discover what motivates their sense of humor.

CLIENT FACTORS: FUNCTIONAL IMPLICATIONS AND OCCUPATIONAL THERAPY INTERVENTION

The previous section provided a basic idea of the ways in which individuals in each category function; this section focuses on the specific functional implications that mental retardation has in relation to client factors (e.g., mental function, sensory function and pain, movement-related functions, and system functions). The client factors are based on the Occupational Therapy Practice Framework.[3] A sampling of how the client factors may be manifested in children and adolescents with mental retardation is presented.

Mental Function

Children and adolescents with mental retardation exhibit the whole range of affective, cognitive, and perceptual functioning. Each client should be assessed in terms of his or her strengths and weaknesses. **Global mental functions** are frequently delayed or absent in children and adolescents with mental retardation. With these functions individuals may lack *orientation* to person, place, time, self, and others. Children with intellectual disabilities may not make eye contact or attend to activities *(consciousness level)*. *Temperament and personality* vary, and clients may experience emotional instability (e.g., quickly change from one emotion to another). Practitioners may find that clients have difficulty choosing activities *(energy and drive)*, have few preferences *(interests)*, or have difficulty with *impulse control.*

Intervention

Intervention is not aimed at improving intelligence (it is not possible to reverse the diagnosis); instead, it is aimed at helping the child or adolescent perform his or her occupations. Toward that end, practitioners focus on the actual occupations the child or adolescent hopes to perform as goals. (See Box 11-1 for sample goals.)

BOX 11-1

Sample Goals Showing a Variety of Functional Levels

- Using a built-up handled spoon, Shawn will feed himself independently at dinner for 2 weeks.
- Kaya will initiate a simple conversation with another adolescent during the school picnic.
- Ali will make a peanut butter and jelly sandwich for his after-school snack (with verbal reminders) within 1 month.
- Within 1 month, Maya will cooperate with dressing by extending her arms and legs on verbal request.
- Sophie will turn her head to identify to the staff her food preferences for each meal within 2 months.

For example, a learning objective of "Helen will learn the five food groups" may be appropriate for a typical second grader. However, the staff at the school would like Helen to eat a proper diet. In fact, Helen eats only sweets. The practitioner rewrote the goal to be "Helen will eat at least one bite of two food groups." In this case, rewriting the goal to include the exact occupational behavior needed is more functional and meaningful to the child and staff. The intervention session would emphasize the importance of consuming at least a small portion of fruits or vegetables, bread, dairy products, or meat. The therapist may decide to use a positive reinforcer (in Helen's case dessert) after she accomplishes this. (It is not wise to use food as a reinforcer in all cases. However, during mealtime it is easy to allow dessert after the meal as a reinforcer.)

Children and adolescents with intellectual disabilities show impairment in **specific mental functions** that may present as the following:

- Shorter *attention* span
- Difficulty storing and retrieving information *(memory)*
- Difficulty recognizing direction and relation of objects to one another *(perception)*
- Slower-learning ability *(thought)*
- Inability to recognize objects or people *(thought)*
- Difficulty making sense of stimuli *(perception)*
- Difficulty with problem solving and critical thinking *(higher-level cognition)*
- Difficulty generalizing information and mastering abstract thinking *(thought)*
- Slow, delayed, or absent *language* skills
- Difficulty with adding and subtracting *(calculations)*
- Poor motor planning *(sequencing complex movements)*
- Inappropriate range and regulation of emotions; self-control *(emotional)*
- Difficulty with body image, self-concept, and self-esteem *(self and time)*

Language Functions

As with physical milestones, it can take longer for children with mental retardation to reach speech and language milestones because of the intellectual delays. For example, shorter memory and attention span could make recalling and retrieving words difficult, whereas difficulties with abstract thinking may make mentally grasping certain concepts a challenge. The language and speech of children with intellectual disabilities may be related to associated physical problems such as inadequate oral-motor muscle tone, which results in unclear articulation and difficulty taking deep breaths or speaking loudly. OT practitioners are responsible for referring children with intellectual disabilities to speech therapists as needed. Frequently the OT practitioner and speech therapist are able to provide intervention together. This benefits the child and family.

Children with severe or profound intellectual disability have numerous global and specific mental functioning deficits. Intervention techniques are individualized to the child or adolescent. In general, children with mental retardation benefit from routine and consistency. Using a reward system (such as a sticker) may be helpful. Children with short attention spans require short sessions with frequent reinforcers. Because children with intellectual disability have difficulty generalizing skills, they benefit by performing the actual occupations being addressed in therapy. Follow-up and consistency by aides help to reinforce the goals. Intervention is modified according to a child's cognitive and physical abilities.

Intervention

The developmental frame of reference, along with the behavioral frame of reference, works well with individuals who have intellectual disabilities. OT intervention requires clear expectations, simple directions, and positive rewards. Furthermore, intervention that replicates the actual context and occupation as close as possible benefits children who are unable to generalize. Sessions that are short, simple (one or two activities), and structured are effective with children and adolescents with mental retardation. Practitioners may be playful in sessions, but be aware that clients with mental retardation may not understand complex humor of the kind that even young children can understand.

Behavioral/Emotional Functions

Children with intellectual disabilities may experience the same range of behavioral issues as their typical peers. However, it may go unnoticed or be more difficult to identify because of the intellectual delay. For example, children with intellectual disability may develop psychosocial disorders of depression, obsessive-compulsive disorder, or attention deficit disorder. Intellectual disability is an associated factor for many genetic syndromes with documented behavioral characteristics, such as Prader-Willi. Children with Prader-Willi syndrome are driven to eat constantly, often non-edible items. They have stereotypical behaviors and features. Children with autism, Down syndrome, and Asperger syndrome may exhibit mental retardation.

Children with intellectual disability may exhibit self-stimulating behaviors (such as hand flapping, biting, and hitting) that make them stand out in typical settings. They may suck on clothing, make repetitive noises, or hop on their toes. Behavioral difficulties associated with mental disabilities include hyperactivity (impulsiveness and excessive activity that result in difficulty functioning in social situations), aggressiveness (e.g., slapping, hitting, kicking, biting, tantrums), excessive shyness (withdrawing during familiar group activities) and distractibility (difficulty paying attention to one task). These behaviors interfere with their functioning and ability to participate in social or academic occupations. During adolescence, children with mental retardation may be socially or sexually inappropriate.

Children with intellectual disabilities attain their social skills later than other children. These children often appear to misbehave or be less mature than their peers. Children with mental disabilities may act much younger than their chronological age.

Intervention

Intervention for emotional issues often uses a behavioral approach. See Box 11-2 for the techniques used in this approach. The OTR and COTA can be instrumental in designing the program. First, data is collected to determine the behaviors that need to be changed. The OTR and COTA use their expertise to describe these behaviors and analyze them for the purpose of determining why they are occurring. They present the individual's strengths and weaknesses so that the team may establish an appropriate award system. The COTA reinforces the system and checks with staff daily to see if they have any new concerns. OT intervention is aimed at reinforcing this as well while working on other established goals.

CLINICAL *Pearl*

Children with intellectual disabilities establish friendships and other relationships. They may experience the full range of emotions, although they may not be able to verbalize these feelings. OT practitioners can help children and adolescents deal with feelings of grief, sadness (when losing someone), intimacy, and love.

CLINICAL *Pearl*

Children with intellectual disabilities may enjoy participation in athletic events, such as the Special Olympics. These events help children develop feelings of success by working toward an athletic goal. Children experience teamwork, achievement, and the benefits of physical activity. Events such as these promote a positive self-concept and self-esteem.

BOX 11-2

Behavioral Modification Techniques

Techniques to diminish behaviors include the following:

- List the behaviors that the child exhibits that interfere with learning, socialization, or engagement in occupations.
- Collect data on each behavior. Record and analyze how often, why, and when the behavior occurs.
- Determine whether the behavior occurs when the child is frustrated by a task that is too difficult or when a certain person or visitor is present.
- Consider the setting in which the behavior occurs. (Is the setting quiet, noisy, dark, etc?)
- Prioritize the behaviors that should be addressed first.
- Behaviors that involve safety issues are priorities.
- OT practitioners may want to prioritize behaviors that may be more easily addressed as a method to build rapport and trust with the child and team.
- Behaviors that are the most upsetting to the staff or in social situations may need to be addressed first. This helps the client engage in social participation.
- With the team (e.g., parent, caregiver, teacher, staff), create a plan to diminish the behavior.
- The OT practitioner provides a task analysis of the behavior. S/he may be able to identify reinforcers or provide insight into why the behaviors are occurring.
- Through the task analysis, the OT practitioner is able to break down the steps to ensure the success of the behavior plan. S/he is able to identify the steps the child is able to achieve.
- The plan must be simple enough to work for a variety of people with limited training.
- Simple plans that are easily incorporated into the child's day are usually successful.
- Behavior plans may include ignoring unwanted behaviors (to diminish them) or providing positive reinforcers for acceptable ones.
- Implement the plan.
- OT practitioners may be responsible for training the staff on the implementation of the plan.
- OT practitioners may adapt or suggest changes to the implementation of the plan after a careful task analysis.
- Collect data on the behavior. Evaluate the outcome and discuss it with the team.
- All team members are responsible for documenting the outcome of the plan.
- Evaluating the success of a plan may include counting behaviors during OT sessions.
- OT practitioners may have to evaluate the use of compensation techniques, assistive technology, or remediation programs designed to diminish the behaviors.

OT, Occupational therapy.

For example, staff from the school requested an OT evaluation of behaviors during breakfast and lunch. The OTR met with the staff, reviewed the files, and observed lunch. The COTA observed breakfast. The COTA and OTR met and compiled observations, discussed possibilities, and brainstormed solutions. The staff was very frustrated with Gianni (the client), who threw his plate of food down at every meal. On observation Gianni sat at a table with three other severely involved students, who required one-on-one assistance to be fed. Gianni fed himself with assistance of set up. He was positioned in his wheelchair at the table. He ate slowly and with a tremor. The staff was busy with the other clients and did not speak to Gianni during the meal. Gianni could not communicate verbally but pointed and grunted to have his needs met. On completion of his meal, he threw the entire tray on the floor. The staff rushed to his side, picked up the tray, threw it away, cleaned up Gianni, and brought him quickly to the classroom.

Although the staff was frustrated with Gianni, they met his needs quickly when he threw his plate down. Therefore, Gianni was reinforced for his behavior. Both the OTR and COTA observed that Gianni looked around right before he threw his plate. The solution was simple. The staff was to look at Gianni periodically, notice when he was finished, take the tray from him, clean him up, and take him to the classroom. In this way Gianni was reinforced for completing his meal (not throwing his plate). Other suggestions to make mealtime more enjoyable were made, such as the following:

- *Limit the number of students (with aides) at the table.*
- *Have the aides sit at eye level.*
- *Limit talk among aides and focus on the clients.*
- *Turn off the music (it was overstimulating) and encourage table conversation.*

The COTA consulted with the staff weekly. Caregivers were willing to try new strategies because the OT clinicians had listened to them, addressed their concerns, and actually made their jobs easier.

CLINICAL *Pearl*

Some clients with mental retardation are not able to feed themselves with spoons or forks but are able to do so with their fingers. Many foods are available that are appropriate to eat with your hands. Instead of spending time trying to teach an older client to use a fork or spoon, instruct the caregiver to serve "finger food" such as pizza, sandwiches, and tacos. This allows the client and caregiver to participate in a pleasant dining experience. The goal may be improved dining habits or social participation during mealtime.

Sensory Function and Pain

Children with intellectual disabilities may have difficulties with *hearing*, *vision*, and *touching*. Screenings and evaluations by professionals will help rule out any problems. The OT practitioner may evaluate the child's reactions to taste, smell, touch, movement, and body position. Children with intellectual disabilities may experience adverse reactions to these sensory experiences and consequently respond unexpectedly in certain situations. For example, a child may not want to eat food of a certain texture. The staff may assume that the child is not hungry when in fact the child does not like the sensory feeling of the food's texture.

Children with *tactile defensiveness* dislike being touched on certain areas of the body or avoid contact with certain textures. Children who have *oral hypersensitivity* may have feeding difficulties; they may dislike certain flavors or textures. Some children have difficulty with the modulation or self-regulation of sensory input that they receive during the day. A sensation that calms one child may alert or disturb another. Frequently, when children cannot handle all of the sensations bombarding them during the day, they might either act out, becoming very active or aggressive, or repress and withdraw, causing them to hide from the situation. Noncompliant or acting-out behaviors may indicate that the child is having difficulty initiating the task because of poor processing of the sensory information, resulting in an inability to carry out, change, or control a motor task.

Intervention

OT practitioners frequently provide teams with information concerning the sensory processing abilities of children with mental retardation. A thorough analysis of the sensory input and responses by the client may provide insight into behaviors interfering with occupations. For example, some children with tactile defensiveness may overreact to bathing. They may dislike the feeling of water on their skin, but the staff or caregivers may interpret this reaction as uncooperative or aggressive behavior. The OT practitioner may be able to prepare the client for the bathing experience by means of a sensory program. This may be something as simple as changing the time of day the bath is given, regulating the temperature of the water, or establishing a brushing protocol before the bath. Other sensory modulation issues may be addressed by providing the caregiver and child more time to accomplish the occupations; frustration arises from both the clients and caregivers when they are rushed.

For example, one staff member at a residential setting was responsible for waking, toileting, dressing, and feeding three adolescents with severe intellectual disabilities before they were transported to school. The staff member stated that breakfast was impossible; the adolescents would not cooperate with her and frequently spat out their food. On observation the COTA realized that the staff member was hurried, the adolescents were stressed, and they were unable to express their food preferences. One adolescent was spitting out food because of a motor deficit (tongue thrusting); the others were being served portions of food that were too large. Intervention consisted of the COTA assisting the staff member in the morning until a routine was established. The COTA modeled the correct feeding techniques. Small-bowled spoons were prescribed so that the staff could not give large portions. The adolescents were instructed on how to show their preferences instead of spitting out the food. A system change was implemented in that two staff members became responsible for the morning routines of three individuals. This was accomplished by having one staff member come in early, which was agreeable to her because of personal/family responsibilities.

Another example of attentiveness to particular sensory input is having an exaggerated reaction (startle reaction) in response to loud noises or other sounds. A startle reaction could cause a child to fall or have a seizure. Children with mental disabilities may also have sensory problems related to body movement and muscle co-

CLINICAL *Pearl*

Children with intellectual disabilities may not be able to express their discomfort in a manner like their typical peers. Practitioners need to be in tune with how they might show this and inform the family and staff.

CLINICAL *Pearl*

Morning routines are difficult under the best of circumstances. OT practitioners can help the staff, caregivers, and clients by providing simplified techniques. Some examples are (1) picking out wrinkle-free clothing, (2) choosing clothing that is easy to get on, (3) providing breakfast finger food if possible so that caregivers can set up the tray for self-feeding, (4) scheduling plenty of time, (5) saving all "treatment" ideas for another time, (6) having the caregiver prepare as much as possible the night before, and (7) encouraging caregivers to take short breaks because stopping and slowing down allows the child to focus on the task. Children who are hurried get frustrated and anxious. Try to train yourself (as a caregiver) to stay with the moment (don't think about being late).

ordination (*vestibular* and *proprioceptive*), which lead to further motor deficits.

Children with mental retardation may not express pain proportionate to the stimuli; therefore, checking in with the child or adolescent and being sensitive to their perceptions is needed. Clients with mental retardation may not understand procedures and may be fearful of new people, making the feelings of pain more intense. Providing comfort in testing or procedural settings from familiar people may help.

Movement-Related Functions

Children with mental disabilities often reach major physical milestones later than usual. In fact, many infants are referred for OT because of developmental delays before being diagnosed with mental retardation. Infants and children with intellectual disabilities typically exhibit low muscle tone. These individuals have inadequate oral-motor muscle tone, which is frequently the cause of referral for OT. Children with intellectual disabilities exhibit a range of motor problems related to brain damage and difficulty learning complex motor tasks.

Intervention

Intervention is aimed at evaluating the movement-related functions of the client and helping him or her adapt to or compensate for the movement problems. Practitioners working on movement-related problems must remember that clients with mental retardation have difficulty finding ways to adapt to the physical challenges and may have more difficulty following through with home programs. Training children with mental retardation to perform movements entails practice, repetition, simple directions, and modification and/or adaptation of the requirements necessary to assure success (see Chapter 20). Specific motor intervention must be designed to address the physical problems associated with secondary diagnoses.

System Functions

COTAs working with clients with intellectual disability must have knowledge of how body systems affect the client's functional ability. These individuals are susceptible to the same conditions as their typical peers, such as those of cardiac, pulmonary, blood, digestive, metabolic, urinary, reproductive, and skin origins. Food allergies and the side effects of medicine may affect clients with intellectual disabilities. Practitioners must be keen observers of behavior and knowledgeable about their clients' medical histories. For example, many syndromes include mental retardation and cardiac problems as associated factors (e.g., Down syndrome).

CLINICAL *Pearl*

Order simple and uncomplicated adaptive/positioning equipment for children and adolescents with mental retardation. These clients may not understand complicated equipment. The staff and family members may misplace these items and become frustrated with the equipment demands along with caregiving.

ROLES OF THE REGISTERED OCCUPATIONAL THERAPIST AND CERTIFIED OCCUPATIONAL THERAPY ASSISTANT

The OTR conducts evaluations of individuals with intellectual disabilities after consultation and sharing of information with the COTA. The evaluation focuses on developing an occupational profile and analysis of the occupational performance (e.g., the ability to carry out ADLs, IADLs, work, play/leisure, education, and social participation).[3,7] The OTR interviews the child's parents, primary caregivers, or teacher to gain information on the child's strengths and weaknesses, goals, and contexts in which the occupations occur (e.g., physical, social, personal, cultural, temporal, spiritual, and virtual environments). The COTA may administer standardized tests after the establishment of service competency and at the discretion of the supervising OTR. The COTA and OTR should work together to evaluate, assess, and provide services for the child.

Infants, children, and adolescents with mental retardation are treated in the home and at daycare centers, outpatient clinics, schools, and residential settings. Knowledge of the contexts, including community resources and environmental support, is essential to the intervention process.

CLINICAL *Pearl*

Remember to communicate and coordinate therapy services if the child receives therapy in the home and at school. For example, consider all environments (school, home, community) before ordering a wheelchair.

CLINICAL *Pearl*

Children with moderate intellectual disability learn through repetitive methods. For example, learning how to put on clothing is best accomplished by setting up the same situation during times that this activity is actually performed.

SUMMARY

Children with intellectual disabilities (mental retardation) exhibit a range of behaviors that interfere with their ability to engage in occupations. OT practitioners working with children who have these disabilities evaluate the child's ability to perform occupations by analyzing the tasks required and associated client factors. Based on this analysis, OT practitioners develop intervention plans designed to maximize the child's strengths and work on the weaknesses. The goal of OT intervention is to help the child or adolescent participate in occupations such as ADLs, IADLs, play/leisure, work, education, and social participation. OT practitioners work with team members and families and must consider the overall goal of increasing the child's ability to participate in occupations. Toward this end the tasks and activities must frequently be adapted and modified, the family and caregivers must provide alternative solutions, and support systems must be established. Therefore, OT practitioners working with children who have intellectual disabilities will need to be aware of community agencies for respite, social opportunities, housing, and assistance. Furthermore, children with intellectual disabilities may experience physical limitations that interfere with their occupations. OT practitioners assist caregivers in taking care of the children.

The role of the OT practitioner in working with children and adolescents with intellectual disabilities is complex. As such, they must use their common sense, creativity, OT knowledge, and life skills to assist children, adolescents, and their families in reaching their goals.

References

1. American Psychiatric Association: *Diagnostic and statistical manual of mental disorders (DSM IV)*, ed 4, Washington, DC, 1994, The Association.
2. American Association on Mental Retardation: *Mental retardation: definition, classification, and system of supports*, ed 9, Washington, DC, 1992, The Association.
3. American Occupational Therapy Association. *Occupational therapy practice framework: domain and process*, Bethesda, Md, 2002, The Association.
4. Case-Smith J: *Pediatric occupational therapy and early intervention*, Stoneham, Mass, 1993, Butterworth-Heinemann.
5. Case-Smith J: *Occupational therapy for children*, ed 5, St Louis, 2005, Mosby.
6. Diffendal J: *A shoebox on a shoestring*, *Advance for Occupational Therapy Practitioners*, King of Prussia, Pa, 2001, Merion Publications.
7. Mader S: *Understanding human anatomy and physiology*, ed 3, Dubuque, Iowa, 1997, William C Brown.
8. Neistadt M, Crepeau E: *Willard and Spackman's occupational therapy*, ed 9, Philadelphia, 1998, Lippincott-Raven.
9. Smith R: *Children with mental retardation: a parent's guide*, Bethesda, Md, 1993, Woodbine House.
10. *Taber's cyclopedic medical dictionary*, ed 19, Philadelphia, 2001, FA Davis.
11. Thompson JR, Bryant B, Campbell EM, et al: *Supports intensity scale*, Washington, DC, 2003, American Association on Mental Retardation.

Recommended Reading

Bradley D: Obsessive-compulsive disorder now recognized in children, *Kansas City Star*, June 5, 2002.

Individual With Disabilities Education Act Final Regulations (1999). Pub L 1205-17, 34 CFR, Part 300, Washington, DC.

Swinth Y, Hanft B: *School-based practice moving beyond 1:1 service delivery*, AOTA, Bethesda, Md, 2002, OT Practice.

RESOURCES

The Association of Retarded Citizens of the United States
1010 Wayne Avenue, Suite 650
Silver Spring, Md
www.thearc.org.

Centers for Disease Control and Prevention
1660 Clifton Road
Atlanta, Ga
http://www.cdc.gov/.

American Association for the Mentally Retarded
444 North Capitol Street
Washington, DC

REVIEW *Questions*

1. Explain how intellectual disability is diagnosed and categorized.
2. Discuss the importance of treating a child with intellectual disabilities as an individual.
3. Explain the way(s) in which multiple disabilities can affect a child with intellectual disabilities.
4. Describe the roles of the registered occupational therapist and certified occupational therapy assistant in intervention for children with intellectual disabilities.
5. Describe how behaviors interfere with learning in children with intellectual disabilities.

SUGGESTED *Activities*

1. Volunteer at a facility that specializes in working with children who have intellectual disabilities.
2. Attend a Down syndrome support group to learn about the challenges faced by the families and caregivers of individuals with this syndrome.
3. Volunteer your time in a school system or early intervention program. Ask to see a sample of the Individual Family Service Plan (IFSP) or Individual Educational Program (IEP).
4. Volunteer to babysit or provide respite care for a child who has developmental delays.
5. Volunteer in a special education classroom that has children with a variety of disabilities.
6. Volunteer in a daycare center and screen the children's developmental skills. Observe the different behaviors.
7. Analyze the tasks of a daily activity to determine the steps.

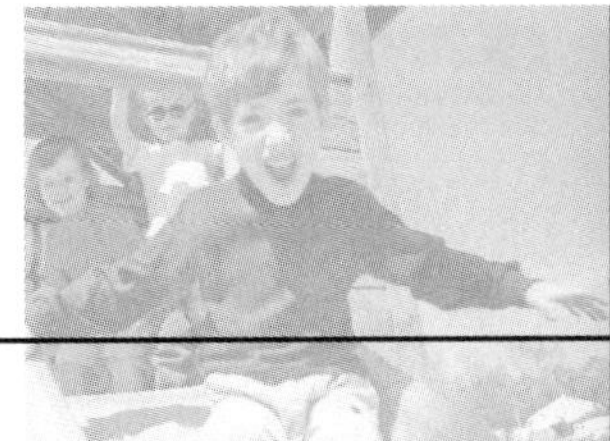

12

Cerebral Palsy

JEAN W. SOLOMON

JANE CLIFFORD O'BRIEN

CHAPTER *Objectives*

After studying this chapter, the reader will be able to accomplish the following:

- Describe the various types of movement disorder labeled cerebral palsy
- Identify and describe the impaired components of normal postural control and movement in children with cerebral palsy
- Explain the ways in which normal and impaired muscle tone influence movement
- Recognize the differences among motor development, motor learning, and motor control
- Identify the role of the certified occupational therapy assistant in the assessment, treatment, and management of individuals with cerebral palsy
- Identify the team members involved in the provision of services to children with cerebral palsy

KEY TERMS

Cerebral palsy
Primitive reflex patterns
Postural mechanism
Righting reactions
Equilibrium reactions
Protective extension reaction
Muscle tone
Spasticity (hypertonicity)
Athetosis
Ataxia
Hypotonicity
Quadriplegia
Diplegia
Hemiplegia

CHAPTER OUTLINE

DEFINITION, DESCRIPTION, AND INCIDENCE

Jeremy, a 12-year-old boy, acquired cerebral palsy at birth when the placenta that connected him to his mother's uterine wall became prematurely dislodged during his delivery. He experienced a lack of oxygen (anoxia) for several minutes. As a result of the anoxia, the parts of his brain that control movement were damaged. Jeremy developed cerebral palsy, affecting all of the muscles in his body, including those that he uses for eating, breathing, and focusing his vision. At age 12, Jeremy has yet to learn to stand or walk independently. He relies on others to assist him with all activities of daily living (ADLs) and attends a school that can accommodate students with physical disabilities. For mobility, Jeremy uses an electric wheelchair that he controls through a switch he activates by tilting his head. Because he cannot easily coordinate his speaking and breathing muscles, his speech is very difficult to understand. Jeremy is now learning to use switches to operate a computer for communication and schoolwork.

Origin

Cerebral palsy, first described by English physician William Little in 1843,[4] is a general term used to describe a variety of postural control and movement disorders that result from a lesion or damage to one or more parts of the central nervous system (CNS). These lesions occur in areas responsible for controlling the quality and quantity of skilled movement (Box 12-1). Cerebral palsy occurs when the sensory, perceptual, and motor areas of the CNS cannot accurately relay and integrate essential information that the brain needs to correctly plan and direct the skilled, efficient movements used in everyday interactions with the environment. The lesion or damage causes impairment in muscle activity to part or all of the body. The muscles shorten and lengthen in uncoordinated, inefficient ways and are unable to work together to create smooth, effective motion. This type of muscle activity is referred to as *impaired coactivation*.

BOX 12-1

Definition of Cerebral Palsy

Cerebral palsy is a disorder of motor functioning caused by a permanent, nonprogressive brain defect or lesion present at or shortly after birth. It causes atypical muscle movements and can affect the muscles controlling breathing, speech, and eye movement.

Progression of Disordered Movement Development

Children who have cerebral palsy demonstrate difficulty in achieving and maintaining normal posture while lying down, sitting, and standing because of impaired muscle coactivation. They also develop abnormal movement compensations, movements, and body postures that evolve as they try to function within their environments. Over time, such movement compensations create barriers to a child's ongoing motor skill development. Instead of freely moving and exploring the world, as the child with a normally developing sensorimotor system does, children who have cerebral palsy may rely on early automatic reflex movement patterns as their primary means of mobility.

Typically, developing infants demonstrate an asymmetrical tonic neck reflex between 1 and 4 months of age.[12] As they turn their heads to one side, the upper extremity on that side extends outward. This early automatic behavior lays the groundwork for the child's future independent ability to visually regard the hand and engage in coordinated eye-hand activities (Figure 12-1).

Children who have cerebral palsy continue to rely on this automatic movement pattern because they are unable to direct their muscles to move successfully in other patterns. The pattern becomes repetitive and fixed

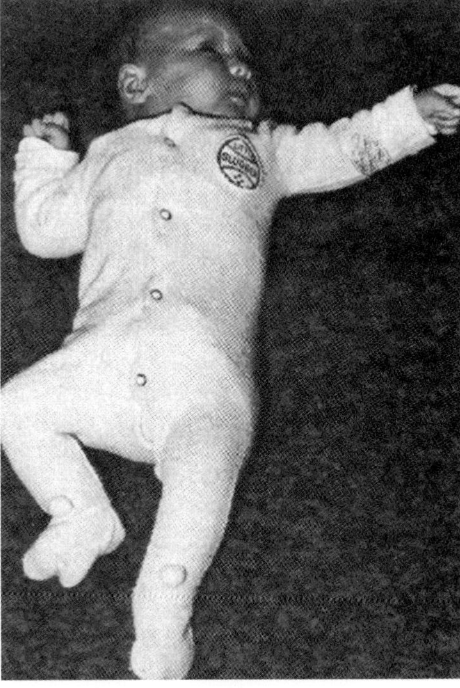

FIGURE 12-1 Normal infant exhibiting asymmetrical tonic neck reflex. (From Case-Smith J: *Occupational therapy for children*, ed 5, St Louis, 2005, Mosby.)

CLINICAL *Pearl*

In the typically developing infant, automatic reflex movement patterns are never obligatory. Therefore, normal infants do not always exhibit the motor responses of the asymmetrical tonic reflexes when their heads are turned to the side.

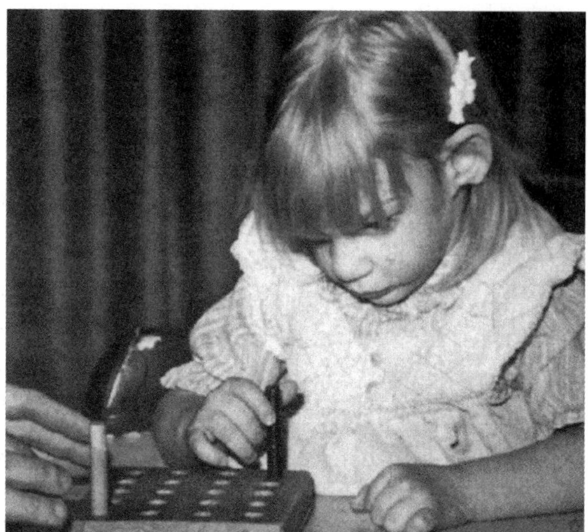

FIGURE 12-2 A child with hemiplegia and spasticity in her left arm and leg. Notice her making a fist with her left hand as she places the peg into the pegboard with her right hand. (From Case-Smith J, Allen AS, Pratt PN: *Occupational therapy for children,* ed 3, St Louis, 1996, Mosby.)

(Figure 12-2). The repetition of the pattern prevents these children from gaining independent voluntary control of their own movements. The use of **primitive reflex patterns** limits the children's access to participation in meaningful activities. The combination of impaired muscle coactivation and the use of reflexively controlled postures may also lead to future contractures in the muscle, tendon, and ligamentous tissues, causing the tissues to become permanently shortened. Bone deformities and alterations of typical shape or alignment may also occur.[6]

The nervous system damage that causes cerebral palsy can occur before or during birth or before a child's second year, the time when myelination of the child's sensory and motor tracts and CNS structures rapidly occurs.[3] Cerebral palsy is described as nonprogressive, nonhereditary, and noncontagious. As a nonprogressive condition, the original defect or lesion occurring in the CNS typically does not worsen or change over time. However, because the lesion occurs in immature brain structures, the progression of the child's motor development may appear to change. Normal nervous system maturation shifts control of voluntary movement toward increasingly higher and more complex areas of the brain. The child who has cerebral palsy exhibits some changes in movement ability that result from the expected progression of motor development skills, but these changes tend to be delayed relative to age and often show much less variety than those seen in the normal child.

Frequency and Causes

Cerebral palsy is diagnosed in 500,000 to 700,000 Americans, or 0.05% of the population, and approximately 1500 babies are born with cerebral palsy in the United States each year.[9] Unfortunately, the exact cause frequently cannot be determined, but known contributing risk factors are prenatal, perinatal, and postnatal. Prenatal factors may include genetic abnormalities or maternal health factors such as stress, malnutrition, exposure to damaging drugs, and pregnancy-induced hypertension. Some gestational conditions of the mother, such as diabetes, may cause perinatal risks to the child as well. Perinatally, children born very prematurely with low birth weights demonstrate an increased risk for cerebral palsy. Medical problems associated with premature birth may directly or indirectly damage the developing sensorimotor areas of the CNS. In particular, respiratory disorders can

BOX 12-2

Risk Factors Associated with the Development of Cerebral Palsy

PRENATAL

- Genetic abnormalities
- Maternal health factors (e.g., chronic stress, malnutrition)
- Teratogenic agents (e.g., drugs, chemical exposure, radiation)

PERINATAL

- Prenatal conditions (e.g., toxemia secondary to maternal diabetes)
- Premature detachment of the placenta
- Medical problems associated with prematurity (e.g., compromised respiration, cardiovascular dysfunction)
- Multiple births

POSTNATAL

- Degenerative disorders (e.g., Tay-Sachs disease)
- Infections (e.g., meningitis, encephalitis)
- Alcohol or drug intoxication transferred while breast-feeding
- Malnutrition
- Trauma
- Anoxia

cause the premature newborn to experience anoxia, which deprives the cells of the oxygen needed to function and survive. Typical postnatal, child-centered conditions that may result in significant damage to the developing CNS may be malnutrition and anoxia but can also stem from infection, trauma, or exposure to environmental toxins. Research also suggests a link between multiple births and an increased risk for cerebral palsy (Box 12-2).[8,14]

POSTURE, POSTURAL CONTROL, AND MOVEMENT

To understand the functional movement problems that develop in children who have cerebral palsy, the occupational therapy (OT) practitioner must be familiar with the ways that people normally control their bodies and execute skilled movements. The term *posture* describes the alignment of the body's parts in relation to each other and the environment. The ability to develop a large repertoire of postures and change them easily during an activity depends on the integration of several automatic, involuntary movement actions referred to as the **postural mechanism.** (See Chapter 5 for a more extensive discussion on the components of normal movement.) The postural mechanism includes several key components.[15]

- Normal muscle tone
- Normal postural tone
- Developmental integration of early, primitive reflex movement patterns
- Emergence of righting, equilibrium, and protective extension reactions
- Intentional, voluntary movements

Disruption in the postural mechanism is a key cause for the movement problems that are seen in cerebral palsy.

Righting, Equilibrium, and Protective Reactions

The functions that aid individuals in maintaining or regaining posture are **righting reactions** and **equilibrium reactions,** often referred to concomitantly as *balance reactions*. These functions can be thought of as static or dynamic. When people are sitting and not engaged in any activity, they are using static balance. When they bend to pick up an object on the floor, they use dynamic balance to right themselves. *Righting* means bringing the body back into "normal" skeletal alignment[5,6] by using only the necessary muscle groups. When righting and equilibrium reactions are not sufficient to regain an upright posture quickly and safely, individuals use another reflexive reaction called the **protective extension reaction.** When people fall they frequently use this reaction, automatically reaching outward from their bodies to catch themselves or break the fall.

CLINICAL *Pearl*

Frequently, children who have cerebral palsy have delayed or absent protective extension responses. These children may move cautiously because of the fear of falling or, as a result of impaired balance, may be at risk for physical injury when moving.

When movement abilities develop normally, children experience and practice many different movements and positions as they work toward mastery of an upright, two-legged stance. Postural stability and the ability to reestablish it through righting and balance reactions evolve developmentally through experimentation and experiences in a variety and combination of positions (e.g., prone, supine, sitting, kneeling, standing). As children refine their control of specific postures through developmental progression, they gain the stable background needed for the infinite variety of skilled, voluntary movements used for environmental interactions. For example, when a person reaches across the dinner table to pass a serving dish, that person must remain stable in the chair while going through several hand and arm motions to lift the dish, move it across the table, and then carefully release it to the person waiting for the dish. Such a task requires the use of the muscles of the trunk and pelvic girdle areas as stabilizers; that is, these areas must do more "holding" as the upper extremity and shoulder girdle muscles perform most of the visible movements. In addition to the different types of muscle activity used for this task, the person must also rely on quick-responding righting and equilibrium reactions and visual perception to remain seated in the chair. The person passing the dish will probably lean to the left or right or forward. In this instance, just as in every executed movement, the leaning or moving from the center of gravity requires shifting of the body's weight. Each time a person shifts weight, righting and equilibrium reactions are used to counterbalance the weight shifts during the movements and help regain an upright posture with body parts correctly realigned. Vision, hearing, and other sensory input also provide perceptual information about whether the person is moving just the right distance when reaching and whether that person is upright in the context of the immediate surroundings.

Muscle Tone

A child's ability to perform sequential movements is supported by the ability of the muscles to maintain the correct amount of tension and elasticity during the movements; the neurophysiological state of the muscle is referred to as **muscle tone.** Best described as a state of continuous mild contraction in the muscle, muscle tone is determined primarily by two factors. First, muscle tone is highly influenced by gravity. The muscle must have enough tone to move against gravity in a smooth, coordinated motion. Second, emotions and mental state, including levels of alertness, fatigue, and excitement, influence muscle tone. Normal muscle tone develops along a continuum, with some variability among members of the normal population.

The muscles' qualities of contractility and elasticity are necessary for an accurate response to the changes in stimuli experienced during movement, an event referred to as *coactivation*. In the previous example a greater degree of force resistance is required for the initial lifting of the serving dish than that required for its actual movement toward a person. It requires more force resistance for a person to carefully lower the dish without dropping it again. Although muscle strength is important for the movement of muscles against an outside force (weight) or gravity, normal muscle tone is also essential. Tone allows the muscles to adapt readily to the changing sensory stimuli resulting from the positional changes of the dish in relation to the arm. The total movement appears smooth and coordinated because normal tone can be sustained in all muscles, including the muscle groups that contract to initiate movement at joints (agonists) and simultaneously relax to allow movement at joints (antagonists). When the agonist muscle group initiates the lifting of the dish, the gradual relaxation and elongation of the opposing antagonist muscle group result in a smooth, directed movement. When the dish is held still for several seconds, the agonist and antagonist muscle groups work with equal force. Cocontraction occurs, resulting in postural stabilization; each muscle group has just the right amount of muscle tone needed for the muscle contractions to keep the joint stable. Individuals with intact sensorimotor functioning can perform an infinite number and variety of movements; all of them require points of postural stability or fixation to provide the stable background for skilled, active movements.[5] Children who have cerebral palsy experience a disorder in the CNS functions that regulate postural control, righting, equilibrium, and muscle tone.[5,6] A certified occupational therapy assistant (COTA) who is planning therapeutic interventions for children who have cerebral palsy must possess an understanding of the ways in which postural control and motor skills develop. This knowledge is imperative for planning functional therapeutic activities that are appropriate for the child's age and physical abilities (Box 12-3).

BOX 12-3

Common Problems of Motor Development in Children with Cerebral Palsy

1. Abnormal muscle tone
   - Hypertonicity: rigid, high tone
   - Hypotonicity: flaccid, floppy, very low tone
   - Fluctuating: rigid, floppy, rigid, floppy
2. Persistence of primitive reflex patterns interfering with voluntary movements
3. Poorly developed normal movement patterns, including balance reactions
4. Distorted body awareness and body scheme because of inaccurate sensory information
5. Joint hypermobility
   - Reduced limb stability
   - Use of postural compensations
6. Muscle weakness
7. Reduced skill development and refinement of movement
8. Decreased exploration of the environment

POSTURAL DEVELOPMENT AND MOTOR CONTROL

As newborns grow, they are continually developing and refining postural control. As with motor skills, the characteristics of posture vary with age. In the past 20 years, much research has been devoted to understanding motor control so that practitioners may provide effective neurological rehabilitation to persons who have cerebral palsy and other neurological disorders. Motor control theory is complex, and detailed explanations are beyond the scope of this text. However, the COTA should recognize the two main schools of thought on motor control. This knowledge can guide the OT practitioner in seeking information that can contribute to implementing effective therapeutic approaches. The theories can be grouped into two models of motor control: the traditional reflex-hierarchical models and the more recent systems models.[7,16]

Reflex-Hierarchical Models

Reflex-hierarchical models propose that purposeful movement is initiated only when the individual experiences a need to move. When the desire to move is stimulated, the person searches long-term memory for a pattern of movement that will accomplish the desired task. The stored movement patterns that the person has practiced the most are the most likely to be used again because they are more embedded in memory. The person prepares to execute the movement, incorporating additional information from the environment to make the movements meet the demands of the task. The previous example of lifting and passing a serving dish can help illustrate this model. From the general experience of lifting and moving objects, an individual can recall from long-term memory the necessary movement patterns. The individual also needs to collect some information from the environment such as the approximate size and weight of the dish. This information helps the individual determine whether both hands are required for the task and what type of grasp should be used to lift and hold on to the dish. Sensory feedback determines whether the individual's movement efforts have been successful (i.e., have met the task demands). With continual repetition, these movement patterns can develop into motor skills. Reflex-hierarchical models support the idea that motor learning optimally occurs when a person engages in repetition of the same task during frequent, regular practice, and breaking down a task into small parts is the most effective way to learn the entire task.[10]

According to reflex models, many children with cerebral palsy use the tonic reflexes controlled by the lower levels of the CNS for managing most of their movements. These movement patterns are "hard wired" into the human nervous system and do not depend on the application of learned patterns for performing tasks. Children with cerebral palsy lack the ability to independently learn to control movement from higher-level brain centers. Their abnormal postural mechanisms and disordered muscle tone cause them to repeatedly use and store in memory those movement patterns that are governed predominantly by the early tonic reflex patterns.

Systems Models

Systems approaches to understanding motor behavior propose that postural control is greatly influenced by an individual's many volitional and functional daily tasks and activities. The sitting posture needed for a person to put on shoes while on a bed is different from that needed when a person is strapped into the seat of an airplane. Systems models purport that posture and movement must be flexible and adaptable so that a person can perform a wide range of daily activities, whereas reflex-hierarchical models state that the control of posture and movement is the outcome or product of a process. Systems models postulate that posture is anticipatory to the initiation of movement. Postural adjustments actually precede movements; they prepare the body to counterbalance the weight shifts that are caused by the movement activity. In this way, less balance disturbance occurs. For example, a person catches two balls, one of which is a small tennis ball and the other a large, heavy medicine ball. Before catching the balls, that person has seen them, used visual perception to make decisions about their sizes and weights, and assumed an appropriate postural stance. This anticipatory process is called *feed forward*.

According to the systems approach, feed forward actions require that posture be highly variable and subject to being affected by all the factors motivating the person to choose to catch the balls. No one right way to execute movement exists; rather, movement is strongly influenced by many variables. This model contrasts with reflex-hierarchical models stating motor development follows a steplike progression, starting with the primitive reflexes and progressing to voluntary movement control through the higher brain centers. The research of the systems theorists has shown that motor activity is most often initiated by the interaction of sensory, perceptual, environmental, and other factors leading to task-focused, goal-directed movement.[7,16]

One other concept from systems model research has important therapeutic implications for the treatment of children with cerebral palsy or other neurologically based disorders. Postural control and movement are at their greatest levels of efficiency, flexibility, and adaptability after randomized practice and repetition.[7,16] Children in elementary school have many opportunities to practice learning to print their names so that the letters will be neatly aligned and a small, equal size. Although children practice printing in school during class, they are also practicing any time they spontaneously write their names during typical childhood activities and games. Over time, this repeated motor pattern develops into a skill; children can adapt the postures and movements used in the activity to fit several different tasks. They can write their names at the top of school papers while seated at their desks or at the bottom of pictures they are drawing while stretched out on the floor. By repeating this task in many different contexts, children gain the skill of motor problem solving. The systems models suggest that children with cerebral palsy need to be challenged with meaningful activities that give them opportunities to solve motor problems and practice their motor strategies in a variety of environments.

CLASSIFICATION AND DISTRIBUTION

Cerebral palsy can be classified according to the location of the lesion in the CNS. For example, a lesion in the motor cortex typically causes increased, or hypertonic, muscle tone during flexor and extensor cocontraction. This increased tone produces **spasticity (hypertonicity);** as a movement is initiated, excessive muscle tone builds up and then rapidly releases, triggering a hyperactive stretch reflex in the muscle. It may show up at the beginning, middle, or end of a movement range, but the result is poor control of voluntary movement and little ability to regulate force of movement. A lesion of the basal ganglia

CLINICAL *Pearl*

Children who have athetosis are often very bright. They also tend to appear physically asymmetrical because they are unable to coordinate the movements of both sides of the body and show significant muscle tightness and a fixed posture on one side. These children assume a fixed, static posture on one side of the body for stability while using the limbs on the opposite side for purposeful actions. For example, a child who has athetosis may stabilize the right arm between crossed legs while reaching with the left arm.

produces a state of widely fluctuating tone called **athetosis.** In athetosis, tone rapidly shifts from normal or hypertonic to unusually low or hypotonic. Movement is very unsteady and appears purposeless and uncontrollable. The person may appear to be swiping at an object or writhing.

Ataxia is a less common tone abnormality. Children who have ataxia also show tonal shifts but to a lesser degree than those with athetosis. These children can be more successful in directing voluntary movements but appear clumsy and may shake involuntarily. They have considerable difficulty with balance, coordination, and maintenance of stable alignment of the head, trunk, shoulders, and pelvis.[16]

Children who have cerebral palsy often show combinations of tone problems. Those who have spastic cerebral palsy move their extremities with abrupt hypertonic motions but may also exhibit marked **hypotonicity** (low muscle tone) in their trunk muscles. Medical and allied health practitioners commonly use two ways to describe each child's movement control problems. One is by the type of movement disorder, which is characterized by the predominant muscle tone observed, and the other is by distribution, which identifies the body parts that are the most affected by the child's movement control problems. The three most common distribution patterns are **quadriplegia,** involving all four extremities; **diplegia,** involving predominantly the lower half of the body; and **hemiplegia,** involving one side of the body.

CLINICAL *Pearl*

The child who has ataxia may use visual fixation to maintain balance while moving toward an object.

CLINICAL *Pearl*

Children who have moderate to severe spastic diplegia have functional limitations in the arms and lower extremities.

Monoplegia and triplegia, which involve one and three extremities, respectively, are rare. In addition to these categories of characteristic tone and topographical distribution, the disorder may also be diagnosed as mild, moderate, or severe. Each level suggests a degree of muscle tone abnormality, types of abnormal reflex activity, the potential for functional activity, and typical associated problems. Knowledge of the degree of muscle tone abnormality and a child's cognitive, sensory, and perceptual status can help the OT practitioner establish realistic and practical therapeutic goals and interventions. A child with mild motor involvement and normal cognition has greater potential to succeed at gaining new motor skills. A child with severe motor involvement and impaired cognition may benefit more from assistive technologies that compensate for the absence of motor skills.

FUNCTIONAL IMPLICATIONS AND ASSOCIATED PROBLEMS

Muscle and Bone Tissue Changes

A host of associated disabilities and health and social problems can be caused by cerebral palsy and influence each person's functional potential. The disorder is nonprogressive in terms of lesion changes in the CNS, but over time the resulting postural disorder may cause muscle tissue contractures, bone deformities, and joint dislocation or misalignment. These changes further limit functional movement, and if they are severe, the child may become highly dependent on others for all ADLs. As the child ages, the potential for painful arthritis in misaligned joints increases. Individuals who are unable to assume more than a few positions or independently shift their weight also risk skin breakdown because body weight is often concentrated over a few joints for prolonged time periods.

Cognition and Language Impairments

More than 60% of children who have cerebral palsy have cognitive and language impairments. The severity of the deficits can range from mild to severe; up to 30% of individuals who have cerebral palsy possess significant communication impairments.[2] Cognitive and linguistic competency can play a significant role in a child's ability to benefit from therapeutic and educational interventions. Children with normal or near-normal cognition can consciously generate problem-solving strategies to perform some functional movement activities that are automatic for most people.

Sensory Problems

Sensory problems are also present in individuals who have cerebral palsy. Visual impairments such as blindness, uncoordinated eye movements, and eye muscle weakness affect as many as 50% of children who have cerebral palsy; auditory reception and processing deficits have an impact on 25%.[2] Additional sensory problems include hypersensitivity (i.e., overreacting to touch, textures, and changes in head position), causing some children to become visibly upset when handled or moved by others. Children with multiple sensory processing problems have more difficulty understanding their environments. Some tactile sensation problems are also linked to abnormal oral movement patterns. Many children dislike certain food textures and may have problems coordinating their chewing, sucking, and swallowing movements. Those with severe problems in this area may be surgically fitted with a gastrostomy tube for feeding. OT practitioners must consider a child's sensory limitations and strengths while setting intervention goals. The practitioner considers each child to determine which sensory experiences are likely to improve occupational performance abilities.

Physical and Behavioral Manifestations

Additional problems can include seizures and other medical conditions not directly related to the child's movement disorder. Abnormal posture and weak muscle activity may compromise cardiac and respiratory functions and prevent these systems from working efficiently. The resulting low endurance and fatigue can influence the child's capacity for activity. The OT practitioner monitors each child's physical endurance and may plan therapeutic goals to increase strength and endurance.

Behavioral problems and social delays are not unusual. Children who have cerebral palsy may become accustomed to receiving assistance from others, and problems such as "learned helplessness" may prevent them from attempting the developmental challenges needed for continued growth and mastery of skills. The inability to manage social and peer interactions can lead to social isolation and immaturity and a repertoire of undesirable social behaviors. The OT practitioner can often assist families and work collaboratively with the child's educational team, which may include teachers, consultants, and administrators, to suggest strategies to enhance the child's social development.

CLINICAL *Pearl*

Because approximately 40% of children who have cerebral palsy have normal or above-normal intelligence, the OT practitioner should not assume that a child is cognitively delayed based on physical appearance or a lack of motor control.

CLINICAL *Pearl*

The OT practitioner working with children who have cerebral palsy offers these children opportunities for a variety of sensory experiences without forcing sensory experiences that a child finds aversive.

ROLES OF THE REGISTERED OCCUPATIONAL THERAPIST AND CERTIFIED OCCUPATIONAL THERAPY ASSISTANT

The registered occupational therapist (OTR) and COTA collaborate to provide services. The individual needs of the child and family and the child's chronological age shape each step in the assessment and intervention process. In infancy and early childhood, OT practitioners focus on family care and management issues such as feeding and bathing, mobility around the home, and family participation. During the early school years the OTR and COTA assist the child with classroom participation, self-care skills, peer socialization, leisure and vocational readiness, and educational and community mobility. For the adolescent who has cerebral palsy, OT services may focus on engagement in work or other productive activities, development of independent living skills, sexual identification and sexual expression, and mobility in the community at large.

Assessment

The OTR and COTA collaboratively assess each individual's needs. Together they evaluate areas of performance, client factors, activity demands, and contexts.[1] The OTR may use one or several standardized tests requiring specialized administration and interpretation skills that can provide the team with specific information about reflex development, sensorimotor functioning, motor skills, and developmental skill levels. The experienced, trained COTA may assist in the administration of some tests. Observation is a crucial part of the assessment process because many children who have cerebral palsy cannot easily follow the directions of standardized tests due to their impaired motor skills. Both practitioners can observe the child's functional abilities at home and in school and leisure activities. Observation of the child's occupational performance provides the practitioner with data on factors influencing the child's muscle tone, reflex activity, gross and fine motor skills, sensory systems, cognition, perception, and psychosocial development. OT practitioners are advised to use a top-down approach to assessment. The Model of Human Occupation Clearinghouse provides a variety of assessments that examine the child's occupational performance.[17] Interviews such as the Pediatric Volitional Questionnaire[5] provide information on the child's motivation. The SCOPE (Short-Children's Occupational Profile Evaluation) provides an overview of the child's volition, roles, habits, and performance within various contexts.[17] The SSI (School Setting Interview) provides information on how the child is functioning at school.[17] These assessments and others explore how the child performs his/her occupations.

The COTA may bring information to plan the most effective OT intervention. The earlier that the patterns of postural abnormality are recognized, the earlier that interventions can be planned to facilitate developmental progress, which minimizes the risk of serious deformities and development of undesirable behaviors.

Assessment data create a "picture" of the child's functioning and indicate his or her strengths and weaknesses. The OTR and COTA use this information (along with parental concerns) to formulate goals to match the child's needs and developmental abilities or potential. Examples include increasing a child's ability to participate in a classroom writing activity and teaching family members to reduce the hypertonicity so that they can bathe or feed him or her. Goals for the adolescent might address accessing public transportation or learning ways to perform homemaking skills. Thorough OT assessment data are essential when working as part of a service delivery team. Classroom teachers may rely on the OT practitioner's expertise to assist in the establishment and implementation of educational goals. Vocational skills trainers need to know the student's physical performance abilities and attitudes toward new tasks. Families may use OT input to select recreational activities for their children.

Intervention

Nathan, a 10-year-old boy who has cerebral palsy, wanted to participate in a special "Day at the Beach" activity with his classmates. The plans included mixing tropical fruit drinks for refreshments. The COTA treating Nathan had already helped him acquire the skills needed to activate a switch-operated computer in his classroom. The COTA then obtained another switch and electronic interface device and attached them to a standard kitchen blender. With the press of a switch, Nathan was able to blend tropical fruit drinks for his classmates.

Individuals who have cerebral palsy and receive OT services can experience a sense of empowerment and control when they successfully perform meaningful occupations, whether it is in the self-care, work, or leisure domain. OT practitioners develop and implement interventions to promote functional performance within each individual's capacities. Through training and consultation, they also assist caregivers and educators in the provision of interventions that facilitate and support the child's occupational performance. Intervention strategies include positioning and handling. The OT practitioner determines the variety of postures a child can assume, maintain, and achieve independently or with physical assistance. Optimum positions are determined for ADLs. Upright sitting positions are needed for most classroom activities, while a relaxed, partially reclined position may be optimal for assisted bathing. Practitioners can also select and recommend specific types of positioning equipment, such as chairs, supine or prone standers, and sidelyers, that support the child during functional activities with the best possible postural alignment, control, and stability. Handling techniques such as slow rocking, slow stroking, imposed rotational movement patterns, and bouncing are used to influence the child's muscle tone, activity level, and ability for independent movement. Techniques such as weight bearing and weight shifting can promote postural alignment and independent movement.[13] A stiff, hypertonic child fixed in a strong extensor posture can be easily positioned in a wheelchair after the practitioner has slowly and alternately rotated the shoulders in a forward and backward motion. Handling relaxes this child's tone throughout the body (Figure 12-3). Each joint can move more easily, and the child can then be placed in the wheelchair with good postural alignment and comfort. Positioning and handling methods are especially important for those individuals who have cerebral palsy and are unable to move independently. These methods also help a child work toward the achievement of performance-area goals such as increased independence in dressing, feeding, playing, and doing schoolwork. An OT practitioner can learn these treatments in special training programs or under the direction of a skilled therapist. The COTA can implement positioning recommendations, teach them to caregivers, and use handling methods to improve the child's functional performance by following the instructions of the OTR.

Persons who have cerebral palsy can achieve greater independence in daily living tasks with assistive and adaptive devices. (See Chapters 18 and 22, respectively, for more information on occupational performance areas and assistive technologies.) The COTA may recommend adapted utensils for the child with limited grasp abilities; suggest a large, weighted pen to aid a student with tremors; or attach a large zipper pull on a child's coat for

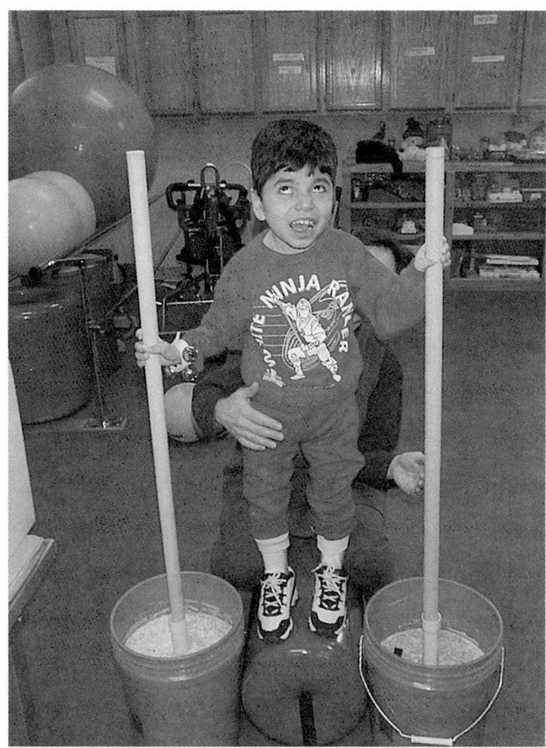

FIGURE 12-3 The occupational therapy practitioner uses specialized positioning and handling techniques to improve the child's ability to act in the environment.

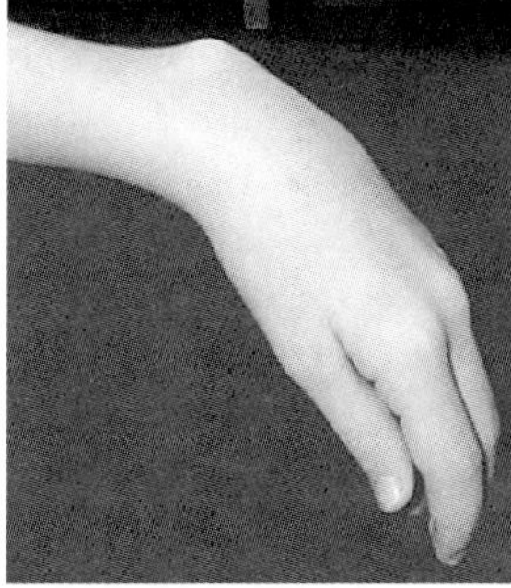

A

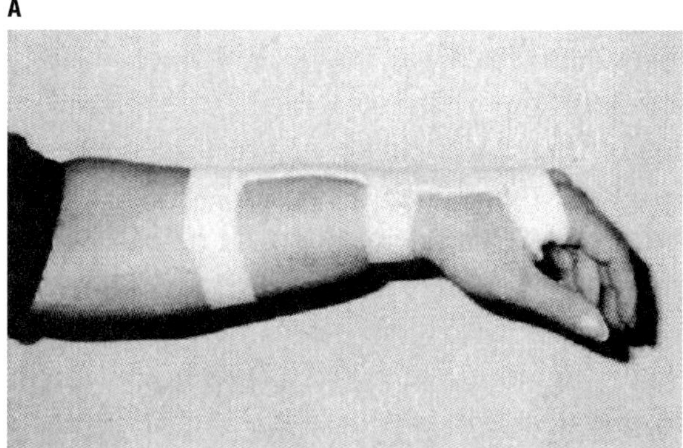

B

FIGURE 12-4 **A**, Unsplinted hand postured inefficiently for function. **B,** Orthotic device that helps keep bones and joints in good alignment and increases the child's ability to use the hand.

a self-dressing activity. The COTA consults with the OTR to determine the safest and most appropriate devices to match each child's abilities. This task is particularly important in the selection of feeding equipment that can influence safe swallowing. The COTA should become familiar with a number of assistive device vendors so that equipment recommendations can be offered for all appropriate occupational performance areas and budget considerations. With a little creative thinking a COTA can often fabricate assistive devices from inexpensive materials. PVC plumbing pipe from a hardware store can be assembled to make an inverted U-shaped frame with suspended toys to be placed in front of a child. For children with limited reaching and grasping abilities, this could be the one way to help them engage in a meaningful play activity.

Many children who have cerebral palsy may benefit from a custom-designed *orthotic device*, a bracing system designed to control, correct, and compensate for bone deformities (Figure 12-4). OT practitioners can design this device to accomplish a variety of goals. A COTA may make a resting orthotic hand splint to decrease or prevent further deformity in a child whose muscle tone abnormalities are causing ulnar deviation. The OT may design an upper extremity orthosis to stabilize wrist and elbow joints so that a student may successfully use a keyboard-typing device at school. Therapists may occasionally help family and school team members solve behavior problems that pose a risk of self-injury by designing appliances to prevent children from biting or otherwise injuring themselves. A COTA who fabricates orthotic devices should have good knowledge of and experience in splinting and work under the supervision of an OTR to devise safe and appropriate wearing schedules while instructing caregivers. The COTA may be required to monitor the application, use, and safety of the fabricated orthosis.

COTAs assist clients who have cerebral palsy in a variety of settings. Intervention programs can occur in the family home, a school setting, or a hospital. In each setting the COTA is part of an interdisciplinary treatment team whose goal is to maximize the child's health, functional capacities, and quality of life. As an occupational specialist the COTA combines knowledge and skill to help each child accomplish purposeful and meaningful daily living tasks within the home, school setting, and community.

CASE *Study*

Missy is a 6-year-old girl. During her birth, she experienced a prolonged period of anoxia that resulted in spastic diplegia. Missy has moderate hypertonia throughout her lower extremities and mild tone problems in her upper extremities. These problems cause difficulties with fine motor and in-hand manipulation tasks such as drawing, writing, and brushing her teeth. Missy demonstrates good balance reactions from her middle trunk area upward but easily loses her balance when seated on a chair without armrests. She frequently topples over when she tries to bend to retrieve something dropped on the floor. Missy is a bright, happy child of normal intelligence and good vision and hearing abilities. From ages 3 to 6 she attended a special preschool and kindergarten program, where she received OT and physical therapy services. Physical therapy practitioners worked with Missy to develop functional mobility skills. She now ambulates independently with a wheeled walker, can lower and raise herself to and from the floor level using an environmental support, and can transfer on and off a preschool-size toilet. OT practitioners helped Missy increase her independence in dressing with the use of Velcro closures and zipper pulls, and they used therapeutic handling and strengthening techniques to improve her manipulation skills with drawing materials and pencils. Because Missy has been so successful in learning self-management skills, her parents and the special education team believe that she is ready to enroll in the regular first grade class of her local elementary school.

OT consultation services are recommended to assist in Missy's successful school transition. Before she starts school, the COTA and OTR participate in a team staffing meeting. Missy's parents, her new first grade teacher, the school's physical education teacher, and the school principal also attend the meeting. The team members decide that the OT team will consult with the classroom teacher to address Missy's seating needs and make sure she can participate in typical first grade activities. The school district OTR reviews the OT documentation from Missy's previous practitioners and then schedules a classroom visit for herself and the COTA, Mike, during the first week of school. During their visit they note that the classroom desks are too high for Missy. She cannot maintain a stable, upright posture on a desk chair and loses her balance whenever she leans sideways. Missy also has difficulty keeping her papers firmly on the desk surface when writing and drawing. The OTR and Mike note two other problems. Because of her lack of developed balance reactions in the lower body, Missy is unable to remove or put on her coat while standing in the coatroom with the other children. At snack time, Missy has difficulty opening her cardboard juice cartons. The teacher also tells Mike that each student is expected to have a daily job, and she would like assistance in selecting one for Missy.

The OTR and Mike review Missy's functional motor skills and tone problems. They note that she sits in a regular chair with her hips rolled back, her knees and toes pointing inward, and her upper body bent forward because of the lack of postural control and stability in the pelvic area and lower extremities. The OTR instructs Mike to locate a smaller chair with armrests for Missy and discusses with him ways to determine a good functional seating position.

The following week Mike and Missy's teacher locate a chair with armrests that provides Missy with good stability. Her feet are flat on the floor, and her hips fit back in the seat with a 90-degree bend. Mike places a piece of Dycem, a nonskid rubbery material, on the seat to provide Missy with additional stability so that she can shift her weight and lean somewhat without significant loss of balance. A desk of a suitable height is found, and nonslip grips are placed under the desk feet so that Missy can reach a standing position easily by pushing on the desk. Mike recommends using removable sticky putty to help Missy keep her papers in place, and he finds a small bench that can be positioned against the wall in the coatroom. Missy can easily manage her coat by sitting on the bench and leaning against the wall. The teacher has learned that Missy enjoys exploring the building but has fewer opportunities to do so than her classmates because she needs additional travel time with her walker. The teacher believes Missy would like the job of taking the daily attendance report to the school office but is not certain how she could accomplish it. Mike suggests strapping an attractive bicycle basket of Missy's choice to her walker. The basket can also be handy for transporting other classroom materials. To solve Missy's snack time drink problem, Mike chooses a small piece of brightly colored splinting material and fashions a ring with a 1-inch-long pencil-like protrusion for Missy's middle finger. She can slide on the ring with the protrusion pointing down from her palm and then use the force of her open hand to punch a hole in the juice carton. The basket and ring enable Missy to be as independent as the other children at snack time.

Mike remembers that the repeated practice of skills in a variety of situations and environments can increase a person's independent motor skill abilities. He contacts Missy's mother, who agrees that Missy can use her ring to manage her drinks at home. After speaking with Mike, the physical education teacher places a bench against a wall in the area where the children change into their gym shoes. Missy can now independently don and doff her Velcro-closure gym shoes.

Mike follows up with Missy's parents and teachers to ensure that she is meeting all the demands. Later, he administers the Pediatric Volitional Questionnaire to ensure that the team has considered Missy's wants.

SUMMARY

Cerebral palsy is a term that encompasses a number of postural control and movement disorders resulting from damage to the areas of the CNS that control movement and balance. Common problems associated with cerebral palsy include limitations in movement options, delays in occupational skill development, muscle tone abnormalities that cause secondary problems such as contractures, and bone or joint deformities. Cerebral palsy can involve total or partial areas of the body, and many individuals who have it experience a number of associated disorders, such as impaired vision, hearing, and communication; below-normal cognition; and seizures.

COTAs can play a vital role in helping children who have cerebral palsy increase their abilities to function independently and expand their repertoire of occupational performance roles. Grounded with an understanding of movement control and skill development, COTAs can apply their knowledge of positioning and handling methods to improve an individual's ability to interact with the environment. COTAs can recommend and instruct in the use of assistive devices and specialized equipment to enable children with cerebral palsy to engage in purposeful activities that match their occupational roles and interests. With guidance from the OTR, COTAs can help children during therapy by using techniques to develop postural control, righting and equilibrium reactions, and controlled movement against gravity. Individual therapy plans incorporate therapeutic interventions that correspond to each child's unique developmental skills and occupational needs. COTAs offer service in many environmental contexts and find creative ways for each child to engage in meaningful activities at home and school and in the community.

References

1. American Occupational Therapy Association: Occupational Therapy Practice Framework: domain and process, *Am J Occup Ther* 56:609, 2002.
2. Batshaw M, Perret Y: *Children with disabilities: a medical primer*, ed 5, Baltimore, 2002, Brookes.
3. Cech D, Martin S: *Functional movement development across the life span*, ed 2, Philadelphia, 2002, Saunders.
4. Connecticut Children's Medical Center: What's new in cerebral palsy, *Pediatric Ortho Update* 2:2, 1990.
5. Geist R, Kielhofner G, Basu S, Kafkes A: The Pediatric Volitional Questionnaire (PVQ) (Version 2.0), Chicago and Model of Human Occupation Clearinghouse, Department of Occupational Therapy, University of Illinois at Chicago, 2002.
6. Horak F: Assumptions underlying motor control for neurological rehabilitation. In Contemporary Management of Motor Control Problems: Proceedings of the II Step Conference, *Found Phys Ther* 1991, Alexandria, Va.
7. Kuban O, Leviton A: Cerebral palsy, *N Engl J Med* 330:188, 1993.
8. Levy S: The developmental disabilities. In Kurtz L, Dowrick P, Levy S, Batshaw M, editors: *Handbook of developmental disabilities*, Gaithersburg, Md, 1996, Aspen.
9. Mathiowetz V, Haugen JB: Evaluation of motor behavior: traditional and contemporary views. In Trombly CA, editor: *Occupational therapy for physical dysfunction*, ed 5, Baltimore, 2002, Williams & Wilkins.
10. Rogers S: Common conditions that influence children's participation. In Case-Smith J, editor: *Occupational therapy for children*, ed 5, St Louis, 2005, Mosby.
11. Scherzer A, Tscharnuter I: *Early diagnosis and therapy in cerebral palsy*, ed 3, New York, 2000, Marcel Dekker.
12. Schoen S, Anderson J: Neurodevelopmental treatment frame of reference. In Kramer P, Hinojosa J, editors: *Frames of reference for pediatric occupational therapy*, ed 2, Baltimore, 1999, Williams & Wilkins.
13. Stanley F, Blair E: Cerebral palsy. In Pless I, editor: *The epidemiology of childhood disorders*, New York, 1994, Oxford University Press.
14. Solomon JW: Evaluation of motor control. In Early MB, editor: *Physical dysfunction practice skills for the occupational therapy assistant*, St Louis, 1998, Mosby.
15. Sugden D, Keogh J: *Problems in movement skill development*, Columbia, SC, 1990, University of South Carolina Press.
16. Vansant A: Motor control and motor learning. In Cech D, Martin S, editors: *Functional movement development across the life span*, ed 2, Philadelphia, 2002, Saunders.
17. http://uic.edu/hsc/acad/cahp/OTMOHOC.

Recommended Reading

Copeland M, Kimmel J: *Evaluation and management of infants and young children with developmental disabilities*, Baltimore, 1989, Brookes.

REVIEW *Questions*

1. Cerebral palsy can be classified by type and distribution over body areas. What are these classifications?
2. How does a COTA incorporate knowledge of motor control theories into treatment approaches for cerebral palsy?
3. What is the postural mechanism, and how is it disrupted in children with cerebral palsy?
4. Describe the ways in which COTAs facilitate function for very young children, school-aged children, and adolescents.
5. Name several physical and psychological conditions that frequently occur in children who have cerebral palsy.
6. Explain the importance of structured observation in the assessment of children who have cerebral palsy.
7. Differentiate between a contracture and a deformity. Explain the therapeutic interventions that the COTA can offer for these problems.

SUGGESTED *Activities*

1. Explore several therapeutic equipment catalogs and identify seating and positioning systems used for children who have cerebral palsy.
2. Challenge your own balance reactions in several positions. For example, try sitting on the edge of a table with your feet off the floor. Notice the way in which your head leads your body toward regaining an upright position. Which muscle groups are needed to make this happen?
3. Walk across a room and observe the way in which weight shifting occurs with each step you take.
4. Sit in a chair at a table. Try assuming a posture in which your hips are rolled back in the chair seat and your legs are extended straight in front of you with your toes pointed inward. Now try to complete a writing task at the table. Notice the tasks that take most of your attention and energy.
5. Visit the Internet website for United Cerebral Palsy at *http://www.ucpa.com*. Explore the information resources that can be helpful to a COTA.

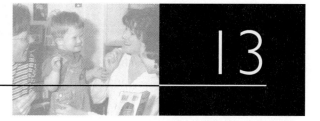

13

Positioning and Handling

JEAN W. SOLOMON
JANE CLIFFORD O'BRIEN

CHAPTER *Objectives*

After studying this chapter, the reader will be able to accomplish the following:

- Define and describe therapeutic positioning and handling techniques
- Explain the benefits of using positioning and handling techniques for children who have movement disorders of the central nervous system
- Identify ways of selecting therapeutic positions
- Describe the advantages and disadvantages of supine, prone, side-lying, and upright antigravity positions
- Describe the types of handling techniques and explain the purpose of each
- Explain the role of positioning and handling techniques in improving occupational performance

KEY TERMS	CHAPTER OUTLINE
Positioning	**BENEFITS**
Handling	**POSITIONING AS A THERAPEUTIC TOOL**
Alignment	General Principles of Positioning
Postural stability	Choosing a Positioning Method
Symmetry	Positioning Methods
Sensory input	**HANDLING AS A THERAPEUTIC TOOL**
Key points of control	Choosing a Handling Technique
Inhibition	Handling Techniques
Facilitation	**INTEGRATING POSITIONING AND HANDLING FOR OCCUPATIONAL PERFORMANCE**
	SUMMARY

Positioning and handling techniques are two tools used by occupational therapy (OT) practitioners to help children perform in school, at home, and during play. **Positioning** is a static process that improves a child's ability to maintain postural control while participating in activities. Positioning techniques can be as simple as holding or placing the child in a particular posture or involve the use of specialized adaptive furniture and equipment. If the positioning is successful, then the child will be able to participate in meaningful activities such as schoolwork, feeding, dressing, and play. **Handling** techniques are dynamic and guide a child's movement by influencing the state of muscle tone or triggering new automatic movement responses that result in functional actions. These methods are used with children whose movement disorders stem from damage to the central nervous system (CNS), such as those who have cerebral palsy. Both methods are adjuncts to therapy and are used as part of the daily intervention plan to increase movement for occupational performance.

BENEFITS

The OT practitioner who uses positioning and handling techniques examines the ways in which these methods create opportunities for children to interact more effectively with the environment. For example, a fifth grade student who has ataxia and cannot stand independently may need positioning assistance to perform classroom activities at the blackboard. A high school freshman who cannot maintain balance while sitting and has poorly integrated primitive postural reflexes may need to establish trunk stability when seated so that s/he can learn computer skills. In each case the practitioner facilitates improved postural control and skilled movement through positioning and handling; the opportunity for improved function ensues. The additional benefits derived from the use of these techniques include the following.

- *Increasing a child's physical comfort and reducing fatigue.* Providing various positioning options for the child who has little independent movement control can eliminate the risk of pressure sores developing or support a state of mental alertness while the body remains relaxed.
- *Promoting skeletal alignment.* Proper **alignment** of the bones and joints minimizes or prevents muscle and connective tissue contractures and bone and joint deformities, thus promoting better movement. A child with hypertonia may use the W-sit position because it provides a wide, stable base of support. However, this position can lead to tightening and contractures in the lower extremity muscle groups as well as hip, knee, and ankle joint malformations. A correct sitting position keeps the bones and joints aligned and moving in their correct planes.
- *Providing the child with a range of sensory experiences that enhance learning.* Children experience the environment differently from different positions. For example, sitting allows them to see things that they may not have observed while lying on their backs. Rolling provides a movement sensation that is not experienced in the prone position. Standing allows the child to experience the sensation of weight bearing throughout the legs and brings objects to a different level.

CLINICAL *Pearl*

Children learn through positioning. They enjoy interacting and exploring in different positions. The OT practitioner could remind parents that equipment may be temporary to give the child the experience.

- *Assisting the child with learning movement.* Handling techniques can facilitate the development of righting reactions and equilibrium reactions. Handling techniques can reduce the strength of primitive reflexes that prevent a child from developing the ability to use both sides of the body in a coordinated manner. Combining handling and positioning establishes a better balance between the pull of spastic muscles so that the body parts can work together for better quality of movement during an activity.

POSITIONING AS A THERAPEUTIC TOOL

The Shankar family is preparing for a traditional Hindu celebration. All the family and friends are expected to partake of a meal while sitting on the floor. Six-year-old Sanjay Shankar has spastic diplegic cerebral palsy, which prevents him from using his arms and hands unless he is sitting with assistance and using supports. Because of his increased muscle tone, his legs extend outward, with his toes pointed in and his hips rolled back so he sits on his sacrum. This sitting position causes his upper body to bend forward. Unless Sanjay uses his arms to brace himself upright, he collapses forward.

The certified occupational therapy assistant (COTA) who treats Sanjay during his outpatient therapy sessions makes a home visit to the Shankar household before the celebration. Mrs. Shankar indicates where the meal will be served. She and the COTA identify a place against the wall where Sanjay can sit. The COTA shows Mrs. Shankar how to position him with his back, shoulders, and hips aligned straight against the wall and his legs folded and crossed in front of him. She suggests placing a low bench or stool in front of Sanjay so that he can easily reach his food without having to hold a plate and can also rest on his arms and elbows to maintain a stable, upright position.

The use of positioning techniques begins as early as possible for children with neuromotor dysfunction because the techniques constitute one of the best ways to help children use any movement abilities they have. Positioning affects all activities, from sleeping, going to the bathroom, traveling, and eating to attending school and playing.[1] No one perfect or ideal position can be used with all children. The positions chosen must enhance the many different kinds of activities in which a child engages. The OT practitioner tries to choose those positions that most closely resemble the typical ones in which activities are performed. As a therapeutic modality, positioning can promote normal development; compensate for the lack of functional abilities; and prevent, minimize, or delay the onset of contractures and deformities that may result in the loss of movement, surgeries, and compromised health.[4]

Positioning equipment may also improve social interaction.[3] For example, brothers and sisters or peers may be more likely to approach a child sitting in a chair than rolling around on his or her back, which is not typical of older children.

General Principles of Positioning

- *Provide support.* Carefully observe the methods children use to independently maintain various positions, such as prone, supine, side-lying, sitting, kneeling, and standing. Use positioning to support only those parts of the body for which they cannot achieve or maintain **postural stability**. The right amount of support allows the arms, hands, and legs to be available for purposeful activity. Too much support stops children from using the movement they already possess.
- *Position for symmetry and skeletal alignment.* Achieve effective and efficient movement of the extremities by keeping the head, neck, trunk, and pelvis aligned. Proper skeletal alignment allows children to shift weight off their center of gravity, which can trigger the righting and equilibrium reactions needed to regain upright postural control. Proper alignment also maintains joint integrity, preventing joints from dislocating or partially dislocating, which is also known as *subluxing*. Positioning **symmetry** helps distribute body weight over bony prominences, thus eliminating the skin breakdown that can develop when a bony area receives constant pressure. Importantly, positioning symmetry allows children to bring their hands to the midline and work with objects using both hands.
- *Offer variety.* People use various positions as they engage in daily activities regardless of their age. The variety of positions stimulates perception as the child makes sense of position in space and views things from different angles. For example, infants' early feeding experiences occur while they are in reclining postures, those of toddlers occur in upright sitting positions, and older children may eat while lying in front of a television. Each new experience broadens children's perceptual and cognitive understanding of the environment. They develop positional preferences that facilitate and enhance the activities they perform. They may enjoy being stretched out on a chaise lounge for recreational reading but find it best to read material for a class while sitting at a desk. OT practitioners offer children enough positioning variety to establish which ones are the best choices for a particular activity and show parents, caregivers, and teachers the positions that work best for them.
- *Consider safety and comfort.* Many factors must be considered when choosing a particular position. Does it prepare a child for a new and unfamiliar activity? If so, can the child remain stable and feel secure in the position? Will the child ever be left unattended or with a minimum of monitoring while in the position? Can the child breathe comfortably in the position? Does the position promote optimum vision and hearing?
- *Select developmentally appropriate positions.* Typically developing children assume many different positions throughout the day. For example, infants sleep on their backs, play on their bellies or sides, eat in a semireclining position, and are carried upright. These positions provide different opportunities and sensory experiences. Children learn from the environment by interacting with it. A small infant is fed in a reclining position, which is appropriate for his or her level of oral-motor skills. Older children must eventually use upright positions to develop mature swallowing, sucking, and chewing movements and for socializing during mealtimes.
- *Determine whether handling interventions are needed to achieve proper positioning.* Handling techniques are needed to balance muscle tone or help a child adjust to an unfamiliar sensory experience that is introduced by a new position. An OT practitioner uses handling to place a child in a desired position. A child should never be forced into a position. Instead, the handling techniques discussed in this chapter should be used to address the neuromotor problems that interfere with proper positioning.

Choosing a Positioning Method

Ward groups positioning methods into the following three approaches.[6]

1. Some activities involve frequent positional changes and weight shifts, such as those required in dressing. During these activities the OT practitioner (or caregiver) may use his or her own body for support.
2. Positioning for activities in which the practitioner's hands need to be free (e.g., to work with a child on skills such as handwriting or feeding) can be accomplished with the use of either standard furniture (appropriate for the child's body size) or by selecting specialized adaptive equipment. Many types of reclining, seating, standing, transport, and mobility systems are available from various manufacturers.
3. Custom approaches are often used when a child has established contractures and deformities and body parts cannot be properly positioned into or supported by the standard equipment.[5] Positioning equipment may be specifically designed to fit the needs of children with severe or multiple disabilities. To create such a customized positioning solution, OT practitioners can couple their knowledge about movement (and its relation to occupational pursuits) with their skills in fabricating supportive equipment.

When selecting a positioning method, the OT practitioner evaluates each child's tolerance for the position, the length of time the child can comfortably maintain the position, the adaptability of the position to the activity it supports, and the age-appropriateness of the position for the particular activity. The OT practitioner keeps documented records and descriptions of successful positions for each child and notes those positions that pose risks for the child, such as compromised respiration. Good record keeping enables the OT practitioner to generate good positioning plans for the child to use at school, at home, or in other environments.

Positioning Methods

Each positioning option offers potential advantages and disadvantages. Infants begin to develop stability and mobility skills in prone, supine, and side-lying postures. For very young children and those with severe movement limitations, these three horizontal positions often make the best use of movements they can elicit independently or with minimal assistance. The choice of positioning method is also determined by the targeted activity. A therapeutic play activity that requires a child to skillfully reach for and manipulate small objects necessitates a positioning technique that gives the child solid support throughout the pelvis and trunk. Reach and manipulation skills demand isolation of small movements; therefore, good proximal support optimizes the child's ability to concentrate on these movements. An additional factor to consider is the spatial relationship influencing the interaction among the child, activity, and other individuals. The position should allow the child to use vision, hearing, and touch to his or her best advantage. A child with strong extensor spasticity may be positioned in a chair that provides flexion at the ankles, knees, and hips; however, if the child must look upward to make eye contact with the person speaking, that small head movement may easily trigger the spasticity and cause him or her to push out of the functional sitting position (Figure 13-1). Always consider whether a child has freedom of movement within a given position. A child who cannot shift weight independently needs assistance from the OT practitioner or caregiver. Generally, a child who is unable to move in and out of positions should not stay in any one position for more than 20 to 30 minutes.

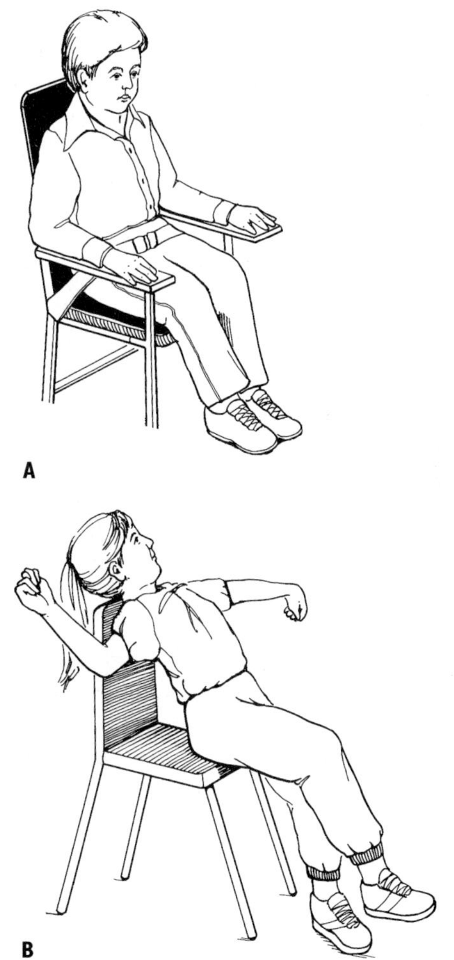

FIGURE 13-1 **A,** Child positioned in stable sitting posture. **B,** Child extends her neck to look up at the teacher, triggering a strong pattern of extensor spasticity. (From Case-Smith J, Allen AS, Pratt PN: *Occupational therapy for children,* ed 3, St Louis, 1996, Mosby.)

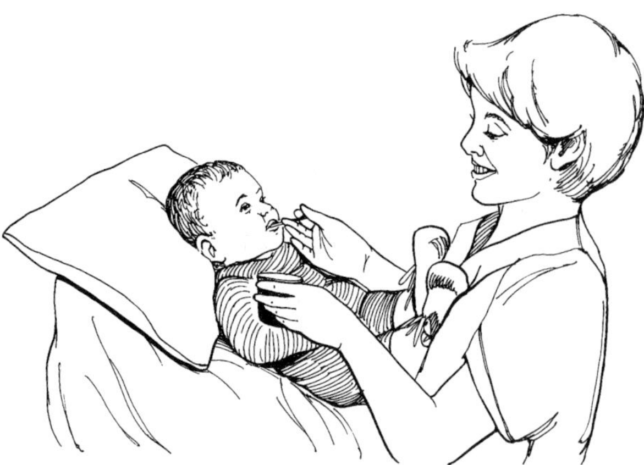

FIGURE 13-2 Supine positioning on a pillow includes maintaining some neck and leg flexion. (From Case-Smith J: *Occupational therapy for children,* ed 5, St Louis, 2005, Mosby.)

BOX 13-1

Advantages and Disadvantages of Supine Position

ADVANTAGES

- Allows children to see environment (e.g., watching television or playing with toys suspended on a mobile)
- It is the easiest position for visual fixation and tracking when head is positioned and supported
- Allows children to actively work to strengthen neck and abdominal flexor muscles
- Provides position of rest and comfort

DISADVANTAGES

- It is the most difficult position from which to raise the arms against gravity.
- It may increase extensor tone.
- It places minimum demands on children to develop head control.
- It encourages shallow abdominal breathing.
- It often elicits an asymmetrical tonic neck reflex.

Supine positioning

Infants spend a great deal of play time in the supine position (on their backs). This position helps infants develop flexor tone and abdominal control as they bring their hands and feet together. The supine position allows them to make eye contact with caregivers and bring their hands together.

Children may be positioned on a flat or inclined surface by using wedges, pillows, rolls, or towels. An important element of supine positioning is that the head be in a midline position and flexed slightly forward (Figure 13-2). Children who exhibit strong extensor muscle tone in this position must also have their hips and knees held in flexed positions. The presence of a strong asymmetrical tonic neck reflex (ATNR) must be counteracted with symmetrical body positioning. Box 13-1 describes the advantages and disadvantages of supine positioning.

Prone positioning

The prone position facilitates hand strength and neck and trunk extension. Infants bear their weight on the hands in the prone position, developing hand arches. Placing a firm foam wedge under the child's upper body, with the edge of the wedge just below the axillary area, can effect the prone position (Figure 13-3). Determine the correct degree of incline according to the child's ability to independently hold the head up during the selected activity. Keep the neck extension below a 45-degree angle to prevent the head movement from triggering hyperextension throughout the body. If the wedge angle is not high enough, the child's head can drop forward toward the floor and trigger too much flexion. A child with contractures in the hip flexor muscles may require pil-

CLINICAL *Pearl*

When you position a child in a supine position, remember the following hints. (1) Support the head in a flexed, forward position. (2) When you work with a baby on your lap or an older child on the floor, keep the knees and hips flexed to minimize the effects of extensor tone and encourage the use of abdominal muscles.

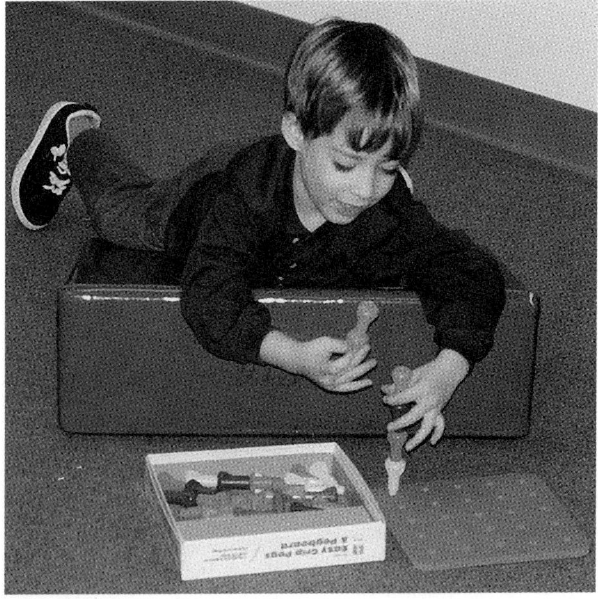

FIGURE 13-3 Child in prone position over a wedge. Note the axillary position, wedge height, and amount of neck extension.

BOX 13-2

Advantages and Disadvantages of Prone Position

ADVANTAGES
- Enables children to practice independent head control
- Provides children with opportunities to stretch hip and knee flexor muscles
- Leads to higher-level motor skills such as elbow propping, crawling, and reaching

DISADVANTAGES
- Children who are unable to independently turn their heads may have trouble breathing.
- Children who are unable to lift their heads or prop their bodies on their arms may have difficulty learning to reach, push up, or use vision properly.

lows under this body area for comfort. Box 13-2 describes the advantages and disadvantages of the prone position.

Side-lying positioning

Most children require external support to maintain alignment in the side-lying position (Figure 13-4). Lying on the side is a good position for children whose muscle tone becomes too high or low in the prone and supine positions. Side-lying positions also give children a stable midline head position and keep their hands in the line of vision. Their hands remain free to reach for and manipulate objects without having to resist the pull of gravity (Box 13-3).

CLINICAL *Pearl*

When you position a child in a prone position, remember the following hints. (1) Place small children or infants in a prone position across your lap for therapeutic dressing and undressing. (2) Make sure the wedges and rolls placed under children are not so high that they cause excessive extensor tone or so low that those with very low tone or strength cannot lift their heads.

BOX 13-3

Advantages and Disadvantages of Side-Lying Position

ADVANTAGES
- Best position to minimize excessive muscle tone; neutral position
- Easiest position in which to align arms, hands, and head in midline, with gravity eliminated
- Little use of asymmetrical tonic neck reflex
- Good for independent play and development of eye-hand coordination

DISADVANTAGES
- Severely affected children are difficult to maintain in this position without the proper equipment.
- This position requires careful positioning of the head to maintain correct alignment of the cervical spine.

Upright antigravity positions

For children to perform a range of tasks, it is sometimes necessary for them to become and remain upright for a given length of time. These tasks can be worked into play, become necessary for schoolwork, or be a part of activities that help them be independent. There are several positions that can aid in their performance.

Sitting

Children begin to sit without assistance around 7 months of age. Sitting requires the child to maintain postural control of the head, trunk, and extremities against the pull of gravity. Once the child assumes a stable sitting posture without having to brace upright using the arms, s/he can

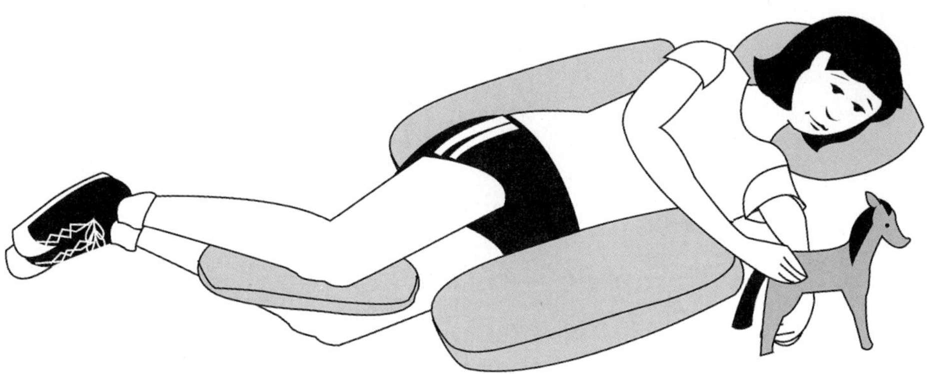

FIGURE 13-4 Side-lying position that provides the child with an opportunity to bring the hands together to play with a toy.

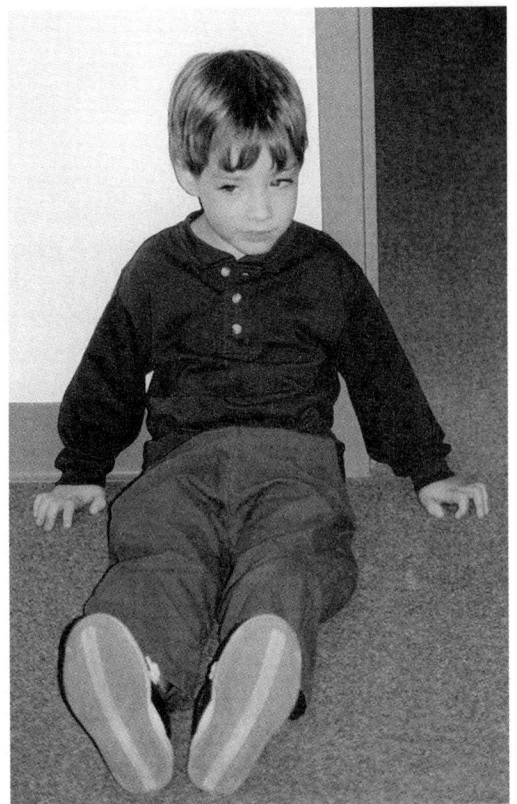

A

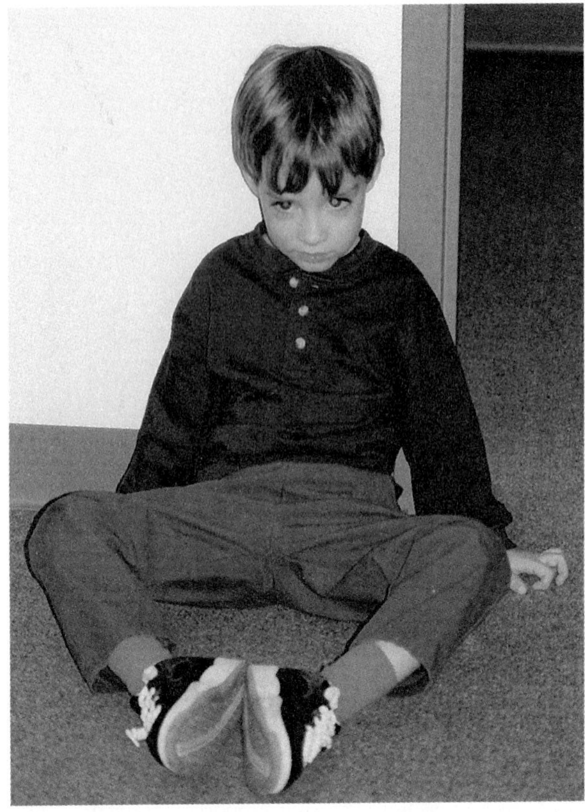

B

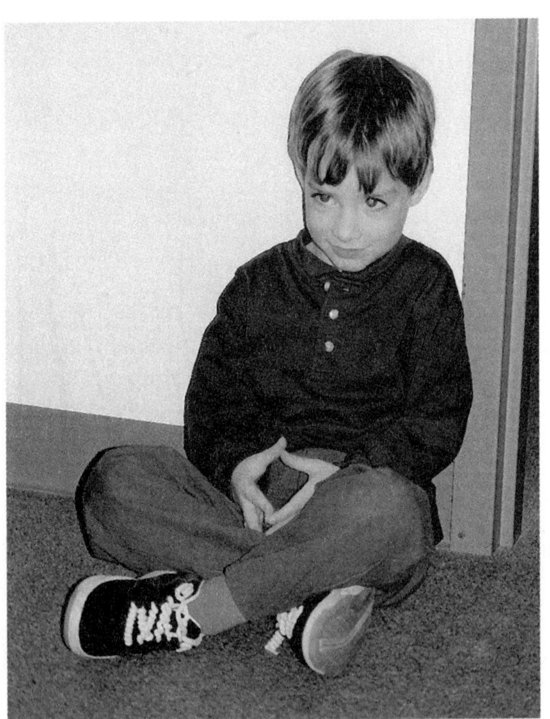

C

FIGURE 13-5 **A,** Long sitting. **B,** Ring sitting. **C,** Crisscross sitting.

shift weight away from the center of gravity to reach, retrieve, and manipulate objects. Sitting provides important visual and kinesthetic experiences that advance the child's perceptual and cognitive development. Skills such as self-feeding, going to the bathroom, doing schoolwork, and play activities require sitting. For children with mus-

CLINICAL *Pearl*

When you position a child in a side-lying posture, remember the following hints. (1) Be sure to alternate sides. (2) Use small rolls or pillows to help the child maintain a position, such as using a towel roll in front of a child who tends to push back into extension in order to allow the child to lean forward and eliminate extensor tone influence. (3) Provide adequate padded surfaces for shoulders and hips to prevent pressure sores and diminished circulation. (4) During play and social interaction, make sure that the toys and individuals are presented well below eye level to encourage flexion and discourage extension.

cle tone abnormalities, assuming a sitting position often requires the use of handling techniques and positioning devices.

There are many sitting positions. Children may long sit (legs straight), ring sit (legs formed in a circle), criss-cross sit (legs bent and crossed), or side sit (legs to one side) (Figure 13-5). The correct sitting position is frequently dependent on the type of chair used (Figure 13-6). Some children can maintain a good sitting position in a standard chair with a few modifications, such as a small, low stool placed under the feet or a rolled towel placed behind the shoulders; other children may need customized seating.

The optimum sitting position emphasizes the following.

- The body is positioned as symmetrically as possible, with the weight evenly distributed on both sides of the body (i.e., on the buttocks, thighs, and feet) and the head aligned with the trunk.
- The head is held in the midline and flexed slightly forward.
- The hips, knees, and ankles are flexed 90 degrees or slightly less.
- The feet are supported in a dorsiflexed position either on the floor or with use of a raised surface.
- The knees are abducted and in good alignment with the hips.
- Any table or lapboard used is at elbow height.

Box 13-4 describes the advantages and disadvantages of the sitting position.

Standing

All children need to experience standing. It involves full weight bearing on the hips and lower extremities and promotes bone development, keeps optimum range of movement in muscle tissue, and maintains good circulation. Children often need positioning assistance to stand with proper postural alignment. Supine and prone standers (Figure 13-7) are used for proper upright standing positions.

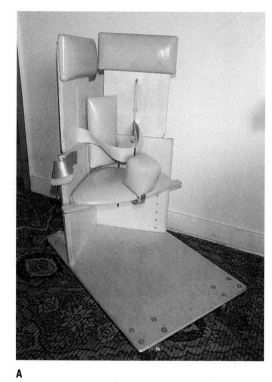

A

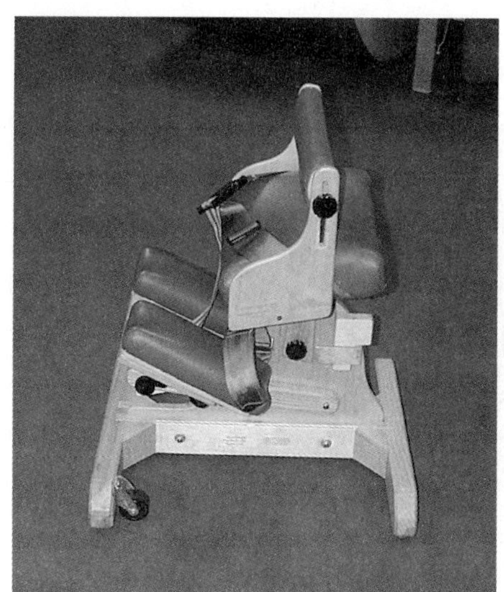

B

FIGURE 13-6 Two examples of adapted seating systems that help inhibit spasticity and compensate for limited postural control.

BOX 13-4

Advantages and Disadvantages of Sitting Position

ADVANTAGES

- Allows children to develop head and trunk control and upper body balance reactions
- Provides an expansive perspective of the environment
- Provides opportunities for midline activities and advanced eye-hand coordination tasks
- Frees the hands for play, self-care, self-help, and communication activities

DISADVANTAGES

- Children with minimum trunk control may try to compensate by using abnormal postures.
- Children who cannot voluntarily shift weight to change positions may have compromised circulation in weight-bearing body areas.
- The sitting position can cause increased contractures in hip flexor and knee flexor muscles.

Standers support the body from either the back or front surface and can be secured in a full vertical tilted position. Reclining a stander can be used to adjust to children's muscle tone and keep their joints properly aligned. Positioning children with the use of standers can be helpful for those with increased extensor tone. Remember to tilt the stander forward just enough to decrease the tone and help the child maintain the head in the midline position. Supine standers that provide support from the lower trunk downward can be helpful for children with diplegia. Using this type of equipment can free the arms and hands. Box 13-5 describes the advantages and disadvantages of the standing position.

CLINICAL *Pearl*

When you position children using standing equipment, remember the following hints. (1) Attach a tray to the front of the stander so that the child's arms and hands can be placed in front, thus giving the child an opportunity to explore objects. (2) Placing two or more children using supine standers close to one another allows them to engage in a game of catch or other similar activity.

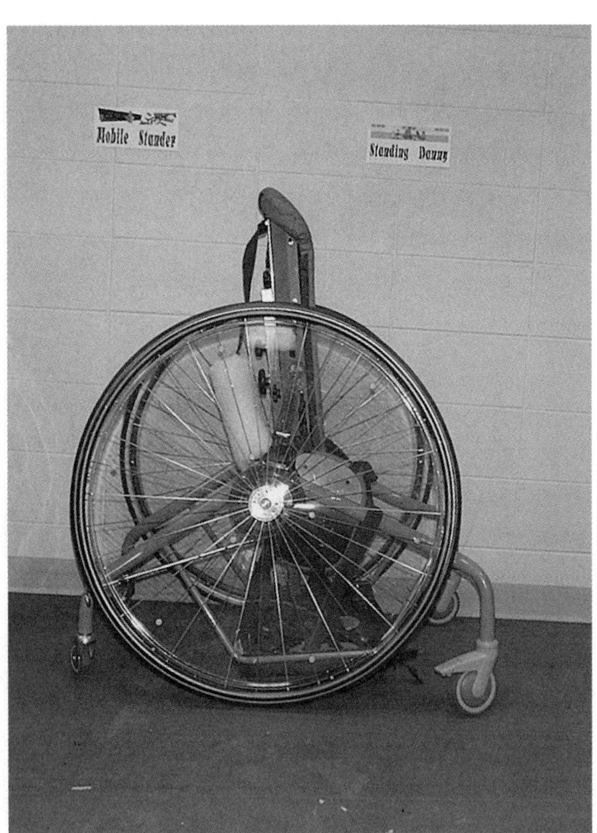

A

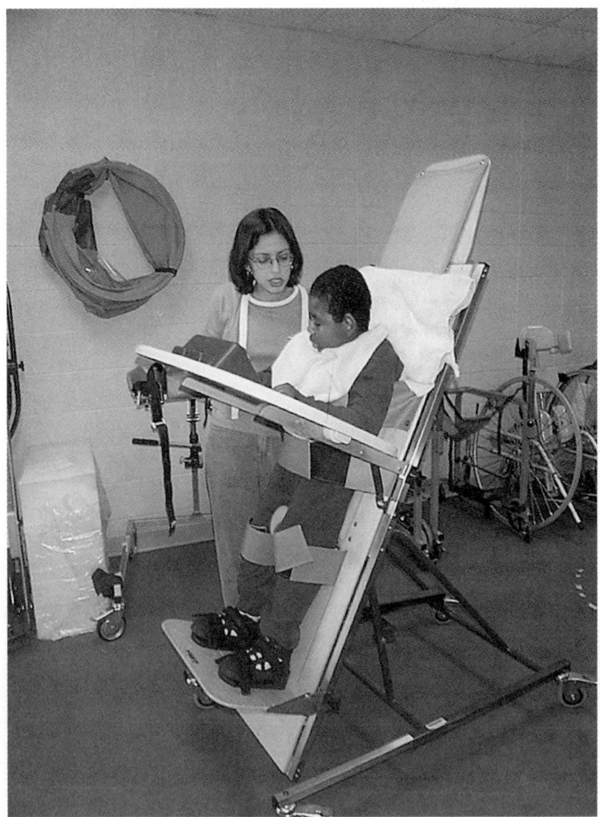

B

FIGURE 13-7 **A,** Mobile prone stander. **B,** Supine stander.

BOX 13-5

Advantages and Disadv[illegible] Position

ADVANTAGES

- Allows child[illegible] upright o[illegible] level
- Act[illegible]eet
- Facilitates the controlled use of the neck and facial muscles used for eating and speaking

DISADVANTAGES

- Older and larger children may require the assistance of two people for positioning in standers.
- Children with little independent postural control may fatigue rapidly when placed in upright antigravity positions.
- Full weight bearing on the hips and lower extremities may be painful for children with muscle contractures or skeletal deformities in these body areas.

Wheelchairs

Wheelchairs provide children with mobility and access to their environment. The OT practitioner, family, and team decide whether the child needs an electric or standard wheelchair. The team makes decisions concerning the other features of the wheelchair, such as the type of frame, push handles, rear wheels, front casters, armrests, [illegible] rests, and wheel locks (Figure 13-8). The appearance [illegible] chair is important, so children may participate in [illegible] the style, fabric, and color.

[illegible]lchairs come in ultralight, light, and heavy-duty [illegible] type of seat selected is important for the fit [illegible] While some children are able to use a solid [illegible] others may require customized seating cushions; still others may be able to use a sling seat.

The rear tires may be solid or filled with air (pneumatic). Air filled tires are easier to push over sandy or rough terrain, yet are not as durable as solid tires. Armrests can be fixed or removable, full length, desk length, or elevating. Removable armrests make it easier to transfer, while full-length armrests provide more stable support for mounting trays or other devices.

It is important for the wheelchair to properly fit the child. Therefore, lending programs may allow children to use a chair for short periods of time while waiting for their

CLINICAL *Pearl*

When you order a chair, consider the modifications that are necessary in order for the child to use the wheelchair at home or school. For example, a large powered wheelchair cannot be carried up the stairs. While the chair may fit the child adequately, the parents need to be able to bring it into the house or apartment. It may be necessary to build a ramp or recommend a different type of chair, depending on the child's environment.

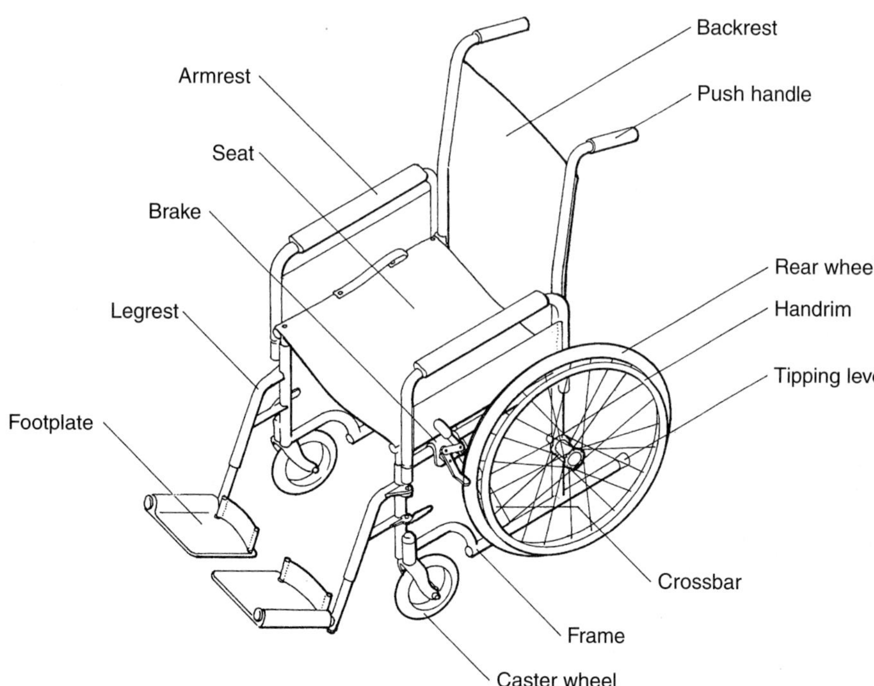

FIGURE 13-8 Conventional wheelchair: the major parts of supporting and propelling structures. (From Ragnarsson RT: Prescription considerations and a comparison of conventional and lightweight wheelchairs, *Rehab Res Dev* 2(suppl):8, 1990.)

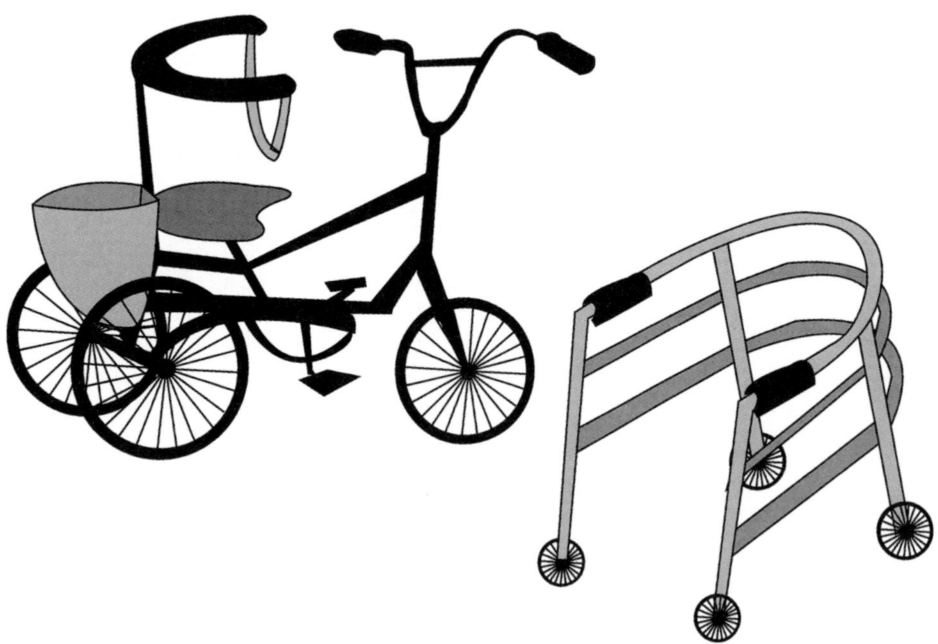

FIGURE 13-9 Types of mobility device.

permanent chairs to arrive. OT practitioners may help parents and families adapt strollers to use as temporary mobility devices for very young children.

Mobility

OT practitioners consider the ability of the child to move around the environment. Children of all ages learn through exploration. For example, infants roll and crawl to investigate their environment; this provides them with new opportunities and experiences to learn and relate to others. OT practitioners may suggest strollers, scooters, adapted tricycles, or other equipment to encourage movement in children (Figure 13-9).

HANDLING AS A THERAPEUTIC TOOL

Two-year-old Lupita Vargas has low muscle tone and overly mobile joints as a result of being born with Down syndrome. Lupita is a very active child. She typically moves around with a "bear walk" (i.e., walking on her hands and feet and locking her elbow and knee joints to support her body weight as she moves forward). Lately, Lupita has been making attempts to stand upright and reach for toys and other objects. She pulls herself up by means of the furniture, but once upright she stands with her feet spaced widely apart. She holds her arms, which are bent at the elbows, away from her body and turned upward for balance. When Lupita attempts to move out of this stance by taking a step or reaching for her toys, she quickly loses her balance and falls.

David, the COTA who is working with Lupita, realizes that she needs to develop increased stability in the muscles and joints throughout her pelvis and trunk to stand up independently. He knows that the increased stability would allow Lupita to move her extremities more freely and help her develop the rotational, diagonal movement patterns and balance reactions needed to interact with her surroundings. During the therapy session, David places his hands over Lupita's hips to give her the pelvic stability she needs to bring her feet closer together.

Following the cues provided by David's hands, Lupita shifts her body weight side to side, forward, and backward over each leg. As she begins feeling stability in the lower part of her body, she is able to use both hands to reach toward her favorite doll, which David has placed on the couch in front of her. He moves the doll to a different place on the couch each time they practice the movement so that Lupita experiences weight shifting in many directions. Each time she moves, she has to use an equilibrium reaction to bring her body back to an upright stance while holding her doll. David continues to use hand placement on Lupita's hips to give her the sensory experience of stability, which helps guide her through movement patterns that she will eventually be able to use more independently. David also helps Lupita's mother learn how to foster the development of her daughter's functional motor skills. Mrs. Vargas is pleased because she realizes that she can incorporate these handling methods many times throughout Lupita's day, such as when she selects her clothes from the closet rack or reaches for her afternoon snack on a small table.

Choosing a Handling Technique

Whereas the goal of positioning techniques is to establish stable functional body postures, handling techniques encompass several active, hands-on interventions. However, just as with positioning, handling is designed to produce an adaptive response from the child so that movements can be more functional, exploratory, and appropriate for a task.[4] Choosing and applying the appropriate handling techniques can be overwhelming to a new or inexperienced COTA. The COTA needs to observe and work alongside an experienced registered occupational therapist (OTR), who can mentor skill development in these methods.

Handling techniques are based on providing specific, graded sensory information to influence the parts of the CNS that govern and produce skilled, automatic movements. The most frequently used types of **sensory input** are vestibular, proprioceptive, and tactile, in addition to the visual input provided by the environment. Therapeutic sensory input is provided at select body locations, which are frequently termed **key points of control.** These key points can be at proximal body areas such as the shoulder girdle, trunk, and pelvis or distal ones such as the extremities.[6] Assisting a child with feeling functional movement integrates the sensory feedback of effective movement. With repeated opportunities, patience, and cognitive training, many children learn to use new motor skills. Box 13-6 describes the indications for the use of handling techniques.

BOX 13-6

Indicators for Use of Inhibition and Facilitation Techniques

INHIBITION
Hypertonicity
Active primitive reflexes
Excessive activity and motion
Behavioral excitation
Excessive sensitivity or reactivity to handling and touch

FACILITATION
Hypotonicity
Inactive primitive reflexes, lack of balance reactions
Excessive relaxation, semiconscious state
Behavioral nonresponsiveness, flat affect
Decreased reactivity to handling and touch

Handling Techniques

Handling techniques can either facilitate or inhibit muscle tone and levels of activity and alertness (Table 13-1). The OT practitioner often uses a combination of these

TABLE 13-1

Selected Neurophysiological Intervention Techniques and Applications

TECHNIQUES	SENSORY METHOD	CLINICAL APPLICATION
FACILITATION TECHNIQUES		
Light-moving touch	Applies tactile input with fingertip or soft object such as cotton swab	Activates superficial muscles
Stretch-muscle tapping	Applies proprioceptive input with three to five taps over muscle belly using fingertips	Promotes holding and maintaining of posture
Heavy joint compression	Applies proprioceptive input manually or with weights through long axis of bone	Promotes holding and maintaining of posture
Battery-operated vibration	Applies tactile and proprioceptive input with the use of battery-operated vibrator over muscle belly	Increases muscle tone and contractions; lasts only while input is being provided
Fast vestibular input	Applies vestibular input by spinning, rocking, or other movements in a quick and irregular way	Increases muscle tone and general arousal state
INHIBITION TECHNIQUES		
Wrapping/neutral warmth	Applies tactile and proprioceptive input as child is being wrapped in blanket	Decreases muscle tone and general arousal state (calms)
Slow stroking of spine while child is in prone position	Applies tactile and proprioceptive input with fingertip pressure	Decreases muscle tone and general arousal state
Slow rocking or rolling	Applies vestibular input slowly and rhythmically	Decreases muscle tone and general arousal state
Applying sustained pressure to tendon	Applies tactile and proprioceptive input	Decreases tone in a specific muscle
Gentle shaking or rocking	Applies vestibular, tactile input slowly and rhythmically	Decreases muscle tone in a specific muscle
Trunk and hip rotation	Applies proprioceptive input	Decreases muscle tone in trunk and throughout

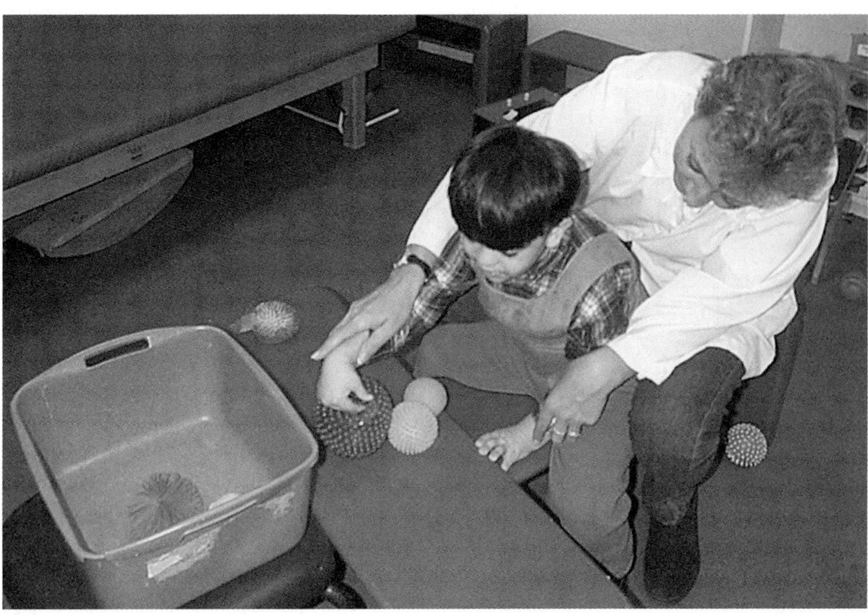

FIGURE 13-10 Slow stroking motions are applied with the whole surface of the palm.

techniques during a therapeutic intervention. Copeland and Kimmel describe the following five **inhibition** handling techniques: neutral warmth, slow stroking, gentle shaking or rocking, trunk and hip rotation, and slow rolling.[1]

Neutral warmth

The OT practitioner gently wraps the child's body in a soft cotton or thermal blanket for 15 to 20 minutes to reduce extreme hypertonicity. Neutral warmth of 96° to 98° F can relax the muscles, thereby reducing muscle tone. The practitioner monitors the child's level of alertness, attempting to create a relaxed physical state while not causing the child to go to sleep. The child should be able to breathe freely and be in a comfortable position, such as supine or lying on the side.

Slow stroking

Using an open palm and the pads of the fingertips only, the practitioner applies a stroking motion with firm but light pressure down the child's back, moving in a cephalocaudal direction. In providing the stroking motion the practitioner uses alternate hands to touch each side of the child's spine, beginning at the base of the skull. Just before lifting one hand from the base of the spine, the practitioner uses the other hand to begin stroking. It is done rhythmically, and the hands never move against the direction of body hair. The typical positions used when applying the strokes are prone, lying on the side, and in a relaxed, sitting position on the floor between the OT practitioner's legs. Three to 5 minutes of stroking is a safe time frame. Slow stroking can also improve abnormal muscle tone in the arms and legs (Figure 13-10).

Gentle shaking or rocking

Shaking is a good technique to reduce tone in an extremity. First, choose a position for the child that is appropriate for the planned activity. Using the flat pads of the fingertips, the practitioner grasps the top portion of the child's body part, such as the arm. The body part is gently and rhythmically shaken while the practitioner's hand moves downward on it. Slow rocking is rhythmical and can include alternating rotational movements, with the practitioner's hands placed at proximal key points such as the shoulders.

Trunk and hip rotation

The practitioner can easily manipulate the trunk and hips using handling techniques while assisting the child with transitioning from one body position to another. The practitioner maintains stability on one side of the body with one hand. With the other hand, the practitioner assists the child with making movements in diagonal planes. Using proximal key points of the trunk and pelvis reduces hypertonicity by inhibiting patterns of total flexion or extension, particularly those elicited by primitive reflex activity (Figure 13-11).

Slow rolling

Slow rolling involves handling primarily the trunk and pelvis. The practitioner places the child in a supine position and slowly rolls him or her from a supine to a side-lying position and then back to a supine position. The practitioner repeats this pattern in the opposite direction and continues alternating the pattern slowly and rhythmically until the child's muscles relax.

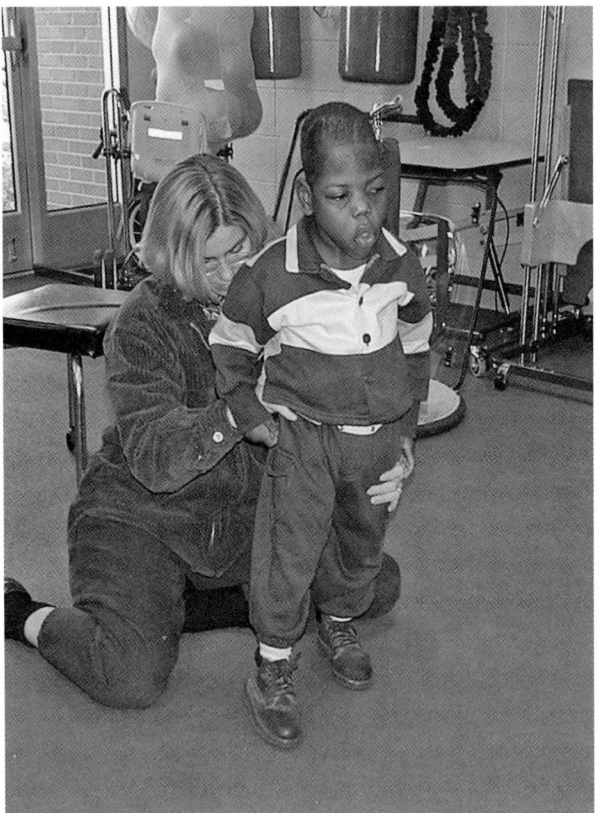

FIGURE 13-11 Handling at key points can facilitate movement.

Facilitation techniques

Although practitioners use inhibitory handling techniques more often than facilitation techniques, facilitation methods are needed to increase low muscle tone, increase levels of alertness, or strengthen the intensity of sensory input to elicit a response. **Facilitation** handling techniques include bouncing, swinging, and rocking in an anterior-posterior movement plane and moving the child into upright antigravity positions (Table 13-2). OT practitioners can use a vast array of equipment, such as therapy balls and vestibular boards, in the service of these facilitation techniques; they can also use themselves as the source of the movements.

OT practitioners should take care to protect from potential dislocation the hypermobile joints of children with particularly low muscle tone. Whether using inhibition or facilitation techniques, OT practitioners must carefully monitor each child's response to the sensory input. Many children with motor system impairments have delayed responses to sensory stimulation or may be experiencing the sensation for the first time. Until OT practitioners become familiar with each child's individual responses, they must proceed slowly. After a minute or so of using a particular facilitation technique, the practitioner should stop and wait a few seconds to assess the way in which the child responds physically and emotionally. When OT practitioners couple their knowledge of positioning and handling methods with sensory integration, they can refine the appropriate type and amount of sensory stimulation needed. Each child's potential response is intertwined with his or her cognitive and perceptual competencies. By working with the OTR, caregivers, and teachers, the COTA can obtain the data needed to integrate good positioning and handling interventions into the child's various daily activities and environments.

INTEGRATING POSITIONING AND HANDLING FOR OCCUPATIONAL PERFORMANCE

Although positioning and handling techniques are important therapeutic tools for the OT practitioner, their use is only part of the process of increasing a child's repertoire of occupational behaviors. Using the principles from the neurodevelopmental treatment approach, Erhardt

TABLE 13-2

Selected Neurodevelopmental Treatment Intervention Techniques

FACILITATION TECHNIQUES	INHIBITION TECHNIQUES
Weight Bearing and Weight Shifting Active movement against gravity promotes increased muscle tone and postural control.	**Weight Bearing and Weight Shifting** Active movement can have an inhibitory effect on spastic muscles.
Joint Compression Gentle compression of well aligned joints promotes muscle activation.	**Rotation** Rotating upper body on lower body can help break up total patterns of movement and decrease the influence of abnormal tone.
Sweeping or Alternate Tapping over Muscles Using cupped hands, the practitioner lightly sweeps or taps the muscle belly to promote activation.	**Oscillation or Hand Vibration** Briskly shaking an extremity for short periods of time or the practitioner shaking a hand over the muscle belly can promote decreased abnormal muscle tone.

outlined three phases, or components, of the treatment process that are used with children who need to develop improved movement skills.[2] The neurodevelopmental principles are included in each phase.

1. *Preparation.* Use positioning and handling techniques to normalize muscle tone and inhibit abnormal reflex activity. Identify the optimum amount of support needed for children to use movement abilities available to them. Use comfortable postures for teaching children new skills.
2. *Facilitation.* Strengthen existing skills and gradually decrease supports as children acquire new skills. Grade activity demands so that children can pay attention to the task itself rather than the way in which the task is done. Allowing children to solve problems during tasks helps produce automatic, spontaneous movements.
3. *Adaptation.* Gradually alter positioning and handling. Vary positions and change sensory cues to increase children's abilities to use skills in a variety of situations.

In the previous scenario, the COTA (David) helps Lupita Vargas achieve stability in a standing position by placing his hands on her hips and then follows this by facilitating weight shifting. David uses facilitation methods to help Lupita repeatedly reach for her doll, which he places in a different location each time. In the facilitation phase of the session, David attempts to grade and strengthen her new reaching skills and balance reactions. When David and Mrs. Vargas explore other ways in which Lupita can use her new abilities, they apply the adaptation phase of the treatment process and continue to strengthen her repertoire of available motor skills.

SUMMARY

Positioning and handling techniques are valuable therapeutic tools used to assist children who have CNS damage. Positioning techniques provide them with stable postural options that can increase their interaction with the environment, facilitate their ability to engage in meaningful activities, and prevent the development of health problems caused by their motor disorders. The COTA recommends positioning approaches and specialized equipment to fit the individual needs of each child. Handling techniques help the child actively engage in activities. By understanding the types of sensory input influencing the nervous system and selecting and grading them, the COTA helps a child engage in the occupations of play, work, and self-care skills.

References

1. Copeland M, Kimmel J: *Evaluation and management of infants and young children with developmental disabilities*, Baltimore, Md, 1989, Brookes.
2. Erhardt RP: *Developmental hand dysfunction: theory, assessment and treatment*, ed 2, San Antonio, Texas, 1994, Therapy Skill Builders.
3. O'Brien JC: Project ARCH: Adaptive Resources for Children with Handicaps. In AOTA *Technology 1990*, Baltimore, Md, 1990, American Occupational Therapy Association.
4. Porter R: Sensory considerations in handling techniques. In Connolly B, Montgomery P, editors: *Therapeutic exercise in developmental disabilities*, Chattanooga, Tenn, 1987, Chattanooga Corporation.
5. Schoen S, Anderson J: Neurodevelopmental treatment frame of reference. In Kramer P, Hinojosa J, editors: *Frames of reference for pediatric occupational therapy*, Baltimore, Md, 1993, Williams & Wilkins.
6. Ward D: *Positioning the handicapped child for function*, ed 2, St Louis, 1984, Phoenix Press.

Recommended Reading

Alexander R, Boehme R, Cupps B: *Normal development of functional motor skills: the first year of life*, San Antonio, Texas, 1993, Therapy Skill Builders.

Bly L: *Motor skills acquisition in the first year of life*, San Antonio, Texas, 1994, Therapy Skill Builders.

Boehme R: *Improving upper body control*, Tucson, Ariz, 1988, Therapy Skill Builders.

Campbell P: *Introduction to neurodevelopmental treatment: application with infants and children with posture and movement disorders*, ed 3, Tallmadge, Ohio, 1990, Children's Hospital Medical Center of Akron.

Dunn Klein M: *Pre-dressing skills*, San Antonio, Texas, 1983, Therapy Skill Builders.

Finnie N: *Handling the young cerebral palsied child at home*, New York, 1975, EP Dutton.

Jaeger L, Gertz J: *Home program instruction sheets for infants and children*, San Antonio, Texas, 1999, Therapy Skill Builders.

Levitt S: *Treatment of cerebral palsy and motor delay*, London, 1977, Blackwell Scientific Publications.

Scherzer A, Tscharnuter I: *Early diagnosis and treatment in cerebral palsy*, ed 2, New York, 1990, Marcel Dekker.

Sheda C, Small C: *Developmental motor activities for therapy: instruction sheets for children*, San Antonio, Texas, 1990, Therapy Skill Builders.

Short-DeGraff M: *Human development for occupational and physical therapists*, Baltimore, Md, 1988, Williams & Wilkins.

REVIEW *Questions*

1. Describe the differences between positioning and handling techniques. What is the primary focus of each?
2. Review each of the benefits that can be achieved through positioning and handling techniques.
3. What are the principles used by the OT practitioner when selecting helpful positions for a child?
4. Why is it important for the COTA to identify more than just one or two positions for a child who has very little independent movement?
5. What are some of the signs that the COTA might observe which suggest that a position poses risks to a child?
6. Therapeutic handling involves using a combination of facilitation and inhibition techniques. What are the indicators for each handling approach?

SUGGESTED *Activities*

1. Choose two or three daily living activities, such as eating, dressing, or performing oral hygiene tasks. Try performing each activity in three different positions; choose both the horizontal and vertical positions. In what ways does the position affect your ability to perform each task? What makes a position comfortable or uncomfortable? With each position, do you notice any changes in the types of sensory input that indicate how to perform the task?
2. Observe normal children of different ages playing. How often do they change or adapt positions? Which positions provide the most stable postures? What do you notice about the ways in which children change from one position to another? Note the qualities of normal movement patterns and think about the way in which these qualities relate to the application of handling techniques.
3. You are a COTA who has been asked to develop a positioning plan for a 5-year-old boy who has spastic diplegia and is entering kindergarten. Suggest positions that would help him participate in activities such as sitting in a reading circle, participating in sand play at floor level, and putting on his jacket to go home. Refer to an adaptive equipment catalog to determine which types of equipment you might recommend for use in his classroom.
4. Find a partner and practice several of the handling techniques described in this chapter. Execute your movements based on the sensory cues you experience while your partner is handling you. Provide verbal feedback about the way that the handling feels.
5. Look at Figure 13-5. In what ways might you use positioning and handling to improve this child's ability to perform the activity?

14

Childhood and Adolescent Psychosocial and Mental Health Disorders

KERRYELLEN G. VROMAN

JANE CLIFFORD O'BRIEN

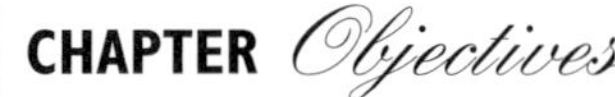

After studying this chapter, the reader will be able to accomplish the following:

- Define psychosocial occupational therapy practice for children and adolescents
- Recognize the signs of behavioral and mental health disorders seen in children and adolescents
- Recognize the symptoms of behavioral and mental health disorders seen in children and adolescents
- Assist in the occupational therapy evaluation process
- Recognize typical assessments used by the occupational therapist and assistant team to develop treatment
- Use evaluation results to guide mental health and psychosocial practice
- Be familiar with types of frames of reference that direct intervention in psychosocial practice
- Select activities that support evidence-based practice
- Be familiar with the types of group intervention for children and adolescents

KEY TERMS

Psychosocial occupational therapy
Disruptive behavior disorders
Tic disorders
Anxiety
Mood disorders
Eating disorders
Substance-related disorders
Substance abuse
Substance dependence
Addiction
Global mental functions
Specific mental functions

CHAPTER OUTLINE

Psychosocial occupational therapy is the area of clinical practice that provides services to children and adolescents with mental health and behavioral problems. This specialty area of practice requires a specific knowledge of the mental health (i.e., mental and behavioral) problems and mental illnesses (psychiatric disorders) diagnosed in childhood and adolescence.

One in five children or adolescents has mental health problems that disrupt the ability to carry out typical age-related everyday activities (Box 14-1). These mental health problems and illnesses can present as difficulties in regulating feelings, organizing thoughts, and demonstrating appropriate behaviors. The diagnoses in children and adolescents include major depression, anxiety disorders, schizophrenia, and substance abuse disorders. Particularly in early adolescence, there is an increased risk of eating disorders, anxiety, depression, and aggressive and antisocial behaviors as well as the onset of substance abuse.[18] These psychiatric conditions, which are usually identified in adolescence, may cause occupational performance problems in adulthood. However, not all mental health disorders in childhood result in adult psychopathology.[19] The therapy needs of children with mental health problems (also referred to as psychiatric disorders) are addressed by multidisciplinary pediatric services in a variety of settings, including psychiatric units in acute-care hospitals, independent psychiatric hospitals, day treatment centers, community mental health centers, and public schools. Services for adolescents are provided in similar settings, but these hospital and community mental health settings frequently overlap with adult services. Furthermore, many adolescents with mental health problems are under the care of either the social welfare or juvenile justice system. These adolescents may be placed in residential facilities or group homes.

The mental health disorders discussed in this chapter include disruptive behavior disorders, anxiety and mood disorders, eating disorders, learning disorders, tic disorders, schizophrenia, and substance-related disorders. This chapter provides information on the impact of these disorders on occupational performance and discusses appropriate occupational therapy (OT) evaluation and the individual and group interventions used. The descriptions of mental health disorders in the first section of this chapter are based on the classifications found in the *Diagnosis and Statistical Manual of Mental Disorders* (DSM-VI-TR).[4] To meet the criteria of mental health disorder the condition has to have symptoms that cause distress and/or affect the individual's social, academic, or everyday functioning.

OVERVIEW OF MENTAL HEALTH DISORDERS

The American Psychiatric Association has developed a comprehensive classification system for the diagnosis of mental health disorders that is published in the DSM-IV-TR.[4] The primary purpose of this classification system is to guide clinical practice. It outlines the clinical criteria for the diagnosis and provides a description of mental health disorders. Each mental health disorder is seen as a biological, behavioral, and psychological dysfunction that has "a clinically significant behavioral or psychological syndrome or pattern that occurs in an individual and is associated with present distress [emotional suffering] or disability [difficulty in functioning in everyday activities] or with a significant increase in suffering death, pain, disability, or loss of freedom (p. xxi)."[4] Therefore, the DSM-VI-TR provides a universal language that health care practitioners use to describe and organize the physical,

BOX 14-1

Quick Facts about Child and Adolescent Mental Health

- One in five children have a diagnosable mental, emotional, or behavioral disorder. However, 70% percent of children do not receive mental health services (Surgeon General's Report on Mental Health, 1999).
- Attention deficit hyperactivity disorder is one of the most common mental disorders in children.
- Autism and related disorders develop in childhood and affect an estimated 1 to 2 per 1000 people (National Institute for Mental Health, 2001).
- Autism is four times more common in boys (National Institute for Mental Health, 2001).
- As many as 1 in every 33 children and 1 in 8 adolescents may have depression (Center for Mental Health Services, 1998).
- Depression is more common in teenage girls than teenage boys (National Institute for Mental Health, 2001).
- Children and teens who have a chronic illness, endure abuse or neglect, or experience other trauma have an increased risk of depression (National Institute for Mental Health, 2000).
- Suicide is the third leading cause of death for 15 to 24 year olds and the sixth leading cause of death for 5 to 14 year olds.
- Twenty percent of the youths in juvenile justice facilities have a serious emotional disturbance, and most have a diagnosable mental disorder. An additional 30% of the youths in these facilities have substance abuse disorders or co-occurring substance abuse disorders (Office of Juvenile Justice and Delinquency Prevention, 2000).

Data from the National Mental Health Association website, www.nmha.org/infoctr/factsheets; National Institute for Mental Health, website www.nimh.nih.gov/publicat/numvbers.cfm.

mental, and behavioral signs and symptoms or patterns of dysfunction. This process of classification helps determine the appropriate interventions and facilitates research into etiology (cause) and treatment effectiveness.

Like physical illness, mental health disorders may have an underlying biological cause requiring medication. However, unlike typical physical illness, children and adults with mental health disorders cope with an additional burden of social stigma. The artist Vincent Van Gogh wrote of his mental illness in a letter to his brother: *"I would not have chosen madness if I had had a choice."* The social isolation of individuals with mental health disorders is a further limitation.

DISRUPTIVE BEHAVIOR DISORDERS

According to DSM-VI, **disruptive behavior disorders** are characterized by socially disruptive behavior that is often more distressing to others than to the individual with the disorder. Attention deficit disorder (ADD), attention deficit hyperactivity disorder (ADHD) (see Chapter 10), conduct disorder, and oppositional defiant disorder are the most frequently encountered disruptive behavior disorders.

Attention Deficit Disorder

Thomas is a 7-year-old boy in a regular second grade classroom. He has always had trouble in school. The kindergarten teacher describes him as "fidgety, restless, and distractible." Now in grade school these symptoms are disrupting his learning. Thomas frequently stares off and has difficulty following multistep verbal directions. At home, his parents report that he needs frequent reminders to follow through with tasks. Thomas is easily frustrated and becomes bored with tasks quickly. For example, he does not adequately brush his teeth or get himself dressed in the morning. Instead, he gets distracted. His parents state that Thomas loses things and often forgets assignments.

Although many children exhibit aspects of these characteristics, Thomas's difficulties persist in all situations (e.g., home, school, and play) and interfere with his ability to participate in daily occupations. He is unable to complete tasks. After a comprehensive evaluation by an experienced team of professionals (a registered occupational therapist [OTR], physical therapist, social worker, psychologist, and developmental pediatrician) and consultation with the teacher, parents, and child, Thomas is diagnosed with ADD. A complete evaluation, including a classroom visit, was required to determine if this diagnosis was correct. The certified occupational therapy assistant (COTA) would have played a role in making classroom observations to establish baseline behavior.

It is important to rule out other reasons that children have difficulty paying attention in class, such as anxiety, sensory difficulties, feeling overwhelmed, fatigue, and boredom. Furthermore, diet and exercise can influence the child's ability to pay attention. A diagnosis of ADD relies on the experience of team members and a determination that the symptoms are interfering with the child's ability to perform everyday activities and are not the result of another medical, psychiatric, or social condition.[6] The behavioral difficulties must occur in a variety of settings, not just in the classroom. Furthermore, the symptoms must be evident before age 7, last for at least 6 months, represent impairment, and not be associated with anxiety disorder.[6] Intervention may include medication, behavioral modification techniques, sensory modulation, and learning strategies. Classroom modifications may help children who have difficulty with attention (Table 14-1).

Attention Deficit Hyperactivity Disorder

Children with attention disorders may exhibit signs of excessive energy (i.e., hyperactivity). Signs of hyperactivity/impulsivity include such things as fidgeting, squirming, talking excessively, difficulty waiting one's turn, and interrupting. Other features associated with ADHD include sleep disorders, emotional lability (fluctuations and mood hypersensitivity), poor self-esteem, and poor frustration tolerance.[19]

Similar to ADD, ADHD is diagnosed by a team of experienced professionals, along with consultation from the teacher, parents, and child. The team gathers information to determine if any other causes for the behaviors exist. The OT practitioner observes the child in the classroom, at home, and during play to provide the team with information on how the child's behaviors affect his or her daily functioning. The OT practitioner may provide strategies and modifications to help the child, teacher, and family. Because the behaviors associated with ADHD may be frustrating to parents and teachers, children may be viewed as "difficult" or "problematic." These negative labels can make children feel inferior and have low self-esteem. The OT practitioner can help by explaining to parents and teachers how to work with the child's behaviors and best meet his or her needs. Some children with ADHD benefit from sensory integration therapy as well as intervention strategies that include accommodations and modifications, behavioral management, cognitive-behavioral therapy, and medication. Both parents and children can benefit from support groups.

TABLE 14-1

Classroom Modifications to Improve Attention

SPECIFIC AREA	MODIFICATIONS
General Strategies	• Use a child's strengths. • Provide structure and clear expectations. • Use short sentences and simple vocabulary. • Provide supportive opportunities for success to help build self-esteem. • Be flexible in classroom procedures (e.g., allowing the use of tape recorders for taking notes and tests when students have trouble with written language). • Make use of self-correcting materials that provide immediate feedback without embarrassment. • Use computers for written work. • Reinforce social skills in school and at home.
Helping with Schoolwork	• Show an interest in the child's homework. • Ask about homework; ask questions that require answers longer than one or two words. • Help the child organize homework materials. • Establish a regular time with child to do homework; develop a schedule. • Find a specific place for the child to do homework that has plenty of light and space to work and is quiet. • Encourage the child to ask questions and look for answers. • Make sure the child justifies answers with facts and evidence. • Practice the skills taught in school and at home. • Relate homework to the child's everyday life (e.g., teach fractions and measurements as you do other therapy activities, such as cooking). • Be a role model: Read a book or newspaper, write a letter with the child, or talk about your experiences of these activities. • Praise the child for both the small steps and big leaps in the right direction.
Language	• Have the child sit where s/he can hear and not be distracted. • Repeat directions; remember gentle cuing and helpful reminders. • Provide visual cues for where to begin tasks and assignments. • NEVER embarrass students. • Phrase questions so that the student may answer "yes" or "no." • Assign shorter written language assignments.
Memory	• Mnemonic strategies: Use rhyming games; allow children to mouth or whisper reading assignments in class. • Allow children to underline in book or circle key words. • Use a tape recorder for taking notes. • Practice memorization before bedtime. • Elaborate on information and relate it to prior knowledge. • Allow children extra time on tests and assignments. • Use visual or verbal learning. • Use active learning such as role-playing and hands-on experiences. • Divide information into categories for the child.
Sensory Integration: Coordination	• Allow the child to move around the classroom. • Ensure that the child goes to recess. • Provide the child with movement experiences. • Provide the child with quiet space when he is overly aroused. • Have the child sit in the back of the room, with few distractions. • Allow for breaks. • Provide noncompetitive games to help make all children successful. • Work on the proximal control needed for handwriting skills. • Provide strengthening and endurance games. • Work on perceptual skills through gross motor activities (e.g., obstacle course).

TABLE 14-1

Classroom Modifications to Improve Attention—cont'd

SPECIFIC AREA	MODIFICATIONS
Sequential Processing	• Repeat instructions slowly and provide word or picture lists of steps. • Allow them to talk through or whisper the order of the steps during a task. • Anticipate difficulties. • Use a whole-word approach to reading.
Visual Processing	• Provide graph paper or grid, which may help the child focus on the page. • Use tactile cues such as raised lines to help the child.
Organizational Skills	• Establish routines. • Provide written as well as verbal instructions for assignments (e.g., a study guide for reading or task completion). • Outline the steps with the child so that s/he can learn the skill. • Develop strategies for taking notes (e.g., highlight key words or tasks). • Make lists and check off the items (e.g., give the child a day planner; electronic day planners can be cool!). • Break long-term projects into small chunks.

CLINICAL *Pearl*

Teachers frequently mention to parents that their children have problems paying attention in class. This alone does not necessarily mean that they have ADD. Children may demonstrate attention problems for a variety of reasons. OT practitioners assist team members in determining if the attention problems are secondary to environmental, social, or sensory conditions. OT practitioners working in school systems play a role in educating teachers concerning the strategies and modifications that help children succeed.

Childhood-Onset Conduct Disorder

Peter is an 8-year-old boy who has difficulty getting along with other children in his class and neighborhood. Both children and adults consider him a bully. Neighbors have complained that Peter throws rocks and fights with other children. Particularly distressing is his cruelty to animals and fascination with fire. At school he was caught stealing money from his teacher's desk. Peter does not listen to his parents and hurts his younger sister. He is doing poorly in the second grade. Next week a parent conference will be held to discuss his aggressive behavior and poor school performance.

Long-standing behaviors that violate the rights of others and the rules of society are the predominant features of conduct disorder. Peter is typical of children with this disorder. The following behaviors characterize conduct disorder.[4]

- Physical aggression toward other people or animals
- Participation in mugging, purse snatching, shoplifting, or burglary
- Destruction of other people's property (e.g., setting fires)
- Breaking of rules (e.g., running away from home or truancy)

Additionally, these major symptoms may be accompanied by the use of addictive substances, recklessness, and temper outbursts. Children diagnosed with conduct disorder lack concern for others and show no feelings of guilt or remorse. Left untreated, a significant number of those suffering from conduct disorder develop antisocial personality disorder as adults and may commit serious crimes including rape, physical assault and battery, and homicide.[4] Despite an image of toughness, conduct disorder is often accompanied by poor self-esteem and symptoms of anxiety, depression, and suicidal thoughts. School performance is typically impaired, especially verbal and reading skills, and is complicated by skipping school and suspension for behavioral problems.[6]

Oppositional Defiant Disorder

Dwayne is a 9-year-old third grade student. He has always been a somewhat "difficult, angry" child, but over the last 19 months he has argued constantly with his parents and younger sister and loses his temper over seemingly trivial issues. A resentful child, he blames others, refuses to obey his parents' rules, and deliberately annoys other people. He says that he hates school and his sister and that his classmates "suck."

CLINICAL *Pearl*

The OT practitioner working with children and early adolescents with disruptive behavior disorders must possess a thorough knowledge of developmental behavior patterns.

The primary symptoms of oppositional defiant disorder are negative, hostile, and defiant behaviors that are more severe than those observed in typical children.[4] Children and early adolescents with oppositional defiant disorder display outbursts of temper, argue, and defy adults. These children may seem angry and resentful of rules, become easily annoyed, and blame others for their mistakes. Oppositional defiant disorder may be an indication of underlying childhood depression or an inability to effectively cope with anger and other uncomfortable feelings.

The normal "difficult" periods of childhood and early adolescence should not be confused with this disorder.[4] Unlike conduct disorder, individuals with this disorder do not seriously violate the rights and ignore the feelings of others. They rarely engage in activities that cause physical harm to others and as a rule do not engage in criminal activity. Their oppositional behavior and stormy relationships with teachers and peers cause these children to have difficulty in school.[6]

LEARNING DISORDERS

Greg is an 8-year-old boy in the third grade who has difficulty with reading and writing. He is cooperative in school but hesitant to ask questions. He avoids writing assignments. During a classroom exercise, the COTA observed that Greg wrote one sentence during "free writing" while his classmates were writing paragraphs. Furthermore, he struggled to complete that sentence. However, the teacher reinforced his effort and said "nice job." An evaluation by the team identified his IQ (intelligence quotient) score as 110, but his performance on writing and reading tasks fell well below that expected of him given his IQ score.

The interdisciplinary team diagnosed Greg with a reading and writing learning disability. The team met with the teacher, parents, and school personnel to develop strategies to assist Greg in school. Greg was allotted extra time on writing assignments, provided extra help with reading, and given permission to have his tests read to him and verbally respond. He was allowed to type out long assignments and not be penalized for spelling or writing errors on tests. The teacher was reminded to keep her expectations clear (e.g., do not accept one sentence if she wants three), while acknowledging that writing and reading were difficult for Greg. Care was taken to match Greg with a teacher who provided clear and consistent expectations for class work the following year.

Approximately 5% of school-aged children experience a learning disability.[6] Specific learning disabilities include *dyslexia* (reading disability), *dysgraphia* (writing disability), and *dyscalculia* (math disability). These disabilities occur in the absence of visual, hearing, or motor difficulties and are not due to mental retardation or an environmental, cultural, or economic disadvantage.[6] Learning disabilities are diagnosed when there is a severe discrepancy between ability and achievement.

OT practitioners help analyze children's learning difficulties. Those with learning disabilities are aware of their difficulties, although they may not understand how to articulate the problems. OT practitioners, parents, teachers, and professionals can help by involving the child in the development of strategies and modifications to be more successful. Strategies may include organization, memory aides, and cuing techniques (see Table 14-1). OT practitioners help children improve performance with assistive devices and adaptive equipment. For example, children with dysgraphia may benefit from using a lap top computer in the classroom. This process may be started as early as the first grade by using typing programs graded at the child's level.

As with any intervention, if children develop their own plans, they are more likely to follow through with the strategies. For example, Greg was given a Day-Timer to keep track of his school assignments and help with his organizational skills. He frequently forgot it and was inconsistent about writing in it. When asked about it he said it was too big, and while he liked the pictures and activities, he did not know where to write. Instead, he decided to use a sheet of paper attached to a clipboard. Each day he wrote the name of the class and the page of the assignment; he crossed the assignment off once it was completed. The system he developed worked much better for him. This is an example of the importance of involving children in problem-solving their own strategies.

TIC DISORDERS

Tic disorders are involuntary, recurrent movements or vocalizations. Common manifestations of motor tics include eye blinking, neck jerking, coughing, shoulder shrugging, facial grimacing, foot stomping, touching objects, and excessive grooming. Signs of vocal tics include throat clearing, grunting, sniffing, snorting, barking, the

CLINICAL *Pearl*

It is important for children to be their own advocates once they are in high school and college. Many colleges make accommodations for students with learning disabilities.

repetition of obscene words *(coprolalia)*, and the repetition of others' words *(echolalia)*. Tics often increase in stressful situations and decrease during sleep or absorbing activities such as computer games.[4] Tourette's syndrome is the most common tic disorder for which treatment is sought.[4,6]

Tourette's Syndrome

Kilian is a 7-year-old third grader. Recently he has started to jerk his neck to the side and make strange faces and grunting noises. These behaviors occur intermittently throughout the day. Kilian is embarrassed that he is unable to control these movements and noises, especially since he has been shouting profanities. Kilian's parents and teacher are concerned by these behaviors, but his classmates are annoyed; when he couldn't stop, they started to avoid him. His school performance is suffering because the jerks and noises distract him.

Tourette's syndrome is a genetic condition in which both motor and vocal tics occur frequently and daily. Symptoms of ADD/ADHD or obsessive-compulsive disorder may be present.[4] Schoolwork, social participation, activities of daily living (ADLs), and play/leisure activities are disrupted by these tics. Kilian's experience, especially his vocal tics, is an example of how socially isolating this disorder can be for children. The strange and obvious nature of verbal and motor tics makes children vulnerable to discrimination.[7] Tourette's syndrome is chronic, although most cases improve during adolescence and early adulthood.[4]

ANXIETY DISORDERS

Anxiety is a normal adaptive response to stress involving feelings of apprehension and arousal of the autonomic nervous system (e.g., palpitations, perspiration, chest pain, stomach discomfort, restlessness, and/or headache).[14] However, anxiety is no longer an adaptive response when these feelings become distressing and interfere with everyday functioning. In a nonadaptive response to stressful events or situations, a child or adolescent will experience cognitive symptoms that include thoughts such as shamefulness, a distorted or inaccurate view of the situation, or feelings of being threatened.[4] In this section the clinical presentations of separation anxiety disorder, phobic and anxiety disorders, and obsessive-compulsive disorder are presented.

Separation Anxiety Disorder

Caitlin is a tentative, shy 7-year-old girl. When at home, where Caitlin prefers to be, she constantly follows her mother while her mother is doing household activities. She will not fall asleep at night unless her mother lies next to her and then awakens during the night with "bad dreams," which have a common theme of finding herself left behind in the supermarket. More recently, Caitlin does not want to go to school. She cries hysterically and becomes so distressed that she becomes physically ill.

Although separation anxiety is normal in infants and very young children, it is not appropriate for those of Caitlin's age. Caitlin's extreme anxiety, associated with anticipating or being separated from home or her mother, is known as *separation anxiety disorder*, a condition experienced by about 4% of children.[18] A child or adolescent with this disorder may experience extreme distress when traveling away from home or may refuse to go to school or visit or sleep over at the homes of friends. These children often cling to familiar adults. The *DSM-VI-TR* diagnostic criteria includes repeated nightmares involving the theme of separation, reluctance or refusal to sleep without a significant person nearby, and persistent worrying about separation or harm to major attachment figures (e.g., the mother or father).[4] Separation or even the anticipation of separation may trigger physical (somatic) symptoms that include headaches, dizziness, palpitations, stomachaches, nausea, and vomiting.[12,14] In severe cases, students may refuse to attend school or participate in social and recreational activities.[4] Therefore, separation anxiety can affect the child's social development.[7] Refusing to attend school or experiencing anxiety while at school can result in poor academic performance. Separation anxiety will usually resolve or decrease in severity, but it may also be a precursor to other conditions, such as panic disorder.

Generalized Anxiety Disorder

The type of generalized anxiety disorder (GAD) that is diagnosed in an estimated 3% of school children and adolescents differs from adult GAD in that the symptoms are more limited.[14,18] As defined by the *DSM-IV-TR*, GAD includes excessive anxiety and worrying (e.g., anticipating future events, school/academic performance) that occurs most days and is not triggered by specific events or social situations.[12,14] Children with GAD cannot control their fears of numerous situations and activities. The associated symptoms of GAD are irritability, tiredness, an inability to relax, restlessness, apprehension and a negative self-image, difficulty concentrating, and disrupted sleep as well as physical symptoms.[14] GAD can occur with other affective disorders (e.g., dysthymia or panic disorder).[14] As with all mental health disorders, the child will have difficulty in school, social situations, and all areas of occupational performance.

Phobic Anxiety Disorder and Social Anxiety Disorder of Childhood

When a child has specific, persistent, and recurring fears that are not features of GAD or some other broader psychological disturbance, such as conduct disorder or pervasive developmental disorder, a phobic anxiety or social anxiety disorder is diagnosed. Children with social and/or phobic disorders exhibit extreme self-consciousness, are easily embarrassed, and are overly concerned about whether they are presenting themselves appropriately in social situations. Consequently, these children withdraw from or avoid social contact thereby disrupting interpersonal relationships with peers. However, social phobias and accompanying symptoms do not occur in situations with family members or familiar people with whom they typically have good social relationships in those contexts.

Obsessive-Compulsive Disorder

Children with obsessive-compulsive disorder (OCD) have recurring disruptive and intrusive thoughts and compulsive, repetitive patterns of behavior.[12,13,24] Obsessive thoughts cause unbearable anxiety, which compulsive behaviors such as ritualistic checking or avoidance (e.g., avoiding cracks) help reduce. However, as these behaviors become essential to the child, they try to resist the action, which then causes further anxiety. Obsessions are expressed as concern and disgust with dirt, germs, or bodily waste; fear of something terrible happening to oneself or a significant other; preoccupation with orderliness; excessive praying; preoccupation with lucky and unlucky numbers; and forbidden yet intrusive (sexual) thoughts or images.[14] The compulsive behaviors of children and adolescents include ordering and rearranging, excessive or ritualistic hand washing or bathing routines, checking locks, and other repetitive ritualistic behaviors that may be undertaken to prevent harm to oneself or others. In severe cases, this disruptive and time-consuming disorder interferes with routine daily activities. Concentration and task completion are also impaired.

MOOD DISORDERS

Mood disorders are emotional disturbances involving either extreme sadness (*dysphoria*, depression with anxiety and/or irritable feelings) or elation (*euphoria*, or an overly elevated mood with an exaggerated sense of well-being).[4] The *DSM-VI-TR* classification includes major depression, dysthymic disorder, premenstrual dysphoria, and bipolar I and II disorders.[4]

Major Depressive Disorder

Wendy is a 10-year-old student in the fifth grade. She lives with her mother and 12-year-old brother. Typically a pleasant, well-behaved child, she has been irritable and withdrawn lately. A good student though somewhat anxious, it has been noticed that over the past several weeks, Wendy's schoolwork has deteriorated and she has stopped spending time with her friends at school. Instead of playing with friends, she comes home after school and often goes to sleep. Her mother has noticed that she is not interested in food, has stopped asking for snacks between meals, and has stopped activities she previously enjoyed (making jewelry and playing computer games). She complains of headaches, stomachaches, and being tired. Wendy's favorite teenage cousin was recently admitted to a hospital after a suicide attempt.

Wendy's presentation is consistent with depression. Depressive disorders (e.g., major and minor depression and brief recurrent depression) represent a common health disorder, particularly in adolescents. The usual symptoms of major depression in children and young adolescents are irritability, somatic (physical) complaints such as headaches and stomachaches, anxiety, and social withdrawal.[24] In older adolescents the symptoms of depression are more consistent with those of adults, such as thoughts of suicide (suicidal ideation), guilt, feelings of worthlessness, and disturbances of sleep and appetite. Wendy is typical of a child or adolescent with depression. She is experiencing an overall state of unhappiness, dissatisfaction with life and feelings of pessimism, a loss of interest and pleasure in almost all activities, and a generalized lack of energy.[21,23] Objective signs of depression are weight change (gain, loss, or failure to maintain normal weight); disturbed sleep (inability to sleep or excessive sleep); slowed motor activity, known as psychomotor retardation or restlessness and agitation. Children and adolescents may also have symptoms such as school phobias, substance abuse, sexual promiscuity, and truancy.[10,13]

Risk factors for depression include family history (especially a mother) as well as those such as abuse or a lack of affection and support. Having other mental health disorders (e.g., ADHD, learning disabilities, or an eating disorder) increases the risk of depression. Likewise, low self-esteem, poor body image, and feelings of a lack of personal control are also associated with depression. Negative events such as sexual abuse, parental divorce, bullying, and the death of a family member also increase the likelihood of depression.

OT practitioners need to be aware that the difficulties associated with depression, which include poor concentration, loss of energy, poor task completion, and

Suicidal Risk Signals

If you can answer "Yes" to any of the following questions about a young person, they may be thinking about suicide. Questions highlighted in bold are particularly concerning and require follow-up from a mental health profession. Be sure to document your concerns and the professionals you notified (e.g., parents, school nurse, or counselor, or teacher). Be sure that the child or adolescent is in a safe supervised situation.

Yes	No	
☐	☐	**Depression:**
—	—	Does this child/adolescent appear sad, irritable, or worthless?
—	—	Is this child/adolescent exhibiting symptoms of depression? (Symptoms of depression include insomnia, anorexia, withdrawn from others, decreased ability to concentrate, and fatigue.)
—	—	Is the child/adolescent acting out or abusing alcohol or drugs? (Depression can be masked by substance abuse, aggressive or risk-taking behavior.)
☐	☐	**Preoccupation with death and dying:**
—	—	Has this child/adolescent been drawing pictures or writing poems or stories about death and suicide?
☐	☐	**Talking about suicide:**
—	—	Has this child/adolescent been expressing a desire to die?
—	—	Has this child/adolescent been making suicidal threats?
—	—	Has this child/adolescent been listening to music with negative themes?
—	—	Has this child/adolescent been joking about suicide?
—	—	Does this child/adolescent have a plan of how he or she would carry out suicide?
☐	☐	**Hopelessness about the future:**
—	—	Can this child/adolescent tell you about plans for the next week or next month?
—	—	Has this child/adolescent been "putting affairs in order?"
—	—	Has this child/adolescent given away special possessions or writen a will?
☐	☐	**Changes in life situation:**
—	—	Have there been any major recent changes such as death of a parent, separation or divorce of parents, school problems, or boyfriend or girlfriend problems?
☐	☐	**Previous suicide attempts:**
—	—	Has this child/adolescent previously attempted to commit suicide?
—	—	Is there evidence of self-injurious behavior (e.g., scratches, cutting)
☐	☐	**Lack of support from family and friends:**
—	—	Has this child/adolescent expressed feeling unloved or unwanted?
☐	☐	**Excessive use of drugs or alcohol:**
—	—	Has this child/adolescent begun or increased use of substances?
☐	☐	**Risk-taking behavior:**
—	—	Does this person engage in dangerous behavior such as driving too fast or walking in the middle of the road rather than on the sidewalk?

FIGURE 14-1 Suicide risk signals. (From Hafen BQ, Frandsen KJ: *Youth suicide: depression and loneliness,* Evergreen, Colo, 1984, Cordillera; Hermes P: *A time to listen: preventing youth suicide,* San Diego, 1987, Harcourt Brace Jovanovich.)

aggression toward others, will lead to academic difficulties. Because of apathy and fatigue, the adolescent may neglect basic ADLs such as personal hygiene. When the child or adolescent loses interest and stops participating in previously enjoyable group activities, the resulting isolation and social withdrawal impair social development.[4,7]

An awareness of the risk of suicide is important. Suicide is the third leading cause of death for 15 to 19 year olds and the fourth leading cause of death among the 10- to 14-year-old age group.[1] A child or adolescent expressing suicidal thoughts or exhibiting a preoccupation with death needs to receive professional psychiatric help immediately and must be closely monitored. Figure 14-1 contains a checklist of suicidal risk signals. If signs of self-mutilating behavior or suicidal ideation are observed, the COTA should immediately report them to the parents or a supervisor or other appropriate team member such as a nurse, psychologist, or mental health counselor as well as document them in the child's chart as soon as possible. Supervision and a safe environment (e.g., no access to medications, harmful tools, guns) are important considerations for OT practitioners working with children who are depressed.

A child or adolescent who has recently started antidepressants may be more at risk of committing suicide than a profoundly lethargic, depressed individual. The therapeutic response to antidepressant medication (e.g., a serotonin specific reuptake inhibitor such as Prozac and Zoloft) usually takes two to three weeks before a marked improvement in mood occurs. There can be an improvement in energy before a significant improvement in mood. The increase in energy may be sufficient for the adolescent who is still depressed to commit suicide.

Children or adolescents who engage in self-mutilating behavior (e.g., cutting or scratching oneself, hair pulling, picking at skin) or appear to suddenly recover from depression are of special concern. Sudden unexplained improvement is known as "flight into health" and can signify that the final decision to end one's life has been made. The OT practitioner should be suspicious of sudden elation and energy in a child or adolescent diagnosed with depression. Other warning signs include getting organized and giving away personal items. These signs may indicate that the child or adolescent has made the decision to commit suicide.

CLINICAL *Pearl*

Depression and depressive symptoms are common and cause occupational performance deficits. Even children and adolescents with subclinical symptoms of depression (i.e., insufficient to meet the criteria for diagnosis) have significant difficulties.[24]

CLINICAL *Pearl*

Depression can also lead to aggressive feelings toward others, including homicidal thoughts. Talking about suicide with adolescents needs to include questions about whether the teen has a desire to hurt other people, such as parents or peers at school. Depression is often an underlying problem in many children who commit violent crimes against family members, teachers, or peers.

CLINICAL *Pearl*

Never be reluctant to ask the child or adolescent in a straightforward manner, "Are you thinking about hurting yourself?" If the answer is affirmative, ask whether s/he has a plan and, if so, the details of the plan. It is important that you ask these questions even at the risk of upsetting the child. If asked directly, a child will be more likely to respond and you can take the necessary steps to make him or her safe.

CLINICAL *Pearl*

Poor school performance and the developmental delays in speech and motor skills that are associated with schizophrenia are not due to mental retardation.[14]

SCHIZOPHRENIA

Schizophrenia is difficult to diagnose because affected children are similar to those with autism or a pervasive developmental disorder in that they also have severely disturbed behavior. This disorder is more common in boys. Furthermore, schizophrenia typically presents in late adolescence or early adulthood, but it can develop as early as 5 or 6 years of age.[4,9,12]

The symptoms of schizophrenia, which include disorganized thought behavior and speech, hallucinations, delusions, and social withdrawal, are similar in children and adults. Adolescents will often have had mental health problems such as withdrawal from activities and social contact before developing an acute psychotic episode marking the onset of schizophrenia. Drug use can also trigger the onset.

This acute psychotic phase of schizophrenia is marked by *positive symptoms* such as hallucinations and delusions. Hallucinations are perceptual disturbances. Auditory hallucinations are internalized voices that are critical or instruct the child to harm or kill himself or herself. Similarly, visual hallucinations (e.g., faces, creatures, or images of the devil) are frightening visual distortions. Unlike those of adults, the delusions and hallucinations of children are not complex. One sign of hallucinations is an inappropriate affect (i.e., expressing emotions that do not match the situation, such as giggling without being able to explain the reason).

The onset of schizophrenia marks a deterioration in function (i.e., occupational performance). The residual, or *negative*, symptoms—lethargy, a blunted affect (i.e., the lack of visible emotional expression in relation to a situation), disorganized thought, poor concentration, and apathy associated with schizophrenia—significantly affect ongoing function and disrupt the normal development and transition from adolescence to adulthood.[4,9,12] As a result of the negative symptoms of schizophrenia, adolescents fail to have the typical experiences of adolescence that are crucial to developing life skills. The result can be chronic disability. Intervention usually involves participation in programs that develop long-term life skills.

EATING DISORDERS

Eating disorders occur primarily in adolescents and young adults and are characterized by dysfunctional eating behaviors that, if untreated, may result in serious physical health problems and even death.[4]

Approximately 10% of teens with anorexia nervosa die from starvation or an electrolyte imbalance.[4]

The most common eating disorders are anorexia nervosa and bulimia nervosa, although the *DSM-IV-TR* classification of these disorders also includes obesity and body dysmorphic disorder. Although, eating disorders are more common in girls, clinical presentation in girls and boys is similar.

Generally, individuals with eating disorders perform well in school and work settings. ADL functioning is intact except for eating and food-related behaviors. However, social functioning becomes impaired because of the preoccupation with weight and fear of rejection. Most teens with eating disorders have low self-esteem; their sense of worth involves an externalized component based on their concerns of how other people judge them and their appearance. Self-evaluation is overly influenced by a perception of their own bodies and body shapes. Teens with eating disorders may spend their leisure time preoccupied with food or weight-reducing activities; they may avoid leisure situations that involve food because of their fear of being discovered or being in a situation of having to eat, which would be stressful.[7,17] In this section we discuss the two most common eating disorders (anorexia nervosa and bulimia) that present in children and adolescents.

Anorexia Nervosa

Jennifer is a 13-year-old girl in junior high school. She makes very good grades and participates in extracurricular activities such as gymnastics and cheerleading, but she exhibits poor self-esteem. During the past 6 months, her parents have become worried about her health. They have noticed that Jennifer skips meals and has become very particular about what she eats. She has lost weight and looks thin even in the baggy clothes she wears. Despite her apparent weight loss, Jennifer thinks she looks fat when she looks at herself in the mirror. She has always been critical of her body, and she says that she started dieting 6 months ago to make the varsity gymnastics squad. She has been taking laxatives every day and does aerobic exercises at least 3 hours daily in addition to her cheerleading and gymnastics practices. Jennifer has not menstruated in more than 4 months.

There are two types of anorexia nervosa: restrictive and binge eating with purging. Jennifer's type shows characteristics of the restrictive type of anorexia nervosa in that she limits her food intake and increases her activity level to lose weight. This disorder typically first develops in early adolescence (approximately 13 years of age).[15] However, it can present in younger children or develop in late adolescence or adulthood. Anorexia nervosa is characterized by an intense fear of being overweight (although most often the child or adolescent is less than the normal weight for age and height), an active pursuit of thinness, and self-denial of weight loss.[4,13,15] Adolescents and children with this disorder have a distorted body image, seeing themselves as overweight in all or some body parts regardless of how thin or emaciated they become. Jennifer is critical of her body and sees herself as fat in the mirror.

Binge eating and vigorous, lengthy exercise sessions are common, and laxatives, diuretics, and purging (self-induced vomiting) may be used to control weight. Adolescents with anorexia nervosa are often preoccupied with food and enjoy preparing meals for others, although they eat little of the food they prepare.[4] Daily food consumed may consist of fat-free yogurt and several diet drinks. When confronted by parents or concerned friends, they deny or minimize the severity of the problem and resist treatment efforts.

Anorexia nervosa can lead to significant medical problems because of malnutrition, ceased menstruation, hypothermia (decreased body temperature), and cardiovascular impairments such as bradycardia, hypotension, and arrhythmia. Renal function can be impaired, and electrolyte imbalance may occur. Repeated vomiting of stomach acid with food can cause dental erosion. Osteoporosis may result from the insufficient intake of calcium- and estrogen-containing foods.

CLINICAL *Pearl*

In cooking and eating activities with clients who have eating disorders, the OT practitioner needs to be aware of problems with food that children or adolescents may have. They may choose to hide food or purge after eating. Be aware of a teen who uses the restroom during or shortly after eating. Individuals with anorexia nervosa may enjoy cooking. It may be a way to feel in control of situations involving food without the pressure of eating, which need not be a requirement for being involved in a cooking group.

Many therapeutic interventions are offered for adolescents with eating disorders, including medication, individual counseling, family therapy, and group programs, a number of which are based on cognitive-behavioral or cognitive models. Intervention aims to address both dysfunctional eating behaviors and associated psychological problems.[15] Therapy programs report treatment success as high as 76%; however, long-term recovery rates are most likely much lower.[15]

Bulimia Nervosa

Kim is a high school junior. She is slightly overweight and does not have a good opinion of herself. Her friends are concerned about her. They have noticed that she vomits in the school bathroom immediately after lunch. Kim buys cookies and other junk food, which she hides. When alone she eats the food rapidly, cramming it into her mouth in big bites. Immediately after she has eaten all she can hold, she is disgusted with herself and goes to the bathroom to make herself vomit. Recently the dental hygienist noted that she had enamel erosion on her teeth and told her that frequent vomiting will cause this to happen.

Bulimia nervosa shares many characteristics with anorexia nervosa except that these adolescents are in the normal weight range for their height or are slightly overweight and they are aware that their eating patterns are abnormal.[15] Kim has many of the primary characteristics of bulimia. She has episodes of binge eating (e.g., eating larger than normal amounts of food, usually very rapidly), which result in her anxiety about gaining weight. She feels unable to control how much or what she eats during binges. Therefore, her binge eating is combined with drastic steps to lose weight such as using laxatives, fasting, excessive exercising, and self-induced vomiting, especially after binging on food.[15] Unlike anorexia nervosa, teens with bulimia do not purge on a regular basis but only after excessive eating.

Psychosocial symptoms associated with bulimia are feelings of inadequacy, low self-worth, and depression. A sense of emptiness leads to eating excessive amounts of food alone or secretly, which then causes feelings of anxiety, shame, guilt, and fear. Purging temporarily eases these feelings and has a calming effect. As a result this pattern of eating and purging becomes a way to regulate mood and cope with emotions. Adolescents with bulimia usually want to stop the pattern of binging and weight loss behaviors but feel unable to change it.

Obesity

Dysfunctional eating behaviors can lead to excessive weight gain.[4] Teens who overeat experience low self-worth and feelings of inadequacy. Eating is used to regulate emotions. However, after binge eating they do not attempt to control their weight (e.g., vomiting or other purging behaviors or exercising). Binge eating results in obesity for these adolescents. Obesity as a result of dysfunctional eating patterns has been proposed as a category of eating disorders in the *DSM-IV-TR*.

SUBSTANCE-RELATED DISORDERS

As defined by the *DSM-IV-TR*, **substance-related disorders** include several categories of disorders resulting from the misuse of drugs, toxins, and medications. The terms *substance abuse* and *dependence* are sometimes used interchangeably; however, they actually refer to two different levels of substance disorder. **Substance abuse** is the classification applied when a pattern of use results in adverse consequences, such as the consumption of alcohol while driving or absence from school. **Substance dependence** is the classification for a more severe disorder involving physical dependency on a substance (e.g., alcohol, cocaine). Residential or hospital programs are often required to help the adolescent safely withdraw from the substance, followed by intensive therapy to change the behavior and psychological dependency of using it. **Addiction,** a common term associated with substance-related disorders, refers to the intense physiological and psychological craving for the substance being abused.[16,23,25] The terms *dependence* and *addiction* are essentially synonymous.

Substance dependence is a pattern of continued use despite serious cognitive, behavioral, and physiological symptoms. According to the *DSM-IV-TR*, the following seven characteristics indicate a substance dependence disorder.

- The development of tolerance (the need to use larger amounts of the substance to obtain the desired effect)
- Unpleasant withdrawal symptoms when use is decreased or stopped
- Use of the substance in increasing amounts or for increasingly longer periods of time
- A desire to stop as well as failed attempts to stop using the substance
- Excessive time spent in acquiring, using, and recovering from the substance
- Neglect and a decline in occupational performance (e.g., work, leisure, ADLs)
- Continued use despite the presence of problems caused by the substance

Although an individual may have all or most of the symptoms listed, at least three of the seven must be present for a diagnosis of substance dependency.[4] Among the many substances abused by children and adolescents are alcohol, amphetamines (uppers), cannabis (marijuana), cocaine, hallucinogens (e.g., LSD), opioids (e.g., heroin), phencyclidines (e.g., PCP, angel dust), sedatives, hypnotics, anxiolytics (e.g., Valium, Librium), steroids, and inhalants (e.g., nitrous oxide, acetone). Young people with substance dependence disorders often spend much of their time acquiring, using, and recovering from the substance.[16] To pay for their substance dependency, adolescents may become involved in illegal activities that often place them at further risk of harm (e.g., prostitution or selling drugs). Furthermore, there are significant health risks. Children and adolescents entering treatment programs have poor physical health and sometimes life-threatening conditions such as human immunodeficiency virus or hepatitis from sharing needles. A strong association exists between alcohol use and suicide.

Substance abuse is a significant area of mental health. The extensive resources available identify specialized interventions for young people with substance abuse and dependency problems. In this chapter we have chosen to highlight inhalant use as one example of substance abuse; it is more common in children and adolescents than adults because inhalants are easily accessible and relatively low in cost.

Inhalant Abuse

Michael, a 15-year-old high school student, was found semiconscious in the local park and was hospitalized. In the 6 months before the hospitalization, Michael's parents noticed changes in his behavior. He had appeared "spaced out and distracted and had become disinterested in his personal hygiene." His mother had noticed a rash around his nose and mouth. He is less outgoing and has avoided being part of family activities. An average student, Michael failed two subjects last term. He no longer plays basketball with neighborhood boys after school and on the weekends; instead, he now spends his time "just hanging." Although he receives a generous allowance, he no longer seems to have money.

Michael's admission to the hospital was the result of respiratory complications from inhalant use. His level of use may have already caused Michael permanent brain damage.

The highest rates of inhalant use are among adolescents and children who live at or below the poverty level, and the majority of emergency room visits for inhalant-related problems are from males.[4] Users call inhaling toxic substances "huffing" or "sniffing." The substances commonly inhaled include gasoline, fingernail polish remover, solvent-based glue, paint thinner, spray paint, dry erasers and permanent markers, correction fluids, and aerosol propellants. Fluid inhalants (e.g., gasoline and paint thinner) are often used with a cloth soaked in the substance that is then held over the mouth and nose during inhalation. This leaves a smell of paint or solvent on the teen's clothes. Aerosol substances are sprayed into a paper or plastic bag, which is then held over the mouth and nose during inhalation.

A common indicator of this type of inhalant abuse is a telltale rash around the nose and mouth and sometimes a runny nose, which was noticed by Michael's mother. The use of inhalants results in rapid absorption of the substance into the bloodstream and creates an almost immediate, intense "high." Psychotic experiences including auditory, visual, and tactile hallucinations (sensory perceptions incompatible with reality, such as the feeling of insects crawling beneath the skin) and delusions (beliefs incompatible with reality, such as users believing they are being poisoned by their parents) may occur. The symptoms of use may include vomiting, dizziness, generalized weakness, and abdominal pains and/or nausea.[4,23] The chronic use of inhalants can cause anxiety; depression; and permanent respiratory, heart, kidney, and liver problems and death resulting from cardiac or respiratory damage.[4,23]

Regardless of the inhalant used, frequent use leads to significant impairment in all areas of occupational performance. Adolescent inhalant users neglect self-care, and there can be decreased attendance and performance in school or work. Previous leisure interests such as dropping out of school activities and spending more time partying or participating in aimless activities such as Michael's description of "just hanging" are typically replaced by activities that revolve around the use of the substance. Socially, the teen may stop spending time with friends who do not use substances and will develop relationships with those peers who abuse them. In severe cases irreversible brain damage with cognitive deficits may occur, causing long-term disability.

IMPACT ON AREAS OF OCCUPATION

Children and adolescents with psychosocial or behavioral disorders experience deficits in one or more areas of occupation (ADLs, instrumental ADLs [IADLs], work, education, social participation, and play/leisure).[2,8] OT practitioners examine *performance patterns* (i.e., habits, routines, and roles) of the occupational performance. For example, does the child or teen engage in self-care, attend school regularly, and participate in extracurricular activities with peers? The examination of performance patterns is combined with analysis of a teen's or child's *performance skills* (i.e., motor, processing, and communication). For example, basic sharing, following rules, and peer communication skills are considered. Table 14-2 describes the effect of specific disorders on occupational performance, which is dependent on intact *client factors* that are divided into mental (global and specific), neuromusculoskeletal, sensory, and systemic (i.e., cardiovascular, hematological, immunological, and respiratory) functions.

The OT practitioner considers the influence of *context* on performance. For example, does the child or adolescent have others with whom to play and a safe environment at home and school? Are the parents supportive physically as well as emotionally and available? In addition to considering the physical and social contexts, it is vital to bear in mind the child's or teen's cultural background. For example, there are differences in individual level of comfort with the therapy and educational system. Extra time may be needed to provide explanations and connect with families so that the parents can participate

TABLE 14-2

Impact of Selected Mental Disorders on Occupational Performance

PSYCHOSOCIAL DISORDER	FUNCTIONING IN ACTIVITIES OF DAILY LIVING	SCHOOL AND WORK FUNCTIONING	PLAY AND LEISURE FUNCTIONING	SOCIAL FUNCTIONING
DISRUPTIVE BEHAVIOR DISORDERS Attention deficit disorder Hyperactivity disorder Conduct disorder Oppositional defiant disorder	Inattention to detail Refuses to comply with rules Difficulty following directions Disorganization and forgetfulness	Tardiness, absence, and neglect of school or work assignments and homework Poor concentration, inattention, and disorganization Restless and off-task behaviors Education potentially disrupted when suspension results from defiant or difficult behavior at school or work (e.g., stealing, bullying)	Poor concentration, inattention, and disorganization Difficulty with activity completion Lack of personal responsibility Engaging in reckless activities (e.g., joining gangs) Lack of constructive leisure activities Physically aggressive or bullying Tendency to defy rules of games or sports Solitary leisure activities may not be affected.	Inability to read social cues Aggressive behavior toward others Destruction of other's property, deceitfulness, and lack of remorse or guilt Annoys others by being argumentative, losing temper, and blaming others for own mistakes
LEARNING DISORDERS	Seldom has problems with ADL skills IADL skills may be disrupted by poor academic skills, disorganization, and the lack of an ability to maintain routines.	Specific disorder deficits (e.g., reading, writing, math) Frustration tolerance Poor self-efficacy in school performance	Associated poor self-esteem Additional time required for academic work Sophisticated games dependent on scholastic abilities; sometimes avoided self-efficacy	Associated poor self-esteem Additional time required for academic work Sophisticated games dependent on scholastic abilities; sometimes avoided due to poor self-efficacy
TIC DISORDERS Tourette's Syndrome	Motor tics Vocal tics (public activities such as shopping may be avoided) Safety considerations	Motor and vocal tics interfering with concentration and visual scanning Motor and vocal tics interfering with participation in group learning activities Difficulty finding an accepting employment setting	Avoidance by others Motor tics interfering with physical abilities Safety considerations Leisure activities that are engrossing and performed alone often unimpaired; in fact, the tics may decrease or disappear	Avoidance by adults and children Socially disruptive nature Embarrassment (self-imposed social withdrawal

Continued

TABLE 14-2

Impact of Selected Mental Disorders on Occupational Performance—cont'd

PSYCHOSOCIAL DISORDER	FUNCTIONING IN ACTIVITIES OF DAILY LIVING	SCHOOL AND WORK FUNCTIONING	PLAY AND LEISURE FUNCTIONING	SOCIAL FUNCTIONING
ANXIETY DISORDERS Separation anxiety disorder Generalized anxiety disorder Phobic and social anxiety disorders Obsessive-compulsive disorder	Anxiety inhibiting beginning ADLs and IADLs Fear of failure Perfectionism Phobias Ritualistic behaviors Inability to attain transition Intrusive thoughts	Anxiety inhibiting beginning tasks Separation anxiety in attending school or work Fear of failure Poor self-efficacy in scholastic activities Perfectionism Phobias Ritualistic behaviors Intrusive thoughts Inability to attain transition Reluctance to take risks	Separation anxiety in attending school or work Reluctance to take risks Anxiety inhibiting the start-up of tasks Fear of failure Poor self-efficacy in scholastic activities Perfectionism Phobias Ritualistic behaviors Intrusive thoughts Inability to attain transition	Limiting relationships to significant and familiar persons Poor social self-efficacy Fear of embarrassment Reluctance to take risks Anxiety initiating social interaction Hypervigilance to social cues or oversensitivity and misinterpretation of them Poor self-esteem Phobias Ritualistic behaviors Intrusive thoughts Lack of spontaneity
MOOD DISORDERS Major depressive disorder	Decreased energy and apathy Sleep and appetite disturbances Difficulty initiating and completing activities Lethargy (psychomotor retardation) Disinterest in appearance Poor self-esteem and self-loathing Somatic (physical) illness	Decreased energy and apathy Sleep and appetite disturbances Difficulty initiating and completing activities Lethargy (psychomotor retardation) Decreased concentration Difficulty with memory and following directions Difficulty with problem solving Somatic (physical) illness	Decreased energy and apathy Sleep and appetite disturbances Difficulty initiating and completing activities Lethargy (psychomotor retardation) Decreased concentration Inability to derive pleasure Lack of spontaneity Lack of adaptive, imaginative playfulness	Decreased energy and apathy Difficulty initiating social contact Self-imposed isolation Lethargy (psychomotor retardation) Decreased concentration Inability to derive pleasure Lack of spontaneity Poor self-esteem Slowed cognitive processing Preoccupation with ruminating thoughts
SCHIZOPHRENIA	Poor concentration and inattention Disorganized thoughts Preoccupation with internal stimuli (e.g., hallucinations) Lack of awareness of reality Distractibility Overall lack of awareness of personal needs	Poor concentration and inattention Disorganized thoughts Preoccupation with internal stimuli (e.g., hallucinations) Lack of awareness of reality Distractibility Tardiness, absence, and neglect of school or work assignments and homework Poor concentration Physical restlessness and agitation Off-task behaviors Gaps in learning Frequent hospitalization	Poor concentration and inattention Disorganized thoughts Preoccupation with internal stimuli (e.g., hallucinations) Lack of awareness of reality Distractibility	Poor concentration and inattention Disorganized thoughts, making conversations difficult Tangential thinking Preoccupation with internal stimuli (e.g., hallucinations) Lack of awareness of reality Distractibility Sometimes inappropriate behavior Inattentive to external cues in social situations

TABLE 14-2

Impact of Selected Mental Disorders on Occupational Performance—cont'd

PSYCHOSOCIAL DISORDER	FUNCTIONING IN ACTIVITIES OF DAILY LIVING	SCHOOL AND WORK FUNCTIONING	PLAY AND LEISURE FUNCTIONING	SOCIAL FUNCTIONING
EATING DISORDERS Anorexia nervosa Bulimia nervosa Obesity	ADL and IADL performance is generally not affected, with the exception of eating Inappropriate food consumption Time spent on health-related behaviors (e.g., dieting, laxative use, exercising)	Performance generally not affected unless physical health is compromised Hospitalization leading to work and school absence Fatigue Poor concentration	Anorexia nervosa causing a focus on weight-controlling behaviors such as exercise Poor body image Overweight teens may restrict sport and leisure activities Lack of cardiovascular fitness	Avoids social contact for fear of having the disorder discovered Poor self-esteem Poor self concept Avoids social events involving food (e.g., going to a restaurant with friends)
SUBSTANCE-RELATED DISORDERS Inhalant abuse	Risky behavior (e.g., use of illegal substances and promiscuity) Apathy about hygiene and appearance Neglect of proper nutrition Time and money spent on substance	Cognitive impairment Tardiness, absence, and neglect of school or work assignments and homework Poor concentration Substance-induced state Consequence of poor physical health (e.g., fatigue, nausea, drug dependency symptoms) Education potentially disrupted when suspension results from criminal activity and use of illegal substances Unreliable in work setting or stealing from employer to support substance use	Replacing activities with individuals who do not use substances with those associated with substance use Dropping out of extracurricular activities to spend time "hanging out" or partying Money spent on substance Substance use dominates activities	Limits social network to substance-using peers Self-imposed social withdrawal from family

ADL(s), Activity(ies) of daily living; *IADL(s),* instrumental ADL(s).

with their children in these settings and use the recommendations. For example, those parents who have not had positive experiences in school or participated in the American school system may be tentative in expressing their needs or knowing what is expected of them and their children. By demonstrating a willingness to listen and taking time for explanations, OT practitioners can help bridge cultural differences and reduce the anxiety of families. Furthermore, by creating an open and trusting relationship, they may find themselves advocates for the children and their families in accessing needed resources and services. The goal is that, with experience and increased knowledge through the COTA's mentoring, parents will become their child's advocate.

While OT practitioners examine all the client factors required to perform occupations, those working with children and teens experiencing psychosocial or mental health disorders pay close attention to *global* and *specific mental functions*. **Global mental functions** refer to consciousness, orientation, sleep, temperament and personality, and energy and drive.[2] **Specific mental functions** refer to attention, memory, perception, thought, higher-level cognition, the mental functions of language, calculation, mental functions of sequencing complex movements, psychomotor ability, emotion, and experiences of self and time.[2]

Children with impairment in global mental functions may present with low self-esteem because of frequent failure or frustration. They may have difficulty expressing themselves through language and may show lability of emotions (frequent fluctuations in mood), which typically affects their social participation. Specific mental functions may be manifested as difficulties with memory needed for academic and ADL tasks. Similarly, specific mental functions are required for organization (e.g., dressing and other ADLs). Children with these impairments may also show poor attention to detail, resulting in errors in academic work.

The OT practitioner analyzes the child's ability to perform the occupation, paying careful attention to the global and specific mental functions that may be interfering with the child's ability to be successful. Using a selected frame of reference, the OT practitioner designs remedial, developmental, and compensatory interventions for these occupational performance problems or deficits.

DATA GATHERING AND EVALUATION

The OTR has the ultimate responsibility of interpreting evaluation information.[3,11] S/he determines the specific areas of evaluation and specific assessment methods and tools. Once a COTA achieves service competency, specific aspects of the information gathering process may be given to him or her, including review of records, interviews, observations, and structured assessments.

Many methods may be used to gather information about the child's or adolescent's current level of functioning. The COTA may be assigned the task of reviewing the client's records. Inpatient and outpatient settings typically maintain medical records that provide information about the client's age, sex, academic level, family situation, cultural background, diagnosis, medical history, psychiatric history, medications, and current symptoms. In the school setting, educational records are reviewed.

CLINICAL *Pearl*

Observation skills are developed by practice. Take every opportunity to observe typical children in their areas of occupation. This provides a comparison for observing children with special needs.

Interviews with the child or adolescent and family members provide information about the individual's home environment, performance of self-care tasks, relationships with family members, and participation in leisure activities. Other members of the treatment team may provide valuable insight (verbally and as documented in the client's records) into the child's or adolescent's occupational performance. For example, in an inpatient setting, nursing staff can identify the client's specific problems with ADLs. In the school setting, teachers may be able to identify specific problems that interfere with learning and academic performance.

Observation is one of the most important evaluation tools of the OT practitioner. Much can be learned about specific client factor deficits by observing the individual's performance in ADLs, IADLs, work, education, leisure/play, and social participation. For example, by observing the child or adolescent during a classroom activity, the OT practitioner can identify specific problems in concentration, attention span, work skills (e.g., neatness and rate of completion), and behavioral deficits that interfere with learning. Observation of the child or adolescent during recess provides information about social skills, including the amount and appropriateness of interaction with peers and participation in available leisure activities. Observation is also the ongoing data gathering process for monitoring improvement. The COTA plays a significant role in the evaluation process because s/he is the practitioner who has regular contact with the child or adolescent.

Structured evaluation tools may be used to assess the occupational performance of children and adolescents.[5,12] For example, the Piers-Harris Scale is used to determine a level of self-concept among children.[17] Many OT departments have developed facility-specific assessments by modifying and combining available tools to meet the needs of the specific setting and client population.

INTERVENTION

Planning

OT is guided by frames of reference and the best practice guidelines for the child or adolescent presenting with occupational performance difficulties (Table 14-3). Intervention planning involves collaborating with the child or adolescent, family, and other individuals, such as the members of a health care or education team. Consistent with the long- and short-term goals, planning considers the strengths and weaknesses of the individual in order to determine interventions (e.g., purposeful activities and strategies or techniques for implementation) as well as frequency and duration of intervention activities. The OT practitioner capitalizes on a child's psychological, social, and behavioral strengths to determine the

TABLE 14-3

Psychosocial Frames of Reference

PSYCHOSOCIAL FRAMES OF REFERENCE	PRINCIPLES	STRATEGIES
Cognitive-Behavioral Therapy Model This frame of reference assumes that maladaptive or faulty thinking patterns adversely influence emotions and contribute to dysfunctional behavior. Examples of this faulty thinking include overgeneralizing (i.e., if it is true in one situation, it is always true) or catastrophizing (i.e., always thinking the worse possible outcome). The greatest improvement occurs when a child or adolescent decreases his or her negative and faulty thinking. This is not achieved by changing negative thoughts to positive ones.	How one thinks and what one believes influence behavior and emotions (e.g., a child's positive or negative view of himself or herself and his or her view of the world as threatening or safe, caring, and supportive). A change in thinking can lead to improvement in function and can reduce emotional distress. The basic core and conditional beliefs are learned and become the personal rules that guide life (e.g., *"if I do this (rule) the consequences are…"*). It is a way of making sense of cause and effect relations. Focusing on the present problems, CBT abuse. Time-limited individual or group therapy focuses on a specific difficulty, condition, or skill acquisition.	Interventions include teaching a person about the relationships among their thinking, behavior, and emotions. Interventions: With the use of media and activities, the following techniques and skills are developed. Identifying patterns of thinking and core beliefs and being aware of how thinking affects feelings and behavior (e.g., "*I always fail*") lead to anxiety in new situations and not trying new activities because of the fear of failure. Cognitive restructuring is also called reframing thinking. This involves changing beliefs and thinking patterns. Self-monitoring and self-talk Learning skills to reduce stress, such as relaxation Developing problem-solving skills to address client-identified problems Homework assignments to consolidate learning and transfer it beyond the therapy setting
Skill Acquisition This frame of reference emphasizes that learning, practicing, and acquiring skills help children and adolescents function in social, academic, work, and family occupations.	Children develop self-efficacy, a sense of success, and skills through practice. Acquiring foundational skills can help children perform in home, school, and community settings. Skill acquisition is based on teaching-learning principles. Learning can be achieved through a therapist's instruction or in an experiential group setting through peer modeling and observation. Skill refinement occurs through specific behavioral feedback. Skills are acquired sequentially (i.e., simple to complex).	Interventions are designed to develop, modify, and refine specific skills for functional occupational performance through instructional methods such as role-playing, experiential skill–based groups, practice and generalization of skill performance, modeling, and feedback on skill performance.
Behavioral This frame of reference changes or develops behaviors required for occupational performance. The OT practitioner identifies target behaviors and shapes these behaviors using reinforcement schedules. Applied behavioral analysis is a widely used frame of reference in health and education.	Children and adolescents exhibit behaviors that can be identified and reinforced. Changing or developing behaviors will improve occupational performance. Behavior can be modified by external forces (e.g., reward or punishment schedules).	Interventions are designed to develop, modify, and refine specific behaviors. Interventions follows strict protocols that are targeted to a specific behavior to be increased or decreased (e.g., increase eye contact from a child with autism or decrease head banging in such a child). Identify behaviors to be shaped, changed, or developed. Teach, demonstrate, and practice behavioral strategies.

Continued

TABLE 14-3

Psychosocial Frames of Reference—cont'd

PSYCHOSOCIAL FRAMES OF REFERENCE	PRINCIPLES	STRATEGIES
		Increase desired behaviors with rewards (e.g., praise, tokens such as stars that can later be redeemed for a toy or an activity of one's choice). Intermittent reinforcement strengthens a behavior.
Psychoeducational The purpose of the psychoeducational group is to share information along a common focus and learn from the experiences and knowledge of group members. This process facilitates change and/or the development of skills. This approach is often used in school-based programs to develop or improve social, communication, or coping skills.	Through knowledge comes change. To develop knowledge and skills for coping with crisis events, developmental transitions, mental health disorders, or current situational challenges (e.g., parental divorce, adolescent difficulties, depression, or bullying) Draws from cognitive-behavioral principles Education is a significant component. Focuses on the here and now Intentional use of group experience for mutual and vicarious (by the examples of others and observation) learning as well as support	Time-limited and theme-focused groups of children and adolescents with similar needs or difficulties A well developed curriculum with sequential instructional sessions in which a variety of teaching methods are used, such as videos, handouts, PowerPoint presentations, and blackboards. Interactive and experiential learning strategies are important components. The techniques consist of brief lectures or presentations, small-group discussions, written exercises, role-playing and behavior rehearsal, peer group modeling and learning from others, and homework tasks to reinforce learning and transfer it to everyday settings.

Data compiled from Furr SR: Structuring the group experience: a format for designing psycho-educational groups, *J Specialists Group Work* 25:29, 2000; Jones KD, Robinson EH: A model for choosing topics and experiences appropriate to group stage, *J Specialists Group Work* 25:356, 2000; Kramer P, Hinojosa J: *Frames of reference for pediatric occupational therapy*, ed 2, Baltimore, Md, 1999, Lippincott, Williams & Wilkins; Sommers-Flanagan R, Barrett-Hakanson T, Clake C, et al: A psycho-educational school-based coping and social skills group for depressed students, *J Specialists Group Work* 55:170, 2000; Stein F, Culter SK: *Psychosocial occupational therapy: a holistic approach*, ed 2, New York, 2002, Delmar.
CBT, Cognitive behavioral therapy; *OT*, occupational therapy.

intervention activities that will meet the therapeutic goals. The goals and activities are based on the client's needs, interests, culture, and environment. The COTA contributes to this intervention planning and implementation.[3]

Long-term psychosocial goals identify the desired treatment outcome, and short-term goals identify the steps necessary to achieve the long-term goals. For example, increased social participation is a common desired outcome of therapy. Such an outcome improves the child's or adolescent's ability to develop competence in age-appropriate occupational roles. Tyrone's story provides an example of one long-term and three short-term goals.

Tyrone is a 9-year-old boy who lives in a foster care home with his two younger brothers after the death of his mother from a drug overdose. He has been extremely withdrawn and fearful for the past 6 months. In school he has been aggressive and socially isolated. His academic performance has dropped significantly. Tyrone has been diagnosed with depression and prescribed Paxil. He attends a before- and after-school program for children at risk.

Long-term Goal: By discharge, Tyrone will demonstrate age-appropriate social participation in peer group activities.

Short-term Goal #1: By the end of Week 1, Tyrone will verbally interact one on one with a peer during a group play activity.

Short-term Goal #2: By the end of Week 2, Tyrone will initiate conversations with peers a minimum of two times during a group activity.

Short-term Goal #3: By the end of Week 1 Tyrone will demonstrate collaborative play behaviors, as demonstrated by sharing materials and taking turns with peers in play activities.

Implementation

Effective intervention follows a set of principles and uses techniques and strategies that are based on the selected frame of reference. The purpose of following a frame of reference is to ensure that the outcomes are related directly to the method of treatment used. For example, medication combined with cognitive-behavioral therapy may be the most effective intervention for the treatment of depression.[21] This combination of interventions relieves symptoms and prevents relapse. Table 14-3 shows some of the frames of reference that direct psychosocial OT interventions.

Most OT intervention with children and adolescents occurs in groups and provides opportunities to learn and practice skills. Well designed OT groups create an optimum environment for achieving the child's or adolescent's goals, facilitating interpersonal interactions, and developing competence in a broad range of skills. Regardless of whether interventions occur individually or in groups, they typically include structure, consistency, and positive experiences.

Intervention activities promote the acquisition of appropriate behavioral skills and address specific areas of occupational performance that children either lack or perform poorly. These activities for children emphasize play and may include toys, games, and crafts that are developmentally appropriate, interesting, fun, and challenging. For adolescents, the activities have a peer group focus and may involve a variety of creative arts and role-playing. The emphasis is often placed on IADLs, self-care, and social activities that are required for transition to adulthood.

Group interventions generally address specific problem areas tailored to a particular age group. For example, in a school setting the OT practitioner may design a task group for children in the first through third grades who have difficulty attending to a task or demonstrate poor work skills. Children can develop or improve the skills needed to complete tasks effectively by working on individual craft projects in a structured small-group setting away from the distractions of the busy classroom. During group sessions, the COTA adapts the planned activities to provide opportunities for success as well as extend the skill level of the children. Additional therapeutic benefits will also be intentionally addressed, such as age-appropriate social skills (e.g., sharing equipment and materials, keeping the work space tidy, and asking for assistance) as well as coping skills (e.g., dealing with frustration). Table 14-4 provides examples of psychosocial OT groups.

For many group interventions there are well developed protocols available. Many of the books and articles in the disciplines of education, social work, OT, outdoor education, and psychology outline specific structured programs that can be implemented. These group protocols have been tried and shown to achieve the identified goals. This is particularly true for areas such as social skills, coping skills, assertiveness training, childhood fitness, and self-esteem and self-awareness programs as well as many others. As an OT practitioner, it is wise to look for and use these resources when planning group interventions.

THERAPEUTIC USE OF SELF

The benefits of an empathic (i.e., conveying to another individual that you have an appreciative sense of that individual's experience), positive relationship between a child or adolescent and adult are well recognized and are the basis of many health and educational mentoring programs (e.g., Big Brothers and Big Sisters). In the OT practitioner and child/adolescent relationship, the interaction and rapport developed is dependent on the practitioner's capacity to effectively facilitate a positive validating relationship and use communication and interpersonal skills in a therapeutic manner.

In a relationship with a child, the challenges include being empathic and consistent and setting boundaries to create a safe and supportive environment while remaining flexible. Implicit in this relationship is respect for the child or adolescent. It is essential to give feedback that makes it clear that the *behavior* is unacceptable or disliked, not the child.

Being conscious and intentional in all interactions is an important dimension of the therapeutic relationship. Realize that all behavior has meaning, including your behavior as the health care practitioner. Children and adolescents will ascribe meaning to your actions. Individuals with poor self-esteem and low self-worth may misinterpret interpersonal cues. For example, if you are consistently late for an appointment, the child may feel that s/he is not important to you. His or her thoughts and feelings are not necessarily obvious or expressed verbally but may be observed in the child's behavior, affect (mood), or response to you as the therapist.

The therapeutic use of self requires that an OT practitioner be self-reflective; open to feedback; and aware of the influence of personal disposition, values, and culture. Although working with children and families is rewarding, it is also emotionally demanding and at times stressful.

TABLE 14-4

Sample Occupational Therapy Groups for Children or Adolescents with Psychosocial Dysfunction

GROUP	PURPOSE	METHODS	OUTCOMES
IMAGINATIVE PLAY GROUP Population/group membership: Children and adolescents with difficulty enjoying or participating in play, interacting with others, problem solving, or feeling good about themselves Imaginative games may help children/adolescents decrease stress and connect with others. Play groups can be used to work on many psychosocial issues. They help children and adolescents learn flexibility and problem solving and may teach clients how to adapt and cope with different situations.	Provide social opportunities to improve the following. • social participation • playfulness • adaptability and flexibility • problem solving • imagination • taking turns • sharing	Develop a "play" in small groups that is later presented. Members discuss the play. Depending on the age of the children, pretend clothing may be used, different scenarios or role-playing. Children may be asked to act out a story or work as a team. Group storytelling Puppetry Props Music	Increased self-expression Increased playfulness (one's approach to activities) Opportunities to role-play may help with reading cues, understanding oneself and others, and dealing with issues. Improved social participation Improved stress reduction
TASK SKILLS GROUP Population/group membership: Children and adolescents experiencing difficulty performing occupations (e.g., ADLs, IADLs, school, work, leisure, social participation) The task skills group helps clients learn, practice, and refine the skills needed to accomplish occupations. The members receive support from the group while developing and refining the skills needed for living.	Provide opportunities to improve the following task skills. Task organization, planning, and implementation such as preparation of materials and cleanup of work area Ability to follow directions On-task behaviors Task completion Recognition of errors and problem-solving skills Ability to work with others Ability to identify steps of projects	Develop a plan as a group and carry out selected tasks. Work together toward completion of the tasks. Engage in group and individual tasks required for ADLs, IADLs, work, education, and leisure/play. Examples of types of groups include meal planning, events (e.g., dance, field trip), crafts, and planning a party.	Improve social participation, sense of belonging, efficacy, and self-confidence through completion of selected tasks as part of a team. Improve the organizational, planning, and problem-solving skills needed to complete selected tasks. Develop skills for ADLs, IADLs, education, work, leisure, and social participation.
LIFE SKILLS Population/group membership: Typical children and adolescents with significant physical or intellectual disabilities living in a residential setting such as a group home.	Teach and promote independence in basic life and self-care skills in the following areas. • Personal care of hygiene, grooming, etc • Dressing • Money management	Methods include task analysis, role-playing, and behavior rehearsal. Educational model advocates teaching, demonstrating, guiding, and practicing with supervision, followed by independent practice.	Develop life skills to promote independence.

TABLE 14-4

Sample Occupational Therapy Groups for Children or Adolescents with Psychosocial Dysfunction—cont'd

GROUP	PURPOSE	METHODS	OUTCOMES
Groups focusing on IADL skills are provided to older adolescents with psychiatric, intellectual, or cognitive disabilities. These adolescents may or may not be in a residential setting. Many may be undergoing transition from the home to a community residential setting such as a group home.	• Functional mobility • Community mobility • Health maintenance • Medication routines • Functional communication • Emergency response • Sexual expression Teach and promote independence in IADLs. These skills overlap with basic life skills but also include the ability to care for oneself and one's environment. These skills include meal preparation, home management, caregiving, care of clothes, more complex money management beyond immediate personal use, and safety procedures.	Experiential learning that involves gradual skill development is a key component in these groups. The setting can be the group home, school, or clinic.	
SOCIAL SKILLS Population/group membership: All children and adolescents The groups work the most effectively if the children or adolescents have similar developmental and cognitive/intellectual levels as well as common problem areas. These groups are often divided into skill areas to include specific groups in communication, relationships and supporting others, problem solving in relationships, and self-monitoring in social situations.	Develop the skills required for interacting and "getting along" with others. Develop the skills required for effective verbal and nonverbal communication. Learn and practice socially appropriate behaviors (e.g., manners, sharing). Learn and practice cooperation and teamwork. Develop positive attitudes toward others (e.g., peers, family, teachers, and authority figures such as the police). Groups can focus on coping with specific problems such as shyness or loneliness.	Concrete activities demonstrate and practice social skills and are often based on a psychoeducational, educational, or social-cognitive model. These structured groups use a variety of learning techniques that combine knowledge and practice of the social skills learned. The methods include pen and paper, role-playing, practical skill demonstration sessions, films, behavior rehearsal, guided practice, homework tasks, experiential learning, and imitation.	Improvement in personal and social relationships Increased verbal participation in classroom setting Positive participation in group activities Increased social interaction with peers Increased inclusion in peer activities Reduction in inappropriate social behavior
COPING SKILLS Population/group membership: Children and adolescents with no significant intellectual disabilities	Provide opportunities to improve or learn coping skills including self-regulation in the following problem areas.	Reflection on the techniques and/or alternatives used to perform occupations helps children and adolescents learn coping skills.	Increased self-esteem and positive self-image Increased self-efficacy in one's ability to manage emotions in a variety of situations

TABLE 14-4

Sample Occupational Therapy Groups for Children or Adolescents with Psychosocial Dysfunction—cont'd

GROUP	PURPOSE	METHODS	OUTCOMES
The groups work the most effectively if the children or adolescents have similar developmental and cognitive/intellectual levels as well as common problem areas.	• Poor impulse control • Excessive motor activity • Distractibility • Low frustration tolerance • Difficulty in delaying gratification • Depression, anxiety, or hostility The groups can focus on coping with specific problems such as grief and stress.	Strategies for working on specific areas may benefit children and adolescents, such as stress management, homework strategies, massage, and writing assignments. The methods include pen and paper, role-playing, practical skill demonstration sessions, films, behavior rehearsal, guided practice, homework tasks, experiential learning, and imitation.	Improvement in one's ability to interact in social settings Improvement in one's ability to share space and materials in a group setting and one on one Decrease in self-destructive behaviors and aggressive or acting-out behaviors
SELF-AWARENESS Population/group membership: Adolescents with no intellectual disabilities Adolescents are able to function in group settings and cope emotionally and cognitively with personal exploration.	Provide activities that increase insight and self-awareness. Facilitate self-reflection and self-evaluation in a supportive and safe context. Facilitate the resolution of inner conflict. Develop a constructive self-concept and build self-esteem.	The methods used in self-awareness groups usually involve an activity after which the product or experience is used in a process of self-reflection. Thoughts and feelings are explored and discussed in the group setting to help the adolescents confront and gain insight into their inner feelings and conflicts. The process of self-discovery leads individuals to make connections between past experiences and current feelings, difficulties, and behaviors. Activities can be group collaborative or competitive exercises and projects as well as individual activities including art, ceramics, sculpture, dance, movement "ropes," courses and/or exercises, games, massage, writing, poetry, and drama.	Reduction in symptoms (e.g., depression) Behavioral change: Reduction in self-destructive, aggressive, or antiauthority behavior Reduction in suicidal thoughts Improvement in self-worth and ongoing development of positive self-concept Improvement in academic performance Improvement in the quality of interpersonal relationships

TABLE 14-4

Sample Occupational Therapy Groups for Children or Adolescents with Psychosocial Dysfunction—cont'd

GROUP	PURPOSE	METHODS	OUTCOMES
		The discussions that are facilitated by the activity can address themes such as *who am I, caring about myself and others, understanding and confronting my problems, taking responsibility for myself, understanding the consequences of my actions,* and *making connections between past events and current feelings.*	

Data compiled from Cara E, MacRae A: *Psychosocial occupational therapy: a clinical practice*, Albany, NY, 2005, Delmar; Stein F, Culter SK: *Psychosocial occupational therapy: a holistic approach*, ed 2, Albany, NY, 2002, Delmar.
ADL(s), Activity(ies) of daily living; *IADL(s)*, instrumental ADL(s).

Therefore, supervision and peer support are beneficial. Having a supportive working environment, participating in professional education, and taking care of one's own well-being will ensure your capacity to have therapeutic relationships with the children or adolescents with whom you work.

SUMMARY

Children and adolescents can have psychosocial and mental disorders that affect areas of occupational performance impeding their development. Knowledge of the signs and symptoms of these disorders helps the OT practitioner design effective intervention. The goal of intervention is to provide the child or adolescent with the tools to engage in occupations. Through engagement in occupations, children and adolescents are able to feel successful and develop their independence. This chapter presents the OT practitioner with practical clinical information for treating children and adolescents with psychosocial and mental health disorders.

References

1. Adults should heed teens' warning signs, *USA Today Magazine* 126:4, 1997.
2. American Occupational Therapy Association: Occupational Therapy Practice Framework: domain and practice, *Am J Occup Ther* 56:609, 2002.
3. American Occupational Therapy Association: Standards of practice for occupational therapy. In American Occupational Therapy Association: *Reference manual of the official documents of the American Occupational Therapy Association*, ed 6, Bethesda, Md, 1996, The Association.
4. American Psychiatric Association: *Diagnostic and statistical manual of mental disorders: DSM-IV-TR*, ed 4, Washington, DC, 2000, American Psychiatric Association.
5. Asher IE: *Occupational therapy assessment tools: an annotated index*, ed 2, Bethesda, Md, 1996, American Occupational Therapy Association.
6. Batshaw ML: *Children with disabilities*, ed 5, Baltimore, Md, 2002, Brooks Publishing.
7. Bonder BR: *Psychopathology and function*, ed 2, Thorofare, NJ, 1995, Slack.
8. Florey L: Psychosocial dysfunction in childhood and adolescence. In Crepeau EB, Cohn ES, Boyt Schell BA, editors: *Willard and Spackman's occupational therapy*, ed 10, Philadelphia, 2003, Lippincott, Williams & Wilkins.
9. Gutkind L: *Stuck in time: the tragedy of childhood mental illness*, New York, 1993, Henry Holt.
10. Hafen BQ, Frandsen KJ: *Youth suicide: depression and loneliness*, Evergreen, Colo, 1984, Cordillera.
11. Hemphill BJ, editor: *The mental health assessment: an integrative approach to the evaluative process*, Thorofare, NJ, 1988, Slack.
12. Kaplan HI, Sadock BJ: *Kaplan and Sadock's synopsis of psychiatry*, ed 8, Baltimore, Md, 1998, Williams & Wilkins.
13. Lambert LW: Mental health of children. In Cara E, MacRae A, editors: *Psychosocial occupational therapy: a clinical practice*, ed 3, Clifton Park, NY, 2005, Thomson Delmar Learning.
14. Masi G, Millepeidi S, Mucci M, et al: Generalized anxiety disorder in referred children and adolescents, *J Am Acad Child Adolesc Psychiatr* 43:752, 2004.

15. Neistein LS, Mackenzie RG: Anorexia nervosa and bulimia nervosa. In Neistein LS, editor: *Adolescent health care: a practical guide*, ed 4, Philadelphia, 2002, Lippincott, Williams & Wilkins.
16. Patton GC, McMorris BJ, Toumboura JW, et al: Puberty and the onset of substance use and abuse, *Pediatrics* 114:e300, 2004.
17. Piers EV: *Piers-Harris children's self-concept scale*, rev ed, Los Angeles, 1984, Western Psychological Service.
18. Robins LN, Regier DA, editors: *Psychiatric disorders in America: the epidemiologic catchments area study*, New York, 1991, The Free Press.
19. Rogers SL: Common conditions that influence children's participation. In Case-Smith J, editor: *Occupational therapy for children*, ed 5, St Louis, 2005, Elsevier Mosby.
20. Sanford M, Offord D, McLeod K, et al: Pathways into the workforce: antecedents of school/workforce status, *J Am Acad Child Adolesc Psychiatr* 33:1036, 1993.
21. Sarles RM, Neistein LS: Adolescent depression. In Neistein LS, editor: *Adolescent health care: a practical guide*, ed 4, Philadelphia, 2002, Lippincott, Williams & Wilkins.
22. Scourfield J, Rice F, Thapar A, et al: Depressive symptoms in children and adolescents: changing etiological influences with development, *J Child Psychol Psychiatr* 44:968, 2003.
23. Sherry CJ: *Inhalants*, New York, 1994, Rosen.
24. Stein F, Culter SK: *Psychosocial occupational therapy: a holistic approach*, ed 2, Albany, NY, 2002, Delmar.
25. Winter PA, editor: *Teen addiction*, San Diego, 1997, Greenhaven.

Recommended Reading

Early MB: *Mental health concepts and techniques for the occupational therapy assistant*, ed 2, New York, 1993, Raven.

REVIEW *Questions*

1. What is a mental disorder?
2. What is the DSM-IV-TR, and how does the OT practitioner use this classification system?
3. Briefly describe three symptoms of each of the following disorders: conduct disorder, oppositional defiant disorder, separation anxiety disorder, Tourette's syndrome, anorexia nervosa, bulimia nervosa, and major depressive disorder.
4. Describe how the symptoms of each of the above disorders affect school performance.
5. What are the principles of psychoeducational groups, and when would you use them?
6. Describe important considerations when designing OT intervention for children with ADHD.

SUGGESTED *Activities*

1. Visit daycare centers and observe children engaged in educational or play activities. Note normal psychosocial behaviors and those that may indicate dysfunction, such as aggression, isolation, and poor attention span.
2. Visit a place where adolescents gather, such as a mall. Note the interaction among adolescents.
3. Many videos that depict mental disorders in children and adolescents are available through campus learning resource centers. Watch videos on the disorders discussed in this chapter and imagine the way you would feel if the child or adolescent were a member of your family. List the questions and concerns that come to mind.
4. Contact the National Alliance for the Mentally Ill (1-800-950-6264) for information on family support.
5. Visit the website of at least three mental health organizations (e.g., depression, attention deficit hyperactivity disorder). Discuss your findings in a small group.

15

Other Common Pediatric Disorders

GRETCHEN EVANS PARKER

CHAPTER *Objectives*

After studying this chapter, the reader will be able to accomplish the following:

- State the importance of having a broad knowledge base of pediatric conditions
- Explain the importance of diagnosis in intervention planning
- Use knowledge of pediatric conditions to plan intervention
- Identify the organ systems that specific conditions affect
- Summarize the ways in which different conditions affect children
- Give examples of the common interventions associated with specific conditions
- Name treatment precautions associated with specific pediatric conditions
- Describe the roles of the certified occupational therapy assistant and registered occupational therapist in the intervention of children with a variety of diagnoses

KEY TERMS

Orthopedic conditions
Amputation
Arthrogryposis
Juvenile rheumatoid arthritis
Genetic conditions
Duchenne muscular dystrophy
Down syndrome
Neurological conditions
Spina bifida
Shaken baby syndrome
Seizures
Sensory system conditions
Vision impairments
Hearing impairments
General sensory disorganization
Fussy baby
Environmentally induced and acquired conditions
Fetal alcohol syndrome
Acquired immunodeficiency syndrome

CHAPTER OUTLINE

This chapter explores pediatric conditions; it is organized by organ systems and the way in which the child acquires the condition being discussed. Its design gives the reader a better understanding of the many types of pediatric conditions encountered by occupational therapy (OT) practitioners and an understanding of the major symptoms and signs of the more common diagnoses. Knowing the basic characteristics of a specific condition serves as a framework for the assessment and intervention of the child. Understanding the characteristics of different pediatric conditions enables the practitioner to be a better equipped member of the child's intervention team.

This chapter focuses on a hypothetical certified occupational therapy assistant (COTA) named Jill as she and her direct supervisor Margaret, a registered occupational therapist (OTR), evaluate and treat children at the clinic where they work.

One day a week, Jill and Margaret visit the school around the corner. There they consult with the teachers who have students with disabilities in their classes. They also help with the vocational readiness program in the class for students with developmental delays. Margaret meets with Jill weekly to review charts and discuss any needed updates to the children's therapy goals. Additionally, Margaret and Jill cotreat the children on Jill's caseload every seventh visit.

Once a month, Margaret indulges her love of horses by consulting at the therapeutic horseback riding program in the neighboring town. There she provides supervision for another COTA, Greg, who is involved in a therapeutic riding class that is focused on children with a variety of health-related problems, including orthopedic conditions and sensory processing problems.

ORTHOPEDIC CONDITIONS

Orthopedic conditions involve bones, joints, and muscles. Frequently, functional deficits are also present in the performance areas of activities of daily living (ADLs), play and leisure, and work and productive skills because of the orthopedic problems.

Amputation

Beth was born with an above-elbow ***amputation*** *(Table 15-1). At the age of 3 months, she had her first OT appointment. Margaret, her OTR, conducted a developmental evaluation at that time and determined that Beth was achieving all her developmental milestones. Margaret and Beth's mother Melanie discussed the pros and cons of fitting Beth with a prosthesis. Margaret told Melanie that most children with congenital upper extremity amputations choose to use a prosthesis as a tool some of the time, but they learn adaptive techniques for performing many activities without it. Small children often use the sensations in their stumps for learning about the environment. Margaret gave Melanie some books as well as the phone numbers of other parents with children who have had congenital upper extremity amputations. She suggested that Melanie and her husband spend some time talking to other people who have experienced raising a child with an upper extremity amputation. After a lot of research, Beth's parents decided to wait to have her fitted with a prosthesis until 2 years of age because she could then begin to understand its use as a tool. They also thought that at 2 years her language skill level would make it easier for her to learn to use the prosthesis. They felt that Beth would gradually learn when to do things with or without it. Her first prosthesis had a friction elbow that did*

TABLE 15-1

Types of Congenital Upper Extremity Amputations

TYPE OF DEFICIENCY	MISSING SKELETAL PARTS
TRANSVERSE AMELIA Forequarter amputation	All or most of the arm is missing from the shoulder and below.
TRANSVERSE HEMIMELIA Below-elbow amputation	All of the arm is missing from the elbow and below.
LONGITUDINAL HEMIMELIA Partial amputation	One of the long bones of the forearm is missing. Fingers or thumb may or may not be missing.
PHOCOMELIA	Bones of the upper or lower arm are missing. All or part of the hand remains.

Data adapted from Rothstein JM, Roy HR, Wolf SL: *The rehabilitation specialist's handbook*, ed 2, Philadelphia, 1998, FA Davis.

not lock and a rubber mitt. Later an adept hand was added. Made of plastic, it had one C-shaped "finger" with an indentation in which the end for the opposing "thumb" fit. The adept hand opened until she chose to close it by pulling on a cable attached to a shoulder harness.

Beth is now 7 years old. She has had two surgeries for the end of the bone in her stump. Every year she has a prosthesis revision, and small details are added or changed. Now that she is older, Beth's parents include her in the decisions for changes. The family has learned that Beth usually knows what works for her better than anyone else on her treatment team. Whenever a change is made, Jill, the COTA, spends a few OT sessions with Beth exploring the new uses and operation of the updated prosthesis. During these sessions, Jill and Margaret work closely together; training requires a specific understanding of the ways in which the prosthesis components work and function. Margaret always directs Beth's and Jill's interactions during these sessions because she has more experience. Jill's role is to implement the therapy goals Margaret has planned. Jill reports Beth's progress to Margaret as well as any needs for a change in treatment.

An infant born missing all or part of a limb has a congenital amputation. A traumatic amputation is the result of an accident, an infection, or cancer. About 2 to 8 children in 10,000 are born each year missing all or part of a limb. The types of amputations vary greatly (see Table 15-1). Thumb and below-elbow amputations are the most common types of upper extremity congenital amputations.[26]

Fitting a prosthesis on a child with a congenital amputation at a very young age allows the child to reach developmental milestones on time. It is less likely to be rejected when the child is older if it becomes a part of the child's body concept early in life. With a less severe congenital amputation a child often does well without a prosthesis until s/he is older. Sometimes the child does not use a prosthesis at all. The use of any prosthesis depends on the severity of the amputation and whether one or both arms are involved. See Box 15-1 for stump and prosthesis care.

CLINICAL *Pearl*

Therapy for an older child who has lost a limb as a result of trauma or surgery is different from therapy for a child with a congenital amputation. A child who loses a limb later in childhood benefits from having a prosthesis fitted as soon as possible for psychological and rehabilitation reasons.

BOX 15-1

Care of the Residual Limb and Prosthesis

Decreased skin surface may result in overheating.
Bandages must be dry and monitored.
Examine stump site each night when prosthesis is removed for excessive redness, irritation, or swelling.
Report any discomfort, redness, or pressure areas to therapist immediately.
Wash limb daily with soap and water, rinse, and dry carefully. Do not soak.
Cleanse limb at night so it can have time to dry thoroughly.
Do not shave or apply lotions or moisturizers to the residual limb.
Check fitting of prosthesis and make sure there are no pressure areas.
Stump socks: Change daily and wash by hand with mild soap and water.
Keep leather parts, liners, and webbing clean and dry.
Inspect for wear.
Check mechanical parts/components frequently.

Adapted from www.monash.edu.au/rehabtech/pub/CARE.HTM; retrieved 7/8/2004.

Arthrogryposis

Courtney is a 4-year-old girl with a beautiful face and a vocabulary that is large for a child of her age. Her arms and legs have a tubular shape; the skin between her fingers and in the folds of her knees and elbows is webbed. During the first 2 years of life, Courtney could not sit on the floor to play because she could not bend her hips and knees, and her feet turned in so much that the soles faced each other (i.e., she had clubbed feet). To get from place to place, she rolled along the floor using the normal movement of her trunk. Her shoulders and forearms turned inward, so the backs of her hands always touched her sides. She currently cannot bend her elbows, and her wrists are permanently bent toward her forearms. Her finger movement is very limited and weak, leaving her with no functional pinching ability. The palms of her hands are narrow and almost fold together.

Because she could not bend her hips and knees, Courtney had surgery at the age of 2 years. Her clubbed feet were also surgically repaired so that she could place the sole of her foot on the floor. Before the surgery, she stood on the sides of her feet; now she can stand for short periods but cannot get to a standing position without help. To keep her legs stable while standing, she wears braces on her knees and ankles. Seated at a table of the right height, Courtney can move toys that are moderately sized and not too heavy. She grasps small things by pressing them between the backs of her wrists.

During Courtney's infancy the COTA, Jill, saw her daily for many months to stretch her muscles and maintain the joint motion she had at birth. The stretching was very painful. Courtney's cries during therapy would often drive her mother from the clinic. To gain maximum increases in joint mobility, the stretching was begun immediately after Courtney was born and continued for several months.[4] Stretching requires great care to avoid damaging joint, muscle, and bone tissue. Jill worked closely with Margaret to determine the amount of stretching to be done. She made resting pan splints for Courtney to wear to encourage functional wrist and hand positioning. Because her triceps constantly pulled her elbows straight, Jill also made soft fabric bands to hold Courtney's elbows bent for 10 to 15 minutes at a time throughout the day, which also helped reduce her elbow extension contractures.

Ongoing therapy is important for helping children with arthrogryposis meet educational, self-care, and play needs. Because of the multiple physical limitations, activities in all areas of their life require adaptations. Technology can provide many play, education, and environmental adaptations (see Chapter 22). Close consultation with family members and school personnel enhances the team approach to treatment and case management.

Arthrogryposis is occasionally genetic but is usually caused by other factors, such as reduced amnionic fluid during gestation or central nervous system (CNS) malformations.[23] In its classic form, all the joints of the extremities are stiff but the spine is not affected. The shoulders are turned in, elbows are straight, and wrists are flexed, with ulnar deviation. The hips may be dislocated and the knees straight with the feet turned in. Arm and leg muscles are small and difficult to see, with webbed skin covering some or all of the joints. The condition is at its worst at birth, so any increases in range of motion (ROM) or joint motion are improvements.[4] In typical cases all the joints of the arms and legs are fixed in one position, which is caused partly by muscle imbalance or lack of muscle development during gestation.

CLINICAL *Pearl*

Parents of a newborn with **arthrogryposis** have a lot to learn in a short period of time. Functional gains are made only in the early months of life. To maintain the gains in joint movement made during therapy, a clearly written home program should be created so that the parents can have easy-to-follow guidelines. The program should include specific exercises, precautions, and a clearly written splint-wearing schedule.

CLINICAL *Pearl*

A dynamic elbow flexion splint for an infant with arthrogryposis can be made with elastic and orthoplast. The elbow straightens against the pull of elastic; the elastic then pulls the elbow into flexion, allowing hand-to-mouth movement. The dynamic elbow flexion splint allows infants to do activities such as eat finger food or blow bubbles.

Juvenile Rheumatoid Arthritis

Five-year-old Amber is a cheerful child who is in kindergarten. She loves riding her bike. Occasionally she becomes irritable, and her mom knows it is time for Amber to take a break from riding the bike. Amber has pauciarticular arthritis, a type of ***juvenile rheumatoid arthritis*** *(JRA) (Table 15-2), and as a result her joints can become painful, hot, and swollen. Once a month Amber visits Jill, the COTA, at the clinic to review her home program of passive and active stretching and strengthening activities. During each visit the OTR, Margaret, measures all of Amber's joints with a goniometer to be sure her ROM is not deteriorating.*

By the time they are adults, 75% of the individuals with JRA have permanent remission.[26] However, these children may have functional limitations due to contractures and deformities.

There are three types of JRA: Still's disease (20% of JRA cases), pauciarticular arthritis (40% of JRA cases), and polyarticular arthritis (40% of JRA cases)[4] (see Table 15-2).[2] Children with JRA experience exacerbations and remissions of symptoms. During exacerbations, or flare-ups, the symptoms worsen and the joints become hot and painful; joint damage can occur. During these flare-ups, children need joint protection (Boxes 15-2 and 15-3). During remissions, or pain-free periods, more normal activities can be resumed. Joint protection efforts should be encouraged even during periods of remission so that their use becomes a habit.

Osteoporosis

Austin has multiple handicaps, is blind, and does not speak. He is 6 years old and can walk if someone holds his hand; he refuses to walk on his own, partly because of his blindness. He cries and falls when he is left standing with no support. Austin prefers to sit and scoot on his bottom, but his hips and knees become stiff from sitting so much. Beginning contractures of the hips and knees limit his ability to stand up straight. Because of his blindness, he constantly alternates between pushing on his eyeballs and mouthing his hands. (See Visual Impairments section in this chapter.) These "blindisms," or self-stimulating behaviors, could cause elbow flexion contractures that would limit his ability to straighten

TABLE 15-2

Three Types of Juvenile Rheumatoid Arthritis

TYPE	LIMB INVOLVEMENT	FUNCTIONAL IMPLICATIONS
PAUCIARTICULAR (FEW JOINTS) Affects four or fewer joints Comprises approximately 40% of JRA cases	Only a few unmatched joints are affected. Leg joints are usually affected, but elbows can also be affected. Children often recover in 1-2 yr. Children can develop an eye inflammation called *iritis* that can lead to blindness unless it is treated early.	Pain and joint stiffness may limit activities. Contractures can develop. Splints may be needed. Work simplification may be needed. Adaptive equipment may be needed. Climbing stairs may be difficult.
POLYARTICULAR (MANY JOINTS) Comprises approximately 30% of JRA cases Five or more joints affected Girls more commonly affected than boys	Onset is fast. The symmetrical joints of legs, wrists, hands, and sometimes the neck are affected.	• Functional implications are the same as those for pauciarticular arthritis but also include the following: Activities can be limited by fatigue. There is difficulty with fine motor activities.
STILL'S DISEASE Affects joints as well as internal organs Comprises approximately 20% of JRA cases	The onset speed and affected limbs are the same as those for polyarticular arthritis. Other organs, such as the spleen and lymph system, may also be affected. Bone damage may affect growth.	• Functional implications are the same as those for polyarticular arthritis but also include the following: • Rash and fever may develop, last for weeks, and require bed confinement.

Data from Case-Smith J: *Occupational therapy for children*, ed 5, St Louis, 2005, Mosby; Arthritis Foundation, www.arthritis.org.
JRA, Juvenile rheumatoid arthritis.

the elbows. His pediatrician thinks that standing independently and walking with a walker for stability would benefit Austin physically as well as make him easier to care for. His doctor has prescribed OT to increase his arm ROM, and the COTA will make elbow splints to maintain the ROM gained during therapy. The splints will also limit the self-stimulation activities. During his first stretching session, Austin's arm bone snapped and broke as Margaret began gentle stretching.

BOX 15-2

Rules of Joint Protection for Children with Juvenile Rheumatoid Arthritis

- If joints are warm and swollen, encourage children to use them carefully during all activities and to continue to do ROM exercises as much as they are able.
- Because tired muscles cannot protect joints, teach children that they should not remain in the same position, such as holding a pencil to write, for long periods without stretching or taking a break.
- Larger muscles are found around big joints, so teach children the way to use big joints for heavy work. For example, they can balance a lunch tray on their forearms, wear a backpack on both shoulders, or carry a purse over a shoulder rather than in a hand.
- If children become tired or are in pain, stop the activity.
- Proper positioning prevents contractures and deformities. Teach children that they should always use good posture.

BOX 15-3

Treatment for Juvenile Rheumatoid Arthritis

Splinting to prevent development of contractures
AROM and PROM exercises to maintain ROM
Careful monitoring of each joint to maintain functional level and prevent deformity
Exercises to maintain or increase strength
Teaching the importance of joint protection during all activities to prevent deformities or contractures

AROM, Active range of motion; *PROM*, passive range of motion; *ROM*, range of motion

CLINICAL *Pearl*

To avoid causing fractures, use care when handling and doing ROM exercises with severely affected, inactive children. Maintaining good joint mobility with daily careful passive stretching and proper positioning that are initiated during infancy helps control osteoporosis.

In children with disabilities, osteoporosis is caused by a lack of weight-bearing activities such as crawling and standing. The bones are weakened as a result of mineral loss; weight-bearing activities and muscles pulling on bones during movement make bones strong. Children who develop osteoporosis are usually severely affected as a result of some other condition such as cerebral palsy. They are usually very inactive and unable to stand; their bones can become so brittle that simple dressing activities could cause a fracture.

GENETIC CONDITIONS

Humans have 23 pairs of chromosomes, which are tiny thread-shaped structures found in each cell of the body. Each chromosome is made up of tiny sections called *genes*. Half of the genes come from the mother through her egg, and the others come from the father through the sperm. The genes are mixed together and determine every aspect of a person's characteristics. Sometimes a gene carrying a specific problem can be passed from one or both parents to the child. Problems can develop when the mother's and father's normal genes mix and match improperly or when an infant receives a gene with a mutation (i.e., a gene that has been damaged or is abnormal in some way). **Genetic conditions** cause characteristic patterns of physical involvement and progression. Knowing whether a child has a genetic condition aids in determining the types of treatment intervention from which the child may benefit. About 30% of developmental disabilities result from inheriting a gene that causes the disability or one that has a particular mutation. Fifty percent of major hearing and vision problems are caused by genetic syndromes.[26] The more common conditions seen by the OT practitioner are discussed in this section. Children with other genetic disorders may occasionally be seen as well. Descriptions for some of the additional genetic disorders are found in Table 15-3.

CLINICAL *Pearl*

With proper joint management, children can be placed in prone or supine standers for weight-bearing activities. Standing is good not only for bone growth and strengthening but also for body functions such as circulation and digestion.

Duchenne Muscular Dystrophy

Kevin has started second grade in a regular classroom, and his teacher is worried. When seated at his desk he looks like the rest of the students in the class, although his arms and legs look chubby. Although he is bright, he has trouble keeping up with his classmates. He struggles to write, and his handwriting is hard to read. Recently he has started to walk his fingers across the desk to get his pencil. It is hard for him to raise his hand to ask a question or get his books out of his desk. When the class goes to other parts of the school for gym or music, Kevin can easily be spotted by his waddling gait. He has lordosis (Figure 15-1); to keep from falling forward, he carries his shoulders and head back. His gait looks like a slow march because he has to pick his feet up high so that his toes do not drag. He falls a lot. To get up from sitting, he "walks" his hands up his legs (Gowers' sign). Kevin has ***Duchenne muscular dystrophy*** *(MD).*

The COTA, Jill, visits Kevin's school weekly. During a recent visit, Kevin's teacher met with Jill to tell her what was happening. Fortunately, Jill already knew Kevin from the clinic and was able to give the teacher suggestions to help meet his classroom needs. Jill suggested that Kevin start using a computer for his written work. She also suggested that he sit at a larger table and have all his books within easy reach rather than sitting at a regular school desk.

Kevin's family brings him to the clinic several times a year so that Jill and Margaret can check on his adaptive equipment needs. Because his ability to move has decreased, Jill has taught the family ROM exercises to keep his joints loose, making it easier to dress and bathe him. She teaches them about proper body positioning to prevent contractures or scoliosis from developing (Figure 15-2). She has also given Kevin a list of strengthening exercises that will help him function independently for as long as possible. Jill knows that usually by the age of 9 years, children with Duchenne MD use a wheelchair at least part of the time.

MD comprises a group of muscle disorders. One of the more common types is Duchenne, or pseudohypertrophic (which literally means "false overgrowth"). In children with Duchenne-type MD, muscle breaks down and is replaced with fat and scar tissue, making the muscles, especially those of the calves, look unusually large. Several other forms of MD also affect boys and girls but usually at a later age. Duchenne-type MD is seen only in boys. About 3 individuals per 100,000 develop the condition.[26] Most children with Duchenne MD survive until they are in their 20s, and a few live until they are in their 30s. The cause of death is usually cardiopulmonary system (heart and lung) complications that lead to pneumonia.

TABLE 15-3

Additional Genetic Conditions

CONDITION AND GENETIC CAUSE	INCIDENCE	COMMON SYMPTOMS AND SIGNS	FUNCTIONAL IMPLICATIONS
TUBEROUS SCLEROSIS Autosomal dominant gene or mutation	1 in 20,000 births[16]	Very mild to severe symptoms Tumors in brain; can cause seizures, mental retardation, delayed language skills, and motor problems, which is rare Tumors in heart, kidneys, eyes, or other organs; can (but may not) cause problems	Possible learning disabilities Possible aggressive or hyperactive behavior Possible inability to speak and need for alternative communication Possible severe delays in gross and fine motor skills Mild to severe delays in self help skill
ANGELMAN SYNDROME Deletion of chromosome 15 from mother[10]	1 in 25,000[13]	Microencephaly (see Table 15-4) Tremors and jerky gait Developmental delays Severe language impairment; nonverbal or severe speech delay Very happy mood (happy puppet syndrome) Possible seizure disorder	Gross and fine motor delays, delayed walking skills Severely delayed self-care skills Inability to speak but possible use of alternative communication Sleep disorders (can be very disruptive to family life) Severe sensory processing problems Behavior problems such as biting, hair pulling, stubbornness, and screaming
PRADER-WILLI SYNDROME Deletion of chromosome 15 from father[19]	1 in 15,000[19]	Growth failure related to poor suck-swallow reflex in infancy Obsessed with food, possibly causing obesity (parents must lock all kitchen cabinets; PRECAUTION: may eat *anything*) Developmental delays, low intelligence Hypotonia and poor reflexes Speech problems related to hypotonia Laid-back attitude but possible stubbornness and violent tantrums Severe stress on families resulting from behavior problems	Obsession with eating (can be dangerous during treatment) Gross and fine motor delays Delayed development of self-help skills Difficulty walking resulting from obesity or low muscle tone May need alternative communication Possible benefits from prevocational and vocational training
RETT SYNDROME Genetic but undetermined[14]	Seen only in girls	Normal or nearly normal development during first 6-18 mo of life Loss of skills and functional use of hands beginning at approximately 18 mo Loss or severely impaired ability to speak Development of repetitive, almost constant hand movements such as hand washing and wringing, clapping, and mouthing Shakiness in trunk and limbs Unsteady, wide-based, stiff-legged walking	Gross and fine motor problems Lacking or delayed self-help skills Difficulty walking or inability to walk Delayed response to requests, possibly taking up to 2 min to respond Possible need for alternative communication

TABLE 15-3

Additional Genetic Conditions—cont'd

CONDITION AND GENETIC CAUSE	INCIDENCE	COMMON SYMPTOMS AND SIGNS	FUNCTIONAL IMPLICATIONS
FRAGILE X SYNDROME Mutation on X chromosome (most common genetic disease in humans)[11]	1 in 2000 males and 1 in 4000 females[1]	Boys more severely affected than girls Possible hyperactivity Low muscle tone Sensory processing problems involving touch and sound Possible autistic behavior Language delays (more common in boys); possible dysfunctional speech Intelligence problems ranging from learning disabilities to severe retardation	Mobility problems; delayed walking skills Gross and fine motor delays Delayed development of self-help skills Possible learning problems ranging from learning disabilities and ADD to mental retardation Possible need for alternative communication in boys (unusual for girls) Possible benefits from prevocational and vocational training

ADD, Attention deficit disorder.

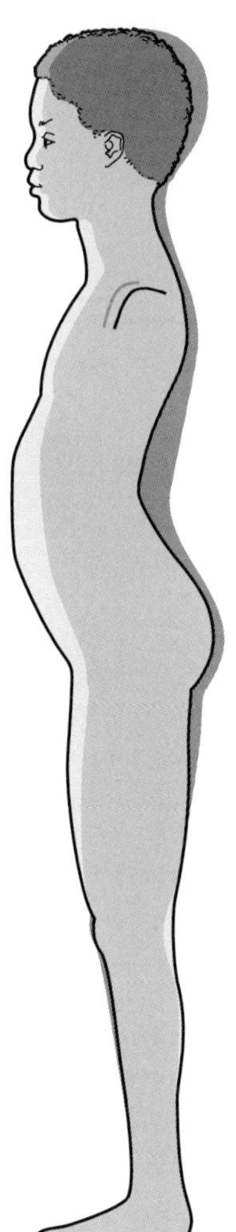

FIGURE 15-1 Lordosis—an increased forward curve of the lower back. The abdomen falls forward and the knees lock backward. The posture shifts weight forward; to balance weight, the child tends to carry the head and shoulders back farther than normal. This posture is common in children with hypotonia.

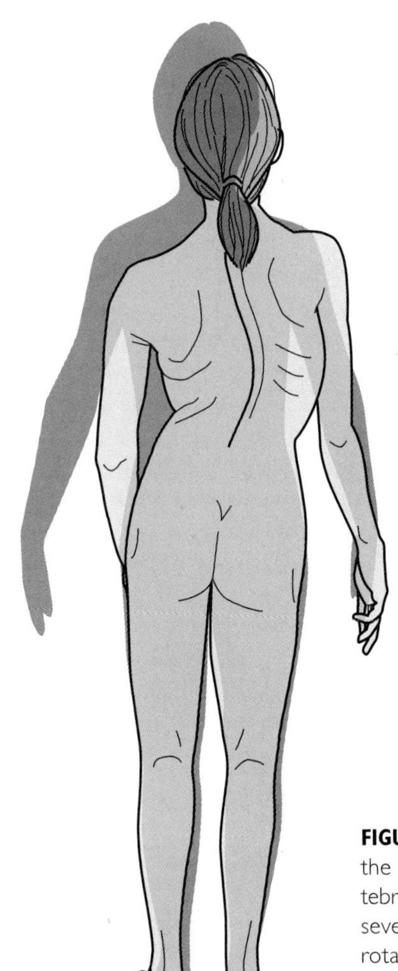

FIGURE 15-2 Scoliosis—the bending of the vertebral column sideways. In severe cases the ribs are rotated, compressing the lungs and reducing their function.

BOX 15-4

Progression of Functional Losses in Children with Duchenne Muscular Dystrophy

LEVEL 1
Initially independent but has progressive functional losses over a period of several years: for example, walks independently but then loses stair-climbing ability and needs leg braces to walk and assistance to get up from a chair

LEVEL 2
In wheelchair: sits erect and is able to roll chair and perform ADLs such as upper extremity dressing, eating, and brushing the teeth in bed or chair

LEVEL 3
In wheelchair: sits erect but is unable to perform ADLs in bed or chair, such as placing equipment conveniently or rolling over without assistance

LEVEL 4
In wheelchair: sits erect with support and can do minimum ADLs such as brushing teeth or eating with adapted equipment

LEVEL 5
In bed: can do no ADLs without assistance

Adapted from Rothstein JM, Roy HR, Wolf SL: *The rehabilitation specialist's handbook,* ed 2, Philadelphia, 1998, FA Davis.
ADLs, Activities of daily living.

The parents of a child who has Duchenne MD usually begin to suspect that something is wrong when the infant begins to walk on his toes at about 1 year of age (Box 15-4). The diagnosis is usually made by the age of 4 after a muscle biopsy is performed. By then the child's calves look large and progressive weakness has begun, especially in the joints closest to the body.

Scoliosis (see Figure 15-2) can develop because of muscle weakness, especially during growth spurts. Proper wheelchair positioning and support are important to prevent scoliosis. Older children with MD may have to use a ventilator, so good body alignment is important for maintaining the vital chest capacity needed for breathing.

Down Syndrome

Dennis has ***Down syndrome.*** *When he was 12 years old, Jill, the COTA, gave him a prevocational assessment at the OTR's request (see Appendix A of this chapter). Based on the results, Jill and Margaret developed a plan of care in which Dennis's prevocational skills could be improved in his vocational readiness classes at school. Dennis is now 15 years old and works as a bagger at the local grocery store for 2 half-days a week. The work is part of the vocational training program run by the local high school. When he carefully sorts and places items in grocery sacks, his short, stubby fingers and hands move slowly. His tongue sometimes protrudes as he works; it seems large for his mouth. His face is full and round. Behind his glasses is a fold of skin on either side of his nose that gives his eyes an Asian appearance. Dennis is about 5 feet 6 inches tall. His chest is round, and his body is chunky (Box 15-5). When he pushes grocery carts to cars, he walks with a wider base of support than normal and his feet roll in. He politely chats with the customers he helps. Dennis is a confident young man and seems to like his work.*

BOX 15-5

Physical Characteristics of Down Syndrome

- Shortened limbs and fingers
- Slanted eye skin fold over nasal corners of eyes
- Small mouth, protruding tongue
- Straight line across palm of hand (simian line)
- Heart defects (congenital, high incidence)
- Mental retardation (usually mild or moderate)
- Atloaxoid instability (important factor for children who engage in sports); can cause quadriplegia after minor neck injuries
- Floppy muscle tone
- Hyperextensibility of hips, limbs, and fingers
- Sensory processing problems
  Diffuse tactile discrimination difficulties
  Tactile sensitivity
  Gravitational insecurity
  Hyperactive postrotary nystagmus
  Poor bilateral motor coordination
- Changes in developmental reflexes in infants (caused by altered sensory processing)
  Reduced suck reflex
- Increased gag reflex (eventually resulting in food selectivity or intolerance and chewing problems)
  Diminished palmar grasp reflex
  Prolonged and exaggerated startle reflex
  Prolonged flexor withdrawal and avoidance reactions in hands and feet
  Delayed placing response in hands and feet
  Lack of primary standing or air response*
  Poor optical righting
  Poor body-on-body righting delayed equilibrium responses, particularly in quadruped and standing

Data from Crepeau EB, Neistadt ME, editors: *Willard and Spackman's occupational therapy,* ed 6, 1998, Philadelphia, JB Lippincott–Raven.
*Normally, when infants' feet touch a supporting surface, they support their body weight against the surface with their feet. Infants with Down syndrome pull their feet away from the supporting surface.

One of 2000 live infants born to women who are less than 40 years of age have Down syndrome; one of 40 infants born to women who are more than 40 has the syndrome. Although inherited abnormal genes or accidental genetic mutations can cause Down syndrome, about 95% of the individuals with this syndrome have an extra twenty-first chromosome. The extra chromosome comes from the father 25% to 30% of the time.[4] Genetic counseling is very important to help parents determine the origin of the syndrome and with future family planning.

Through early intervention and ongoing treatment, OT is an important part of helping children who have Down syndrome reach their maximum potential. Recent research indicates that early intervention, including teaching families the ways to enrich their children's environment, helps reduce developmental delays.[21] Constant monitoring and changes in treatment also help children's developmental progress.

Chronic Fatigue Immune Dysfunction Syndrome and Fibromyalgia

In the past, 14-year-old Rachel had some growing pains and felt under the weather. Lately she has been waking up tired every morning. Her symptoms started with a flulike illness and sore throat that would not go away. Now she has tremendous difficulty just getting through each day; she falls asleep every time she sits down. Despite her fatigue, she cannot sleep more than 1 or 2 hours at night before muscle jerks awaken her and she is covered with sweat. Every morning she gets out of bed feeling shaky. On some days she experiences sudden weak spells and sweats. Sometimes she feels like she will pass out. At other times her heart races and she feels like she is having a panic attack. She has been having problems with an irritable bowel and alternates between having constipation and loose stools. She has also started having trouble with bladder infections and reduced bladder control. On many days her muscles feel stiff and sore. Nothing the family doctor tried has helped her.

One day her brother found a website describing Rachel's condition perfectly; it was called fibromyalgia syndrome (FMS). The family doctor agreed with the diagnosis and said that Rachel was also one of the 40% of people with chronic fatigue immune dysfunction syndrome (CFIDS) and FMS (CFIDS/FMS) who also had reactive hypoglycemia. Hypoglycemia is a low blood glucose level; this caused Rachel's panic attacks, sweats, shakiness, and feelings of weakness.

Realizing that Rachel fatigued easily and repetitive motions such as those used for writing could be painful, the doctor recommended an OT consultation. Margaret met with Rachel's teacher and recommended that Rachel write less by photocopying a classmate's notes. Rachel was given a second set of books for home use and an elevator pass so that she would not have to climb the stairs. Margaret also ordered Rachel a built-up pen to help reduce her muscle fatigue while she is writing.

More children are beginning to be recognized as having CFIDS, FMS, or CFIDS/FMS. Emerging research indicates that these conditions are similar enough to have the same cause, with the only difference being some of the symptoms.[3] The exact diagnosis (i.e., CFIDS, FMS, or CFIDS/FMS) given to a child may depend more on the specialist who is making the diagnosis than on the child's symptoms because the symptoms of the diseases are very similar. These symptoms (Box 15-6) can develop gradually or linger after a case of the flu. Suspect CFIDS/FMS in a child if a parent has been identified as having one of the syndromes. At least half of the children born to parents with one of the syndromes are suspected to also be affected.

BOX 15-6

Symptoms of Chronic Fatigue Immune Dysfunction Syndrome and Fibromyalgia

- Children may have several or all of the following symptoms or conditions:
- Growing pains
- Frequent periods of not feeling well
- ADD
- Sleep disturbances or insomnia
- Irritable bowel syndrome
  - Gas or bloating
  - Periods of alternating constipation and diarrhea or loose stools
- Urinary tract problems
  - Reduced bladder control
  - Bladder infections
  - Painful urination
- Deep aches in calves and other muscles
- Frequent and severe headaches
- Lack of stamina
- Short-term memory loss
- Neurological problems
  - Shooting leg pains
  - Restless leg syndrome (feeling a constant need to move the legs)
  - Muscle tics or twitches
  - Numbness
- Reactive hypoglycemia
  - Racing heartbeat
  - Shakiness
  - Blacking out
  - Sweats
  - Anxiety or panic attacks

From St Amand RP: *What your doctor may not tell you about pediatric fibromyalgia,* New York, 2002, Warner Books.

BOX 15-7

Characteristics of Children with Attention Deficit Disorder or Attention Deficit Hyperactivity Disorder

Very active or fidgety
Impulsive; act without thinking of consequences
Have racing thoughts
Inattentive during activities they consider boring or unexciting (which often include doing schoolwork)
Slow to wake up in the morning; are disorganized or grumpy unless anticipating an exciting activity
Slow to fall asleep
Spatially dyslexic (write mirror-image reversals of letters; have difficulty with left-right discrimination; have difficulty properly sequencing letters, words, or numbers)
Have episodic temper tantrums that include hitting, biting, and kicking
Bed wetters
Inexplicably emotionally negative

Adapted from Fact Sheet on Attention Deficit Hyperactivity Disorder (adhd/add): http://add.org/content/abc/factsheet.htm.

TABLE 15-4

Other Common Central Nervous System Conditions

CONDITION	SYMPTOMS OR SIGNS
AGENESIS OF THE CORPUS CALLOSUM Absence or poor development of the central part of the brain that connects the two hemispheres	Deficits ranging from mild learning problems to severe physical and mental problems Possible vision or hearing problems Possible sensory processing problems Possible eye-hand coordination problems Mental retardation and epilepsy (common)
MICROENCEPHALY Literally, "small head"	Head that appears small for body Moderate to severe mental retardation Moderate to severe motor problems Possible seizure disorder

Forty percent of people with CFIDS/FMS also have reactive hypoglycemia.[24] Hypoglycemia can cause individuals to feel like they are having panic attacks or like they are simply anxious. It can also cause the heart to race, shakiness, and fatigue.[24] A promising medical treatment is being developed that puts this combination of conditions into remission in both children and adults.*

Children with CFIDS/FMS may be referred to OT for the treatment of attention deficit disorder (ADD) or attention deficit hyperactivity disorder (ADHD) (Box 15-7). The ADD or ADHD associated with CFIDS/FMS is probably caused more by the pain and fatigue characteristic of CFIDS/FMS than the sensory processing deficits and difficulties typical of children with true ADD or ADHD. Children who have had pain for a long period of time may not consider it abnormal. The pain or fatigue may cause them to move around more than others to alleviate the pain or wake up. The constant pain and need to move may distract them from their schoolwork and activities.[24]

Children with CFIDS/FMS often need help with work simplification, self-care skills, or adaptive equipment because of fatigue, cognitive problems, or pain. Once the condition is identified, children may benefit from using built-up pencils to ease finger pain and fatigue. Fatigue and pain interfere with the performance of repetitive activities and may cause writing to become difficult.

*See www.FibromyalgiaTreatment.com

NEUROLOGICAL CONDITIONS

Children born with problems in the brain or spine (the CNS) have congenital **neurological conditions.** They may also be acquired from trauma or infection at the time of birth or in the early months of life. Neurological conditions may affect the CNS or the peripheral nerves (the nerves outside of the brain and spinal cord). The more common neurological conditions seen by the OT practitioner are discussed in depth. Table 15-4 describes other CNS conditions.

Spina Bifida

Yesterday 10-year-old Niki was on the school playground playing catch when she began to feel ill. Today she is in the hospital recovering from surgery to repair a shunt that was previously placed to control her hydrocephalus. Her father rushed her to the emergency room when she got off the bus with a fever and headache (Box 15-8). Niki was born with ***spina bifida*** *and has had many surgeries, most of which were to repair her shunt. Others were to repair the hole in her back and her congenital clubbed feet. Her legs are paralyzed, and she has no bowel or bladder control. She has*

BOX 15-8

Signs of a Blocked Shunt

Headache
Nausea or vomiting
Irritability
Changes in behavior or school performance
Temperature elevation
Pallor
Visual perception difficulties

learned to use a catheter to empty her bladder and uses a special bowel program to eliminate. When she was younger, Niki walked with crutches and braces but was always frightened of being on her feet. As she got older, she gained weight, which made it hard to walk. Now Niki uses a manual wheelchair to move around.

There are three types of spina bifida classification: (1) occulta, (2) meningocele, and (3) myelomeningocele (Figure 15-3). Spina bifida, a condition in which one or more of the vertebrae are not formed properly, is the most common type of congenital spinal abnormality.[6] The meninges (the covering of the spinal cord) or the meninges *and* the spinal cord push out through an abnormal opening in the vertebra in the meningocele and myelomeningocele types, respectively. The amount of resulting disability can range from minimal, as it is in individuals with spina bifida occulta, to severe, as it is in individuals who have a myelomeningocele. The OT practitioner typically sees children with the myelomeningocele type because their limitations and disabilities are the most severe of the three. (NOTE: The terms *spina bifida* and *myelomeningocele* are used synonymously in the remainder of this section.)

Spina bifida occurs in about 1 of 1000 births. Its cause may be genetic or result from high maternal temperatures or insufficient folic acid in the mother's diet. The amount of resulting physical disability is related to the size and location of the defect.[26] The higher the level of the spinal opening, the greater the disability (see Figure 15-3). Eighty percent of children born with spina bifida have hydrocephalus caused by excess cerebrospinal fluid. To drain the fluid, a shunt is placed in the ventricles of the brain. The tube (which is similar to small aquarium tubing) runs down the neck to the abdomen, where the extra fluid drains. Scoliosis or kyphosis may be present at birth or develop later (see Figures 15-2 and 15-4), and

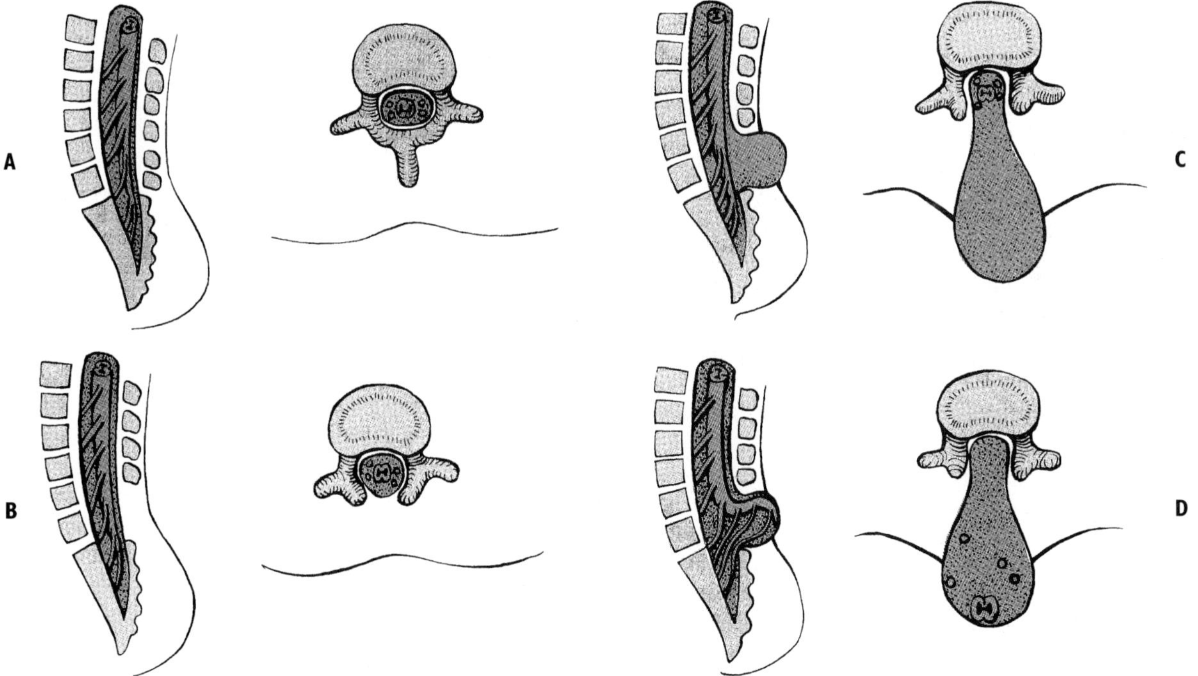

FIGURE 15-3 Normal vertebral column and three forms of spina bifida. **A,** Normal: intact vertebral column, meninges, and spinal cord. **B,** Spina bifida occulta: bony defect in vertebral column. This type of spina bifida can be diagnosed only by x-ray and often goes undetected. **C,** Meningocele: bony defect in which meninges fill with spinal fluid and protrude through an opening in the vertebral column. **D,** Myelomeningocele: bony defect in which meninges fill with spinal fluid and a portion of the spinal cord with its nerves protrude through an opening in the vertebral column. This type of spina bifida is the most severe and can be detected at birth. (From Wong DL: *Whaley and Wong's nursing care of infants and children,* ed 6, 1999, St Louis, Mosby.)

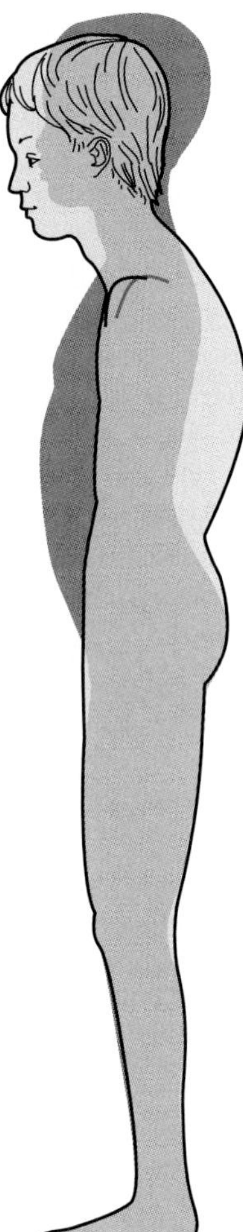

FIGURE 15-4 Congenital kyphosis—a backward rounding of the spine in the chest area that can be caused by malformed vertebrae. Changes in the spine cause the head and shoulders to be carried forward. The front of the body bends forward, compressing the internal organs.[27]

both conditions are difficult to treat. In the early months, proper positioning of the paralyzed legs is important to prevent the development of contractures. Because of the lack of mobility, children are not able to engage in the normal developmental sensorimotor experiences. This is an important area of treatment in OT for older infants. The lack of sensorimotor experience may contribute to poor development of body concept, fear of movement, tactile sensitivity, poor eye-hand control, and poor motor planning. Infants and toddlers with spina bifida benefit from a good home program of sensory enrichment that is related to the therapy provided in the clinic.

Shaken Baby Syndrome

The young parents of 7-month-old Tony sat nervously in the hospital waiting room wondering how a day that had started so normally could be ending like this. That morning Tony's mother had been called in to work unexpectedly; she had not had time to take him to his regular sitter, so she called her neighbor to watch him.

When Tony's mother got home that afternoon, she found him in a deep sleep. When she finally woke him, he forcefully vomited his lunch. She became very frightened when she noticed that his left arm and leg seemed floppy. When his whole body suddenly began to jerk uncontrollably, she frantically called 911 and the paramedics carried him by ambulance to the nearest hospital.

When the physician finally spoke with Tony's parents, he told them that Tony had received an emergency tracheotomy, a surgical procedure in which a hole is made in the throat to allow an individual to breathe. After a computerized axial tomography (CAT) scan of the head had showed bleeding on one side of the brain, the doctor gave Tony phenobarbital to stop his seizures. The bleeding is what had caused his arm and leg to seem hemiplegic (floppy). Tony had received head trauma caused by an extremely rapid, forceful movement. His brain had started to swell, and the pressure inside his head was dangerously high (Box 15-9). A neurosurgeon put a drain in his head to control the pressure. An ophthalmologist confirmed that Tony had bleeding behind both eyes. The physician told his parents that usually the eyes heal with time but that sometimes shaken infants can become completely blind.

Tony's mother was stunned to hear that her child had been shaken. The police soon arrived to question her. She told them that her neighbor had cared for Tony that day. A background check at the police station revealed that the neighbor had been previously charged with shaking her own grandchild.

Infants who are violently shaken by adults sustain serious brain damage. **Shaken baby syndrome** causes the brain to hit the inside of the skull so hard that it bruises the brain or causes bleeding. The damage caused by shaking is proportional to the size of the child; larger children are harder to shake. To give a proportional size com-

BOX 15-9

Possible Injuries from Shaken Baby Syndrome

- Injuries inside the brain
- Brain swelling
- Diffuse nerve cell damage
- Shear injury
- Bleeding
- Injuries outside the brain
- Retinal bleeding (75% to 90%)
- Rib fractures
- Bruises
- Abdominal injuries

Adapted from Alexander RC, Smith WL: Shaken baby syndrome, *Inf Young Childr* 10:3, 1998.

parison, an adult shaking a child is similar to a 2000-lb gorilla shaking a grown man.[1] The exact number of shaken baby cases is not known because of a lack of information in general about child abuse cases. Subtle cases may go undetected. Many cases show that the children have suffered previous abuse. Men are responsible for 60% of these cases; 15% involve baby sitters of either sex. However, mothers may also be at high risk for shaking a baby too hard. Members of lower socioeconomic groups and younger adults are more likely to shake infants too hard, and the person shaking the infant has usually been previously abused. Most of the cases of shaken baby syndrome involve children less than 2 years of age; about 25% of these children die. Only a small percentage of infants who survive a severe shaking return to an almost normal condition after the abuse.[1] Children with disabilities are at greater risk for being abused and neglected; they are at least twice as likely to be mistreated as children without disabilities. Another major risk factor involves the number of caregivers an infant has. A normal child averages three caregivers besides the parents, but an infant with disabilities could have as many as 27.[7]

Children with shaken baby syndrome can have developmental delays, visual impairments, and neurological damage, which can result in mild learning problems or profound mental impairments. Brain injuries usually involve bleeding or lack of oxygen. Loss of muscle control or cerebral palsy is a common result (see Chapter 12). The eyes often heal within weeks or months if the retinas remain attached. If the brain is damaged in the area involving vision, visual impairments or cortical blindness can result. Because the eyes are not actually damaged in children with cortical blindness, they see images as if they were looking through several layers of plastic wrap.

The treatment of children with shaken baby syndrome involves monitoring for developmental delays to ensure that their development continues and is progressing at an age-appropriate level. Assessment of vision begins with clinical observations to determine whether the children require large objects or specific color contrasts to interact with their surroundings. As the children develop, they may need to learn the many skills used by individuals who are legally blind to improve independence (see "Vision Impairments" section in this chapter). When children have motor impairments or cerebral palsy caused by the brain damage from being shaken, a careful assessment of normal and abnormal movement patterns must be made. Parents, teachers, and caregivers can learn to inhibit or prevent abnormal movement patterns by handling the child properly, allowing more normal movements to develop (see Chapter 13).

CLINICAL *Pearl*

It is not unusual for children with cortical blindness to need corrective lenses or glasses because they are nearsighted or farsighted. A developmental optometrist can determine whether glasses would be beneficial.

Erb's Palsy

As her anxious father watched, Kira's mother Debbie laid the sleeping 7-day-old infant on the mat in the clinic. When Debbie unwrapped the receiving blanket, Kira began to awaken, gave a lusty yawn, and stretched. Her right arm reached out as her back arched and she awakened. The other arm lay lifelessly at her side, and her left shoulder fell back against the mat. As she finished stretching, her right arm flexed against her chest, bringing her fist under her chin; the left one still did not move.

Kira's birth had been difficult. Weighing more than 9 lb, she became lodged in the birth canal because her shoulders were too wide for Debbie's narrow pelvis. The left shoulder was stuck, which stretched the nerve roots of the brachial plexus (the nerves from the neck area of the spinal cord that supply the arm). As the OTR, Margaret, examined Kira's arm, it felt limp in her hands and had no muscle tone. Her left fingers did not reflexively curl around Margaret's finger as Margaret laid her finger across Kira's palm. Gentle pinches on her left arm showed that she felt nothing. The infant quietly watched Margaret as she moved Kira's arm through its ROM. No joint tightness or limitations were present. Margaret would have referred Kira for x-rays had she begun crying; Margaret knew that Kira would experience pain if she had an undetected fracture of the humerus or clavicle or any tissue tearing in the shoulder joint.

Erb's palsy occurs in about 2% of births.[20] During birth, stretching or tearing of the peripheral nerves that supply the arm and shoulder can cause Erb's palsy. Infants who are born feet first or are too large for the birth canal are at risk for this type of injury. Erb's palsy can generally be diagnosed in the first 24 hours after birth. The paralysis usually goes away untreated in a few days or weeks. During the first 2 weeks of life, 40% of infants recover; 35% worsen by the time they are 18 months old. By 18 months, gross and fine motor skill development are also delayed.[20] Infants who have not been treated in the early months of life develop elbow flexion contractures, and the affected arm is noticeably shorter than the other one.

Older children who have not had good early care or have not completely recovered may benefit from instruction in ADL skills. A residual strength assessment may indicate that a home strengthening program would be beneficial. Designing strengthening programs for children requires creativity and diversity to engage them and keep their interest long enough to yield benefits. Any home program must include attention to active ROM (AROM) and passive ROM (PROM). Until full and balanced muscle strength or full growth is attained, contracture development is possible.

After assessing Kira's function, the parents were taught ways in which to physically handle her at home to prevent further damage. The therapist showed them how to support her arm so that it would not flop away from her body as they picked her up. They were taught how to use ROM exercises with all of the left-arm joints, including the shoulder, to prevent stiffness and increase mobility. While Margaret was finishing Kira's assessment, Jill made a small sling to make holding Kira easier; soft cotton tubing was placed over her arm and pinned to her shirt, a design that worked well (Figure 15-5). The sling should not be used when Kira is sleeping because it may pose a risk for strangulation.

In addition to helping the parents hold Kira, the sling actually served another function. Because Kira felt almost no sensation in her affected arm, Jill positioned the sling so that her left hand rested under her chin next to her right hand. This allowed Kira to explore her hands and become accustomed to having a left hand. As children with brachial plexus injuries grow, they often ignore the affected hand and arm because they feel little or no physical sensation. The therapist instructed the parents to talk to Kira about her two hands and to hold them together to help her touch and feel them. Infants begin to explore their physical bodies by mouthing their hands. By placing an affected hand in the mouth, they begin to explore the shapes of their fingers with their tongues. This also helps the mouth to become accustomed to feeling new sensations. Margaret encouraged the parents to put Kira's hands in her mouth.

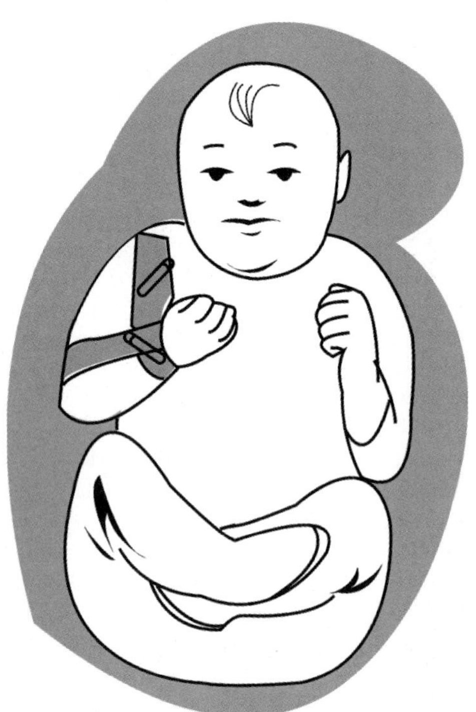

FIGURE 15-5 Sling for infant with Erb's palsy. It is made of a cotton stockinette and safety pins. It is pinned to the infant's shirt at the houlder in a position that keeps the affected hand near the infant's face.

As Kira grew older and stronger, Margaret checked for the return of muscle activity every week. The shoulder was the first to show tiny movements. By then Kira could hold up her head to play while on her tummy with a rolled towel under her shoulders. During her therapy sessions Kira was placed in supported, upper extremity weight-bearing positions to encourage the use of her returning strength and facilitate bone growth and improved bone density, reducing the chance of developing osteoporosis in the arm. By putting Kira in upper extremity weight-bearing positions, the practitioner hoped to avoid noticeable growth differences between the two arms as Kira got older. When her biceps became active, Kira was encouraged to bend her elbow in order to suck on her left fingers and hold them in her mouth independently. The parents were instructed to put bits of food Kira liked on her left hand while gently restraining her right arm to encourage her to bring her left hand to her mouth. As each muscle group began to show activity, new and appropriate weight-bearing and play activities were introduced to Kira's home program to encourage her to strengthen her left arm (see Chapter 13).

At 1 year of age, Kira had movement of muscles throughout her entire arm. The shoulder and elbow muscles were the strongest, but all of the muscle groups remained unbalanced and weaker than those in the right arm. At the age of 2 the parents enrolled Kira in a parent-toddler gymnastics class to encourage her to use her affected arm in bilateral activities. The parents were very knowledgeable by then and found an instructor who was willing to meet her needs. To make the classes even more productive, Margaret met with the teacher to discuss Kira's needs and limitations. Gymnastics was very motivating to her, and in the attempt to keep up with the class, her strength continued to improve. The gymnastic routines stretched her tight joints as well. Kira is now 6 years old; although her left arm is a little smaller than her right and she has mild weakness in her elbow and the muscles below it, her left arm weakness is not noticeable to those unaware of her problem. Because bone grows faster than muscle, Margaret continues to monitor Kira's progress every few months to ensure that no further contractures are developing and to adjust her home program.

Seizures

Ryan is a 6 year old diagnosed with right hemiplegic cerebral palsy and a seizure disorder. During a busy day in the clinic, Ryan and Jill, his COTA, were working on putting on a shirt. Ryan had just gotten tangled up in the shirt when he gave a high-pitched cry, his head went back, and he fell off his stool. Jill knew Ryan had a history of uncontrolled ***seizures*** *and knew right away what had happened (Box 15-10). She immediately removed the stool from the area so that he would not bump it with his flailing arms and legs. She turned his head to the side and tucked a cushion under it. She carefully watched his breathing and skin color, timed the seizure, and waited for it to subside. In a few minutes, Ryan began to regain consciousness but was groggy. Jill knew that the OT session for that day was over and that Ryan needed a nap. She documented the time of the seizure and informed the parents and physician about it.*

BOX 15-10

Caring for a Child Who Is Having a Seizure

If the child is flailing, make sure nothing is close by that could cause an injury if hit with his or her body.
Place something soft under the head.
Do not place anything in the mouth; it may damage the teeth.
Do not put a finger in the mouth. It will be bitten—hard.
Roll the child on the side to avoid inhaling vomit.
Call for emergency medical help if the child's skin begins to turn blue.

About 2% of the general population experience seizures of some type.[4] One fourth of those have ongoing repeated seizures or epilepsy. Epilepsy occurs more often in children than adults, and many children outgrow their

TABLE 15-5

Seizures

TYPE OF SEIZURE	CHARACTERISTICS
Grand mal seizures	Possible crying out or mood change before the seizure
	Loss of consciousness for 2-5 min
	Fall; shaking of arms, legs, and body
	Possible loss of control of bowels and bladder
	Afterward, possible deep sleep, headache, or muscle soreness
Absence (petit mal) seizures	Mostly in children
	Most likely to occur many times a day
	Brief loss of consciousness (10-30 s)
	Possible eye or muscle fluttering
	No loss of muscle tone
	Sudden cessation of activity; restarts a few seconds later
Febrile seizures	Mostly in children 3 mo-5 yr
	Most common in children with existing neurological problems
	In individuals with fever but no brain infection
	Varying duration; brief or up to 15 minutes
Infantile spasms (salaam seizures)	Seen in children under 3 yr with obvious brain damage
	A few seconds in duration but occur several times each day
	Sudden flexion of arms, extension of legs, and forward flexion of the trunk
Akinetic or drop seizures	Brief and sudden
	Complete loss of consciousness and muscle tone
	Danger of head injury because child will suddenly fall to the ground

Data from Berkow R, editor: *The Merck manual*, ed 17, Rahway, NJ, 1999, Merck.

seizures.[4] Most people with seizures have only one type, which is usually grand mal (Table 15-5). About a third have both grand mal and petit mal types.[4] Children with congenital brain damage, including those with cerebral palsy (particularly hemiplegia), spina bifida, and microcephaly, may have seizures.

SENSORY SYSTEM CONDITIONS

Sensory system conditions include those involving **vision impairments** (seeing impairments) and auditory system impairments **(hearing impairments).** Children may also have processing problems or deficits in other sensory systems, including the tactile (touch) system, the vestibular (balance and movement) system, and the proprioceptive (position sense) system (see Chapter 21).

Vision Impairments

Evan was born 3 weeks late and weighed 8½ lb. During the first 12 months he was a happy, busy baby and met all his developmental milestones on schedule. By his first birthday, he had shown no interest in walking. If placed on his feet with nothing to hold on to, Evan would scream from fear and drop down to his bottom immediately. His grandmother assumed that his ankles were weak and bought him ankle-high leather shoes. Evan still had no interest in walking. At 18 months he finally began walking, and at the same time the "terrible two's" began. His cheerful personality disappeared, and he was frustrated most of the time. He seemed happy only when left sitting quietly in his room playing with his construction toys. He hated playing on playground equipment; merry-go-rounds terrified him. Evan remained fearful and stubborn long past the "terrible two's" stage. At 4 years of age he still could climb stairs only one at a time. Temper tantrums were a daily event. He refused to join the neighborhood boys in gross motor play. He could not catch a ball but loved his big-wheel tricycle. He could not hop or even stand on one foot, and his running was clumsy. Interactions with other children his age always turned into confrontations. He still sat for hours playing with building toys. His mother had never noticed that one eye turned in slightly or that he always sat very close to the television to watch videos.

One day, when he was almost 5, Evan's vision was tested at his cooperative nursery. His mother was shocked to learn that he could not pass even a simple distance vision test. She immediately made an appointment with a developmental optometrist (a children's eye doctor) and was even more shocked to find out that Evan was legally blind. The doctor explained that he had used his normal intelligence to compensate for poor vision. Because he was born with poor eyesight, Evan did not know what normal vision was. He had started walking later than normal because when he stood up he could no longer see the floor. He could not catch a ball because he could not see it coming. He was frustrated all the time because he knew that he was not as capable as his friends of playing neighborhood games.

The day that Evan put on his first pair of glasses, he stood at the kitchen window and was amazed that he could see the garden. Almost five of the most precious years of gross motor and social development had been severely affected by his lack of clear vision. Those lost visual experiences continued to affect his development in later years. He always had trouble interpreting the emotional expressions on people's faces and understanding nonverbal language. Sports were never among his favorite activities and it took time for his gross motor skills to catch up to his chronological age, but he loved his first computer and excelled in school.

About 1 in 4000 children is legally blind. One in 20 has significant but less severe vision problems. Thirty percent of children with multiple handicaps have some sort of vision problem.[26] Because a large proportion of children who have handicaps also have vision problems, the vision of all children with special needs should be monitored closely (Box 15-11). Discovering vision problems early can alert practitioners and family members to the need for appropriate intervention. Glasses may ease developmental and motor delays if the problem is detected early. Children who are identified early as having a vision problem may be referred to special organizations for help (see Appendix B of this chapter).

CLINICAL *Pearl*

All children should have their eyes examined by age 3. A visual evoked response test that detects brain activity during visual stimulation can be administered for infants who are suspected of having vision problems.

BOX 15-11

Signs of Undetected Visual Problems

- Parents notice the child does not focus on his/her face or toys.
- The child holds objects close to his face.
- Gross and fine motor skills are poor.
- The child has crossed eyes or jerky eye movements.
- The child closes one eye to focus on an object.
- The child tilts his head while looking at specific objects.
- The older child performs poorly in school.

Data from Case-Smith J: *Occupational therapy for children*, ed 5, St Louis, 2005, Mosby.

Children who are legally blind may be able to see objects if they are close enough. People who are totally blind have no perception of light. Children with cortical blindness have physically functional eyes, but the visual processing part of their brain has been damaged in some way, resulting in images that look as if they are being seen through several layers of plastic wrap. Less severe vision problems must also be considered during therapy. Visual perception is the understanding of what is being seen. It can affect eye-hand coordination. Crossed eyes cause double vision because the image seen by each eye does not fuse into one image. A lazy eye can affect depth perception because only one eye at a time is working. Many of the more minor problems can be improved by performing eye exercises prescribed by a developmental optometrist. These minor problems are identified in 80% of children with reading problems.[18]

The treatment plan for children who have vision impairments depends on the severity of the impairment (Table 15-6). Legally blind children may be able to see quite well with corrective lenses; many of the interventions used for totally blind children also often benefit these children. If the impairment has been discovered after late infancy (i.e., after about 18 months), legally blind children may have problems with sensory integration, particularly with tactile defensiveness (being extremely sensitive to certain textures) and vestibular processing. It can be assumed that totally blind children will have these problems as well. Playing with various textured materials helps to normalize the feeling of different textures in the hands and reduce the aversion to touch.

Opportunities to experience movement are important. To help children who are blind tolerate movement, start with gross motor activities that involve little movement and increase the amount of movement slowly. Many playground toys can be adapted for this purpose by the practitioner. Blind infants and younger children do not know to reach out for objects in the environment. By tying toys to strollers, chairs, or cribs and teaching the infants to feel for objects with their hands, they learn to "look" for objects around them. Teaching children to look for objects in increasingly larger areas can enhance this skill.

Vision is a learned skill. Any residual vision a child has should be used. The more a child uses the visual pathways, the better the vision becomes. Treating a child in a darkened room with a spotlight on the activity helps the child see better by reducing other visual distractions. Emphasizing the visual contrasts between or among the surfaces of objects also increases the child's ability to see. For example, outlining a container's opening with a dark marker, sewing a bright ribbon around the neck and arm openings of a shirt, and reducing clutter on a desk surface are ways to improve contrast.

Children with total blindness often fill the void left by a lack of visual stimulation with other forms of sensory

TABLE 15-6

Suggestions for Working with Blind and Low-Vision Children

METHOD TO USE	PURPOSE OF THE APPROACH
Use the children's names.	Helps reduce the feeling of isolation; alerts children that they are included in what is going on around them
Explain what is going to occur.	Helps to create a relationship as well as helps them understand what is going on
Describe the room.	Helps children associate sounds, smells, and shapes
Walk the children to locations when possible.	Helps children develop space perception
Reduce extra noise.	Helps children identify sound clues
Use touch to introduce new things; brush objects on the back of the hand first.	Helps identify location and function of objects; helps develop independence and teach children that their actions have a cause and effect.
Explain new activities and surroundings.	Helps calm children who do not understand a new activity; helps them understand what is going to happen
Talk to the child, not about them.	Helps prevent you from underestimating children's ability to understand what is said to them
Never assume that children with vision impairments see something.	Helps prevent you from assuming that children can see and understand you

Data from Harrell L: *Touch the baby. Blind and visually impaired children as patients: helping them respond to care,* New York, 1984, American Foundation for the Blind.

CLINICAL *Pearl*

A fun and useful game for children with vision impairments is "flashlight hide-and-seek." Darken a room and "hide" toys around the room. Shine a flashlight on one of the toys, and ask a child to go get it. The team who finds the most toys wins. This is a great competitive game and a good way to stimulate children's visual pathways.

self-stimulation called *blindisms*. Blindisms are consistent, repetitive movements that are proportional to the degree of blindness. Blindisms can take the form of body rocking or head shaking, which stimulates the vestibular system, or eye poking, which stimulates the optic nerve. These activities can become socially unacceptable, so more accepted forms of stimulation should be taught to these children.

Hearing Impairments

Eighteen-month-old Sam was born with a genetic syndrome and was developmentally delayed. For that reason he was attending weekly OT sessions. The COTA, Jill, was always exhausted after his treatment sessions because he never followed directions and was hyperactive and distractible. His genetic syndrome made speech difficult, so the therapist was beginning to use age-appropriate sign language to help him identify objects and express his needs. His parents found that using sign language at home reduced his frustration.

Everyone working with Sam feared he could have mental retardation, yet when shown a complex age-appropriate game he could play it well. Sam's mother was frustrated because he was frequently stubborn. Sometimes he would withdraw to his room for hours and play alone; at other times he would scream in frustration as he tried to communicate his desires.

One day Sam was playing in the yard near the driveway when his teenage brother started his car. The car backfired loudly, and Sam's mother was so startled that she jumped and dropped what she was holding. She rushed to Sam, assuming that he was also frightened. She was shocked to find him playing in the sandbox, unaware that anything had happened. That night the family reflected on Sam's response and began to suspect that he had a hearing loss.

Sam was soon fitted with hearing aids for both ears. He began learning to understand spoken language extremely rapidly. His development quickly began to catch up to that of his peers. Because his genetic condition had limited his speech, Sam continued to learn sign language, but his family was amazed at how quickly he learned to understand what was said to him.

Sam had a considerable developmental delay because of his undetected lack of hearing. His progress needed to be continually followed to monitor and update his OT program. Although he seemed to have mental retardation when he was first brought to the clinic, once his hearing improved Sam began to perform more age-appropriate tasks with less frustration.

CLINICAL *Pearl*

It may be helpful to attach a child's hearing aids to the back of his or her shirt or blouse with clear fishing line and a safety pin to keep the child from losing them.

About 28 million Americans have a hearing loss, and about 2 million are profoundly deaf.[25] Few occupational therapists work with people who are deaf unless those individuals have other disabling conditions. Hearing loss accompanies many other developmental problems and can be caused by maternal infection during pregnancy. An undetected hearing loss causes developmental delays. Because a critical period exists for the acquisition of language skills, early detection of a hearing loss is very important.

Most OT services for individuals with hearing impairments address the related developmental delays. The first 4 years of life are the most important for language development. Impaired language skills affect all other areas

BOX 15-12

Possible Indications of Hearing Loss in Infants and Children

Newborn has no startle reflex when hearing a loud noise.
Three month old does not turn head toward toys that make noise.
Infant stops babbling around 6 months of age.
Infants between 8 and 12 months old do not turn toward sounds coming from behind.
Two year old does not use words.
Two year old does not respond to requests such as "show me the ball."
Three year old's speech is mostly unintelligible.
Three year old skips beginning consonants of words.
Three year old does not use two- or three-word sentences.
Three year old uses mostly vowels.
Child of any age speaks too loudly or too softly; voice has poor quality.
Child always sounds like a person who has a cold.

Adapted from Case-Smith J: *Occupational therapy for children*, ed 5, St Louis, 2005, Mosby.

of development, including social and environmental interactions and identification of objects. Early detection and treatment of hearing loss are essential for normal development in these areas.[17] A vigilant therapist is aware of and able to identify the signs of hearing loss in children (Box 15-12). Parents often begin to suspect that their infant has a hearing loss when s/he is not awakened by loud noises or does not turn toward a noisy toy. Older infants who do not hear well will not pay attention to simple commands or give feedback to questions. Any infant or child who is suspected of having a hearing loss should be referred for hearing testing. Younger infants can be given an evoked response audiometry test, which is a record of brain waves that occur in response to test sounds.

Several methods of communication can be used with the deaf. "Total communication" includes lip reading, using oral speech, signing, and using gestures (Box 15-13). In the book *Signing Exact English*, Tom Spradley states that "language is something that is caught, not taught."[12] American sign language (ASL) is a rich and unique language but is often difficult for hearing parents to learn. Tom Spradley recommends that deaf children "catch" ASL from deaf friends at school and "catch" English from parents by signing exact English (SEE), which is completely different from ASL.[12] Learning the seemingly foreign language of ASL is a huge task for new parents of deaf children. While they are learning it, the vocabulary available from SEE enables communication between parent and child. Parents who know their infants have hearing impairments can begin using SEE in the early months of life. This allows the infant to "catch" English from the parents, making the infant bilingual as ASL is learned. OT aids this process by using the signs taught in the home and introducing new signs for identifying new objects or activities during therapy. The signs chosen should relate to items or ideas the child understands, such as objects the child can see or touch or actions such as eating and dressing. Constant communication between the practitioner and parents is vital to prevent confusion and foster language growth for the child and everyone who is working with the child.

BOX 15-13

Suggestions for Total Communication

Face the child at eye level.
Be directly in front of the child so that your face and hands can be easily seen.
Get the child's attention.
Use good overhead lighting.
Speak in a normal tone of voice.
Say a word and sign it at the same time.
Use appropriate pauses.
Sit close to the child.
Keep instructions simple.
Be consistent.
Talk to the child. Deaf children need to "hear" the same amount of language as an average child.

Adapted from Case-Smith J: *Occupational therapy for children*, ed 5, St Louis, 2005, Mosby

Helping a child to accept using a new hearing aid may be difficult because of tactile defensiveness (a physical and tactile overreaction to objects). The head is often the most sensitive part of a child's body. The younger a child is fitted with hearing aids, the easier it is for the child to accept them. The aids must be thought of as clothing—necessary items that are put on each morning. An older child may need to start using new hearing aids during quiet times in speech-related activities. Hearing aids have recently undergone significant changes. Audiologists can now make more precise fittings to accommodate certain types of hearing loss. The aids are programmable and can be adjusted for factors such as background noise or voice levels. Because hearing aids are sensitive pieces of equipment, practitioners must be able to recognize their common malfunctions. Batteries often expire in approximately a week, depending on how much they are used. Batteries can also stop working because of corrosion or incorrect installation. An audible squeal coming from the hearing aid can be caused by a loose ear mold or incorrectly set switches. Ear molds often become plugged with wax, which block sound transmission.

GENERAL SENSORY DISORGANIZATION

In some conditions all of the child's sensory systems transmit information poorly, causing the perception of the world to be frightening. Changes in any one of the sensory systems affect development, making it difficult for children to make sense of gross or fine motor activities or even their surroundings. For example, one way that infants learn about their mothers is through the sense of touch; if the perception of touch is not normal, the infants may perceive touch as painful or frightening. If the vestibular system (which detects movement) is not responsive, infants may be happy only when they are moving or someone is holding them while walking. If several sensory systems are not functioning properly, behavior and development can be adversely affected as well as the relationship between infants and their parents or caregivers.

Fussy Baby

Leigh was born 3 weeks early. By the time she was 3 months of age, she would scream for hours at a time. Leigh was happy only when her mother Gayle held her and walked

around. No one but Gayle could calm her; she was tired and frustrated. After Gayle took Leigh to the pediatrician several times, the doctor concluded that nothing was seriously wrong; she just had colic. All of Leigh's tests were normal, and changing her formula and prescribing medication did nothing. The only assurance the doctor could give Gayle was that Leigh would grow out of the screaming episodes.

At 8 months Leigh still cried most of the time. She could be comforted only by being tucked into a fabric baby carrier on Gayle's shoulders. During a well-baby checkup, the doctor told Gayle that she and Leigh may not have bonded. Gayle adored Leigh and knew that bonding was not the problem.

Long after Leigh should have grown accustomed to eating solid food, it still made her gag. Leigh hated fuzzy toys and shivered when she touched one. The noise from squeaky toys made her jump and scream in fear. Leigh would become startled and scream when she was picked up from behind. She did not walk until she was 14 months old, and even then she fell more than normal. When she learned to run her gait was clumsy, and she did not like climbing on playground toys. Temper tantrums were Leigh's way of showing that she did not want to do something.

The tantrums continued well into her elementary-school years. Although Leigh did well in school, at home she was stubborn and refused to cooperate with anyone. When she became a teenager her grades fell sharply; she began to use drugs and alcohol and skip classes in school. Leigh was almost killed several times in car wrecks. In desperation her parents took her to a psychologist, who finally diagnosed attention deficit disorder (ADD) (see Box 15-7).

Infants can be fussy for many reasons, including maternal drug or alcohol abuse during pregnancy. (See sections titled "Effects of Cocaine Use" and "Fetal Alcohol Syndrome" in this chapter.) Infants with genetic problems such as Down or Angelman syndrome may have **general sensory disorganization.** Children with a history of ADD, ADHD, or learning disabilities were often fussy infants. Those with autism are often also fussy infants (Box 15-14). Families who already have members with learning disabilities, ADD, or ADHD (see Box 15-7) are more likely to have fussy infants.[4,8,9]

The formal assessment for a **fussy baby** who is between the ages of 4 and 18 months is the test of sensory functions in infants (TSFI). The TSFI measures infants' reactions to touch or movement and their use of vision to locate the source of touch or respond to objects in their visual field. The test also evaluates their ability to move the body while playing. The results indicate how well infants use sensation to understand their environments and bodies. The level of functioning in the tested areas can affect all areas of learning throughout life.

BOX 15-14

Signs of Autism or Pervasive Developmental Disorder

INFANTS

Stiffen when picked up or do not physically conform to the adult's body when held
Do not calm when held; may prefer to lay in the crib
Startle easily when touched or bed is bumped
Hate baths, dressing, or diaper changing
Have poor sucking ability or are hard to feed
Have poor muscle tone; bodies feel floppy
Do not have age-appropriate head control or age-appropriate ability to sit, crawl, or walk

CHILDREN

Seem unaware of surroundings
Do not make eye contact
Have general learning problems
Do not relate to others
Only eat certain food textures
Refuse to touch certain textures (e.g., mud and sand)
Have sleep problems such as difficulty getting to sleep or staying asleep
Are hyperactive
Are withdrawn, miserable, anxious, or afraid
Display repetitive behavior or speech patterns
Fixate on one object or body part
Compulsively touch smooth objects
Show fascination with lights
Flap arms when excited
Frequently jump, rock, or spin self or objects
Walk on tiptoes
Giggle or scream for no apparent reason
Eat strange substances (e.g., soil, paper, toothpaste, soap, rubber)

Infants who cry constantly, particularly past the age of 3 months, may have problems with sensory regulation (see Chapter 21) and not colic. Some characteristics of fussy babies are listed in Box 15-15. If these characteristics are recognized early, treatment can help the infant become calmer. The results from the TSFI give a good indication of the level at which treatment should begin, but observing infants who are less than 4 months old and questioning their parents is also helpful. In some cases, trial and error coupled with educated guessing is the only method to determine the way to calm an infant (Table 15-7).

Language Delay and Language Impairments

As Jill, the COTA, was taking a case history during Tommy's first visit to the clinic, a look that he gave her caused her to question the diagnosis. His mother Nancy had

BOX 15-15

Characteristics of a Fussy Baby

Sleep problems
Infant takes more than 20 minutes to fall asleep and wakes up several times a night.
Difficult to calm
Infant cannot calm self by putting hand in mouth or by looking at or listening to toys such as an infant mobile or music boxes.
Infant is difficult to calm, and mother spends many hours doing so during the day.
Feeding problems
Infant has no eating schedule.
Infant vomits, refuses food, or has other problems unrelated to allergies.
Overarousal
New types of stimulation or situations cause the infant to become overwhelmed and appear intense, wide eyed, or jittery.

Data from DeGangi GA, Greenspan SI: *Test of sensory functions in infants,* Los Angeles, 1989, Western Psychological Services.

BOX 15-16

Pervasive Developmental Disorder

A child is given the diagnosis of PDD when the precise diagnosis is not clear. A child given this diagnosis may not receive valuable treatments that are appropriate for the actual undiagnosed condition. Subgroups and related conditions that may not be diagnosed in a child who is identified as having PDD include the following:

- Angelman syndrome
- Apraxia
- Asperger syndrome
- Attention deficit disorder
- Fragile X syndrome
- Landau-Kleffner syndrome
- Language delay
- Prader-Willi syndrome
- Rett syndrome

Adapted from Autism Research Institute: 1998, *www.autism.org/; www.info.med.yale.edu/chldstudy/autism/PDDINFO.html; www.med.umich.edu/1LIBR/yourchild/autism.htm.*
PDD, Pervasive developmental disorder.

TABLE 15-7

Common Problems and Ideas to Try for Fussy Babies

REACTION (PROBLEM)	POSSIBLE CAUSE	TREATMENT
Pulls away from the nipple	Very sensitive to touch in mouth	Use infant's fingers to rub lips, working into mouth and to gums and tongue. Eventually begins using own finger or a cloth to do same procedure.
Flails arms and legs and screams	Frightened by movement	Swaddle infant with baby blanket.
Hates wind-up swing, stroller, or other moving things; has a strong startle reaction to movement during activities such as dressing; Scares self when moving independently	Frightened by movement	Swing the infant in "blanket hammock." Start with tiny swings and build up slowly to larger ones. Sit on a therapy ball, hold infant snuggly against chest facing you, and bounce or roll the ball slowly under hips. Start with tiny movements and increase slowly to larger ones.
Wants bottle but is not hungry	Reduced feeling of sensation in mouth	Offer pacifier or heavily textured toys for chewing. Touch gums and tongue with pressure using cloth-wrapped finger.
Seems frightened or gags when touching some things with hands or feet	Feels the sensation too strongly or not strongly enough	Play in large pans of various materials like rice or beans. First allow infant to watch play. Slowly encourage infant to touch items in pan. Goal is to get infant's entire body into pan.

just been told that he had pervasive developmental disorder (PDD) (Box 15-16), a condition that is very much like autism. Nancy stated that Tommy, who was almost 3 years old, did not speak at all (even in single words). He was frustrated all the time. He would throw a tantrum when a person interrupted anything he was doing. His only play activity was lining cars end to end. He would lie on his mother's bed for hours and trace the stripes on the sheets with his finger. He always had a toy car in each hand wherever he went. He preferred to wear only a diaper but would wear one particular sweat suit when his mother insisted. When a person other than a family member came near him, he would begin screaming. Nancy said her house was in a shambles because Tommy never stopped running, climbing, jumping, and throwing. The only thing that calmed him was country music videos; he insisted that the television volume be extremely loud all day. He refused to eat most foods and was very small for his age. Nancy could force him to eat yogurt or animal crackers in small portions.

When Tommy looked at Jill as she was taking the history, he seemed to be trying to communicate. His OT evaluation indicated that he had a severe sensory processing disorder and showed tactile defensiveness all over his body. His mouth was so sensitive to touch that he could not eat because he could not stand the feel of food in his mouth. He carried cars so that he did not have to touch other things. He liked the country music to be loud because it blocked out other sounds that confused him. He lined up cars and traced stripes to give himself some sort of visual organization and control. Tommy progressed using a combination of sensory integration therapy, speech therapy, horseback riding therapy, intervention from a preschool teacher who was knowledgeable about sensory processing problems, and a good home program. At the age of 6, his speech was labored and not always clear but improving. He also began to relate to people other than family members as his social skills improved.

Children develop language problems for many reasons. Some do eventually learn to talk, others may learn only a few sentences, and still others may never learn any words at all. Children are often nonverbal because of other developmental problems caused by genetic disorders or because of neurological conditions such as cerebral palsy. Major language delays seem to occur more often in boys, who often have several areas of sensory processing problems. Children with language delays can develop learning problems later.

Always be patient with children who do not talk or have trouble understanding speech. Most children use "prelanguage" before they start using speech as a form of communication: they point to an object to indicate that they want it or pull a parent to the cookie jar to indicate they want a cookie. Children who are physically unable to move their limbs may indicate their needs with a smile or an eye gaze. Language comprehension develops before a child's ability to express himself or herself in words.

CLINICAL *Pearl*

Adding spices to food often reduces oral defensiveness. Decreasing the texture of food by blending it or adding texture by including crisp cereal could make it easier for children to tolerate the food.

Other forms of communication can be used to reduce frustration while verbal skills are developing. Children with fair or good hand control can learn words in ASL to aid in communication. Using signs during therapy sessions and at home may be the most convenient way for children to communicate. Choose signs that have meaning in the child's everyday life. Another alternative for communication is a simple poster board to which pictures are taped of people and objects commonly encountered in a particular child's everyday life. For young children colored shapes of green and red could be substituted for the words "yes" and "no," which are important for indicating choices. A more portable communication system can be created by using a small photo album with single pictures on each page.

Facilitated communication

The administrators at Aaron's school recommended that he be placed in a class for children with multiple handicaps because he seemed to understand little of what was said to him and was nonverbal. Aaron's parents knew he could understand everything that was said to him. They insisted that he be placed with students his own age in a regular classroom. To avoid a potential lawsuit by the parents, the school administrators placed Aaron in a regular classroom and moved him up a grade each year. Aaron sat in class every day doing no written work but seeming to listen. When he was 13 years old, he learned to use facilitated communication with a tiny keyboard communicator to express his thoughts. He began relating amazing perceptions about his past, classmates, and family as well as current events. His teachers were finally able to administer tests and discovered that Aaron was reading and doing math at his appropriate grade level.

Facilitated communication is a method of assisting children with severe communication delays by emotionally and physically supporting the child while s/he tries to point. With the help of another person (a facilitator), children can point to letters, words, or pictures on a computer or some other communicative device.[5] Children using facilitated communication have the facilitator help them point a finger, control tremors, and slow down movements. The approach is controversial because the facilitators have the ability to influence the children, which could cause them to communicate the facilitators' thoughts instead of their own. Under the right circumstances and with a trustworthy facilitator, this method of communication is the only way in which some nonver-

BOX 15-17

Developmental Dyspraxia

Developmental dyspraxia is a disorder characterized by an impairment in the ability to plan and carry out sensory and motor tasks. Children with this problem may have trouble starting or stopping a movement. They may be able to do routine activities but have trouble with new ones. Sometimes the force of their movement is too strong or weak to be effective, or they may have trouble with balance, vision, or short-term memory, for example.

Adapted from http://www.ninds.nih.gov/disorders/dyspraxia/dyspraxia.htm.

bal but intelligent children can express themselves. It is used for some children with developmental dyspraxia (Box 15-17) or autism (see Box 15-14).

ENVIRONMENTALLY INDUCED AND ACQUIRED CONDITIONS

Environmentally induced and acquired conditions can develop before or after birth and are directly related to factors found in the environment. Contributing factors include drugs, toxic chemicals, allergens, and viruses.

Failure to Thrive

Nathan was born 5 weeks early and weighed only 3 lb. He was resuscitated twice in the delivery room because his breathing had stopped. He left the delivery room in an incubator, and on his arrival in the neonatal intensive care unit (NICU) he was put on a respirator. Because he was too weak to suckle, he was fed through the nose by a tube that went to his stomach (a nasogastric [NG] tube). Wires were taped to his chest to monitor his heartbeat and to his head to measure brain activity. When Nathan was born he was too ill to be held by anyone, including his parents. Four weeks after he was born Nathan had not grown in length and had gained only a few ounces. After consulting with the medical team, the parents agreed to remove Nathan from the respirator because they were told that he had no chance of survival. After all his equipment was removed, Nathan was handed to his mother for the first time. She rocked and sang to him in the NICU. Two months later, after his parents had spent every day touching, rocking, and talking to him, Nathan weighed 4½ lb and was able to go home with his parents.

BOX 15-18

Signs of Possible Failure to Thrive

Weight persistently less than 3% on growth charts
Weight less than 80% of ideal for height and age
Progressive loss of weight to below third percentile
Decrease in expected growth rate compared with previous pattern

Data from Berkow R, editor: *The Merck manual,* ed 17, Rahway, NJ, 1999, Merck.

Failure to thrive (FTT) can be a symptom of another acute or chronic condition or can be a condition in its own right. When FTT is a symptom of another condition, it is usually obvious by the age of 6 months. Weight gain is the most accurate indicator of an infant's nutritional status. Delayed growth in height usually indicates more severe and prolonged poor nutrition. A reduced head growth rate suggests severe malnutrition because the body provides energy to the brain before any other organ (Box 15-18).[4]

When infants fail to thrive but have no other physical conditions (i.e., they are physically normal at birth and have contracted no illnesses after birth), the problem is caused by neglect or a lack of appropriate stimulation. This type of FTT can occur at any age. Hospitalized infants or children may fail to thrive because of a lack of social stimulation; an infant of a parent who is depressed or has poor parenting skills may fail to thrive, as may a fussy baby whose mother is under significant stress or mentally ill.

Another group of infants who may experience FTT includes those who are premature and those with feeding problems caused by neurological or orthopedic factors (such as cleft palate) or poor sucking ability caused by cerebral palsy or sensory problems.

Children with FTT present with feeding issues such as poor suck-swallow-breathe, tactile sensitivity, delayed oral-motor skills, and decreased variability in their diets. OT personnel must evaluate and intervene in these areas. An important aspect of the treatment of FTT includes parental or caregiver training on feeding issues. Children trying to gain weight may require frequent high-calorie snacks throughout the day. Therefore, consultation with a nutritionist or dietitian may be warranted. Children with FTT may require intervention aimed at improving sensory modulation and development. Therapists must work closely with families and caregivers to help children with FTT.

Fetal Alcohol Syndrome

The use of alcohol during pregnancy is the most common cause of birth defects. **Fetal alcohol syndrome** (FAS) occurs in 2 to 6 births out of 1000.[26] The infants of chronic drinkers are the most severely affected. Alcohol consumption during pregnancy causes mental retardation, microencephaly, small facial features, poor development of the corpus callosum (see Table 15-4), and heart defects. Characteristic facial features include a turned-up nose and small jaw; a cleft lip or palate may also develop. Children with FAS may also experience an FTT and be fussy. One or more of these problems can result in a developmental delay. Hyperactivity can develop and adversely affect attention span and learning. Children with FAS are frequently hypotonic, have poor coordination, and may have sensory processing difficulties.[26] Infants or children with milder cases of FAS may be referred for OT treatment of hyperactivity caused by a sensory processing disorder. The infants may also have related learning problems as they grow older. Fine motor and visual perception skills must be assessed before the treatment intervention plan can be determined.

Effects of Cocaine Use

Cocaine use during pregnancy can produce malformations of the fetus's arms, legs, bowel, bladder, and genitals. It can cause poor blood flow to the placenta, causing a miscarriage or neurological damage to developing infants. Some may experience bleeding in the brain at birth. The infants of mothers who used cocaine near the time of birth will go through withdrawal after birth. Symptoms of withdrawal include vomiting and diarrhea, irritability, sweating, convulsions, and hyperventilation. Wrapping these infants tightly and feeding them frequently to calm them can help alleviate the symptoms of mild withdrawal.[4]

Infants who have been exposed to cocaine before birth can be unpredictable. A careful assessment of all developmental areas must be done to determine the areas needing intervention. Because of the possible neurological involvement, sensory integration evaluation and monitoring should be included. Treatment is highly individualized so that it can meet each child's unique needs. Long-term follow-up clarifies whether the child will develop learning disabilities or emotional/behavioral difficulties.

Human Immunodeficiency Virus

The human immunodeficiency virus (HIV) causes the immune system to break down, resulting in many different problems as early as the first 1 or 2 years of life. Early symptoms may be FTT, fever, and diarrhea. Half of all HIV-infected infants develop full-blown **acquired immunodeficiency syndrome** (AIDS) by the age of 3.[4] A woman infected with HIV can pass the virus on to her infant during pregnancy, birth, or breast-feeding. Infants born to women who are infected before or during pregnancy and receive no medical treatment have about one chance in four of being born with the HIV infection. Medical treatment with zidovudine (AZT) during pregnancy and labor may reduce the risk of infant infection to about 1 in 12. HIV-infected mothers *must not* breast-feed. Treating infants with AZT for the first several weeks of life can reduce but not prevent the risk of infection.[4]

Children with AIDS may have delayed motor or cognitive development. They may not meet developmental milestones or attain certain intellectual skills and may develop microencephaly.[15] The loss of social skills and language occurs in about 20% of children with AIDS. Paralysis, tremors, spasticity, and balance problems can also develop; major organ systems are damaged. Half of the infants born with AIDS develop pneumonia by 15 months, a common cause of death.[4] Children with AIDS-related

BOX 15-19

Precautions for Working with Children Who Have Infectious Diseases

Wear gloves when coming into contact with blood or secretions.
Mix 1 oz of bleach with 10 oz of water and disinfect surfaces.
Bandage all cuts and sores.
Wash hands and/or body parts immediately after contact with blood.
Use sharp instruments only when necessary.

Adapted from the Centers for Disease Control: http://www.cdc.gov/mmwr/preview/mmwrhtml/00001583.htm.

BOX 15-20

Transmission of Human Immunodeficiency Virus

HIV does not survive well in the environment. Simply drying a surface contaminated with HIV kills 90% to 99% of the virus. HIV exists in different concentrations in the blood, semen, vaginal fluid, breast milk, saliva, and tears. Infection occurs when blood or body secretions that could contain visible blood, such as urine, vomit, or feces, come into contact with an open wound or mucous membranes, which are found inside the mouth, nose, eyes, vagina, and rectum. The concentration of the virus in saliva, sweat, and tears is low, and no case of HIV infection through these fluids has been documented.

Adapted from the Centers for Disease Control: http://www.niaid.nih.gov/newsroom/simple/background.htm#A.

CLINICAL *Pearl*

Monitoring for developmental delays is one of the main goals of OT for children with AIDS. Because their mothers are frequently ill as well, the occupational therapist coordinates care for the mothers and their children.

complex (ARC) are infected with HIV and have some symptoms but have not had serious infections.[4] In the United States, 2% of all individuals with AIDS are children or adolescents. In 90% of pediatric AIDS cases, children have gotten the virus at birth from their mother. From 1993 to 1996, 4325 children had AIDS or an HIV infection that was acquired at birth. By 1996 the Centers for Disease Control (CDC) reported 7476 cases of AIDS in children (Boxes 15-19 and 15-20).[26]

Latex Allergy

Children with spina bifida, those who need frequent surgery, and those who must use catheters for congenital urinary tract problems are the most likely ones to become allergic to latex. Between 18% and 40% of the mentioned children will develop sensitivity to latex.[22] However, anyone who has frequent exposure to latex through work or surgery can develop an allergy. A reaction can occur after breathing latex dust from an open package or contact between latex and skin, mucous membranes, open lesions, or blood. Coming into contact with a person or object that has just been in contact with latex can cause a reaction. Symptoms include watery eyes, wheezing, hives, rash, and swelling. Severe reactions can result in anaphylaxis, a system-wide body reaction that affects heart rate and the ability to breathe; it can be fatal.[22]

The number of observed children who have or develop an allergy to latex is increasing for several reasons. Universal precautions require the use of latex gloves to prevent the spread of infection; latex is also used in many health care products, such as tape, bottle nipples, and catheters.

To avoid developing a latex allergy, try to use it as little as possible. During play activities, substitute Mylar balloons for latex balloons. Vinyl gloves can be used instead of latex gloves. Check the labels of tapes or any other substances that may contain rubber products. During assessments always ask parents or caregivers about possible allergies, which not only makes the rehabilitation team aware of possible problems but also teaches the parents about symptoms to be aware of should an allergy develop.

CLINICAL *Pearl*

Children who are allergic to latex may also be allergic to bananas, avocados, and kiwi fruit because they are all from the same plant family as latex. Being around latex and consuming any of these fruits may heighten the reaction.

Lead Poisoning

It is estimated that about 4 million children in the United States have high enough lead levels to slow their development.[13] Although many environmental toxins exist, lead is the one that most commonly affects children. Children living in older homes have a greater risk of exposure to peeling paint containing lead (which children sometimes eat) and lead used in plumbing. Lead is no longer used in these materials; however, children can eat or breathe lead from contaminated air, food, water, and soil as well. Some industries, such as battery manufacturing, produce higher air and dust levels of lead than other industries. Parents working in these industries can carry lead home from work on their clothing. Mothers with high lead levels can pass it on to their infants during gestation. Mild toxicity produces muscle aches and fatigue, and moderate levels cause fatigue, headaches, cramping, vomiting, and weight loss. High toxicity levels cause mental retardation, behavior problems, seizures, and sometimes death. Even low toxicity levels can affect intelligence and behavior.[26]

Allergies to Food and Chemicals

The use of art supplies, construction materials, and food during pediatric therapy should be carefully assessed so that children's developing bodies are not unnecessarily exposed to toxic chemicals, toxic materials, and allergy-

BOX 15-21

Most Common Foods Associated with Food Allergies

- Wheat
- Soy
- Corn
- Eggs
- Peanuts
- Milk
- Citrus foods
- Tree nuts
- Shellfish

Adapted from University of Maryland Medicine: http://www.umm.edu/pediatric-info/food.htm.

CLINICAL *Pearl*

Styrofoam packing peanuts are fun to play with but can emit formaldehyde fumes or be accidentally eaten. Never allow children to play in a pile so large that they could immerse their bodies or heads. Styrofoam peanuts are very lightweight and can be easily inhaled and block breathing.

producing food. Always check with parents or guardians about their children's food allergies before using food for an art project or feeding therapy (Box 15-21). Toxic chemical fumes or materials may cause asthma, skin irritation, anaphylaxis, or other unseen damage that can accumulate over time. Always ensure that the materials used in therapy are nontoxic. Avoid using latex products when another substitute is available.

ROLE OF THE CERTIFIED OCCUPATIONAL THERAPY ASSISTANT AND REGISTERED OCCUPATIONAL THERAPIST IN ASSESSMENT AND INTERVENTION

Greg has been a COTA for 10 years. He is also a certified riding instructor for the North American Riding for the Handicapped Association (NARHA), which has a therapeutic riding program in his town. He has ridden all his life and shows horses as often as he can. In his therapeutic riding sessions, he uses horses to treat children with sensory processing problems and motor delays. By analyzing all of the activities involved in caring for and riding horses, Greg has developed a comprehensive treatment program for each child he treats. Margaret, the OTR, is not certified by NARHA. She has her own horse and loves to ride. Margaret has a contract with the riding program to supervise Greg monthly.*

Six-year-old Emily was referred to the riding program by her pediatrician. The doctor's referral indicated that he suspected Emily had ADD (see Box 15-6), sensory processing problems, and a possible learning disability. Based on the pediatrician's referral, Margaret asked Greg to administer the Miller Preschool Assessment (see Appendix A of this chapter). Margaret and Greg will discuss the results of the test during their next monthly meeting. Together they will write a plan of care for Greg to follow. Greg will use the plan to choose the activities that Emily will be engaged in for her horseback riding therapy sessions.

*NARHA provides information on and sets standards for therapeutic riding and certifies therapists as horseback riding instructors (see Appendix B of this chapter).

An OTR must supervise a COTA in any work setting where a COTA provides OT services to infants and children. The level of supervision required depends on many variables. The OTR is responsible for the provision of OT services (which includes the assessment and intervention processes) while working with children and adolescents with physical dysfunctions. The COTA assists the OTR in data collection and evaluation during the assessment process using standardized or simply structured tests and interviews.

The COTA directly provides services for children with physical dysfunctions. The OT practitioners work together to develop a plan of care. While providing services to a child or adolescent, the COTA follows a documented care plan under the supervision of the OTR. The level of supervision depends on the COTA's level of experience and service competency.

SUMMARY

Working with children can be a rewarding experience for OT practitioners. Meeting the needs of children is a complex task. Not only must practitioners meet the needs of their clients but they must also educate the family and caregivers. The role of OT practitioners takes on an added dimension when they join a school's educational team to treat school-age children. Knowing the common characteristics of children's conditions helps practitioners provide a focus for the initial assessment and treatment plan. These two components reveal that although the various conditions have common characteristics, the needs of children and their families are unique and must be addressed.

References

1. Alexander RC, Smith WL: Shaken baby syndrome, *Inf Young Childr* 10:1, 1998.
2. Arthritis Foundation: *www.arthritis.org*.
3. Bell DS, Bell KM, Cheney PR, et al: Primary juvenile fibromyalgia syndrome and chronic fatigue syndrome in adolescents, *Clin Infect Dis* 18:21, 1994.
4. Berkow R, editor: *The Merck manual*, ed 17, Rahway, NJ, 1999, Merck. http://www.merck.com/mrkshared/mmanual/home.jsp.
5. Biklen D: Questions and answers about facilitated communication, *Facil Comm Dig* 2:10, 1993.
6. Case-Smith J: *Occupational therapy for children*, ed 5, St Louis, 2005, Mosby.
7. Crosse SB, Kaye E, Ratnofsky AC: *Report on the maltreatment of children with disabilities*, National Center on Child Abuse and Neglect, Washington, DC, 1993, US Department of Health and Human Services.
8. DeGangi GA, Greenspan SI: *Test of sensory functions in infants*, Los Angeles, 1990, Western Psychological Services.

9. Edelson SM: *Angelman syndrome*, Angelman Syndrome Foundation, 1995, Aurora, Ill, http://www.autism.org/angel.html.
10. Facts About Angelman Syndrome: http://www.margaretkay.com/Angelman_Syndrome.htm.
11. Fragile-X Research Foundation: www.fraxa.org
12. Gustason G, Zawolkow E, Pfetzing D, Lopez L: *Signing exact English*, Los Alamitos, Calif, 1994, Modern Signs Press.
13. Haan MN, Gerson M, Zishka BA: Identification of children at risk for lead poisoning: an evaluation of routine pediatric blood lead screening in an HMO-insured population, *Am Acad Pediatr* 97:84, 1996.
14. International Rett Syndrome Association: http://www.rettsyndrome.org/main/overview.htm.
15. National Institute of Allergy and Infectious Diseases: http://www.niaid.nih.gov/newsroom/simple/background.htm#A.
16. National Institute of Neurological Disorders and Stroke: www.ninds.nih.gov.
17. Neistadt ME, Crepeau EB, editors: *Willard and Spackman's occupational therapy*, ed 10, 2003, Philadelphia, JB Lippincott–Raven.
18. Optometrists Network: http://www.children-special-needs.org/vision_therapy/what_is_vision_therapy.html.
19. Prader-Willi Syndrome Association: www.pwsausa.org.
20. Pronsati MP: Erb's palsy, *Adv Occup Ther* 7:19, 1991.
21. Pueschel SM: *A parent's guide to Down syndrome: toward a brighter future*, ed 2, Baltimore, 2001, PH Brookes Publishing.
22. Romanczuk A: Latex use with infants and children: it can cause problems, *Matern Child Nurs* 18:208, 1993.
23. Shriners Hospitals for Children: http://www.shrinershq.org/patientedu/arthrogryposis.html.
24. St Amand RP: *What your doctor may not tell you about pediatric fibromyalgia*, New York, 2002, Warner Books.
25. Stancliff B: Silent services: treating deaf clients, *OT Practice* 3:27, 1998.
26. Wallace HM, Biehl RF, MacQueen JC, Blackman JA, editors: *Mosby's resource guide to children with disabilities and chronic illness*, St Louis, 1997, Mosby.
27. Your Orthopedic Connection, American Academy of Orthopedic Surgeons: http://orthoinfo.aaos.org/fact/thr_report.cfm?Thread_ID=247&topcategory=Spine.

Recommended Reading

American Occupational Therapy Association: *Rheumatoid arthritis: caring for your hands*, 1995, Bethesda, Md, The Association.

Bruni M: *Fine motor skills in children with Down syndrome*, Bethesda, Md, 1998, Woodbine House.

Corn KN: *Idiopathic scoliosis: potential interaction of neurological variables as causation*, Master's thesis, Modesto, Calif, 1998, University of the Pacific.

Dunn MK: *Pre-sign language skills*, San Antonio, Texas, 1982, Therapy Skill Builders.

Erhardt RP: *Developmental visual dysfunction*, San Antonio, Texas, 1993, Therapy Skill Builders.

Frick SM, Frick R, Oetter P, Richter EW: *Out of the mouths of babes*, San Antonio, Texas, 1998, The Psychological Corporation, USA.

Gross MA: *The ADD brain: diagnosis, treatment and science of attention deficit disorder (ADD/ADHD) in adults, teenagers and children*, 1997, Nova Science Publishers.

Puttkammer CH: *Working with substance exposed children*, San Antonio, Texas, 1994, Therapy Skill Builders.

Williams MS, Shellenberger S: *How does your engine run?* Albuquerque, NM, 1994, Therapy Works.

REVIEW *Questions*

1. Explain the difference between a central and a peripheral nervous system condition.
2. What are the three types of juvenile rheumatoid arthritis? Describe them. Which functional limitations do each cause?
3. Name the four spine conditions discussed in this chapter. In what way does each affect the functional performance of the child?
4. Describe the reason a COTA must have a good understanding of the symptoms and signs of a child's condition before doing the initial assessment. In what way does this aid in treatment?
5. Describe two genetic syndromes. Explain the ways they affect the child's ADL skills.
6. Using information you have learned about the sensory systems, explain why it is so important to treat sensory system problems early.
7. What are the differences among legal blindness, total blindness, and cortical blindness? In what ways are they the same? In what ways can you make learning easier for a child who has vision impairments?
8. In what ways does an undetected hearing loss affect a child's early development?
9. Name three avoidable environmental factors that affect infants either before or after birth. Explain how these factors can cause developmental delays.
10. Describe arthrogryposis. In what ways can it affect the child's daily functioning?
11. Why is it important to watch for signs of abuse in children who are disabled?
12. What is total communication? In what ways could it be used during a therapy session?

SUGGESTED *Activities*

1. Visit a classroom for children who have special needs and observe the children at work. During your visit, observe and keep a list of the way each child's condition affects the ability to do schoolwork. Later, make a list of suggestions you think might improve each child's ability to do schoolwork.
2. Spend some time at an outpatient clinic observing the children receiving OT services. Make a list of characteristics observed in individual children. Later, try to identify each child's possible condition or which of the systems is/are involved.
3. Spend some time observing a child with a disability playing. Write down ways that the child's specific condition affects the ability to play.
4. Interview a COTA who works in a school system. Ask in what ways the COTA's knowledge of a student's condition helps decide what information to obtain during the evaluation and intervention processes. Make notes during your visit; later, come up with ideas of your own to add to the list.
5. Talk with a family who has a child with a disability. Before the interview, use the knowledge you have gained from this chapter to make a list of the way(s) you would expect the child's disability to affect the family. During the interview, make notes about the family's comments. Later, compare your initial list with the family's comments. How accurate were your expectations?

CHAPTER 15 APPENDIX A

Commonly Used Pediatric Assessments

TEST NAME	AREAS TESTED	AGES
Alberta Infant Motor Scale (AIMS)	*Motor:* Assesses postural control in supine, prone, sitting, and standing positions	0-18 mo
Ayres Clinical Observations	*Sensory and motor:* Assesses postural and motor control and planning and sensory reactions	3-18 yr
Bayley Scales of Infant Development II	*Developmental:* Assesses mental, motor, and behavioral development	0-42 mo
Bruininks-Oseretsky Test of Motor Proficiency	*Developmental:* Assesses gross and fine motor proficiency and upper limb coordination	$4^1/_2$-$14^1/_2$ yr
The Carolina Curriculum for Infants and Toddlers with Special Needs	*Behavioral:* Assesses mental, communication, self-help, and gross and fine motor skills	0-36 yr
DeGangi-Berk Test of Sensory Integration (TSI)	*Sensory:* Assesses underlying sensorimotor mechanisms; postural control, bilateral motor integration, reflex integration	3-5 yr
Denver II	*Developmental:* Detects possible developmental problems in gross and fine motor, language, and personal social skills	2 wk-6 yr
Developmental Test of Visual-Motor Integration (VMI)	*Developmental:* Assesses visual-motor skills	2-15 yr
Erhardt Developmental Prehension Assessment	*Developmental:* Describes details of grip patterns, involuntary hand and arm patterns, early voluntary hand and arm movements, and prewriting skills	0-15 mo
Erhardt Developmental Vision Assessment	*Developmental:* Assesses involuntary and voluntary eye control	0-teens
Functional Independence Measure for Children (Wee-FIM)	*Functional:* Measures severity of disability; assesses self-care, mobility, gross and fine motor, language, and social skills	6 mo-7 yr
Gesell Preschool Assessment	*Developmental:* Assesses motor, adaptive, language, and personal social skills	$2^1/_2$-6 yr
Hawaii Early Learning Profile (HELP)	*Behavioral:* Determines developmental level; assesses cognitive, language, gross and fine motor, social, and self-help skills	0-3 yr
Miller Assessment of Preschoolers (MAP)	*Developmental:* Identifies children with mild to moderate delays; assesses sensorimotor and cognitive skills	33-68 mo
National Children's Medical Center Prevocational Capabilities Assessment	*Developmental and sensorimotor:* Assesses cognition, gross and fine motor function, and sensory processing	12-19 yr
Peabody Developmental Motor Scales	*Developmental:* Assesses reflexes and gross and fine motor skills	0-83 mo
Sensory Integration and Praxis Test (SIPT)	*Sensorimotor:* Assesses general sensory organization, coordination of right and left, motor planning, visual-motor coordination, and perception	4-8 yr

CHAPTER 15 APPENDIX A—cont'd

Commonly Used Pediatric Assessments

TEST NAME	AREAS TESTED	AGES
Test of Sensory Functions in Infants (TSFI)	*Sensory:* Assesses tactile and deep pressure functions, visual-tactile integration, adaptive motor function, oculomotor function, and reactivity to vestibular stimulation	4-18 mo
Test of Visual-Perceptual Skills (TVPS) (nonmotor)	*Developmental:* Assesses visual form discrimination, memory, spatial relationships, form constancy, sequencing, and figure-ground discrimination.	4-13 yr
Transdisciplinary Play-Based Assessment	*Developmental:* Determines developmental skill level, learning style, and interaction through structured play; assesses cognitive, communication; sensorimotor, and social skills.	6 mo-6 yr

Adapted from Rothstein JM, Roy SH, Wolf SL: *The rehabilitation specialist's handbook,* Philadelphia, 1998, FA Davis.

CHAPTER 15 APPENDIX B

Organizations and Websites

Attention Deficit Disorder Association
PO Box 543
Pottstown, PA 19464
(484) 945-2101
Fax: (610) 970-7520

The Agenesis of the Corpus Callosum (ACC) Network
5749 Merrill Hall, Room 18
University of Maine
Orono, ME 04469-5749
(207) 581-3159
Fax: (207) 581-3120
Website: *http://www.kumc.edu/gec/support/agenesis.html*

American Foundation for the Blind (AFB)
AFB Headquarters
15 Penn Plaza, Suite 300
New York, NY 10001
(212) 502-7600
Fax: (212) 502-7777
e-mail: *afbinfo@afb.net*
Website: *http://www.afb.org/*

Angelman's Syndrome Foundation
3015 East New York Street
Suite A2265
Aurora, IL 60504
(800) 432-6435 or (630) 978-4245
e-mail: *info@angelman.org*
Website: *http://www.angelman.org/*

The Arc of the United States
1010 Wayne Avenue, Suite 650
Silver Spring, MD 20910
(301) 565-3842
Fax: (301) 565-3843 or (301) 565-5342
Website: *http://thearc.org*

Arthritis Foundation
1330 West Peachtree Street
Atlanta, GA 30309
(404) 872-7100
Arthritis Answers:
(800) 283-7800
Website: *http://www.arthritis.org/*

Autism Research Institute
4182 Adams Avenue
San Diego, CA 92156
Fax: (619) 563-6840
Website: *http://www.autism.com/ari*

Autism Society of America
7910 Woodmont Avenue, Suite 300
Bethesda, MD 20814
(800) 328-8476
Website: *http://www.autism-society.org/*

Centers for Disease Control (CDC): CDC National Prevention Information Network
PO Box 6003
Rockville, MD 20849-6003
e-mail: *info@cdcnpin.org*
(800) 458-5231
(301) 562-1098 International
(800) 243-7012 TTY
CDC National AIDS Hotline
(800) 342-AIDS (2437)
Spanish: (800) 344-SIDA (7432)
Deaf: (800) 243-7889
Website: *http://www.cdcnpin.org/scripts/hiv/index.asp*

Children and Adults with Attention-Deficit/ Hyperactivity Disorder (CHADD)
8181 Professional Place, Suite 150
Landover, MD 20785
(800) 233 4050
Website: *http://www.chadd.org/*

Epilepsy Foundation
4351 Garden City Drive
Landover, MD 20785
(800) 332-1000
Website: *http://www.efa.org/*

Facilitated Communication Institute
370 Huntington Hall
Syracuse University
Syracuse, NY 13244-2340
(315) 443-9657
Fax: (315) 443-2274
Website: *http://soeweb.syr.edu/thefci/*

CHAPTER 15 APPENDIX B—cont'd

Organizations and Websites

Foundation for Blind Children
1235 East Harmont Drive
Phoenix, AZ 85020
http://www.the-fbc.org

International Rett Syndrome Association
9121 Piscataway Road, Suite 2-B
Clinton, MD 20735
(301) 856-3334
(800) 818-RETT
Fax: (301) 856-3336
e-mail: *irsa@rettsyndrome.org*
Website: *http://www.rettsyndrome.org/*

Muscular Dystrophy Association
3300 East Sunrise Drive
Tucson, AZ 85718
(800) 572-1717
Website: *http://www.mdausa.org/*

The National Brachial Plexus/Erb's Palsy Association, Inc
PO Box 23
Larsen, WI 54947
(920) 836-2151
Website: *http://www.nbpepa.org/*

National Council on Disability
1331 F Street, NW, Suite 850
Washington, DC 20004
(202) 272-2004 (voice)
Fax: (202) 272-2022
TTY: (202) 272-2074
e-mail: *mquigley@ncd.gov*
Website: *http://www.ncd.gov/*

National Down Syndrome Congress
1370 Center Drive, Suite 102
Atlanta, GA 30338
(800) 232-6372
e-mail: *info@ndsccenter.org*
Website: *http://www.ndsccenter.org/*

National Down Syndrome Society
666 Broadway
New York, NY 10012
(800) 221-4602
e-mail: *info@ndss.org*
Website: *http://www.ndss.org/*

National Fragile X Foundation
PO Box 190488
San Francisco, CA 94159
(800) 688-8765
(925) 938-9300
Website: *http://www.fragilex.org/home.htm*

National Information Center for Children and Youth with Disabilities
PO Box 1492
Washington, DC 20013-1492
(800) 695-0285 (voice/TT)
(202) 884-8200 (voice/TT)
(800) 999-5599
Website: *http://www.kidsource.com/NICHCY/index.html*

National Institute on Deafness and Other Communication Disorders
National Institutes of Health
31 Center Drive, MSC 2320
Bethesda, MD 20892-2320
(800) 241-1044
(800) 241-1055 TTY
e-mail: *nidcdinfo@nidcd.nih.gov*
Website: *http://www.nidcd.nih.gov/*

National Organization for Rare Disorders, Inc
55 Kenosia Avenue
PO Box 1968
Danbury, CT 06813-1968
(203) 744-0100
(800) 999-6673 (voice)
(203) 797-9590 (TDD)
e-mail: *orphan@rarediseases.org*
Website: *http://www.rarediseases.org/*

National Tuberous Sclerosis Alliance
801 Roeder Road
Suite 750
Silver Spring, MD 20910
(800) 225-6872
Fax: (301) 562-9870
Website: *http://www.tsalliance.org*

CHAPTER 15 APPENDIX B—cont'd

Organizations and Websites

North American Riding for the Handicapped Association (NARHA)
PO Box 33150
Denver, CO 80233
(800) 369-RIDE (7433)
(303) 452-1212
Fax: (303) 252-4610
e-mail: *NARHA@NARHA.ORG*
Website: *http://www.NARHA.org/*

The Prader-Willi Syndrome Association (USA)
5700 Midnight Pass Road
Sarasota, FL 34242
(800) 926-4797
(941) 312-0400
Fax: (941) 312-0142
Website: *http://www.pwsausa.org*

Spina Bifida Association of America
4590 MacArthur Boulevard, NW
Suite 250
Washington, DC 20007
(800) 621-3141
(202) 944-3285
e-mail: *sbaa@sbaa.org*
Website: *http://www.sbaa.org*

United Cerebral Palsy Association
1660 L Street, NW
Suite 700
Washington, DC 20036
(800) 872-5827
(202) 776-0406
202-973-7197 TTY
Website: *http://www.ucp.org/*

16

Therapeutic Media: Activity with Purpose

NADINE KUZYK HANNER
ANGELA CHINNERS MARSH
RANDI CARLSON NEIDEFFER

CHAPTER *Objectives*

After studying this chapter, the reader will be able to accomplish the following:

- Describe considerations necessary when selecting media
- Describe the role of the certified occupational therapy assistant in choosing therapeutic media
- Select developmentally appropriate therapeutic media for children in different age groups
- Describe gradation of therapeutic activities based on client factors and activity demands
- Explain the importance of the impact of contextual (i.e., cultural, physical, social, personal, spiritual, temporal, and virtual) conditions when choosing therapeutic media

KEY TERMS

Media
Method
Therapeutic media
Grading
Activity demands
Client factors
Grading activities
Adapting activities
Collaboration
Service competency
Cultural considerations

CHAPTER OUTLINE

This chapter introduces the entry-level certified occupational therapy assistant (COTA) to the definition, background, and application of therapeutic media.

Media, the plural of medium, is defined as "an intervening substance through which something else is transmitted or carried on; an agency by which something is accomplished, conveyed, or transferred."[1] **Method** refers to "a means or manner of procedure, especially a regular and systematic way of accomplishing something."[1]

To further clarify these terms in the context of the occupational therapy (OT) profession, a purposeful activity is chosen to produce desired outcomes for a client and carried out with the use of selected media. The media and method are chosen for their therapeutic value and individualized for each child's specific needs.

BACKGROUND AND RATIONALE OF THERAPEUTIC MEDIA

In the early days of OT, arts and crafts were the primary therapeutic activities used by OT practitioners. As social and economic times changed and technology rapidly grew, the repertoire of media used in the OT profession expanded and evolved to meet the changing needs of clients. However, craft activities continue to be used in various practice settings and are of particular value in the treatment of the pediatric population. Children can acquire and practice the skills necessary for them to function in their occupations through the use of crafts as **therapeutic media.** Furthermore, engagement in crafts is typically an occupation of childhood. This chapter describes the selection and use of traditional and nontraditional therapeutic media as an intervention for children.

SELECTION OF THERAPEUTIC MEDIA

COTAs use clinical reasoning skills when choosing therapeutic media for their clients. Specifically, activities that are meaningful and motivating to clients and address their goals are deemed therapeutic. The COTA considers the client's interests, therapy goals, client factors, performance skills, performance patterns, and contexts. For example, the COTA considers and respects the beliefs and traditions of the child's culture when planning activities. **Grading** of the media and **activity demands** are important aspects to be reviewed before selecting media.

Activities carried out in group settings must be easily **graded** and adapted to meet the "just right" challenge for individuals. The following discussion will help facilitate the thought process necessary in successful media selection for intervention planning and implementation.

CLINICAL *Pearl*

As defined by the Occupational Therapy Practice Framework, activity demands are "the aspects of an activity which include the objects used and their properties, space demands, social demands, sequencing and timing, required actions, required body functions, and required body structures needed to carry out the activity."[2]

Occupations

The following questions may help the OT practitioner select meaningful, motivating, and age-appropriate media for children and adolescents:

1. Are the media relevant to the client's age and occupational role (e.g., student, sibling, worker)?
2. Are the media related to the client's current interests and hobbies, or can they possibly spark his or her interest to pursue a new leisure activity (e.g., drawing, computers, photography, needlecraft)?
3. Has the child or adolescent experience with the media?

Goals

The following questions may help the OT practitioner select activities and media based on the client's goals:

1. What specific goals will be addressed?
2. How will the activity (media and method) facilitate the attainment of the client's goals?
3. Can the chosen media facilitate the desired outcomes?

Client Factors and Performance Skills

The goal of OT intervention is for clients to work toward their goals while feeling successful and safe. The COTA analyzes activities in terms of **client factors** (i.e., mental functions; sensory functions and pain; and neuromusculoskeletal, cardiovascular, hematological, immunological, and respiratory system functions) to design intervention so that the client's goals can be met. The following questions may be useful in guiding the OT practitioner:

1. What physical requirements (i.e., neuromusculoskeletal and movement-related functions) are needed to complete the activity or use the media (e.g., range of motion, strength, bilateral hand use)?
2. What specific mental functions (e.g., attention, organization, awareness, memory, perception) must the client possess to successfully work with the selected media?

3. What are the performance skills (i.e., motor, process, communication/interaction) required to successfully complete this activity?
4. What are the safety issues surrounding the use of the media? Does the client possess the safety awareness to handle the media or participate in the activity without risk (e.g., impulsiveness, allergies)?
5. What sensory functions are required for the client to participate in the activity or with the media (e.g., visual acuity, balance, tactile discrimination)?

Contexts

Context comprises all the conditions surrounding the client.[2] Contexts include physical, social, personal, cultural, temporal, spiritual, and virtual aspects.[2] The context in which an activity occurs can influence the client's motivation for, the meaning derived from, and successful completion of the activity. OT practitioners consider context(s) when selecting intervention activities for clients. The following questions serve to highlight contextual influence in activity selection:

1. Is the therapeutic activity consistent with the client's cultural, social, spiritual, and personal backgrounds?
2. What are the social (e.g., political, economic, institutional) conditions surrounding the activity?
3. What are the personal characteristics of the client, and how will they affect activity selection (e.g., age, gender, socioeconomic status, educational status)?
4. Does this activity have any spiritual aspects that must be considered?
5. What are the temporal aspects (e.g., stage of life, time of day, time of year, duration) of the activity? How will this influence the selection of media?
6. What are the physical characteristics of the activity? Where does it take place?
7. How long will the activity take?

Grading and Adapting

Therapeutic activities may need to be changed to promote success. The following questions may assist the OT practitioner in **grading activities** (changing the degree of difficulty of the activity) and **adapting activities** (changing how the activity is to be performed):

1. Can the level of complexity of the activity be increased or decreased according to the client's thought processing level (e.g., decreasing steps, taught by backward chaining, fading assistance)?
2. Can the provided media be modified if necessary for the client's physical skills (e.g., less or more resistance, larger or smaller objects)?
3. Can the media be changed for the client's sensory function requirements (e.g., placing media on bright backgrounds to increase the contrast for low-vision clients or changing the texture of materials to accommodate the client's tactile needs)?
4. Are the media versatile enough to be individualized within a group activity?
5. If it is determined that there is a need for adaptive equipment to enhance the client's performance, is it available at the treatment setting?

Activity Demands

The successful planning of an activity requires that the OT practitioner of analyze activity demands. The term *activity demands* refers to the objects and their properties, space demands, social demands, sequence and timing, required actions, and required body functions and structures.[2] Analysis of the activity demands helps the OT practitioner select appropriate activities and media. The following questions may guide the OT practitioner:

1. Are the tools and equipment necessary to use the media available and in good condition?
2. Are there adequate tools and materials for the number of clients?
3. Is there an adequate working surface, open space, and lighting for the activity?
4. What are the social and communication skills needed to participate in the activity?
5. What are the steps, sequence, and timing of the activity? Will there be enough time to complete it?
6. What are the skills required to successfully complete the activity?
7. What body structures are needed to complete the activity?
8. How can the activity be changed for clients who have difficulties?
9. What are the safety precautions?
10. What is the cost of the activity?
11. Where can the activity take place?

ROLE OF THE CERTIFIED OCCUPATIONAL THERAPY ASSISTANT AND REGISTERED OCCUPATIONAL THERAPIST IN SELECTING THERAPEUTIC MEDIA

Collaboration refers to cooperating with others to meet a mutual goal.[3] Under the supervision of and in collaboration with the registered occupational therapist (OTR), COTAs deliver OT services. It is the legal and ethical responsibility of both the OTR and COTA to ensure that the COTA establish the service competency necessary to choose the media that are relevant to the client's occupational goals.

CLINICAL *Pearl*

Service competency ensures that one therapist be able to obtain the same results from a procedure or activity as another. Two examples of establishing service competency are videotaping treatment techniques to be critiqued by an experienced therapist and reviewing standardized test results to ensure correct administration procedures and accurate scoring. Another method is the use of competency checkoffs for skills such as range of motion (measured with the goniometer), manual muscle testing, and safe transfer techniques.

COTAs who do not practice within close proximity of other therapists (such as those working in some school systems or home health care) can establish service competency and expand their skills by seeking an experienced mentor. Pediatric focus groups provide opportunities to collaborate with other OT practitioners and discuss intervention strategies. Furthermore, COTAs may discover new intervention strategies and uses of media by attending professional conferences and continuing education. Commercial companies offer online resources for media projects and supplies that may prove helpful to OT practitioners.

USE OF THERAPEUTIC MEDIA

The OT practitioner uses therapeutic media during the intervention process. The media may be used within the context of a purposeful activity (i.e., one that directly relates to the client's goals and occupational role) or as a preparatory activity (i.e., one that addresses client factors and the underlying skills necessary to achieve these goals).

Kevin is a 7-year-old boy with juvenile rheumatoid arthritis who is in the 2nd grade. He enjoys art class but has difficulty painting when his joints are inflamed. He also has difficulty holding the paint brush (Figure 16-1, A). The COTA decided to work on Kevin's goal to improve fine motor skills for academic work by using a painting activity. As preparation, Kevin and the COTA completed some stretching exercises (both passive and active). The COTA set up a painting activity similar to the one that would be conducted in art class later that week. Since Kevin takes longer than the other children to complete his work, the art teacher was thrilled that the COTA could break down the steps and allow Kevin to get a head start. Furthermore, it allowed the COTA to determine what types of adaptation work best with Kevin. She provided Kevin with a built-up handled paintbrush and an easel positioned close to him and lowered so that he would not have to raise his arm as high as the other children. Kevin enjoyed painting and was looking forward to finishing his project in art class later that week (Figure 16-1, B).

In this scenario, painting was the goal (fine motor skills to participate in school) and the media as well (to work on increasing fine motor skills). The COTA was able to help Kevin achieve success in a meaningful activity that is part of his occupational role as a student. The preparatory activity in this case was the stretching and

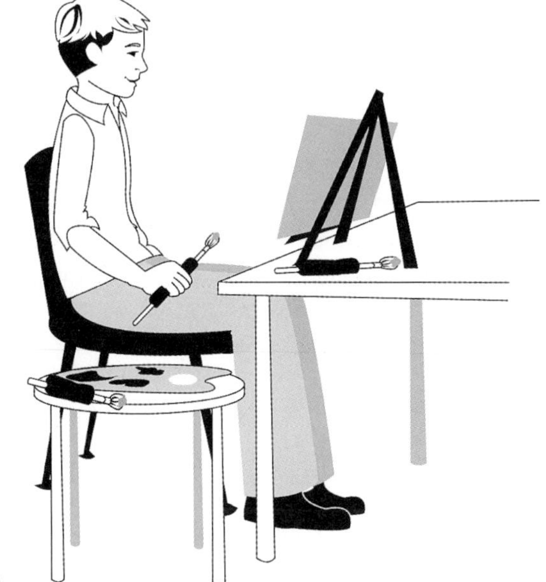
A

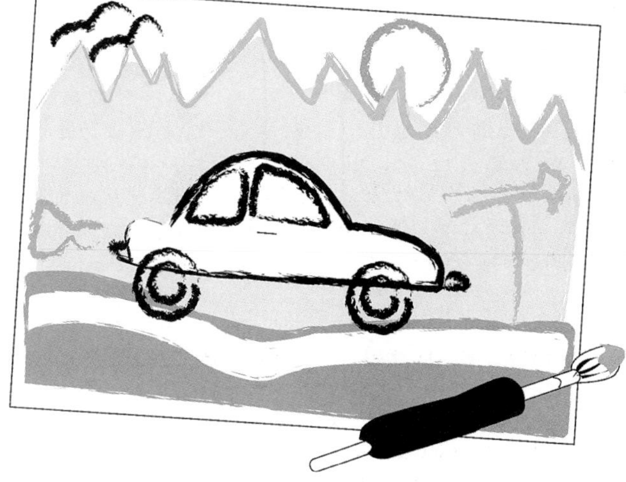
B

FIGURE 16-1 **A,** Kevin has difficulty holding a paintbrush. **B,** Kevin's finished artwork after his paintbrush and easel have been adapted.

exercising required before beginning the painting. The COTA provided the child with adaptations (e.g., built-up handled paintbrush) to ensure success in art class. The child became invested in the painting activity and was motivated to continue it in art class later that week.

The COTA recognized the importance of using media and activities that were occupation based and meaningful to the child.

ACTIVITIES

The following section provides examples of how the COTA chooses meaningful and therapeutic activities. Each scenario provides a client profile, a description of the media and method chosen, suggestions for grading and adapting the activity, and an overview of the required client factors specific to the case. Tables 16-1 through 16-4 provide commonly used therapeutic media for each age group.

TABLE 16-1

Examples of Activities for Infants

ACTIVITY	BRIEF DESCRIPTION OF ACTIVITY OR PRODUCT
Handprint wreath	Arrange cutout or painted handprints in wreath pattern.
Body awareness: Dressing/bathing games	Use lotion, soap, powder, and movement while naming body parts during bathing and dressing.
Bubbles	Adult blows bubbles while providing infant with cues to visually track, reach, and pop.
Multitexture mat	This item can be homemade or purchased for infant to crawl over, walk on, and explore textures
Cardboard box play	Push/pull infant (sitting inside box) across floor for vestibular input.
Hand/foot games	Some examples are Peek-A-Boo, Patty Cake, and This Little Piggy.
Scooping/pouring activities	Use various media, such as water, sand, dirt, and rice.
Music with pots and pans	Use various sizes of pots, pans, plastic bowls, and wooden spoons.
Commercially available developmental toys	Some specific types include cause and effect, sequencing, push/pull toys, stuffed animals, and texture books. Some examples are nesting toys, push lawnmower toys, and See and Say.

TABLE 16-2

Examples of Activities for Early Childhood

ACTIVITY	BRIEF DESCRIPTION OF ACTIVITY OR PRODUCT
Paper bag puppets	Use paper lunch bags; Cut, glue, or color puppet features onto bag.
Marshmallow people	Use pretzel stick to connect marshmallow body parts.
Birdfeeder	Roll pine cone in peanut butter and birdseed.
Sorting games	Use pincer grasp or tweezers/tongs to pick up small manipulative objects for sorting.
Tissue paper collage	Have child crumple up precut squares of tissue paper with fingers and place on glue dots within a defined space.
Parachute	Great group activity! Incorporate songs; emphasize up, down, and around; and toss items onto parachute or sheet.
Loop cereal or noodle jewelry	String items on such implements as a curling ribbon, plastic craft lace, and pipe cleaner.
Painting	Some examples are finger painting and sponge painting.
Body movement games	Some examples are I'm a Little Teapot; Head, Shoulder, Knees, and Toes; and Row, Row, Row Your Boat.
Commercial games/toys	Some examples are Don't Spill the Beans, Barrel of Monkeys, Candy Land, Hi Ho Cheerio, Memory, Ants in the Pants, Don't Break the Ice, Mr. Potato Head, Shape Sorter, Counting Bears, and nesting items.

TABLE 16-3

Examples of Activities for Middle Childhood

ACTIVITY	BRIEF DESCRIPTION OF ACTIVITY OR PRODUCT
Paper chains	Have child cut strips of paper or use precut strips. Attach by various means, such as a paperclip, staples, or glue. Vary colors. Consider cultural differences.
Windsocks	Roll construction paper to form cylinder and secure with staples or tape. Attach crepe paper streamers along bottom edge. Punch holes and thread yarn for hanger. Use markers, stickers, or other items to decorate.
Gingerbread house	Buy a ready-made kit or use pint-size milk carton, graham crackers, stiff icing, and candies to decorate.
Sun catchers	Melt crayon shavings between 2 pieces of wax paper using iron. Have child make a frame out of popsicle sticks, construction paper, or other items.
Papier-mâché piñata	Use a thin box. Dip tissue or newspaper strips into a flour and water mixture (consistency of thin white glue) and drape over box in layers. Allow to dry completely. Adult slits a hole in the box to fill with candy. Child decorates with paint, stickers, or other items.
Body movement games	Some examples are Red Light/Green Light, Simon Says, Hopscotch, and Animal Walks.
Commercial games/toys	Some examples are Bop It, Hungry Hippo, Connect Four, Tiddily Winks, Legos, Mega Links, Uno, Go Fish, Barrel of Monkeys, and Pick Up Sticks.

TABLE 16-4

Examples of Activities for Adolescence

ACTIVITY	BRIEF DESCRIPTION OF ACTIVITY OR PRODUCT
Origami	Fold paper to form 3-D shapes; may use purchased kits or craft book.
Flowerpot decoupage	Cut out pictures from magazines, greeting cards, or old books. Brush decoupage glue on back of picture. Apply picture to flowerpot. Apply additional decoupage glue, covering picture and surface completely until entire area is smooth and uniform.
Picture frame	Cover an old picture frame using various media (e.g., seashells, puzzle pieces, twigs, gemstones).
T-shirt painting/tie-dye	Use various fabric paints, stencils, sponges, or brushes on T-shirt. Buy commercial tie-dye kits or follow instructions available in craft books (see References).
Collage	Cut out pictures from magazines or catalogs of interest to clients and glue onto poster board. Add decorative accents as desired (e.g., glitter bows, stickers).
CD mobile	Decorate and hang promotional or unwanted CDs with fishing line from coat hanger, driftwood, or other items or locations.
Rubbings	Rub crayons, charcoal pencils, pastels, or other similar items onto thin paper placed over embossed surfaces (e.g., building cornerstones, carved wood, coins).
Rubber stamping	Create cards, gift tags, and stationary by using commercial rubber stamps and stamp pads.
Commercial games	Some examples are dominoes, Mancala, Pictionary, Jenga, card games, Backgammon, Simon, and Perfection.

Infancy: Birth through 18 Months

MIGUEL'S WATER PLAY SESSION. *Miguel is a 12-month-old boy with a diagnosis of Down syndrome. He receives outpatient OT and PT (physical therapy) services once a week. The goals for OT include working to improve Miguel's physical endurance and hand skills for play. During therapy sessions the COTA works on increasing postural stability for independent sitting as well as improving reaching and grasping skills. This week the COTA and PTA (physical therapy assistant) have collaborated and planned activities to address Miguel's OT and PT goals in the pool at the clinic. The COTA discussed the upcoming session with Miguel's parents, who reported that he loves to play in the water and they would like for him to develop preswimming skills (Figure 16-2). Miguel will wear a swimsuit with an attached flotation device for safety while in the pool. To prepare him for the water and increase body awareness, the therapist will rub his arms, legs, and back with water while naming each body part.*

The media and/or materials needed are as follows.

- Water
- Kick board
- Small water toys requiring hand skill (e.g., plastic fish, simple squirt toys)
- Sponge balls
- Beach ball

The method used comprises the following components:

1. Set the environment. Have all materials within the therapist's reach.
2. Miguel is positioned on the edge of the pool, with the PTA providing support at the trunk level as necessary for safety. The COTA, who is positioned in front of Miguel, holds up pool toys at various planes to facilitate reaching up, down, and across the midline. The COTA carefully monitors his facial expressions for signs of fear and provides positive feedback while facilitating the "just right" challenge. Once she has ensured his comfort level, she asks him to kick a large ball positioned in front of him.
3. Once he becomes more comfortable, Miguel is positioned prone on the kick board in the pool, with the PTA facilitating trunk stability in the prone-extension position. He works on head and trunk control in this position and is encouraged to kick through the water to move forward so that he can reach the toys placed in front of him. The COTA holds a sponge ball just below the surface of the water for Miguel to grasp and pull toward him. This movement simulates the dog paddle motion which is needed for swimming. To improve hand strength, the COTA shows him how to squeeze the water out of the ball to sink a small toy boat.

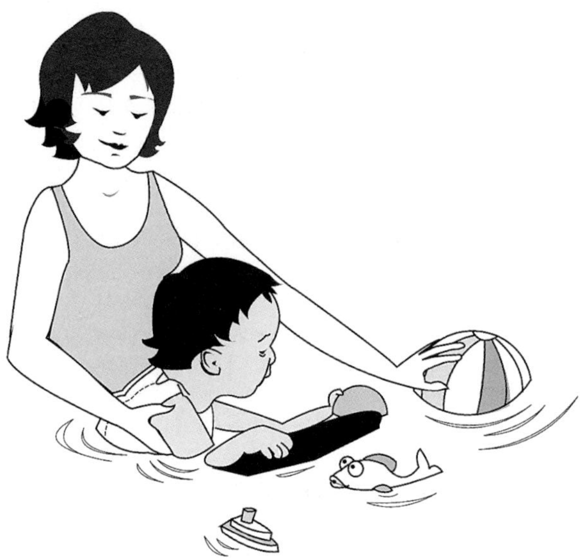

FIGURE 16-2 Miguel is active in the swimming pool.

CLINICAL *Pearl*

Working while in a prone position strengthens cervical, trunk, and scapular musculature. Strengthening these muscle groups increases overall postural stability.

The client factors addressed and considered for Miguel during this activity are as follows:

Mental functions

Global: Miguel was interested and motivated by his enjoyment of water play.

Neuromusculoskeletal and movement-related functions

- Joints and bones: Miguel reached to various planes with both the upper and lower extremities, which required mobility and stability of the joints.
- Muscle: Although Miguel had low muscle tone, the buoyancy of the water allowed efficient use of his strength and endurance as he moved his arms and legs against the resistance of the water.
- Movement: Miguel needed control of voluntary movement for reaching, grasping, eye-hand coordination, and eye-foot coordination to complete the activity. He also used bilateral integration while reaching across the midline for toys.

Skin and related structure functions

- Skin: Miguel had intact skin integrity, as evidenced by the absence of open wounds and abrasions. This was an important consideration when engaging in water play in a public pool.

Suggestions for grading and adapting the activity are as follows:

- Use a variety of positions and surfaces (edge of pool for stable surface and kick board or raft for unstable surface).
- If a pool is not available, these or similar activities can be carried out with a water table or in a bathtub.
- Vary the distance and height when presenting objects for reaching and grasping.
- The level of assistance can be increased or decreased according to the client's needs.
- Simulate swimming activities to help prepare the child for the occupation of swimming. For example, blowing bubbles, kicking feet, reaching forward, and cupping water are all prerequisite swimming skills.

The COTA selected water as a motivating medium based on the parents' report of Miguel's enjoyment of water play. Through collaboration, both disciplines were able to safely address Miguel's PT and OT goals by working in the pool. Furthermore, swimming is an occupation of childhood in which the child and parents were interested.

JESSICA'S HANDPRINT/FOOTPRINT BUTTERFLY. Jessica is an 18-month-old child who receives early-intervention OT services at her daycare center two times a week. She has a diagnosis of agenesis of the corpus callosum and hypotonia. Jessica's mother would like her to be able to sit independently and tolerate sensory input during a bath. The COTA addresses these aspects of the Individual Family Service Plan (IFSP) by providing controlled sensory input to decrease Jessica's tactile sensitivity and working to improve trunk stability. The COTA and preschool teacher collaborate by planning a group activity for Mother's Day that can be adapted to Jessica's needs (a handprint/footprint butterfly) (Figure 16-3). As a preparatory activity, the COTA brushes Jessica's hands on both sides as well as the soles of her feet. She then facilitates transitional movements to various positions to maximize trunk stability and upper extremity weight bearing.

The media and/or materials needed are as follows:

- Several colors of nontoxic paint in pie tins
- Poster board

CLINICAL *Pearl*

Many therapists use the Wilbarger Brushing Protocol for decreasing tactile sensitivity with the pediatric population.[4] This is a powerful tool and should be used only after training has been completed and service competency is established for this technique.

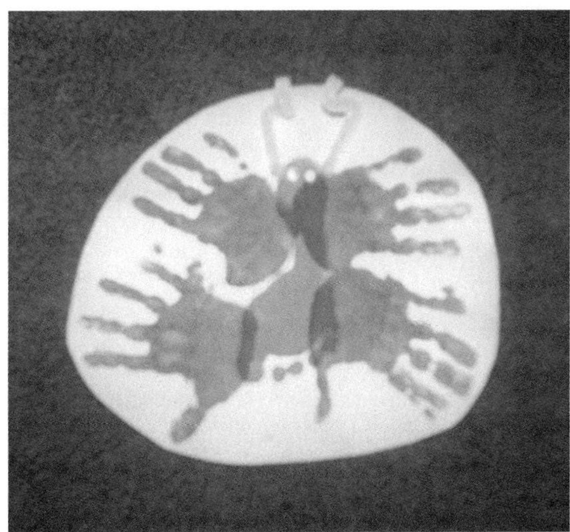

FIGURE 16-3 Butterfly print.

- Soft-bristle paintbrush
- Pipe cleaner (preformed)
- Protective covering for floor
- Glue
- Paper towels

The method used comprises the following elements:

1. Set the environment. Cover the floor, place all materials nearby, and position the poster board.
2. The COTA sits on the floor in back of Jessica to provide supported sitting.
3. Jessica's foot is brushed with paint and pressed onto the poster board to form the body of the butterfly. The paper is rotated one-half turn and Jessica's hand is brushed with paint. The COTA presses Jessica's hand onto one side of the body at the top and bottom. The procedure is repeated with the opposite hand on the other side of the body. This forms the wings. Additional paint is added with the paintbrush as needed for detail. The COTA dabs Jessica's index finger into the paint and daubs the top of the body to form the eyes.
4. After the paint dries the antennae (pipe cleaners) are glued on by an adult.

Suggestions for grading and adapting the activity are as follows:

- Complete in more than one session.
- Provide adapted positioning for external trunk support (i.e., adaptive chair, adult assistance, environmental support).
- Add various media to the paint to provide increased tactile input (i.e., sand, uncooked rice, cornmeal).

- Thin paint with water to change tactile input.
- Dip hand into paint instead of brushing it onto palm.
- Apply paint on hand with a cotton ball.
- If tactile input is not tolerated, trace the shape of the hand and have the child use a paintbrush to fill in the shape. Use hand-over-hand assistance as needed.

The client factors addressed and considered for Jessica during this activity are as follows:

Mental functions

Global: Jessica needed an appropriate level of arousal in order to participate in the activity. She was motivated by the playful way in which the activity was presented.

Sensory functions

Proprioception was required for Jessica to sustain various positions, such as sitting upright and upper extremity weight bearing. Jessica's visual functions were stimulated by the bright colors of the paint, and vestibular functions were necessary for her to sustain balance in upright sitting. She used tactile functions to discriminate between the sensation of the COTA's hand and the texture of the paint.

Neuromusculoskeletal and movement-related functions

- Muscle: Although Jessica had low muscle tone, she had sufficient strength and endurance to sustain upright sitting and transition to various postures with assistance.
- Movement: Righting reactions were required to re-establish the midline after placing her painted palm onto the surface of the paper. With minimum assistance, Jessica was able to initiate the voluntary movement of her hands and fingers to press her painted palms onto the paper.

The COTA chose the activity based on Jessica's IFSP goals and integrated it into the classroom. Making Mother's Day projects is an important occupation for children of all ages. By considering the demands of the activity, the COTA was able to work on the IFSP goals of stabilizing the trunk and decreasing tactile sensitivity while working in the least restrictive environment. See Table 16-1 for other commonly used therapeutic media for infants.

Early Childhood: 18 Months through 5 Years

ALLIE'S PUDDING PAINTING. *Allie is a 36-month-old child with a diagnosis of autism. She receives OT services from a home health agency twice a week. OT sessions focus on improving self-feeding, manipulating objects with her hands for play and dressing (fine motor skills), and improving visual motor skills through imitation of age-appropriate prewriting strokes. She is noted to have oral sensitivity. Allie's mother requested activities that she can do easily with her at home during play. The COTA will model a pudding painting activity that the mother can do with Allie. To prepare Allie for the activity, she will squeeze and manipulate Play-Doh, which improves hand strength and digit isolation.*

The media and/or materials needed are as follows:

- One snack-size pudding cup (choose a flavor and color that the child will like)
- Flat surface such as a cookie sheet or paper plate
- Large pullover shirt that can get messy
- Spoon
- Napkin

The method used comprises the following elements:

1. Set the environment. Since this activity is messy, cover the work surface. Have materials close by.
2. Allie dons a pullover shirt, with help as needed.
3. Allie and the COTA open the pudding cup. Allie scoops the pudding onto a cookie sheet with assistance to sustain grasp or reposition as needed. She spreads the pudding with her hand.
4. The COTA assists Allie in establishing index finger isolation and provides occasional assistance as needed during the activity. Allie imitates prewriting strokes in pudding (vertical and horizontal lines, circle, and cross) as demonstrated by the COTA.
5. Once the prewriting activity is over and cleaned up, Allie's mother gives her a new pudding cup. With the COTA's assistance, Allie eats the pudding with a spoon as a snack.

The client factors addressed and considered for Allie during this activity are as follows:

Mental functions

- Global: Allie was motivated by the new experience of completing prewriting strokes in the pudding. She showed an interest in the new activity. Allie turned when her name was called throughout the activity, showing orientation to person.
- Specific: Allie needed sustained attention for 3-minute periods to complete both the visual motor and self-feeding tasks. Visuospatial perception skills were used throughout the prewriting activity to imitate the strokes. Allie used tactile functions while working with the texture of the pudding during the prewriting activity.

Sensory functions

- Hearing and vestibular: Allie engaged in vestibular functions to sustain dynamic sitting balance while reaching to complete prewriting strokes.
- Additional: Kinesthesia and the sense of joint position were used to manipulate the pudding and reach and move fingers through the pudding. Tactile functions were required as Allie accepted the texture of the pudding both through her fingertips and in her mouth while eating the pudding.

Neuromusculoskeletal and movement-related functions

- Joints and bones: Functional range of motion of the upper extremities was needed to don the pullover shirt.
- Movement: Allie needed to establish control of voluntary movement, specifically eye-hand coordination for both the fine motor and self-care aspects of the session.

Suggestions for grading and adapting the activity are as follows:

- Use thicker or thinner food textures as needed to change resistance.
- Use items such as pretzel sticks, carrot sticks, and marshmallows for the child to write with if they are tactile defensive.
- Increase or decrease the level of difficulty as needed by having the child imitate, copy, or write from memory.
- Use adaptive equipment such as a scoop bowl or adaptive spoon to increase independence with self-feeding.
- Use nonfood items to practice prewriting and writing skills (e.g., shaving cream, sand, lotion, finger paint).
- Vary the working position (e.g., supported sitting, prone on floor, standing).

After the session is over, the COTA and mother discuss the process and outcome of the activity. The COTA suggests similar activities with different food items and other prewriting activities so that the mother can participate fully in helping Allie reach the goals.

CARRIE'S CLOTHESPIN CATERPILLAR MAGNETS. *Carrie is a 4-year-old child who attends the Early Childhood Diagnostic Program (ECDP) in a public elementary school. She receives weekly OT services in this setting to support the educational goals in her Individual Education Plan (IEP) (see Chapter 4). The goals of OT services include addressing difficulties with fine motor, visual perception, and sensory processing. The class thematic unit this week is insects. The COTA has planned to have the children make clothespin caterpillar magnets (Figure 16-4, A). As a preparatory activity, the children will participate in a music and movement group. In addition, Carrie will string large beads onto a pipe cleaner (Figure 16-4, B)as a fine motor warm-up and search for small plastic items hidden in a rice bowl to decrease tactile sensitivity (Figure 16-4, C).*

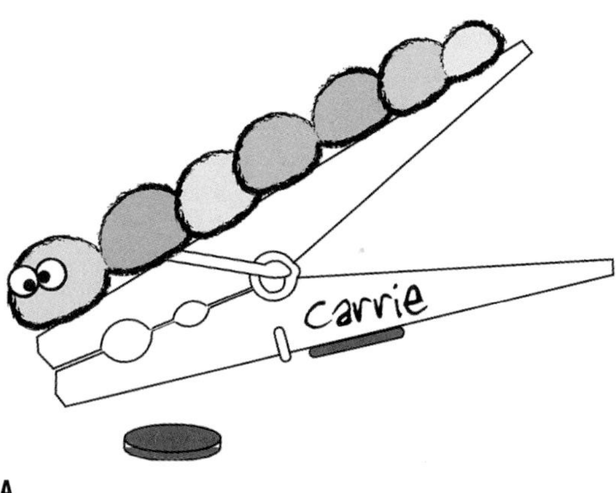

A

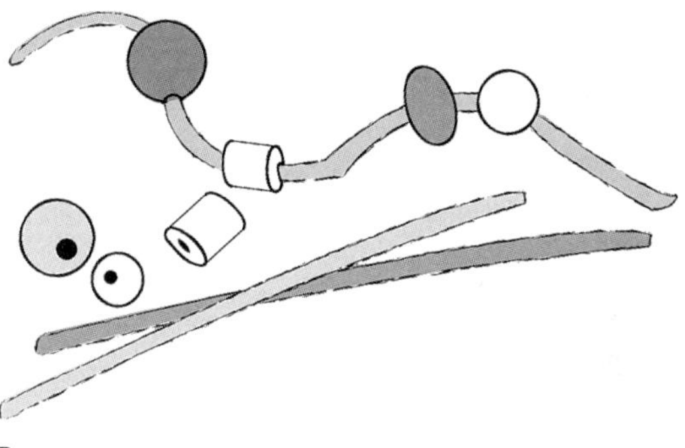

B

C

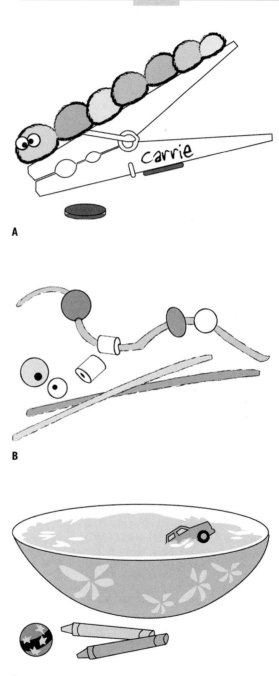

FIGURE 16-4 **A,** Carrie's clothespin caterpillar magnet. **B,** Carrie strings large beads onto pipe cleaners. **C,** She searches for small plastic items hidden in a rice bowl.

CLINICAL *Pearl*

Preparatory activities can be thought of as warm-up techniques to prepare the client for a specific desired action. Activities such as a gross motor movement group can increase motor planning for tasks such as handwriting. Hand musculature may be developed by upper extremity weight bearing that occurs during activities such as crawling through a tunnel. Likewise, bead stringing can be used to facilitate the pincer grasp needed to hold a pencil for handwriting.

The media and/or materials needed are as follows:

- One standard-size wooden clothespin
- Craft glue or wood glue
- Six multicolored pom-poms (about $^1/_2$ inch)
- One chenille stick (pipe cleaner) about 4 inches long
- Two small wiggle eyes
- 2-inch piece of magnet with adhesive backing
- Cotton swabs
- Small dish or paper plate
- Tweezers

The method used comprises the following elements:

1. Set the environment. Make sure that the table and chair are the appropriate height. Have all materials on the table within reach.
2. Follow the simple color pattern of a completed caterpillar model.
3. Providing assistance as needed, squeeze glue from the bottle onto a small dish.
4. Using a cotton swab to dip into the glue, spread it onto one side of the clothespin. As tolerated, use the index finger to spread the glue evenly.
5. Following the model for color pattern, pick out the needed pom-poms from a large assortment.
6. Use tweezers to pick up and place pom-poms onto glue following the color pattern.
7. Use a cotton swab to apply two drops of glue to the caterpillar's head (first pom-pom) for the eyes. Place two wiggle eyes onto the drops of glue.
8. Providing assistance as needed, twist the pipe cleaner around the side of the clothespin, behind the head of the caterpillar, to form the antennae.
9. Peel the adhesive backing from the magnet and place it onto the back of the clothespin, providing assistance as needed.

The client factors addressed and considered for Carrie during this activity are as follows.

CLINICAL *Pearl*

Provide adequate supervision at all times when using small materials to ensure the safety of the child. Many children have poor impulse control and safety awareness and may use materials inappropriately.

Mental functions

- Specific: Visuospatial perception was needed to line the pom-poms on the clothespin as shown in the model. Interpretation of sensory stimuli (tactile) was required whenever Carrie spread the glue with her fingertips. Choosing the color and size of the pom-poms required recognition and categorization skills to follow the given pattern of the model.

Sensory functions and pain

Additional: Proprioceptive functions provided the feedback necessary for her to sustain adequate pressure while using the tweezers to pick up, move, and place the pom-poms without dropping them. Although Carrie's tactile functions were hypersensitive, she tolerated a limited amount of input from the glue.

Neuromusculoskeletal and movement-related functions

Movement: Control of voluntary movement functions was needed during those aspects of the activity that required eye-hand coordination to place pom-poms matching the given pattern.

Suggestions for grading and adapting the activity are as follows:

- Use larger or smaller clothespins and pom-poms as needed.
- When decreased fine motor skills are present, use tongs instead of tweezers.
- Use hot glue, with child placing pom-poms.
- Give more or less assistance, depending on the child's abilities.
- Instead of twisting pipe cleaner for the antennae, the child can glue on a paper antenna.
- Adjust the complexity of the color pattern, depending on the child's abilities.
- Adapt the environment. For example, increase or decrease the group size, reduce the amount of materials presented at a time, or choose an area that offers the fewest visual stimuli.

The COTA conducted this activity in Carrie's least restrictive environment (classroom). In working with the teacher, the COTA was able to design, develop, and implement a therapeutic activity, relating it to both the weekly thematic unit and Carrie's goals.

See Table 16-2 for other commonly used therapeutic media for the early childhood age group.

Middle Childhood: 6 Years until Onset of Puberty

DAVID'S BIRTHDAY CROWN. *David is a 6-year-old boy in kindergarten with a diagnosis of ADHD. He has difficulty completing cutting and handwriting tasks; the teacher notes that he struggles with puzzles and becomes frustrated easily. David receives school-based OT services once a week to address fine motor and visual perceptual difficulties that interfere with classroom activities. His teacher asked the COTA to help David make a "birthday crown" to celebrate his birthday. The COTA is excited to work with David on this activity because it addresses both of his goals. As a preparatory activity, the COTA has David manipulate firm therapy putty to retrieve beads. The COTA also provides an air-filled cushion for him to sit on during this activity to increase his attention.*

CLINICAL *Pearl*

There are various products on the market, such as air-filled cushions and ball chairs, to help clients increase their attention by providing them with vestibular input controlled by their movements.

The media and/or materials needed are as follows:

- Poster board
- Small items for decoration (e.g., stickers, sequins, buttons)
- Scissors
- Glue
- Cotton swabs
- Stencils (letters and shapes)
- Markers, crayons
- Stapler
- Glitter

The method used comprises the following elements:

1. Set the environment. Make sure the chair and table are appropriate heights. Have the materials within reach. Reduce the amount of visual and auditory stimuli. Make sure that the lighting is adequate.
2. The COTA draws a crown pattern on the poster board, and David cuts the pattern.
3. The COTA measures David's head and marks the crown for him to staple later.
4. David decorates the crown (Figure 16-5, A). He uses letter stencils to write his name with the correct formation, receiving verbal cues from the COTA for direction. He practices in-hand manipulation with buttons and sequins to place on the crown. David also works on pincer grasp by using a cotton swab to spread the glue.
5. David staples the crown where the COTA previously marked, and he places the crown on his head.
6. David and the COTA clean up the area.

The client factors addressed and considered for David during this activity are as follows:

Mental functions

- Global: David was motivated to make the crown for his birthday. As most children do, he values the celebration of personal holidays. He was able to modulate his level of arousal to carry the task through to its completion.
- Specific: David was able to sustain attention to complete the multistep task. Perceptual functions were used to place the stencils in a linear aspect and in the correct sequence to write his name. He was able to implement problem-solving skills to identify and correct errors in the project. David had to regulate his emotional functions to control his impulsiveness. His self-esteem was raised as he completed and wore the crown in celebration of his special day.

Neuromusculoskeletal and movement-related functions

- Muscle: David's muscle tone and strength allowed him to sustain a grasp on the scissors, hold the pencil correctly, and depress the stapler.
- Movement: Control of voluntary movement for bilateral integration and eye-hand coordination allowed David to stabilize the stencil with the nondominant hand as he wrote with his dominant hand.

Sensory functions and pain

- Additional: Kinesthesia and a sense of joint position were required for David to grade movement and use the stapler without tearing the paper. These functions also allowed him to advance the scissors through the paper in a smooth and controlled fashion.

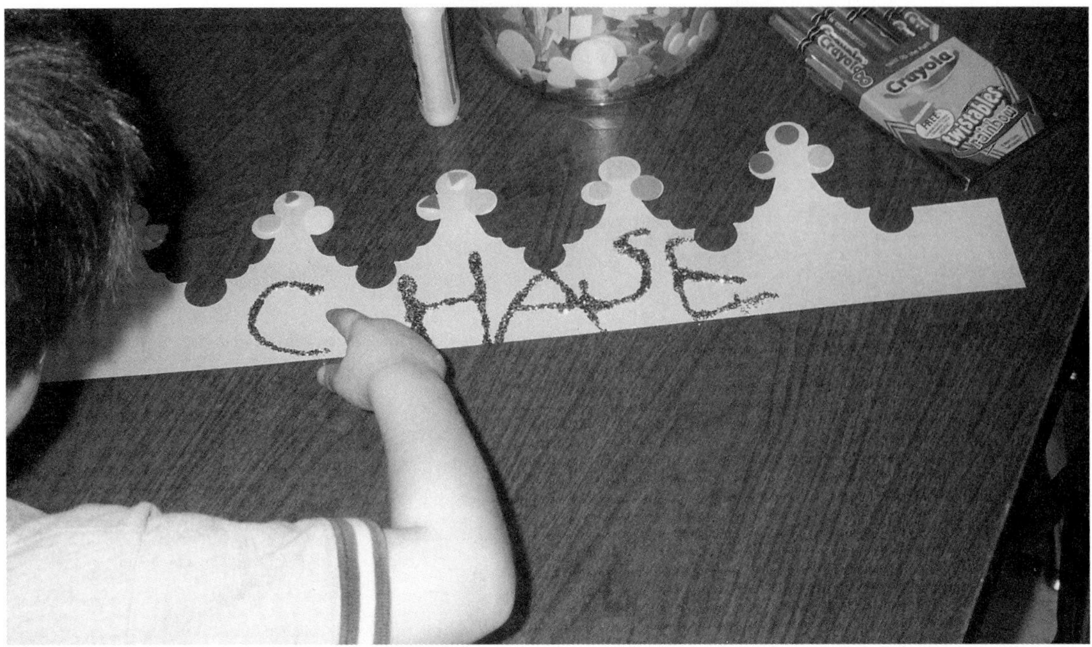

A

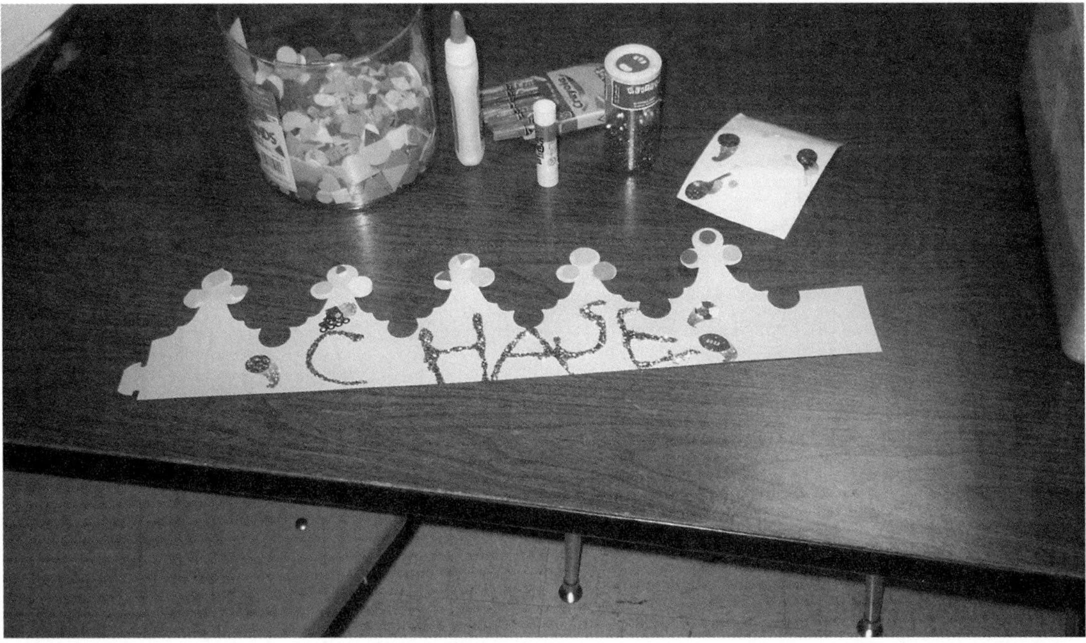

B

FIGURE 16-5 **A,** Boy with crown. **B,** Completed crown on table.

Suggestions for grading and adapting the activity are as follows:

- Provide a model.
- Use tape rather than a stapler if safety is a concern or if strength is poor.
- Use glue sticks, squeeze glue from a bottle, or use other items to spread glue (e.g., paintbrush, cotton ball).
- Give wider or thinner lines as needed to cut.
- Increase or decrease the difficulty of the crown pattern as needed for cutting.

- Break activity up over several treatment sessions, depending on attentiveness as well as other factors.

The COTA made the activity meaningful by centering it on David's birthday. She chose preparatory activities that would increase his ability to succeed with the functional activity of making the birthday crown. The COTA considered David's difficulty attending to tasks and adapted the environment by providing an air-filled cushion for David to sit upon (Figure 16-5, *B*).

CASEY'S CRISPY RICE CEREAL TREATS. *Casey is a 13-year-old moderately intellectually delayed student in a self-contained class at the local middle school. His class often engages in cooking activities to work on their independent living and transitional job training skills. Casey has a short attention span, and the teacher and COTA have often discussed his inability to carry out multistep tasks to completion. These are the areas that the COTA targets during OT sessions. The students are going to host a fall luncheon for their parents. They have compiled a shopping list and purchased the ingredients on a community-based field trip. The classroom has a full kitchen, and the students will be preparing side dishes for the meal. Casey is making the dessert, a pumpkin-shaped crispy rice cereal treat. After a discussion about the various cultures within the classroom, the teacher and the COTA decide that it would be more appropriate to make a generic pumpkin motif than a jack-o-lantern. The COTA decided to incorporate the activity within the OT session. She prepares him for the activity by carefully reviewing the rules of the session and showing him the finished product.*

The media and/or materials needed are as follows:

- 6 cups of crispy rice cereal
- 1 bag of marshmallows
- 2 tablespoons of margarine
- Orange decorative sprinkles
- Raisins, chocolate chips, and chocolate-covered candies
- Spearmint gumdrop leaves
- Pretzel sticks
- Large mixing bowl (microwave safe)
- Large spoon
- Wax paper

The method used comprises the following elements:

1. Set the environment. Gather together all the ingredients and have cooking utensils within reach. Casey washes and dries his hands.
2. Open the bag of marshmallows (with the COTA's supervision). Empty the contents into the bowl along with the margarine. Put the bowl in the microwave for 1 minute. Stir the mixture and microwave for an additional minute. (Verbal cues are provided to assist Casey in setting and attending to the microwave timer.)
3. Using potholders, remove the bowl from the microwave.
4. Measure six cups of cereal (with the COTA providing cues as needed).
5. Pour the cereal into the bowl and mix it thoroughly with the melted marshmallow and margarine mixture by using a large spoon.
6. Wash and dry hands before handling the food.
7. The COTA demonstrates how to obtain an adequate amount of cereal mixture to form a round-shaped ball. Roll the cereal ball in the orange decorative sprinkles and place each one on a sheet of wax paper.
8. Add features to the pumpkin with raisins, chocolate chips, and chocolate-covered candies, and push a pretzel stick into the top and place spearmint candy leaves on each side to resemble the stem of a pumpkin.
9. Wash all the items used in warm, soapy water; rinse and dry them; and clean the countertops.

The client factors addressed and considered for Casey during this activity are as follows:

Mental functions

- Global: Casey was motivated to complete this activity because the guests would include his parents.
- Specific: Casey demonstrated sustained attention for approximately 30 minutes with frequent cues and verbal directions. He used higher-level cognitive functions for good judgment, adhering to safety precautions when using the scissors and handling hot cooking utensils. Casey had to visually interpret sensory stimuli and use calculation functions to measure the ingredients. He also had to accurately motor-plan several steps, such as pouring ingredients into the measuring containers and emptying them into a bowl without spillage.

Neuromusculoskeletal and movement-related functions

- Movement: Asymmetrical bilateral skills were needed for Casey to stabilize a mixing bowl while stirring the ingredients and form the rice crispy mixture into a ball. Symmetrical bilateral skills were used while Casey was using both hands to remove the bowl from the microwave.

Suggestions for grading and adapting the activity are as follows:

- If tactile defensiveness is a concern, insert hands into sandwich bags to decrease the feeling of the mixture or pour the mixture into a flat container and pat down with a nonstick spatula.
- Adult completes more of the activity (i.e., touching mixture), and student does pouring and stirring.
- Use Dycem under the bowl to increase its stability on the flat surface.
- Adapt the spoon as needed.
- Use thicker pretzel rods that will not break as easily.
- Use tongs or tweezers to place features.
- Provide visual aids to break down the sequence of the activity.
- Substitute another dry cereal to change the consistency of the mixture (input to hands).
- Use large visual timers, which are available from adapted-equipment catalogs, to provide temporal cues.

Taking into consideration Casey's short attention span, the COTA adapted the activity by providing verbal cues and redirection as needed. She coordinated Casey's treatment around the classroom activity so that he could remain in the least restrictive environment and fulfill his role as a student. After discussing the activity with the teacher, the COTA decided to make a pumpkin shaped dessert for the fall season rather than a Halloween jack-o-lantern. Some children in the class did not celebrate Halloween, therefore, **cultural considerations** were respected.

Adolescence: Puberty until Onset of Adulthood

SARAH'S SCRAPBOOK SESSION. *Sarah is a 13-year-old girl with a diagnosis of cerebral palsy, spastic hemiplegia type. She receives OT services in an outpatient clinic once a week to address difficulties with self-care and leisure due to the limited use of her right arm. In a previous session, Sarah and the COTA talked about making a scrapbook containing photographs of what she did over the recent winter holidays. Sarah agreed that she would like to work on such a project (Figure 16-6). She brought in selected photographs of a family get-together during their Hanukah celebration. Sarah began the session with preparatory activities to increase sensory awareness and active range of motion of her right arm before starting the scrapbook session.*

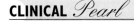

CLINICAL *Pearl*

Many children who have difficulty following verbally issued directions for multistep tasks benefit from visual sequence cards or a visual schedule.

CLINICAL *Pearl*

Before working with food products, determine that the client has no allergies to items such as wheat or peanuts. Also consider religious or other dietary restrictions (e.g., gluten-free diets, lactose intolerance).

The media and/or materials needed are as follows:

- Card stock (culturally appropriate colors and varying thicknesses)
- Scrapbook pages
- Glue
- Adapted cutting equipment
- Stamps and stamp pads
- Hole punch
- String
- Scissors with varied cutting designs
- Stickers, cropping stencils, markers or colored pencils

The method used comprises the following elements:

1. Set the environment. Gather the materials and adjust the chair and table to the appropriate heights to provide support for postural control. Position the materials to facilitate reaching and crossing the midline as well as other extension movements.
2. Organize pictures in the desired pages. Cut card stock to frame pictures with the use of adaptive equipment as needed. Stamp phrases or motifs onto the back-

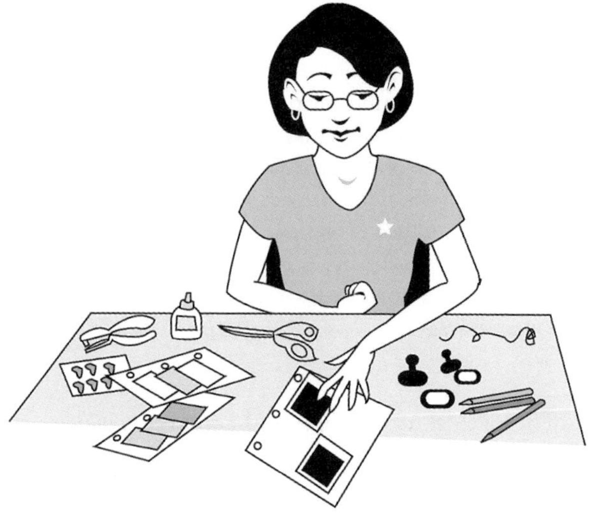

FIGURE 16-6 Sarah works on her scrapbook.

ground of scrapbook pages, place stickers there, and use cropping stencils.

3. Decorate a cover for the book with card stock, stickers, and drawings. Punch holes with a hole puncher, and secure the book by tying it with a string.
4. The COTA and Sarah clean up the work area. Sarah discusses the family activities shown in thepictures.

CLINICAL *Pearl*

Optimum seating posture for completing fine motor activities is obtained by sitting with the hips, knees, and ankles at 90 degrees of flexion. Both feet should be flat on the floor and the pelvis at a slight posterior tilt. The tabletop height should be 2 inches below the elbow crease when the client's arms are positioned vertically at the side of the body (anatomical position).

The client factors addressed and considered for Sarah during this activity are as follows:

Mental functions

- Global: Sarah was motivated to complete the project because it reiterated the importance of her family's values and religious traditions. She was aware of person, place, time, self, and others, which was observed in her description of the events.
- Specific: Thought functions such as recognition were needed to choose the appropriate tools to complete the project. Sarah applied categorization skills as well as perceptual skills to complete such tasks as sorting and placing the pictures on the pages, decorating the pages with the stamps, and cutting the borders to frame the pictures. Higher-level cognitive functions such as time management were used to complete the project within the given time frame of the therapy session.

Sensory functions and pain

- Visual: Acuity and field functions were necessary for Sarah to visually locate and discriminate among the materials on the table surface.
- Additional sensory functions: Kinesthesia and a sense of joint position were enhanced through preparatory activities and then used to retrieve the tools and materials with her affected arm.

Neuromusculoskeletal and movement-related functions

- Joints and bones: Sarah needed to sustain postural alignment while working in and crossing through the midline. Range of motion was needed for all reaching and grasping.
- Muscle: Muscle tone (spasticity) was inhibited for purposeful movement. Muscle power functions were used for Sarah to sustain a sufficient grasp on the scissors, hole puncher, and stamps.
- Movement: The asymmetrical tonic neck reflex was integrated well enough to allow Sarah to turn toward the needed materials without abnormal movement patterns impeding the use of her bilateral upper extremities. Eye-hand coordination was intact for cropping and similar tasks.

Suggestions for grading and adapting the activity are as follows:

- Vary the thickness of the paper to be cut (thicker paper or card stock is easier to hold and gives more sensory feedback during cutting).
- Vary the type of scissors used.
- Use adaptive equipment for stabilizing the paper to be cut if the child is unsuccessful in adequately securing and manipulating the paper.
- Have a completed scrapbook to use as a model if needed.
- Provide assistance and withhold it as appropriate.
- Increase or decrease time constraints as needed (i.e., two sessions in contrast to one).

The COTA addressed Sarah's goal to increase the functional use of her right arm. She considered the areas of occupation because Sarah may follow through with this at home and participate in making scrapbooks as a leisure activity. The COTA adapted the activity to ensure a "just right" challenge for her client.

HARRY'S WOODWORKING PROJECT. Harry is a 17-year-old individual who is moderately mentally disabled and is getting ready to make the transition from a self-contained classroom in high school to a sheltered workshop. It is felt that Harry could complete simple woodworking projects successfully in the workshop. The COTA has been treating Harry once a week for 30 minutes by consulting with his teacher and working toward goals such as improving motor planning to complete multistep activities as well as monitoring and supplying adapted equipment for fine motor activities. Harry's interdisciplinary team, including the school psychologist, job coach, teacher, COTA, speech therapist, and parents, have agreed that it is in Harry's best interests to become familiar with the materials he will be using at the workshop and consider possible adapted equipment needs. The COTA has spoken with personnel involved in the workshop and knows what Harry's tasks will entail. Later she will consult with them regarding Harry's abilities and needs. When he is given a choice, Harry decides to make a small wooden jewelry box as an end-of-year present for his teacher. The COTA consults with the speech therapist, who provides her with sequence cards to increase Harry's independence in completing the task. The COTA gathers supplies such as a built-up handled paintbrush and a sanding block because Harry has a weak grasp. Using the workshop within the school, the COTA carefully set up the environment in consideration of Harry's decreased attention span and distractibility. The COTA and Harry reviewed the plans of the project and decided that it would have to be completed in two sessions.

The media and/or materials needed are as follows:

- A small wooden box obtained from a craft supply store
- Paint and a built-up handled paintbrush
- Sandpaper and a sanding block
- A facemask to wear during sanding
- Decorations (e.g., faux jewels, shells, colored tiles, stencils)
- Glue
- Cloth
- Picture sequence cards

The method used comprises the following elements:

1. Set the environment. Consider the lighting, seating, height of work surface, positioning of materials, and visual and auditory distractions. Protect the work surface with a newspaper or drop cloth. Set up the sequence cards on the work surface.
2. Don the mask in preparation for sanding. Use the sanding block to sand the box.
3. Clean all wood surfaces with a soft cloth.
4. Apply the paint and let it dry.
5. Choose decorations and apply with glue.

The client factors addressed and considered for Harry during this activity are as follows:

CLINICAL *Pearl*

When working with pediatric clients, use low-odor paints and finishes in a well ventilated area. Also consider any skin allergies that may exist and take the necessary precautions, such as using gloves. When using tools and potentially hazardous materials, determine that the client has good safety awareness and provide proper supervision.

Mental functions

- Global: Harry demonstrated conscientiousness in following the rules of the workshop.
- Specific: Sustained attention for 30 minutes enabled Harry to complete the multistep process and safely work with the materials. He needed to use retrospective memory for the safety rules that were reviewed at the start of the project. Perceptual functions such as interpretation of tactile and visual information were important as Harry worked with the sanding block and the paint. Harry also used interpretation of olfactory stimuli as he was aware of the odors of the paint and the freshly sanded wood. Harry was required to use good judgment and problem-solving skills throughout the project. Visual cards aided his ability to sequence the steps, and motor planning was needed to carry them out. His intact sense of self-esteem was reinforced as he carried out the process of choosing the project, constructing it, and presenting it to his teacher.

Neuromusculoskeletal and movement-related functions

- Muscle: Harry was able to initiate and sustain sufficient grasp on the surface of the sanding block and adapted paintbrush despite the decreased strength in his hands.
- Movement: Control of voluntary movement functions was needed to keep the paint in the correct areas and apply the small objects used for decorating the jewelry box as well as opening, closing, and manipulating the containers of spillable contents.

Skin and related structure functions

Protective: The integrity of the skin was required as protection against getting sawdust or paint residue into open wounds or abrasions.

Suggestions for grading and adapting the activity are as follows:

- Adaptive equipment can be used to increase the client's independence, such as a sanding block in Harry's case. Another example would be Dycem or a jig for stabilizing materials.
- Break up the task into several sessions.
- Use written or pictorial sequence cards as needed.
- Allow the client to gather, clean, and put away supplies as feasible.

The COTA considered client factors as well as social and occupational issues while choosing and setting up the activity. Harry felt invested in the project; he was given choices and successfully performed the work with little intervention because of the COTA's careful consideration of activity demands.

SUMMARY

Therapeutic media are important components in OT treatment and have changed with time and technology, varying according to the culture. Media are used within the context of functional activities as well as a preparatory tool to enhance skills and reach therapy goals. The collaboration between the OTR and COTA is best served once the COTA has established service competency and sound clinical reasoning skills. With these skills the COTA can choose media that facilitate the goals and are meaningful to the client. Other important considerations include the selection of media that are developmentally relevant to the client and may be graded according to client factors and activity demands. As explained throughout this chapter, the COTA can design, develop, and implement treatment activities that present the "just right" challenge for each client.

References

1. *American heritage dictionary of the English language*, ed 4, New York, 2000, Houghton Mifflin Company.
2. American Occupational Therapy Association: Occupational therapy practice framework: domain and practice, *Am J Occup Ther* 56:609, 2002.
3. Punwar AJ, Peloquin SM: *Occupational therapy: principles and practice*, ed 2, Baltimore, 2000, Lippincott, Williams & Wilkins.
4. Wilbarger P: Planning an adequate sensory diet: application of sensory processing theory during the first year of life, *Zero to Three* 5:7, 1984.

Recommended Reading

Drake M: *Crafts in therapy and rehabilitation*, ed 2, Thorofare, NJ, 1998, Slack.

Johnson C, Lobdell K, Nesbitt J, Clare M: *Therapeutic crafts: a practical approach*, Thorofare, NJ, 1996, Slack.

Kuffner T: *The children's busy book*, Minnetonka, Minn, 2001, Meadowbrook Press.

Kuffner T: *The preschooler's busy book*, Minnetonka, Minn, 1998, Meadowbrook Press.

Kuffner T: *The toddler's busy book*, Minnetonka, Minn, 1999, Meadowbrook Press.

Wilbarger P: *The sensory diet: activity programs based on sensory processing theory*, American Occupational Therapy Association Sensory Integration Special Interest Section Newsletter, 18:1, 1995.

Wilbarger J, Stackhouse TM: Sensory modulation: a review of the literature. Occupational Therapy Innovations. www.ot-innovations.com/sensory_modulation.html.

Catalogs

S & S
Southpaw
Integrations
Childcraft
Lakeshore

Retail

Michael's
AC Moore
Wal-Mart

Internet

www.craftsforkids.com
www.creativekidsathome.com
www.kidsdomain.com
www.crayola.com
www.theideabox.com
For other current websites, search with the keywords "crafts, kids."

REVIEW *Questions*

1. What should you consider when selecting media?
2. What is the role of the COTA in selecting therapeutic media?
3. Describe why choosing appropriate therapeutic media for different age groups is important.
4. What cultural considerations need to be made during treatment planning?
5. Explain the principle of grading therapeutic activities.
6. What purposes do craft activities in the pediatric population serve?
7. Compare and contrast preparatory activities with functional activities.

SUGGESTED *Activities*

1. Visit a daycare center or preschool during a group craft activity. Observe the media used, activity demands, and method used. Did you notice the staff using any preparatory activities? Based on the results you observed, do you think preparatory activities would have made a difference in the results that were obtained? Would the end result have been different with OT intervention?
2. Choose a medium and formulate five different activities using the same one.
3. Consider one of the above activities and adapt and grade it for various client factors (refer to the Occupational Therapy Practice Framework), age groups, and culture as outlined in this chapter.
4. Plan a craft activity or game considering the following questions. What materials do you need? How much time will it take to prepare the materials? Can you use items on hand or do you have to buy specific ones (e.g., a playground ball and recycled water bottles rather than a purchased bowling game)? Which option is more cost effective?
5. With your planned craft activity or game resulting from the above questions, list the activity demands required to complete it. (Refer to the section on activity demands from the Occupational Therapy Practice Framework.)

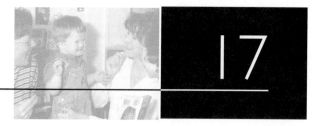

17

Play and Playfulness

JANE CLIFFORD O'BRIEN

CHAPTER *Objectives*

After studying this chapter, the reader will be able to accomplish the following:

- Describe the characteristics of play and playfulness and differentiate between the two
- Describe ways to facilitate play and playfulness in children with special needs
- Describe the way that play is used as a tool in therapy sessions to increase skills
- Describe how play is used as a goal of occupational therapy
- Identify occupational therapy assessments used to evaluate play and playfulness
- Describe techniques that promote play and playfulness

KEY TERMS

Play
Intrinsic motivation
Internal control
Freedom to suspend reality
Pretend play
Playfulness
Spontaneity
Play goals
Play assessment
Play environment
Play adaptations

CHAPTER OUTLINE

Think about a time in your childhood when you were playing.

What were you doing?
Who was with you?
Where were you?
How did you feel?
What was the expression on your face?
What did you learn?
Was playing an important aspect of your day?

Perhaps you are thinking about a time you and your friends sat on your grandmother's porch and played house. Maybe you were playing school. Recalling these moments brings many happy memories to mind. People remember laughing, making friends, learning and testing skills such as who could jump the highest, problem solving, and negotiating. These skills are critical to a child's development and provide a foundation for the future.

Children learn motor, social-emotional, language, and cognitive skills through play.[16,22,25,38,39] To illustrate this fact, consider a 12-month-old girl playing in the water sprinkler. The child bends down to feel the cool water in her hands. She is practicing motor planning, squatting, and balancing while receiving a tactile sensation of the water on her hands. As she cups her hands on the sprinkler, she must coordinate her tiny fingers to grasp the nozzle. Cognitively, she pays attention to the water and tries to figure out what happens when she changes her hand position. She is learning the ways in which liquid differs from the solid ground on which she stands. She problem-solves to keep the water in her hands and tries to understand the reason it leaks through. Orally, she feels the water on her tongue and swallows the droplets. She sticks her tongue out and gathers the liquid in her throat to swallow it. Her 4-year-old brother joins the play activity, and now she must share the sprinkler. He laughs and jumps. She watches and smiles and tries to imitate his skills. She is developing social skills. The children repeat the play activities. By watching them it becomes clear that play requires many skills.

Children learn and refine skills during play.[1,4,5,11,14,20] This is demonstrated as children show off feats of strength and agility, problem-solve to play a game or perform a motor skill, and work out problems that arise. They communicate to satisfy their needs and decide on rules for the activities by negotiating with group members. Often children spend the entire play time deciding on the rules of the game or the way the story will unfold. They use their language skills and must become keen observers of nonverbal communication.[5,8]

Maximizing a child's ability to play interests occupational therapy (OT) practitioners because it is the primary occupation of childhood and critical to the development of skills.[8,21,28] To appreciate its importance, imagine life without play. Life would certainly be lacking without play. Parham and Primeau underscored the importance of play by stating that it may reveal what makes life worth living.[34]

With this appreciation of its importance, imagine making a difference in a child's ability to play. Developing a child's play skills comprehensively affects both the child and his or her family. The child is better able to interact with friends, family members, and the environment.

OT practitioners work with children to enhance their ability to play and therefore make a difference in their lives.

PLAY

Most adults smile when asked to remember a time they were playing. They reminisce about childhood memories of favorite toys and activities. They laugh and relate humorous stories such as the time they attempted to jump over a ditch and failed and fell into the mud. They remember being lost in the woods, falling into the water, having mud fights, and conducting elaborate neighborhood play events. Adults recall historic events such as pretending they were astronauts landing on the moon. They are able to describe the activities, feelings, and skills they gained during play. Most agree that play was and still is fun!

Play is generally defined as a pleasurable, self-initiated activity of which the child is in control. **Intrinsic motivation** is the self-initiation or drive to action that is rewarded by the activity itself rather than some external reward.[8] Intrinsic motivation is demonstrated when children repeat activities over and over.[8] **Internal control** is the extent to which the child is in control of the actions and to some degree the outcome of an activity.[8] Internal control is observed when children spontaneously change the play (e.g., when a 6-year-old boy declares in the middle of a pretend game, "Now I am going to be the good guy."). Intrinsic motivation and internal control are important for the development of problem solving, learning, and socialization skills.

Another element of play is the **freedom to suspend reality,** which is sometimes seen as the ability to participate in make-believe activities, or **pretend play**[8] (Figure 17-1). Pretend play develops as children are able to engage in higher cognitive functioning.[38] They begin by role playing simple everyday actions such as feeding a doll. They are able to engage in elaborate make-believe scenarios as their language and cognitive skills develop.

Freedom to suspend reality also includes teasing, joking, mischief, and bending the rules.[8] Children turn old games into new ones by changing the rules, creating new situations, and using objects imaginatively during play.

A

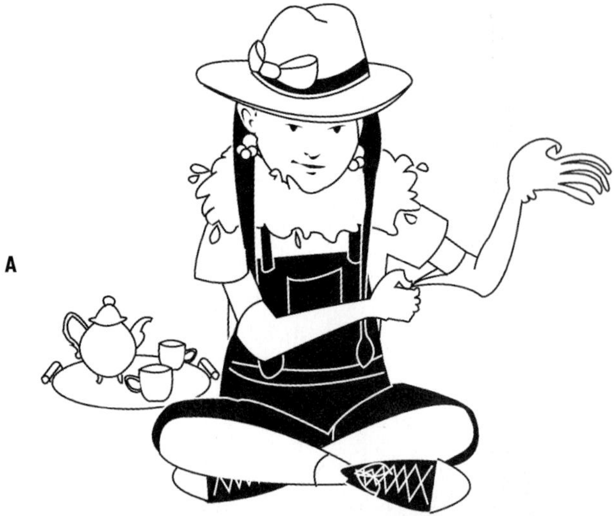

B

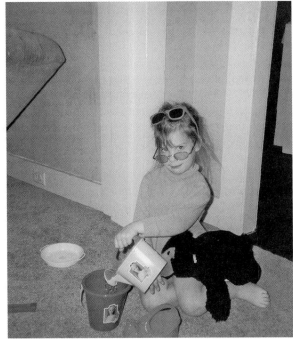

FIGURE 17-1 **A,** Pretend play allows children to break free from rules. **B,** Alison plants a garden with her bear.

Play is the primary occupation of children and a medium for intervention.* Play affords skillful OT practitioners unlimited opportunities to teach, refine, and enable more successful functioning and play.

PLAYFULNESS

Playfulness is the disposition to play.[4,9] It is a style individuals use to flexibly approach problems and can be regarded as an aspect of a child's personality.[9] Playfulness, like play, encompasses intrinsic motivation, internal control, and freedom to suspend reality, all of which occur on a continuum.[8,16,25,28]

*References 9, 16, 20, 27, 32, 33.

CLINICAL *Pearl*

OT practitioners can evaluate the characteristics of play to design intervention. Emphasis is placed on using the child's strengths to improve weak areas. For example, a child who is highly motivated to play but lacks the needed physical skills may be encouraged to perform activities in an alternative way. A child who focuses on the end product versus the process of play (e.g., winning the game) may benefit from participating in play activities that have no end product, such as imaginative play.

Children who are engaged in the play process are intrinsically motivated. They show signs of enjoyment and seem to be having fun.[8,10] Internal control is evidenced in sharing, playing with others, entering new play situations, initiating play, deciding, modifying activities, and challenging themselves.[8,10] Children who use objects creatively or in unconventional ways, tease, and pretend show the element of freedom to suspend reality [8,10] (Figure 17-2).

Children lacking playfulness exhibit problems fulfilling their roles as players. For example, Sam is a 6-year-old boy with sensory integrative dysfunction. He has difficulty with motor tasks and does not play well with friends. Sam is not spontaneous in activities. He requires time to plan the way he will accomplish motor tasks. Sam becomes very upset when he does not get his way. He does not like the rules to change and has trouble changing pace once he is involved in an activity. Moreover, he does not read the other children's cues and frequently plays roughly. He shows poor body awareness by getting too close to the other children. Sam does not initiate play with his peers. His slow and awkward movements cause him to lag behind. During the OT evaluation, Sam states that he has no friends and no one likes him. His parents are worried that Sam does not have any friends. The goal of his OT sessions is to improve his playfulness so that he can interact with friends at home, at school, and in the community.

The OT practitioner works to develop rapport with Sam and plans fun and playful activities. Sam does not initiate play activities but is cooperative and attempts all of them. The OT practitioner strives to see him have fun and be spontaneous during the therapy sessions, hoping that this behavior extends to the home and school.

During one session the OT practitioner and Sam engage in a game of Star Wars. *Sam, playing Darth Vader, runs after the practitioner, saying, "I will get you, Luke." The*

A

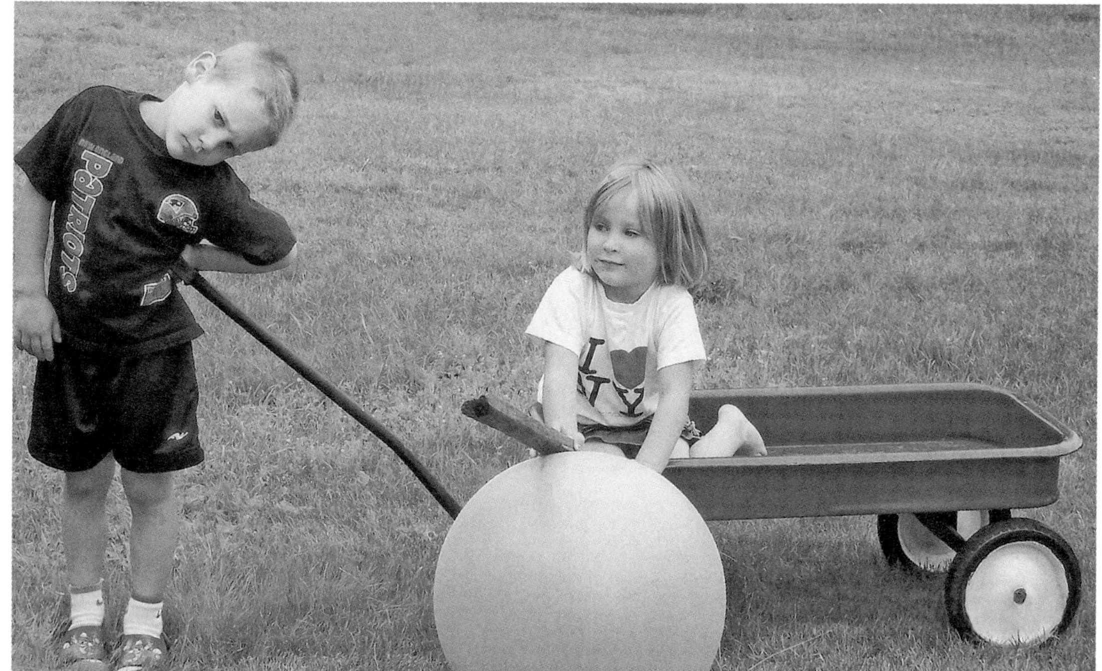

B

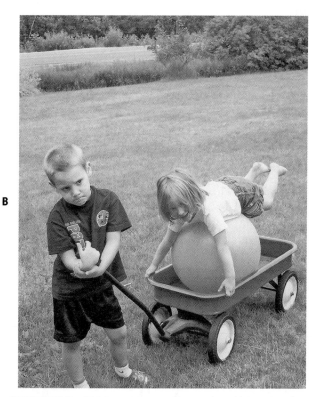

FIGURE 17-2 Children must negotiate and problem-solve during play. **A,** Max and Molly spend time figuring out what to do with the large ball, stick, and wagon. They must negotiate who will pull the wagon. **B,** Max pulls the wagon while Molly is holding on tight. They challenge their motor skills (e.g., balancing on the large ball). Using objects in unconventional ways (e.g., lying on the ball in the wagon) is part of playfulness.

OT practitioner is thrilled that Sam is initiating play. However, shortly thereafter Sam stops playing, looks at the practitioner, and says, "Is it time to go yet?"

Sam exhibits a low level of playfulness. He is not engaged in sustained, intense enjoyment. He focuses on the end product (completing therapy) rather than being intrinsically motivated to play. Poor internal control is characterized by an inability to enter new play situations, initiate play with peers, share, decide what to do, and challenge himself. Sam is able to engage in pretend play when acting out Star Wars *with the OT practitioner but has difficulty reading others' cues, which is evident when he plays too roughly and gets too close to his peers during interactions.*

Considering Sam's limitations and the long-term goal that he be able to play with peers, his therapy objectives include the following.

---

1. Spontaneously initiate a change in activity at least three times during a 45-minute supervised play situation.
2. Respond positively (smile, cooperate with the OT practitioner) when he does not get his way at least three times during a supervised play situation.
3. Enter a group of peers already playing on the playground and participate in the activity without interrupting the play at least three times a week.

4. Engage in a motor challenge during play at least three times during a supervised play situation.

Framing situations as play allows children to know what play is so that they may interact accordingly. They are free to pretend, challenge each other, and tease without malice. All of these actions require that children read nonverbal and verbal cues. Reading nonverbal cues allows children to realize when they have pushed a boundary too far during play.

Scott and Alison are playing in a sandbox, pouring sand on each other. They laugh and watch for cues from each other that say, "This is okay. We are still playing." The game continues, and Alison begins to pour sand on Scott's head. She receives a serious look from Scott. The nonverbal cue says, "Hey, that is a little too close to my eyes. I do not like that." Alison responds with a smile that says, "Oops! I'm sorry," and pours sand on Scott's arm instead. Her nonverbal response says, "Okay, I'll be more careful." This exchange of cues allows the play to continue while they learn to be attentive to each other. They are learning the rules and boundaries of play.

Assessment of a child's playfulness provides information about the way the child processes, problem-solves, and manages emotional stress. These skills are important to the child's development and social well-being.

NATURE OF PLAY AND PLAYFULNESS

OT practitioners must understand the nature of play and playfulness in order to use it effectively as an intervention technique. When children play and are playful they may laugh, smile, and be active. They may also be serious, quiet, and totally absorbed in play, depending on the activity (Figure 17-3). Play can be frustrating, and it can involve failures. The flexible and spontaneous nature of play and playfulness is demonstrated when children change themes or use toys in unpredictable ways.

The process (doing) rather than the product (outcome) provides the primary source of reward in play activities.[8] Children engage in play for its own sake.[9,10] Playful children discover, create, and explore. Therefore, no way of playing is right or wrong. It is a safe outlet for children to challenge themselves and helps them develop skills.

OT practitioners must remember to maintain the nature of play and playfulness during therapy. Children with special needs may require additional assistance to play.[24,36] OT practitioners are knowledgeable about the abilities of children with special needs and are therefore in an ideal position to promote play and playfulness.

CONSIDERATIONS FOR PLAY

The normal sequence for the development of play is often delayed in children with special needs.* (See Chapter 7 for a discussion of this sequence.) This may be the result of limited physical, cognitive, or social-emotional skills.[20,22,26] For example, a young girl who is unable to bring her hands to her mouth has trouble exploring her environment. Children who are unable to experience sensations in a normal manner often require intervention to engage in normal play opportunities, which stimulate their growth and development. If they are not afforded these opportunities, they may exhibit poor play skills.[26,30,36] Children with special needs may require environmental and play adaptations and intervention to provide them with these experiences.[26,29,30] For example, children who are unable to sit independently may benefit from sitting in an adapted chair. In this way they can interact and play at the same level as their peers without fear of falling over.[30]

Children with special needs require time to develop their abilities. They may take longer to respond, make less obvious responses, initiate activities less frequently, and be less interactive than other children.[24,29] Researchers and theorists report that children with special needs are often passive in their play.[22,24,26] In cases involving children with mental retardation, they have been described as exhibiting a restricted repertoire of play and language, decreased attention span, and less social interaction during play.[22,24,26] In cases involving children with autism, they are described as demonstrating more stereotypical movements and less diversity in play.[22,36] Children with visual impairments are less interested in reaching out to explore and engage in social exchanges during play.[22] Children with hearing impairments show less symbolic and less organized play.[22]

Children with special needs require assistance in order to meet developmental challenges and learn ways to play.[19,22,24,26,29] OT practitioners must understand typical play patterns and support children when teaching skills and facilitating play. For example, OT practitioners can increase **spontaneity** in children by allowing them to discover play materials that have been hidden or placed within reach.[12,26,29,36]

CLINICAL *Pearl*

Children play in various positions. OT practitioners make sure that children with special needs spend time in many positions, such as supine, quadruped, sitting, and standing. Play time is not the time to work on positioning. Children should be free to use their arms and hands and feel safe.

*References 18, 20, 22, 24, 26, 29.

A

B

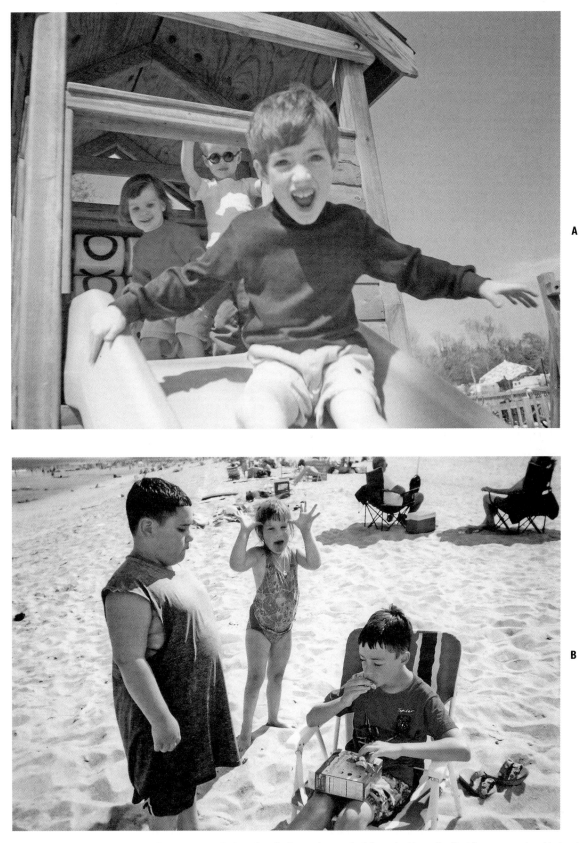

FIGURE 17-3 Playful children may be silly or serious during play. **A,** Scott shows playfulness by his smile. **B,** Alison teases her big brother Scott.

Continued

C

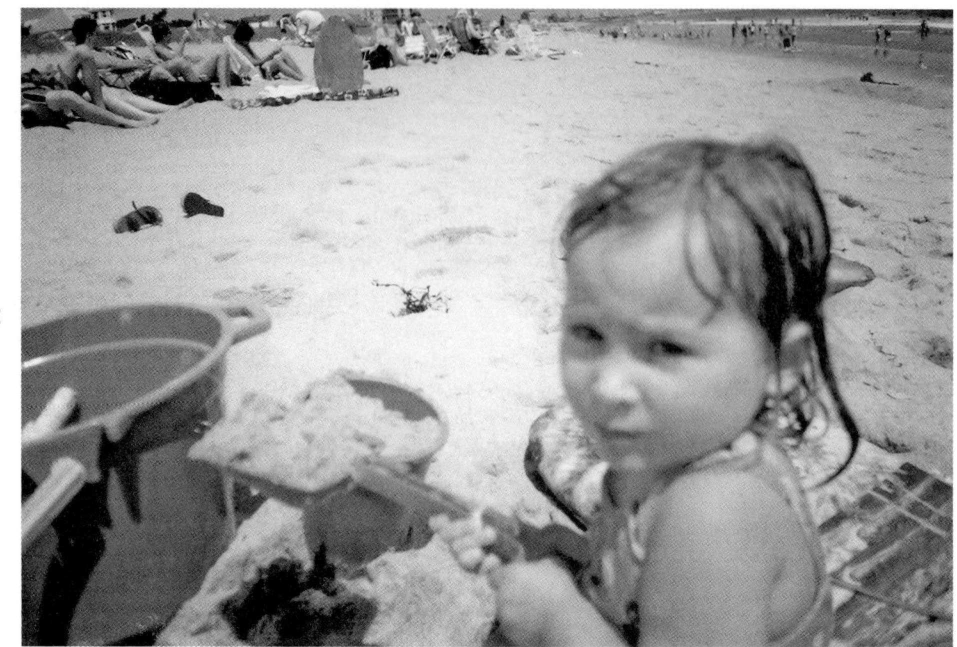

FIGURE 17-3, cont'd **C,** Molly is quite serious while building a sandcastle.

OT practitioners must identify the child's strengths and weaknesses, as well as those of the family, to design effective intervention. Capitalizing on strengths can increase the success of therapy and facilitate advanced play skills.

CLINICAL *Pearl*

Observe the child's movements when deciding where to position a switch. Place the switch where the child can activate it by using movement patterns he uses automatically. This promotes play and provides the child with control and immediate success.

RELEVANCE OF PLAY

Twelve-month-old Frankie cannot sit up because of hydrocephalus and poor trunk tone. He is nonverbal. He can move his arms but is unable to reach and grasp objects. He occasionally smiles and laughs. His vision is poor. The OT practitioner places a mercury switch attached to a flashlight on his arm after positioning him. If he raises his arm, the flashlight lights up in his face. Frankie raises his arm soon after the switch is placed on his arm and smiles when the flashlight lights up in his face. He puts his arm down and the light turns off. Frankie laughs and laughs. He repeats this activity numerous times. It is evident that he realizes he is in control of the light. His mother has tears in her eyes. She turns to the practitioner and says, "Frankie is playing."

OT changed this family's perception of Frankie by showing them his ability to play, which is both a powerful tool and an important outcome in OT.

OT practitioners work with families, educators, and other professionals to improve the quality of life for children and their families. Play is vital to a child's development and an important outcome of intervention. OT practitioners who use play may be faced with parents and professionals who do not take them seriously.[7,9,17] Engaging the parents in discussions from the beginning educates them about the importance of play during therapy sessions. Practitioners should discuss with parents how the session went and the progress made toward the goals. OT practitioners who recognize that the parents do not value play as a goal may decide to emphasize the use of play as a tool to increase the child's skills in other areas. Professionals may take OT practitioners more seriously once they see the progress a child makes in therapy. Practitioners may frequently need to educate parents and professionals on the purpose of the use of play.

Activities recommended for the home should be limited to those that are fun and nonthreatening for the child in order to promote play and playfulness. The child can engage in activities in which he can show off his abilities to his parents. This is motivating for both the child and the parents. OT practitioners investigate the role of play in the children's lives and focus on providing them with a means to play.

Play as a Tool

Play is often used as a tool to increase skill development. Therapy is designed around play activities that will increase skills such as strength, motor planning, problem solving, grasping, and handwriting, which are necessary for the child to function. Using play as a tool to improve a child's ability to function has many advantages. Children typically cooperate and readily engage in play. Most goals can be addressed during a play session because play encompasses a variety of activities.

The characteristics of play (i.e., intrinsic motivation, internal control, and suspension of reality) need to be present when play is used as a tool to improve a child's skills. These characteristics occur within the framework of a play setting. The OT practitioner arranges the environment so that children can choose activities that help meet their goals while having fun. The practitioner allows the child to tease, engage in mischief, and face challenges.

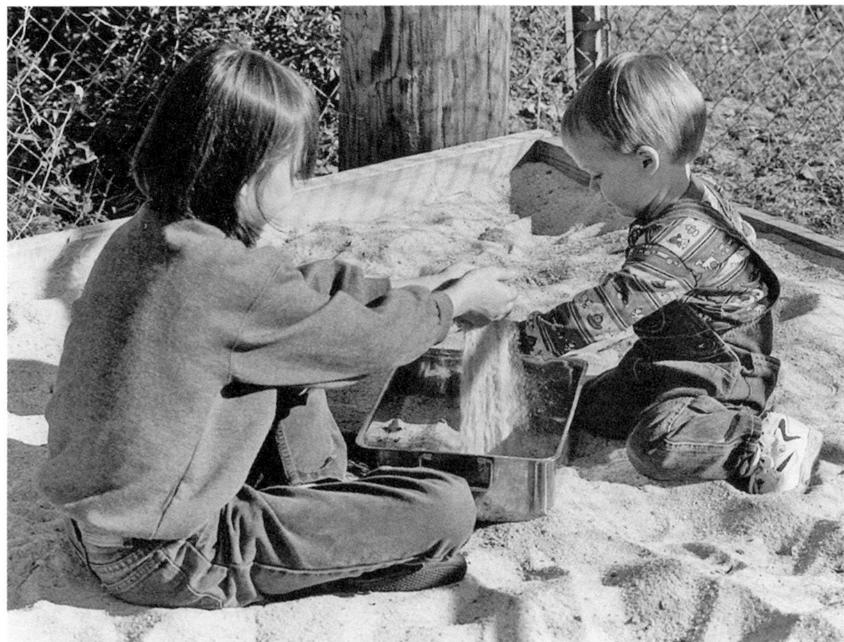

A

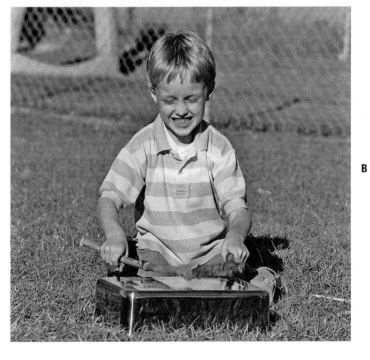

B

FIGURE 17-4 Everyday household objects allow for pretend play and creativity. **A,** A brother and sister are using a stainless steel cake pan to build sandcastles. **B,** The same cake pan is turned upside down and, with some sticks from the yard, is being used as a drum.

CLINICAL *Pearl*

Many household items make novel toys for the clinic and can also be used at home. Pots and pans can be musical instruments, containers, or even hats. They promote pretend play. Use cardboard boxes, grocery bags, and laundry baskets for a variety of play activities. Bring them into the clinic to allow children to explore and create with them (Figure 17-4).

Making therapy sessions fun through play is not always easy. OT practitioners must set up an environment to encourage the child to choose activities that foster therapy goals. This is considered the *art* of therapy.[2,9] The OT practitioner sets up *just* the *right* challenge, which is one that is neither too hard nor too easy.[2,9] The OT practitioner must know the child's strengths and weaknesses to do this effectively. Some children are competitive and enjoy such games. Others fear failure and may be easily intimidated by competitive games. Some children enjoy roughhousing and others do not. Making a therapy session fun means observing a child's subtle cues and spontaneously adapting the session to maintain a level of excitement and motivation.

A physically and emotionally safe environment allows the child to feel in control. The OT practitioner designs activities to target specific skills. The child is only aware that the activity is fun. Often the practitioner may need to discreetly change the way the task is performed to get the maximum benefit from the activity. This must be done playfully to keep the flow of the play session going.[16] Sometimes the practice of a skill takes priority over playing.

A critical element of play is for activities to be free from rules. This does not mean that rules are not present in play activities but that they are negotiable. Children may make up new rules and change them during play. OT practitioners should provide enough rules for children to feel secure and safe without imposing so many that they do not feel free to play. Both the child and practitioner must have the freedom to change the activity. Therefore, if a child is performing an activity that does not promote the therapy goals, the practitioner can modify the challenge. This is illustrated in a therapy session challenging David's balance.

David is kneeling on a platform swing and propelling it forward and backward. The practitioner increases the skill level required by saying, "Oh, here come the asteroids," and throwing large balls under the swing. David looks at the OT practitioner, smiles, and says, "Hey, no fair. I didn't know that was coming." The practitioner responds, "The asteroids came out of nowhere! Luckily, you are Superman and were able to stay on the spaceship!" The changes are skillfully made so that the session remains playful.

CLINICAL *Pearl*

Children love to swing. Remember that swings are not just for children with sensory integrative dysfunction. Many children benefit from the sensations and movement patterns that accompany swinging.

Children can imagine a therapy session to be a spaceship ride, an Olympic quest, a deep sea diving expedition, a skiing event, or a leisurely stroll down the alley. Through pretend play the child gains skills in imagination, verbalization, and communication. Pretend play allows the practitioner to use the same equipment in countless ways that tap into the child's imagination. Teasing, joking, and mischief are parts of play. The child may teasingly throw a softball to hit the practitioner's head. They may joke that the OT practitioner cannot perform a skill. Children develop their sense of humor during play.

Play provides an excellent tool for intervention when used correctly because children are highly motivated to participate.*

Angie is a 2-year-old girl with hemiplegia on the right side of her body. She lives with her two brothers, ages 8 and 9, and her parents. Angie attends day care daily. She receives OT services for 1 hour weekly. Her parents report that she does not play well with other children. She grabs their toys, pushes them, and screams to have her needs met. She does not like to be touched on her right side and does little weight bearing on that side. Angie has a difficult time engaging in play activities. She screams and cries when the practitioner touches her on the right arm. She does not initiate play. Angie exhibits decreased active range of motion (AROM) in her right arm.

The OT practitioner designs treatment that involves play to increase Angie's use of her right side. (See Chapter 7 for a description of the sequence and development of typical play and useful information for designing this type of intervention.) The OT practitioner considers Angie's age when choosing the play activities. Based on his or her knowledge of 2-year-old children, the practitioner chooses busy and messy play activities. According to Parten, 2 year olds usually participate in solitary play but do make an effort to interact with other children.[35,37] The practitioner notes that 2-year-old children enjoy sensory activities such as playing in sandboxes, water play, and working with Play-

*References 9, 11, 12, 17, 22, 27, 29.

Doh. They also enjoy manipulative toys such as Legos, pop-up toys, and blocks and gross motor toys such as balls, riding toys, and swings. Table 17-1 includes a list of suitable toys and activities for various ages.

The child's age and gender, the setting, and the concerns of the parents must be considered when writing the goals and objectives of therapy. The OT practitioner considers the child's physical capabilities and the factors interfering with

TABLE 17-1

Toys and Play Activities Designed to Target Selected Client Factors

CLIENT FACTOR	TOYS AND ACTIVITIES
Sensory Function	
Sensory awareness and sensory processing	
Tactile	Water play, massage, Play Doh, koosh balls, glue, beans, sand play, tactile boards, brushing, lotion games, stickers
Proprioceptive	Trampolines, jumping, pulling on ropes, climbing ladders, tug-of-war, pulling a wagon, wheelbarrow walking, pushing
Vestibular	Riding a bike, skateboarding, see-saw, sliding, swinging, Sit and Spin, rocking horse
Visual	Mobiles, toys that move, bright-colored rattles and toys, mirrors
Auditory	Musical toys, bells, rattles, tape recorders, songs
Gustatory	Food, gum, candy
Olfactory	Smelly markers, Play Doh, smelly stickers, food
Neuromusculoskeletal and Movement-Related Functions	
Strength	Ball games, bike riding, manipulative games, jump rope, Red Rover, London Bridge, swimming, sports
Endurance	Repetitive games, walking, sports, hiking, swimming, bike riding, climbing
Postural control	Trampolines, bike riding, sports, swimming, climbing, walking on an uneven trail
Gross coordination	Outdoor playground equipment, bikes, sports, water, outdoor play
Fine motor	Manipulative, arts and crafts, small toys, figurines, dolls, dress-up, sewing, coloring, cutting
Oral motor	Musical instruments, whistles, bubble blowers, pinwheels
Mental Functions (Affective, Cognitive, Perceptual)	
Affective	
Psychological	Self-esteem board games, art projects, motor challenges
Interpersonal	Pictionary, team games, Twister, new games
Self-expression	Arts and crafts, pottery, clay, dance
Self-management	
Coping skills	Monopoly, life skills game, role playing
Cognitive	
Memory, sequencing	Board games (e.g., Memory, Clue, Monopoly, Candy Land)
Categorization	Card games (e.g., Hearts, Go Fish), sorting, matching games
Spatial operations	Puzzles, models, arts and crafts, Legos, Lincoln Logs
Problem solving	Board games, card games, arts and crafts, puzzles
Perceptual	
Perceptual processing	Puzzles, building blocks, doll houses, farms, building logs, model cars and airplanes, paper dolls, coloring books, mazes, computer games, dress-up, obstacle courses, Simon Says, Follow-the-Leader

Adapted from the American Occupational Therapy Association: Uniform terminology for occupational therapy, *Am J Occup Ther* 48:1047, 1994; American Occupational Therapy Association: Occupational therapy practice framework: domain and process, *Am J Occup Ther* 56:609, 2002.

her ability to play. Angie has right-sided hypersensitivity. She does not bear weight on the right side. Considering Angie's limitations and the long-term goal that she will use her right hand spontaneously for bimanual activities, Angie's therapy objectives include the following:

1. *She will spontaneously reach for objects placed above her head with her right hand at least five times during a 45-minute therapy session.*
2. *Using two hands, she will catch a 20-inch ball tossed underhand from two feet away at least three times in a 45-minute session.*
3. *She will walk at least 10 feet while holding on with both hands to a push toy such as a shopping cart.*
4. *She will use both hands to take apart small objects such as pop beads.*

Box 17-1 contains sample objectives involving play as a tool for OT intervention.

The practitioner designs play activities that incorporate the use of Angie's right side. She plays games rolling a large ball, wheelbarrow racing, and climbing a ladder. She pulls pop beads apart, dresses baby dolls, pours sand and water into containers, and makes confetti out of newspaper. All these activities require Angie to use both arms. The practitioner stages the activities so that Angie is successful. The OT practitioner frequently provides Angie with hand-over-hand assistance. S/he watches for cues from Angie when placing a hand on her arms. The practitioner uses humor and laughter to keep the session playful. Treatment focuses on keeping the atmosphere fun and playful while increasing the functional use of Angie's right arm. The emphasis of the treatment session is to promote bilateral hand skill development. The OT practitioner assists Angie in using her right hand during play.

BOX 17-1

Sample Objectives When Play Is the Tool for Occupational Therapy Intervention

- Child will catch a large object such as a beach ball with both hands at least five times when it is thrown directly to him or her from 3 feet away.
- Child will utilize a neat pincer grip to pick up ten small objects for use in daily activities.
- Child will ride a bike at least 20 yards in a straight line without falling.
- Child will make at least three out of ten baskets from the free-throw line.
- Child will put on and button a shirt independently.

CLINICAL *Pearl*

Children love little packages. Wrap little items in small boxes and allow the children to unwrap them to work on fine motor skills through play. Have them wrap up surprises for other children as a fun way to work on hand skills.

Table 17-1 lists toys associated with the development of specific client factors. Angie's case demonstrates the use of play as a tool to improve a child's physical skills. The practitioner uses play activities to increase the ability of the child to use her right side.

Play as a Goal

OT practitioners must be careful to avoid "teaching" play. They model play, cultivate the skills needed for play, and set up the environment to facilitate play. OT practitioners must ensure that play is enjoyable. Increasing the skills required for play is important and beneficial to the child.

OT practitioners must maintain the quality of play.[9,21,37] A child who has the skills needed for play but does not engage in spontaneous and intrinsically motivated activity is at risk. That child may show deficits in play that will carry over to the school, home, and community. Play deficits in childhood may inhibit a child's ability to gain the needed skills for adulthood.[11,13-15,20,23,37] Therefore, it is important for OT practitioners to target play as a goal of therapy.

The OT practitioner emphasizes the child's approach to activities and the manner in which the child plays when play itself is the goal of therapy. If play is viewed as a goal of therapy rather than merely a tool of intervention, the practitioner notices the way Angie engages in play, not just whether she uses her right hand to manipulate a toy. A short-term objective to increase Angie's play might be for her to spontaneously initiate play with a peer at least three times during an adult-supervised play session. Box 17-2 contains sample objectives when play is the goal of OT intervention.

Angie's OT sessions include playmates because she needs assistance playing with others. The practitioner designs the environment to encourage Angie to respond to changes and be spontaneous. Angie participates in bilateral activities such as playing with balls, wheelbarrow racing, and ladder climbing. The practitioner provides a playful attitude while allowing Angie to pick the activities and choose the way she

BOX 17-2

Sample Objectives When Play or Playfulness Is the Intended Outcome of Occupational Therapy Intervention

- Child will initiate one new activity during an adult-supervised play session.
- Child will enter into a play activity (already in progress) without disrupting the group during an adult-supervised play session.
- Child will stay with the same basic play theme for at least 15 minutes during an adult-supervised play session.
- Child will use an object in an unconventional manner spontaneously at least once during an adult-supervised play session.
- Child will share toys with another child (trading toys at least three times) during a 15-minute play session.

will perform them. The practitioner facilitates sharing, negotiating, and taking turns. The OT practitioner encourages the child's parents and teachers to facilitate the skills of sharing, negotiating, and taking turns at home and school, providing Angie with many opportunities to improve her play skills.

CLINICAL *Pearl*

Invite another child or practitioner to keep the play sessions exciting. This is a great way to learn new activities and methods of playing.

Angie's second session differs from the first, which targeted the use of her right hand, in that the emphasis is now on both interaction and motor skills as opposed to motor skills alone. The OT practitioner pays close attention to Angie's ability to engage in spontaneous activity, choose a variety of tasks, initiate changes, and read the cues of her peers. The Test of Playfulness (ToP) is used as a framework for the observation, evaluation, and documentation of playfulness.[8] (O'Brien and colleagues were able to design ***play goals*** *after a parental interview and a 30-minute observation of free play using the ToP as a guide.[31])*

It is possible to use play as both a tool for therapy and a goal of therapy sessions. In Angie's case, it would be appropriate to work on increasing the use of her right side as well as improving play. This takes skill on the part of the OT practitioner, who must have the trust of the child and read his or her cues very carefully to maintain the child's engagement in play.

ROLE OF THE REGISTERED OCCUPATIONAL THERAPIST AND CERTIFIED OCCUPATIONAL THERAPY ASSISTANT DURING PLAY ASSESSMENT

The observation of children during play provides OT practitioners with important information. **Play assessment,** in combination with parent, child, and teacher interviews, provides the practitioner with necessary information. Bryze supports the contributions of narratives in collecting information on play.[6] These narratives focus on the interviews of parents, caregivers, and children.

OT practitioners use a variety of play assessments when working with children with special needs. (See Appendix A of Chapter 17 for descriptions of several play assessments.) The registered occupational therapist (OTR) is responsible for the evaluation and analysis of information when evaluating play but can delegate portions of the assessment to the certified occupational therapy assistant (COTA), who can assist in interviewing the teachers and caregivers and observing the children during play. The OT practitioner uses the results of the play assessments to design therapy goals and provide effective intervention. Play assessments provide a foundation for organizing information.

It is not always possible to evaluate children with moderate to severe physical and cognitive disabilities through standardized testing. However, play evaluations may be administered to all children. These evaluations provide the flexibility needed to assess children and give measurable information concerning a child's strengths and weaknesses. For example, the ToP has been found to be reliable in measuring playfulness in children with mental retardation; the Knox Preschool Play Scale (PPS) is reliable in measuring play skills in children with multiple handicaps. The Transdisciplinary Play-Based Assessment (TPBA) is designed to be used with all children and includes an accompanying intervention manual (Transdisciplinary Play-Based Intervention [TPBI]) to assist therapists in intervention planning. The findings obtained from play evaluations are easily translated into measurable goals for therapy sessions that allow clinicians to organize intervention more deliberately, thereby benefiting the children they treat.

TECHNIQUES TO PROMOTE PLAY AND PLAYFULNESS

There is an art and science to fully utilizing play in OT practice. Just as with any treatment, OT practitioners must practice the techniques. The science of using play involves understanding the characteristics, components, and settings that facilitate it. OT practitioners must identify the desired outcome of therapy and evaluate the motor, psychological, and/or social factors interfering with the child's ability to play.

Creating a therapeutic environment involves analyzing a child's skills and determining the way(s) to adapt activities. Knowledge of the development of the motor, cognitive, language, social-emotional, and play skills of children is essential to designing effective treatment. Examination of the environment and knowledge of the child's culture help OT practitioners determine appropriate play activities.

Therapy using play requires the OT practitioner to find the child within himself or herself. Playful practitioners practice play and are able to support the child's playful nature. Clinical expertise in the therapeutic use of self is important for understanding the way(s) to evoke play in children and is considered part of the art of therapy. OT practitioners engage in the art of therapy when they connect with the child. Skillful practitioners play effortlessly with children while challenging them to acquire and master new skills. The art of therapy involves weaving clinical judgment, skill, and individual style into successful therapy sessions.

Examples of How to Improve Playfulness

- Practitioners set up the environment to facilitate playfulness in children and adolescents. The environment can be easily modified to promote playfulness.
- Set up a playful environment. Spaces can be modified to meet the needs of the child.
- Set up a "tea party" theme by adding a small table, tea set, and pink table cloth.
- Use curtains or dividers to separate children's and adults' spaces if sharing the clinic.
- Change themes of space through paintings or party items (e.g., birds, piñatas, or other decorations)
- Keep the space child friendly.
- Music adds a playful nature to the space.
- Introduce the child's favorite toys. You may ask them to bring one or two to the session.
- Add an element of "pretend" to the session.
- Change the demands of the task to provide the *just right* challenge.

CLINICAL *Pearl*

Get in touch with your playful side. Spend a day with a child to remember the way it feels to play. Let the child lead you and show you how to play.

- Magnetic blocks are easier for children with coordination difficulties.
- Adaptive toys allow children to hit a switch or pull a lever to activate a toy.
- Puppets come in all sizes so that they can be easily graded.
- Limiting the directions to games makes it easier for children.
- Change the rules to make children more successful, or bring the target closer.
- Finger painting is easier than using a brush.
- Sitting in adapted chairs allows children to use their hands better.
- Allow for a variety of positions during play.
- Remember that eye contact may be overwhelming to some children. In addition, it is not imperative that children smile to have fun.
- Allow the child to make changes to the activity.

Characteristics of Playful Occupational Therapy Practitioners

OT practitioners can cultivate specific characteristics in themselves that promote play (Box 17-3). They must be playful themselves if they wish to treat children effectively and facilitate play and playfulness. Children view a happy, smiling practitioner, one who is able to interact joyfully with them, as playful.

It is important for the practitioner to establish goals and structure the treatment setting. However, the OT practitioner must be flexible enough to change the activity based on the child's responses. S/he needs to be skillful in planning and setting up a playful environment so that the child will choose activities that further the therapeutic goals. This ensures that therapy will be fun for the child. Facilitating play requires that the practitioner keep goals clearly in mind while structuring the environment and adjusting the mode of interaction.[17,22]

OT practitioners acting as play facilitators attend to a child's interests, elaborate on his or her verbalizations, and model play behaviors.[22] If an activity is not challenging to a child but s/he is enjoying it, the practitioner may decide to continue the activity before increasing the skill required. The child may need to practice the task to gain mastery.[37] Children need to be challenged in all areas of development. OT practitioners need to provide social, cognitive, and motor challenges.

Practitioners need to be creative to spark children's imaginations during play sessions. (See Appendix B of Chapter 17 for a resource list of play ideas.) A sense of humor is vital; practitioners may have to act silly, make mistakes, and even act as a peer to encourage a child to play. From the child's point of view, the practitioner may seem to demand that s/he perform tasks that seem much

BOX 17-3

Characteristics of Occupational Therapy Practitioners That Promote Play and Playfulness in Children

- *Playfulness.* Have warm, inviting, and sincere personalities
- *Flexibility, creativity, and spontaneity.* Change activities and pace based on the needs of the child. Able to stop activities and create new ones if needed
- *Child friendliness.* Interact at the child's level and are familiar with child's terms and current trends, such as *Dalmatians, Power Rangers, Barney,* and *Teletubbies*
- *Sense of humor.* Try out silly things and laugh at themselves
- *Intuition.* Are able to read child's cues (nonverbal and verbal) and are aware of signs of boredom, fatigue, or frustration
- *Positive reinforcement.* Offer sincere praise when child has performed well, has tried very hard, or is in need of support
- *Patience.* Allow child to experience some frustration. Help the child work on frustration tolerance through play
- *Observational skills.* Able to watch and not intervene at every turn. Allow the child to be in control
- *Openness.* Learn new games and play activities from children. Watch children in many settings to keep activities novel
- *Fun.* Smile, laugh, and play with the child

harder to them than to the adult. When a child asks to play the role of the practitioner and then says, "Okay, now stand on your head and clap your hands together behind your back three times. I will time you," this suggests that the degree of challenge the child has experienced during treatment sessions is too much.

Reading a child's verbal and nonverbal cues provides OT practitioners with information that may change the play activities. This is important in gaining the trust of the child. Children need to feel that someone is listening to them. Skillful OT practitioners use the child's cues as indicators of stress and emotion. They can assist children in learning to listen to and give cues by nodding and listening to their nonverbal and verbal feedback.

Praising children is highly effective if done properly. They appreciate honest and specific praise. They realize that play can be frustrating and not always successful. OT practitioners need to allow children with special needs to feel frustration and experience failure sometimes.

Playful practitioners allow children to make mistakes occasionally. Some of the most playful sessions are those in which the children make mistakes along the way. It is the process that is important.

CLINICAL *Pearl*

Provide children with a theme for play activities. Ask them to bring in something from home and use it during therapy.

An obstacle course in the clinic is difficult for Jon to climb on without falling. He tries numerous times and each time falls into the pillows laughing. He is determined to succeed. He works on this activity until he succeeds in doing it properly. Once he masters the task he moves on to something new. For Jon, falling into the pillows is almost as fun as staying on the course.

Practitioners must have a sense of humor. They must take into consideration the setting and the play frame. Therefore, if the child says, "I have a laser gun," during a pretend game, the practitioner does not become alarmed. However, a child may be crying out for help during play. OT practitioners should take these opportunities to reach out to the child. Perhaps the most important characteristic of playful practitioners is that they have fun. Children learn the way to play from practitioners who get involved in it. They smile, laugh, and enjoy playing.

BOX 17-4

Characteristics of Optimum Play Environment

- *Playful.* Provides cheerful, warm, and safe feeling
- *Fun and inviting.* Is child friendly; is decorated in such a way that children enjoy being there
- *Safe.* Keeps children physically and emotionally safe so that they can feel free to explore and play; has mats available
- *Novel.* Provides various new toys and challenges
- *Flexible and creative.* Allows children to play in different ways with the toys; is arranged to promote a variety of play activities
- *Encouraging.* Includes adults who facilitate play, are not directive, ensure that the children are safe, assist when needed, and disappear when appropriate
- *Creative.* Materials and supplies are available to promote creativity and do not necessarily have an end product. Children enjoy sand, water, clay, and Play-Doh
- *Quiet.* Allows children some space to be alone if they desire

Characteristics of Optimum Play Environment

The optimum **play environment** has specific characteristics (Box 17-4); first and foremost is a safe environment.[3,38]

Children must be and feel physically and emotionally safe. The environment should have a variety of age-appropriate toys from which the child can choose.[3,12,17,22,29] These toys need not be expensive; children enjoy playing with household items such as pots and pans.

The OT practitioner should design an environment that promotes novelty, the opportunity for exploration, repetition, and the imitation of competent role models.[16] Novelty makes the session fun and enjoyable, fosters creativity, and creates arousal. Providing an environment that allows for exploration requires arranging toys so that children can look for them, reach them, and investigate the surroundings. They learn from repetition and should be allowed to do this during play. Repetition is encouraged by the initiation of the same activity with a different theme, goal, or object. For example, the practitioner may ask a child to throw a ball at a new target to continue the activity. Being a competent role model requires the practitioner to demonstrate playful behavior. Parents and professionals need to give children space to work out play scenarios, and this space must be safe (Box 17-5).

BOX 17-5

Safety in the Play Environment

THE BEST SAFETY PRECAUTION IS TO WATCH ALL CHILDREN CAREFULLY AT ALL TIMES

- Plug all electrical outlets with safety caps.
- Ensure that bookshelves are sturdy and will not topple. Anchor to the wall at the top.
- Do not place toys so that they will fall on toddlers' heads when they pull them down.
- Cut all cords so that children cannot get caught in them.
- Have plenty of mats under equipment.
- Pad corners of walls and furniture.
- Know infant CPR.
- Be sure that cleaning supplies and medications are out of reach.
- Be sure that water tables are closed when not in use.
- Watch for and mop up slippery surfaces.
- Have a first-aid kit available and review emergency procedures.
- Check out all equipment periodically to ensure that it is in good working order.
- Clean and disinfect toys and surfaces after each use.
- Follow universal precautions for cleaning up spills.

The play space should be arranged to promote a variety of types of play[1,3] (see Chapter 7). The ways to promote different types of play include the following.

1. *Pretend play.* This type of play promotes make-believe and may include the kitchen table, play food, puppets, and dress-up clothes.
2. *Constructive play.* This type of play is designed to allow children to build and create things and includes blocks, Legos, Lincoln Logs, and various other building toys; arts and crafts, paper; crayons, clay, markers, paint, chalk, and scissors; and wind-up toys, beads, and small manipulative toys.
3. *Reflective or reading area.* This is a quiet area where children can go to read and/or write. Items included in this area may include books, audiotapes, videotapes, paper, and pencils.
4. *Sensorimotor area.* This area is for major motor movements. Toys and equipment present in this area include mats, balls, bikes, swings, balance beams, and trampolines.
5. *Exploratory play.* This type of play includes water, sand, and other tactile play activities.
6. *Computer play.* This play area includes a computer with a variety of games.
7. *Musical play.* This type of play promotes music and includes whistles, rattles, drums, pianos, rhythm games, singing, and tapes.

The OT practitioner should allow children to express creativity and spontaneity. Toys have many uses in addition to those suggested by the manufacturer. Unless the children are being harmful to others or themselves, allow them to use toys in different ways. Some children are not aware of the way the toy is typically used. After they have taken some time to explore it, the practitioner may demonstrate the expected way without imposing only one method of playing with the toy.

Many children enjoy roughhousing. Children with special needs may also enjoy this. Gentle roughhousing can provide sensory input to them and is often therapeutic and fun. Children of all ages learn through physical contact, and therapy sessions can provide a safe environment for this type of contact. Children may push each other playfully, and adults do not always need to intervene.

CLINICAL *Pearl*

Musical games are fun and playful ways to help a child become more attentive to verbal directions. The child must pay attention to the words of the song or beat of the music to follow along.

Playful environments take advantage of themes and are decorated for the occasion. Make sure that the play environment is not too stimulating. Use warm colors such as pinks, melons, and yellows.[2] The temperature of the room should be warm, not too hot or cold. Children enjoy being outdoors, so they should be able to play in outdoor settings as well. They should have places for quiet time and concentration.

The best way to promote play and playfulness in children is to be a playful adult in a playful environment. Arranging the play environment helps OT practitioners become skillful at utilizing the environment therapeutically.

SUMMARY

OT practitioners view play as the major occupation of childhood and believe it is crucial to a child's development. They facilitate the development of play in children with special needs. Therefore, they must understand the characteristics of play if they wish to make significant changes in the play of the children they treat. Practitioners play an important role in helping parents, teachers, and peers play with children with special needs. They may be able to make simple **play adaptations** that allow these children to be included with their peers in play.

Play is a fun, spontaneous, internally motivated, and self-directed activity that is free from rigid rules. *Playfulness* is defined as an individual's disposition to play. OT practitioners typically use play as a tool to improve a child's skills and a goal for therapy.

OT practitioners should expand their use of play by exploring its characteristics and practicing these techniques in the treatment of children. They can have a tremendous impact on the lives of children and their families through fun, creative, enjoyable, and spontaneous activities, allowing children to develop play skills that will carry over to the home, school, and community and help prepare them for adult roles.

References

1. Axline VM: Play therapy procedures and results. In Schaefer C, editor: *The therapeutic use of play*, New York, 1976, Jason Aronson.
2. Ayres AJ: *Sensory integration and learning disorders*, Los Angeles, 1972, Western Psychological Services.
3. Bantz DL, Siktberg L: Teaching families to evaluate age-appropriate toys, *J Pediatr Health Care* 7:111, 1993.
4. Barnett LA: The adaptive powers of being playful. In Duncan MC, Chick G, Aycock A, editors: *Play and culture studies*, vol 1, Greenwich, Conn, 1998, Ablex Publishing.
5. Berger KS: *The developing person through the lifespan*, ed 3, New York, 1994, Worth Publishers.
6. Bryze KC: Narrative contributions to the play history. In Parham LD, Fazio LS, editors: *Play in occupational therapy for children*, St Louis, 1997, Mosby.
7. Bundy AC: Assessment of play and leisure: delineation of the problem, *Am Occup Ther* 47:217, 1993.
8. Bundy AC: Play and playfulness: what to look for. In Parham LD, Fazio LS, editors: *Play in occupational therapy for children*, St Louis, 1997, Mosby.
9. Bundy AC: Play theory and sensory integration. In Fisher AG, Murray EA, Bundy AC, editors: *Sensory integration: theory and practice*, Philadelphia, 1991, FA Davis.
10. Bundy AC, Nelson L, Metzger P, Bingaman K: Reliability and validity of a test of playfulness, *Occup J Res 21*:276, 2001.
11. Carlson BW, Ginglend DR: *Play activities for the retarded child: how to help him grow and learn through music, games, handicrafts, and other play activities*, New York, 1961, Abingdon Press.
12. Cass JE: *The significance of children's play*, London, 1971, Batsford.
13. Clifford JM, Bundy AC: Play preference and play performance in normal boys and boys with sensory integrative dysfunction, *Am J Occup Ther* 9:202, 1989.
14. Cohen D: *The development of play*, New York, 1987, New York University Press.
15. Coster W: Occupation-centered assessment of children, *Am J Occup Ther* 52:337, 1998.
16. Csikszentmihalyi M: Beyond boredom and anxiety, ed 1, San Francisco, 1975, Jossey-Bass.
17. Florey L: Development through play. In Schaefer C, editor: *The therapeutic use of play*, New York, 1976, Jason Aronson.
18. Greenstein DB: It's child's play. In Galvin J, editor: *Evaluating, selecting, and using appropriate assistive technology*, Gaithersburg, Md, 1996, Aspen.
19. Hart R: *Therapeutic play activities for hospitalized children*, St Louis, 1992, Mosby.
20. Jernberg AM: *Theraplay: a new treatment using structured play for problem children and their families*, San Francisco, 1979, Jossey-Bass.
21. Kielhofner G, editor: *A model of human occupation*, Baltimore, 1985, Williams & Wilkins.
22. Linder TW, editor: *Transdisciplinary play based assessment*, Baltimore, 1990, Paul H Brookes.
23. Llorens LA: *Application of a developmental theory for health and rehabilitation*, Bethesda, Md, 1976, American Occupational Therapy Association.
24. Marfo K, editor: *Parent-child interaction and developmental disabilities*, New York, 1988, Praeger.
25. Millar S: *The psychology of play*, New York, 1974, Aronson.
26. Moran JM, Kalakian LH: *Movement experiences for the mentally retarded or emotionally disturbed child*, Minneapolis, 1974, Burgess.
27. Morrison CD, Bundy AC, Fisher AG: The contribution of motor skills and playfulness to the play performance of pre-schoolers, *Am J Occup Ther* 45:687, 1991.
28. Morrison CD, Metzger P, Pratt P: Play. In Case-Smith J, Allen A, Pratt PN, editors: *Occupational therapy for children*, ed 3, St Louis, 1996, Mosby.

29. Musselwhite CR: *Adaptive play for special needs children*, San Diego, 1986, College-Hill Press.
30. O'Brien JC, Boatwright T, Chaplin J, et al: The impact of positioning equipment on play skills of physically impaired children. In Duncan MC, Chick G, Aycock A, editors: *Play and culture studies*, vol 1, Greenwich, Conn, 1998, Ablex Publishing.
31. O'Brien JC, CoRer P, Lynn R, et al: The impact of occupational therapy on a child's playfulness, *Occup Ther Healthcare* 12:39, 1999.
32. O'Brien JC, Shirley R: Does playfulness change over time: a preliminary look using the Test of Playfulness, *Occup Ther J Res* 21:132, 2001.
33. Okimoto AM, Bundy AC, Hanzlik J: Playfulness in children with and without disability: Measurement and intervention. *Am J Occup Ther* 54:73, 2000.
34. Parham LD, Primeau L: Play and occupational therapy. In Parham LD, Fazio LS, editors: *Play in occupational therapy for children*, St Louis, 1997, Mosby.
35. Parten M: Social play among pre-school children, *J Abnorm Soc Psychol* 28:136, 1933.
36. Reed CN, Dunbar SB, Bundy AC: The effects of an inclusive preschool experience on the playfulness of children with and without autism, *Phys Occup Ther Pediatr* 19:73, 2000.
37. Reilly M, editor: *Play as exploratory learning: studies in curiosity behavior*, Beverly Hills, Calif, 1974, Sage.
38. Rubin K, Fein GG, Vandenberg B: Play. In Mussen PH, editor: *Handbook of child psychology*, ed 4, New York, 1983, Wiley.
39. Sutton-Smith B: Play in cognitive development. In Schaefer C, editor: *The therapeutic use of play*, New York, 1976, Jason Aronson.

Recommended Reading

Britton L, Turner S: *Montessori play and learn: a parent's guide to purposeful play from two to six*, New York, 1993, Crown Publishers.

Featherstone H: *A difference in the family: life with a disabled child*, New York, 1980, Basic Books.

Florey L: Studies of play: implications for growth, development and clinical practice, *Am J Occup Ther* 35:519.

Linder T: *Transdisciplinary play based intervention*, Baltimore, 1993, Paul H Brookes.

Singer D, Singer J: *Partners in play: a step by step guide to imaginative play in children*, New York, 1977, Harper & Row.

Sutton-Smith B: *The ambiguity of play*, Boston, 1998, Harvard University Press.

Young S: *Movement is fun*, Torrance, Calif, 1988, Sensory Integration International.

REVIEW *Questions*

1. Describe the characteristics of play and playfulness.
2. What is the difference between play and playfulness?
3. How would you facilitate play and playfulness in children with special needs?
4. What characteristics do you possess that would promote play and playfulness in children with special needs?
5. How is play used as a tool in the treatment of children?
6. Describe the way(s) that play can be the goal of therapy.
7. List three play assessments used by OT practitioners. Describe the ways they are administered and the information you gain from them.
8. How can the environment stimulate play and playfulness?

SUGGESTED *Activities*

1. Volunteer to baby-sit for a child with special needs. Play with the child. Reflect on the experience by writing a one-page composition describing the way you felt about the time you spent with the child.
2. Plan and participate in an activity you enjoy with others. Describe the activity, materials needed, and environment. How did you feel during the activity?
3. In a small group, discuss your favorite childhood games and playmates. What types of skills did you learn as a child during play? What feelings do these memories bring to mind?
4. In a small group, role-play the characteristics of OT practitioners that promote playfulness in children.

CHAPTER 17 APPENDIX A

Play Assessments

KNOX PRESCHOOL PLAY SCALE[5]

The Knox Preschool Play Scale (PPS) provides a developmental description of play behavior in four domains: space management, materials management, imitation, and participation. It is designed for children 0 to 6 years old. The Knox PPS is easy to administer and score. It requires two 30-minute observations of free play (indoors and outdoors). The revised scale provides age equivalencies to 6 months for children 0 to 3 years of age and yearly for children 3 to 5 years of age.[7]

TEST OF PLAYFULNESS[2,3]

The Test of Playfulness (ToP) provides an objective measurement of playfulness. Children are observed playing in familiar environments suitable for that purpose with peers for 15 minutes inside and 15 minutes outside. Administration of the scale requires training by viewing videotapes of children playing and scoring them according to ToP guidelines. Occupational therapy (OT) practitioners can use the information to systematically examine playfulness in children.[3]

TRANSDISCIPLINARY PLAY-BASED ASSESSMENT[6]

The Transdisciplinary Play-Based Assessment (TPBA) is a procedure for administering a comprehensive transdisciplinary assessment for children 0 to 3 years of age. The TPBA provides structured guidelines for performing this assessment. Clinicians can use this procedure to design intervention. The TPBA is an observational assessment that may take as long as 1½ hours to administer. Team members participate in the assessment. Information is gained in cognitive, social-emotional, communication and language, and motor skills.[6]

PLAY HISTORY[7,8]

A play history is a semistructured interview designed to obtain information about the child's behavior. The play history is based on the developmental progression of play and examines behaviors in five developmental phases: (1) sensorimotor, (2) symbolic and simple constructive, (3) dramatic and complex constructive, (4) games, and (5) recreational. Practitioners using this scale must have a firm knowledge of the normal progression of play. The scale provides a framework for gathering information on it.[8]

CHILDREN'S PLAYFULNESS SCALE[1]

The Children's Playfulness Scale* scale consists of 23 Likert-type format items and uses a five-point response/scoring system: "sounds exactly like the child," "sounds a lot like the child," "sounds somewhat like the child," "sounds a little like the child," and "does not sound at all like the child." Children receive a playfulness score. This scale is efficient and inexpensive and requires no direct observation of the child. Bundy and Clifton questioned the use of this scale for children with disabilities.[4]

Appendix References

1. Barnett LA: Playfulness: definition, design, and measurement, *Play Culture* 3:319, 1990.
2. Bundy AC: Play and playfulness: what to look for. In Parham LD, Fazio LS, editors: *Play in occupational therapy for children*, St Louis, 1997, Mosby.
3. Bundy AC: *Test of playfulness (ToP) version 3.5*, Fort Collins, Colo, 2000, Colorado State University Press.
4. Bundy AC, Clifton JL: Construct validity of the children's playfulness scale. In Duncan MC, Chick G, Aycock A, editors: *Play and culture studies*, vol 1, Greenwich, Conn, 1998, Ablex Publishing.
5. Knox S: Development and current use of the Knox preschool play scale. In Parham LD, Fazio LS, editors: *Play in occupational therapy*, St. Louis, 1997, Mosby–Year Book
6. Linder TW, editor: *Transdisciplinary play-based assessment*, Baltimore, 1990, Paul H Brookes.
7. Reilly M, editor: *Play as exploratory learning*, Beverly Hills, Calif, 1974, Sage.
8. Takata N: Play as a prescription. In Reilly M, editor: *Play as exploratory learning*, Beverly Hills, Calif, 1974, Sage.

*Scales that may be administered by COTAs on establishing service competency with supervising OTR.

CHAPTER 17 APPENDIX B

Resources for Play Activity Ideas

PUBLICATIONS

Burkhart LJ: *More homemade battery devices for severely handicapped children with suggested activities*, College Park, Md, 1982, Linda J Burkhart.

Cole J, Tiergreen A, Calmenson S: *Eentsy, weentsy spider: fingerplays and action rhymes*, New York, 1991, Mulberry Books.

Coleman K, McNairn P, Shioleno C: *Quick tech magic music-based literacy activities*, Solana, Calif, 2004, Mayer-Johnson Company.

Dexter S: *Joyful play with toddlers: recipes for fun with odds and ends (tool for everyday parenting series)*, Seattle, 1996, Parenting Press.

Hamilton L: *Child's play around the world: 170 crafts, games and projects for 2-6 year olds*, New York, 1996, Beverly.

Judith G, Ellison S: *365 days of creative play for children 2 years and up*, Trabuco Canyon, Calif, 1995, Sourcebooks.

Kranowitz CS: *101 activities for kids in tight spaces: at the doctor's office; on car, train, and plane trips; and home sick in bed*, New York, 1995, St Martin's Press.

Miller K: *Things to do with toddlers and twos*, West Palm Beach, Fla, 1984, Telshare.

Morris LR, Schultz L: *Creative play activities for children with disabilities: a resource book for teachers and parents*, ed 2, Champaign, Ill, 1989, Human Kinetic Books.

Munger EM, Bowden SJ: *Beyond peek-a-boo and pat-a-cake: activities for baby's first twenty-four months*, ed 3, Clinton, NJ, 1993, New Win Pub.

Nipp S, Beall PC: *Wee sing children's songs and fingerplays (audiocassette)*, New York, 1994, Price Stern Sloan Audio.

Nolan A: *Great explorations: 100 creative play ideas for parents and preschoolers from playspace at the children's museum*, Boston, 1997, Pocket Books.

Silberg J: *300 3-minute games: quick and easy activities for 2–5 year olds*, Beltsville, Md, 1997, Gryphon House.

Totline Staff: *1001 rhymes and fingerplays*, Pomona, Calif, 1994, Warren Publishing House.

Ulene A, Shelov S: *Discovery play: loving and learning with your baby*, Berkeley, Calif, 1994, Ulyss Press.

Wright C, Nomura M: *From toys to computers: access for the physically disabled child*, San Jose, Calif, 1990, C Wright.

WEBSITE GAMES, ACTIVITIES, AND PRINTABLES FOR CHILDREN

www.brighting.com
Activities, experiments with science explanations, coloring pages

www.childfun.com
Printables, crafts, themes

www.Disneyland.com
Games, printables

www.Kidwizard.com
Crafts, games

www.Learningplanet.com
Educational activities, printables, games

www.PrimaryGames.com
Online games, coloring pages, mazes

www.School.discovery.com
School activities, awards, certificates

www.Teachervision.com
Teacher lessons, certificates, behavior management forms, printables, articles

COMPANIES AND PUBLICATIONS HELPFUL IN ADAPTING PLAY FOR CHILDREN WITH SPECIAL NEEDS

Ablenet
1091 Tenth Avenue, Southeast
Minneapolis, MN 55414-1312
(800) 322-0956

Linda Burkhart
8503 Rhode Island Avenue
College Park, MD 20740
(301) 345-9152

Crestwood Company
6625 North Sidney Place
Milwaukee, WI 53209-3259
(414) 352-5678

Exceptional Parent Magazine
PO Box 5446
Pittsfield, MA 01203-9321
(800) 247-8080

Don Johnston
PO Box 639
Wauconda, IL 60084-0639
(800) 999-4660

CHAPTER 17 APPENDIX B—cont'd

Resources for Play Activity Ideas

National Therapeutic Recreation Society
2775 South Quincy Street, Suite 300
Arlington, VA 22206
(703) 820-4940

Toys for Special Children
385 Warburton Avenue
Hastings-on-Hudson, NY 10706

18

Activities of Daily Living and Instrumental Activities of Daily Living

LISE M.W. JONES

PEGGY ZAKS MACHOVER*

CHAPTER *Objectives*

After studying this chapter, the reader will be able to accomplish the following:

- Describe therapeutic activities that the certified occupational therapy assistant might use to address a variety of problems related to activities of daily living: feeding, dressing, toileting, hygiene, grooming, functional mobility, personal device care, and sleep and rest
- Describe therapeutic activities that the certified occupational therapy assistant might use to address a variety of problems related to instrumental activities of daily living: communication device use, financial management, safety procedures and emergency responses, health management and maintenance, community mobility, financial management, shopping, meal preparation and cleanup, and home management
- Apply the occupational therapy tools of analyzing, grading, and adapting activities of daily living and instrumental activities of daily living for specific children
- Give examples of the ways in which reading the child in context from moment to moment guides an intervention session
- Identify the ways in which the certified occupational therapy assistant works with parents, caregivers, registered occupational therapist supervisors, agency administrators, and team members to address activities of daily living and instrumental activities of daily living for the child

*We thank the following talented certified occupational therapy assistants (COTAs) and registered occupational therapists (OTRs) who have worked with us in pediatric occupational therapy and brought their enthusiasm, intelligence, ideas, and caring to the field and creation of this chapter: Alexandra Aristizabal, Dottie Bade (OTR), Andrea Brown, Andrea D'Aquino, Laura Falco, Darlie Faustin, Petal Fletcher, Louise Lear Greene, Doreen Torres Grey (OTR), Marge Lesser, Gloria Monroy, Felicity Reimold, and Barbara Vaccaro (OTR). We also thank Ike and Alexandra Machover, Anna and Jesse Guterman, and Julia Eidson for all their help.

KEY TERMS

Occupations
Activities
Activities of daily living
Instrumental activities of daily living
Whole skills
Motor plan
Cognitive memory
Motor memory
Eating
Feeding
Suck-swallow-breathe synchrony
Oral defensiveness
Spasticity
Tongue thrust
Pica behavior
Proprioceptive feedback
Grading activities
Forward chaining
Backward chaining
Fading assistance
Splinter skill
Stereognosis
Level of arousal

CHAPTER OUTLINE

The occupational therapy (OT) practitioner's primary goal is to help people engage in occupations to support participation in life. **Occupations** are activities that have unique meaning and purpose for a person. **Activities** are goal-directed actions. Engaging in occupations is central to one's personal identity, health, and sense of well-being.

Occupational performance is defined as the ability to carry out activities in daily life. The domain of OT divides performance into seven areas of occupation.[1] This chapter addresses the role of the certified occupational therapy assistant (COTA) during intervention in two areas of occupation: activities of daily living and instrumental activities of daily living.

Activities of daily living (ADLs) are also referred to as basic ADLs (BADLs) or personal ADLs (PADLs). ADLs are the means by which individuals care for and use their own bodies every day. The OT framework identifies the ADLs as eating, feeding, bowel and bladder management, toilet hygiene, bathing and showering, personal hygiene and grooming, dressing, personal device care, sexual activity, sleep and rest, and functional mobility.

Instrumental activities of daily living (IADLs) include communication device use, health management, care of pets, shopping in the community, food preparation, laundry, financial management, and medication routines. IADLs tend to be more complex than ADLs and require more cognitive skills, problem solving, and judgment.

IADLs may be optional for some children or performed by caregivers. Before working on a specific ADL or IADL in intervention, foundation skills and the patterns needed to perform an activity are usually addressed. It may be necessary to adapt or modify the ADL or IADL to promote success. Whenever possible, the specific ADL or IADL is addressed at the time when it naturally occurs. Children tend to remember strategies the best and new methods are the most meaningful when taught at routine times in natural contexts.

In general, when you eat, dress, wash hands, bathe, or wash dishes, you do so without thinking about how to do the occupations or activities. Borrowing from the field of psychology, we can refer to these skills as being automatic or **whole.** The occupations or activities become engrained and part of who we are. Over time we practice and refine our performance of one or more of these skills so that eventually little thought is required to realize smooth performance. COTAs consider this question: "How do we help clients reach the outcome of performing independent ADLs and IADLs?" They help clients learn each component of an activity, put them together into smooth sequences, and remember them for use in daily life. For example, tying shoes requires a multitude of sequenced steps leading to a comprehensive **motor plan.** The motor plan of tying shoes includes (1) the idea—"I have the idea that I want to tie my shoe," (2) the plan—"I have to think through the sequence of steps required to tie my shoe," and (3) the action—"I have to execute the physical sequence of steps to tie my shoe."

As an individual's **cognitive memory** (recall of thought) of the plan becomes quicker, the **motor memory** (recall of action patterns in body structures like muscles and joints) also becomes more fluid. Little by little, the concentration on each tiny step of the plan is relaxed. Each step of the sequence leading to the motor plan merges with those previously learned. The plan and motor sequencing become integrated into the smooth flow of the whole skill of tying shoes. Once the steps and motor sequence are learned and you have integrated them, you have acquired the *whole skill.*

Children treated in OT may have trouble with some part of the motor plan or motor memory. Some may have acquired whole skills but do not use them regularly, which results in forgetting the plan and motor memory deficits.

For skills to become whole, children need practice, review, and regular use in daily life contexts. Several factors that can interfere with cognitive or motor memory are learning disabilities, low muscle tone, neurological or physical injury, disease, and poor discrimination of tactile and muscle-joint sensations. Intervention is aimed at developing whole skills.

CLINICAL *Pearl*

Try to schedule therapy for a child during snack time or mealtime to address eating, feeding, and hand-washing goals. Allot extra time at the end of a session to work on putting on a jacket and operating fasteners before the child goes outside. Children tend to remember strategies the best and new methods are the most meaningful when they happen at the regular time.

ACTIVITIES OF DAILY LIVING

Eating and Feeding

Eating is the ability to keep food and fluids in the mouth, move them around inside the mouth, and swallow them. **Feeding** is the process of bringing food and fluids to the mouth from containers such as plates, bowls, and cups. The activities of eating and feeding are presented together due to the natural and continual interplay between the two.

Suck-swallow-breathe synchrony

At birth the infant must coordinate sucking, swallowing, and breathing to survive. When the newborn begins to suckle the mother's breast or nipple of a bottle, the actions of sucking, swallowing, and breathing become rhythmically synchronized so that the infant can receive adequate nutrition. This **suck-swallow-breathe synchrony** (s-s-b synchrony) is a skill used continuously throughout life.[12] The s-s-b synchrony allows individuals to breathe while simultaneously and unconsciously sucking in and swallowing food, drink, and saliva. The infant's strong sucking action develops the sensory discrimination and muscle control needed later for eating solid foods and talking without concentrating, suffocating, or drooling. A disruption in s-s-b synchrony can interfere with development.

Any noticeable problems in s-s-b synchrony are addressed in a multidisciplinary manner. The COTA consults with the registered occupational therapist (OTR), speech/language pathologist (SLP), doctor, nurse, and caregivers. The goal is to work toward automatic, smooth, and rhythmic sucking, swallowing, and breathing (Box 18-1).

The following three signs are common indicators of inefficient s-s-b synchrony:

BOX 18-1

Activities to Promote Breathing

- Proper breathing can be facilitated by performing activities in a prone position, in which the stomach is resting on soft, bouncy or elastic surfaces.[26,27] Try swinging the child on an inner tube swing or rocking him or her on a soft therapy ball. These activities help activate and strengthen the diaphragm (the muscle that pushes air out of the lungs), leading to deeper breathing.
- To promote deep breathing for toddlers and children, use a variety of blowing toys and activities such as blowing bubbles, pinwheels, whistles, feathers, cotton balls, Ping-Pong balls, and drops of paint on paper.[27] These activities will also increase lip seal by developing strength and sensation in the lips and cheeks and strength in the diaphragm. Older children may prefer to play harmonicas or other wind instruments, blow up balloons, or blow bubbles with bubble gum. Singing is beneficial for all ages.
- Sitting in a partially supine position makes it somewhat easier for children with weakness to activate the diaphragm. Therefore, sitting on a beanbag or leaning back on a pile of pillows can help a child gain enough force to breathe deeply and blow or suck hard.[12]

1. *Inadequate lip seal while sucking or blowing.* Typically, when a child sucks on a bottle or straw, no air or liquid escapes through the sides of the mouth. The lips need to fit tightly around a nipple or straw to create suction. The lips also need to fit tightly around whistles, balloons, and other blow toys to operate them. Therefore, lip seal can be observed during sucking or blowing. A break in the lip seal is often noted by a hissing or sputtering noise. If this break is repeatedly observed or heard, intervention is recommended. Many children with low muscle tone, facial weakness, poor motor planning, or incoordination have trouble with the lip seal. These children also often have speech problems.
2. *Gasping for air while sucking or eating.* An infant who has s-s-b synchrony displays smooth, rhythmic breathing through the nose when sucking liquids or eating from a spoon. Gasping for air indicates that breathing, sucking, and swallowing are not synchronized, and the child may be uncomfortable. A child who gasps for air but does not have a cold requires treatment for s-s-b synchrony.
3. *Excessive drooling when not being fed.* Typically, drooling is seen when an infant is teething or a toddler is concentrating on learning new activities. By about 2 years of age, drooling usually subsides. Initiate intervention if drooling is excessive.

The COTA addresses oral-motor problems under the close supervision of the OTR and after medical problems have been ruled out. The following techniques are used to improve s-s-b synchrony:

- To facilitate efficient swallowing while breathing, keep the child's head and neck vertical or somewhat flexed (bent forward). If the child's head is hyperextended (curved back), the child may aspirate (inhale food into the esophagus) and choke. "Bird feeding," which is feeding a child while the child's head is hyperextended, is unsafe and should not be practiced (Figure 18-1; Box 18-2).
- Swallowing may be facilitated by slowly stroking upward on the lateral muscles (side muscles) of the throat. Avoid touching the trachea (breathing tube running down the center of the neck). In theory, when the swallowing muscles sense that they are being gently pulled upward, they will react by resisting with a downward swallow.
- Sour tastes can improve lip pursing and swallowing in children.[29] Try using tiny amounts of lemonade powder, frozen lemonade or limeade concentrate, or slices of fresh lemon. Children can be encouraged but should never be forced to taste anything.

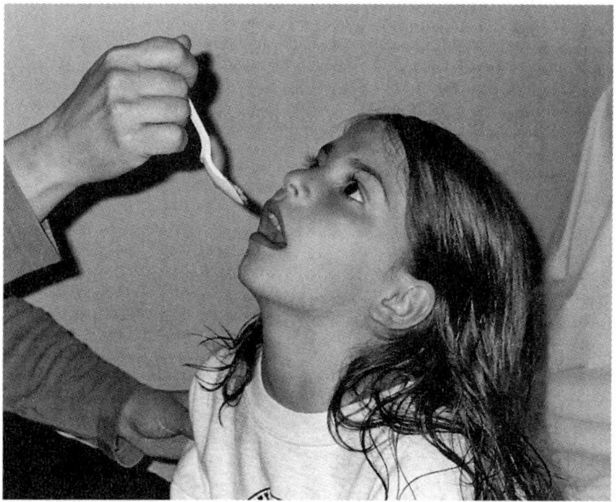

FIGURE 18-1 "Bird feeding," in which the head is abnormally hyperextended, is dangerous and can cause choking.

BOX 18-2

Proper Feeding Positions

- Swallowing is easiest with the head in a slightly flexed position.
- Even if a child constantly spits or drips food out of the mouth, maintain the head and neck in a safe, neutral or slightly flexed position at all times to facilitate proper breathing and prevent aspiration (i.e., food going down the windpipe into the lungs).
- Position children in an upright, stable posture with feet on the floor.

- Straws are great tools to facilitate the lip seal and strengthen the lip and cheek muscles needed for drinking, eating, and speaking. Straws come in a variety of materials, including soft and hard plastic, latex, and rubber. A short, narrow straw requires less strength to sip from than a long, wide one. Thin liquids like water and juice require less strength to sip than thick liquids like mild shakes or puréed soup. Flexible tubing or bendable plastic straws (Figure 18-2) may be used with children who have some of the following issues: severely weak neck muscles, trouble positioning the head, need to stay in bed to drink, and/or trouble positioning the cup or straw for any reason. (**Precaution:** Walking and running while drinking from a straw are unsafe; be sure that the child is sitting in a stable position before s/he uses a straw.)

Transition from bottle to cup

The transition from a bottle to a cup is negotiated with parents and team members. The COTA consults with the OTR about guidelines and coordinates activities with the child, caregivers, and other team members, like the SLP, nurse, and/or doctor. Team members determine the developmental and physical readiness of the child, the proper time and place for the transition, and the way in which straw or other specialized cups will be used to aid the transition.

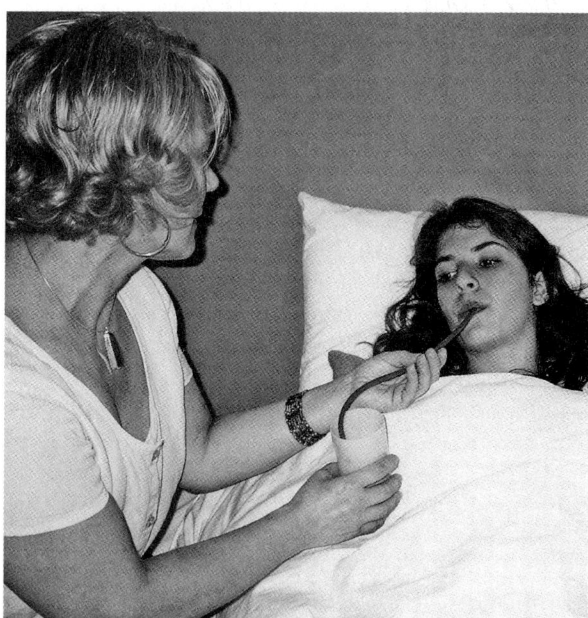

FIGURE 18-2 The girl can lean back to drink when sipping through a bendable straw or flexible tubing.

The strong sucking action of an infant prepares the muscles of the jaw, tongue, cheeks, and throat for drinking from a cup, chewing, and talking. The actual transition from sucking on a nipple to drinking from a cup

BOX 18-3

Oral-Motor Activities

Oral-motor activities should be fun and rewarding for children. Do not force oral-motor activities.

- As with all eating and feeding activities, take extreme care to prevent discomfort and injury.
- If an infant or child resists participating in an activity, s/he may be trying to tell the practitioner that it is not the right activity. Consult the registered occupational therapist.
- If a child has a head cold and a runny nose, limit blowing activities until the cold has subsided. Forceful blowing can cause fluids or air to back up in the eustachian tube, resulting in excess pressure behind the eardrum, which could burst.

can be problematic and stressful for some children and parents (Box 18-3).

The child may resist the change from the nipple to the cup for a variety of reasons. (1) Sucking provides a calming, nurturing feeling, so the child may prefer to continue this action rather than change to a different style of drinking. (2) Drinking from a cup introduces unfamiliar sensations that the child may not find satisfying initially. (3) Abnormal muscle tone, whether it is hypertonicity (high muscle tone, or tight muscles and joints) or hypotonicity (low muscle tone, or loose muscles and joints), in the face and body can prevent proper lip and mouth control. (4) Other neuromotor or physical problems can interfere with the muscle control needed to drink from a cup. (5) **Oral defensiveness** (i.e., aversion to harmless oral sensations) can make a child resist any change.

A number of basic skills are needed for successful transition from a bottle to a cup.

1. *Muscle tone needs to be adequate (i.e., not too low and not too high)*. Inhibition techniques (calming, slowing, reducing) for high muscle tone and facilitation techniques (exciting, speeding, increasing) for low muscle tone are used to improve tone in the trunk, upper extremities, neck, and face to make drinking (and eating) skills easier for the child.[25]
2. *Efficient and proper lip closure*. Intervention strategies that promote oral-motor control require comfortable positioning for both the therapist and child. The child's postural stability and alignment are essential for proper oral-motor function.[5,10,25] To promote lip closure around a bottle, cup, or spoon when working with a child who has significant physical limitations, use the positioning seen in Figure 18-3. The child is seated in a chair with equal weight bearing on both hips; the trunk and head are centered on the midline position. The shoulders are not too retracted (pulled back) or too protracted (rounded forward). The head is in a neutral (straight up) position or is slightly flexed (bent forward) and never hyperextended. To keep the head and shoulders positioned properly, the OT practitioner's nondominant arm is placed around the child's shoulders and neck for support. The nondominant hand helps control the jaw, cheeks, and lips. With the use of the index and middle fingers, gentle but firm pressure is applied just above the upper lip and just below the lower lip. The OT practitioner's dominant hand is free to control the bottle, cup, straw, spoon, or fork. The dominant hand introduces a drink or food into the child's mouth.

- The lip seal may increase with the use of different sizes of nipples, spouts, straws, or cutout cups.[27] Finding the right nipple or spout may improve lip closure and sucking (with its accompanying frustration and inadequate nutrition) and functional eating.

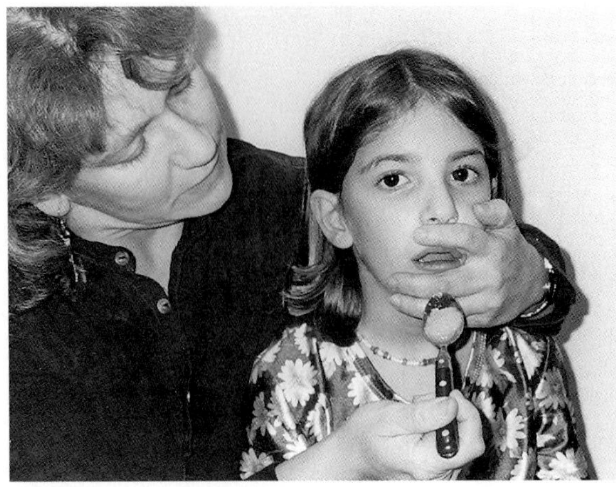

FIGURE 18-3 The therapist supports the child's head, shoulders, jaw, and lips in the proper position to aid oral-motor control.

CLINICAL *Pearl*

Consult with the SLP when choosing a cup. Some speech therapists report that "sippy cups" with flat, wide spouts foster improper tongue placement and immature sucking patterns. If a child is at risk of reverting to immature sucking and drinking patterns, it may be best to avoid using cups with flat, wide spouts (Figure 18-4, A). A straw cup, which requires an adequate lip seal and promotes proper tongue placement and sucking patterns, is an excellent alternative (Figure 18-4, B).

- To promote lip closure, place a straw at the midline of the body, centered between the child's lips. Watch for children who move the straw to the side of the mouth, push it too far back in the mouth, or chew on it. These children may have weakness or poor touch-pressure discrimination in the mouth or jaw. Placing the straw in the midline position promotes lip closure as well as strength and coordination of the lip, tongue, and cheek muscles.
- Lip closure can sometimes be facilitated by applying two light downward strokes to the sensitive area of skin between the nose and upper lip (Figure 18-5).[27] The lip closure response may be delayed. If this stroking method is used too frequently within a short period, the child may stop responding for a while. The OT practitioner can wait and try again. If the child has significant physical problems like cerebral palsy with **spasticity** (involuntary overtightening of muscles,

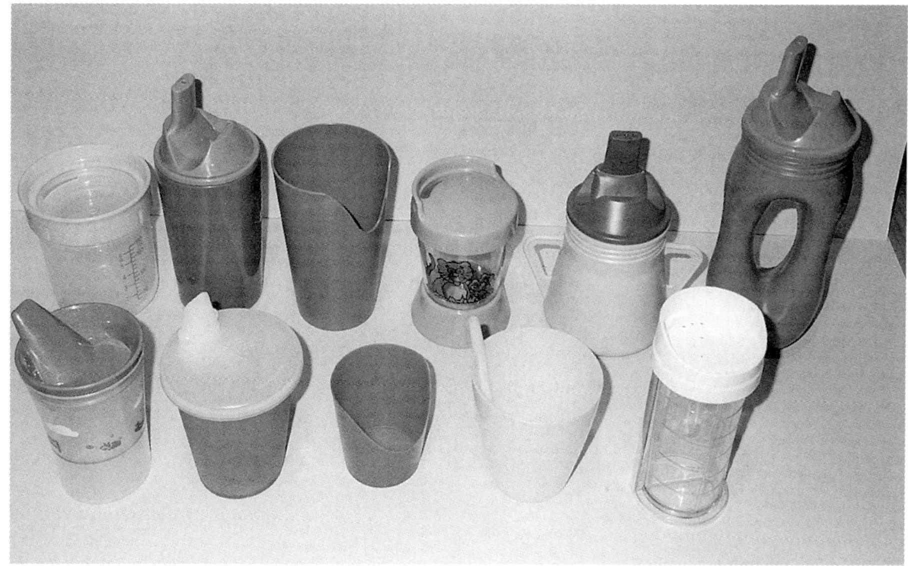

A

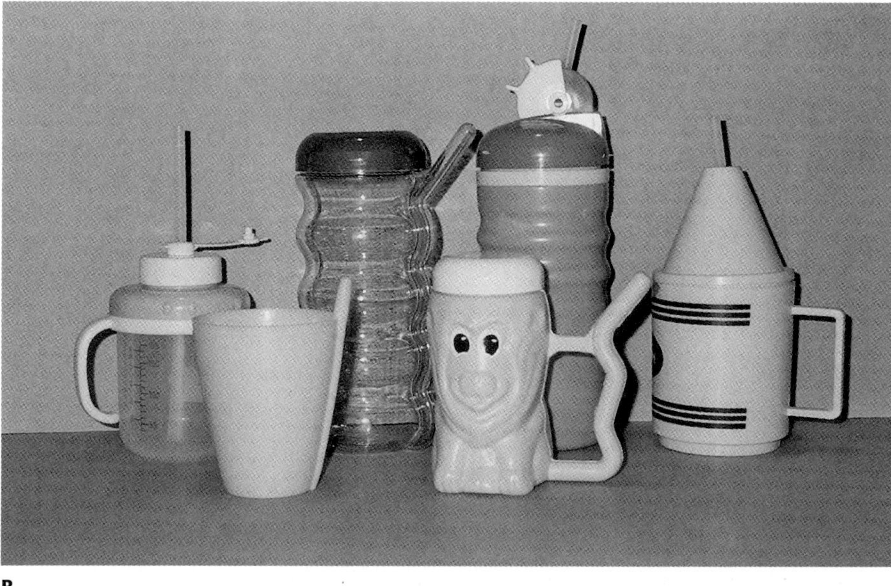

B

FIGURE 18-4 **A,** Cups with spouts, cutouts, and different handholds can facilitate the transition from a bottle to a cup. **B,** Numerous straw cups that are available.

causing stiff movements), this light stroking may produce the opposite effect, causing the mouth to open.

3. *Specialized transition cups.* A variety of attractive transition, straw, or spout cups can be obtained through catalogs or stores once the team determines that the child is ready for the transition from a bottle to a cup. Some cups have two handles so that children with limited grasping ability, strength, or coordination can lift the cups more securely. Some have weighted bottoms that prevent tipping over. Certain transition cups have detachable nipples that can be replaced with a straw when the child is ready. For children who have poor s-s-b synchrony, some cups have a stopper button that the therapist, caregiver, or child can press to stop and start the flow of liquid. Simply being able to choose between several appealing cups or straws may ease the transition.
   - Cutout cups are helpful for children with mild to moderate motor problems. One side is cut out in a U shape. As the cup is placed on the child's lower lip and tipped for drinking, the cutout portion fits around the child's nose. S/he drinks more easily because the head does not have to tip backward.
4. *Reduce oral defensiveness.* A child's resistance to using a cup may be partially caused by oral defensiveness (i.e., aversion to harmless oral sensations). Several techniques can help increase a child's tolerance to different tastes, textures, and temperatures. The

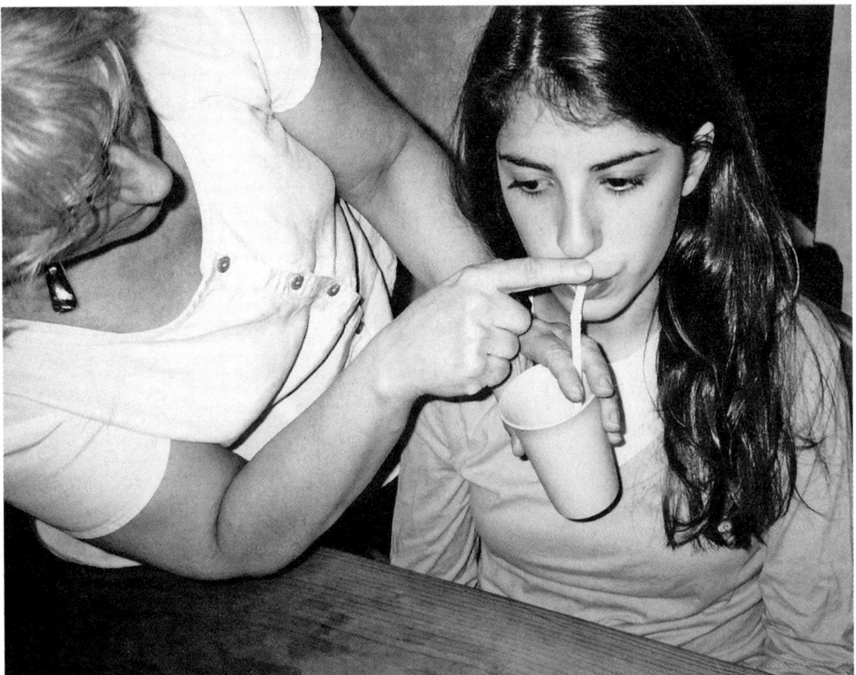

FIGURE 18-5 The straw is placed at the midline and just inside the child's lips, not too far back and not on the side of the mouth. To promote lip closure around the straw, the occupational therapy practitioner applies two light downward strokes between the nose and upper lip.

Wilbarger intraoral (inside the mouth) technique for oral defensiveness can be learned in a continuing education course or from a person who has attended the course.[38] When administered correctly it may increase tolerance for different textures, temperatures, and shapes in the mouth.

- The jaw tug technique[27] involves placing a thumb or two fingers on the lower teeth and gently but firmly tugging downward on the lower jaw 10 times. Some children can be taught to perform this technique on themselves before eating (Figure 18-6). It can provide temporary inhibition of defensive reactions.
- Other deep pressure techniques used in and around the mouth can increase tolerance for oral sensations as well as sensory awareness and motor control. One involves gently but firmly pressing the cheeks and gradually moving deep pressure to areas around the lips and then pressing directly on the mouth.

OT practitioners involved in feeding programs benefit from attending continuing education classes to learn the details about oral-motor and respiratory treatment and intervention techniques, including positioning and handling for feeding (Box 18-4).

BOX 18-4

Dealing with the Demands of a Child with Sensory Defensiveness

- Carefully gauge proximity (closeness) to the child. Hair or clothing may accidentally touch him or her, causing an aversive response.
- Grade the volume of speech being used. A regular speaking voice may be too loud for the child.
- Watch for signs that the child may have trouble listening and working at the same time. Speaking while the child is working may be confusing or overwhelming to him or her.

Chewing: transitioning from liquids to solids

For children with mild oral-motor planning problems and/or jaw weakness, several strategies are recommended for facilitating chewing. (Refer to recommended readings for additional resources).

1. Add small amounts of a thick-textured substance such as pudding, wheat germ, or Thicket (a commercial product available from Milani Foods) to liquids. Gradually increase the liquid's consistency.
2. Add small amounts of chewable food, such as chunks of cooked and skinned apple, to puréed food such as applesauce. Put a few noodles or cooked carrots in a vegetable purée.
3. Use food that dissolves easily in saliva, such as oat, corn, or rice cereal. When mixed with milk, the cereal soon becomes a lumpy-textured mixture that is chewable yet safe and easy to swallow.
4. Place food that dissolves easily in saliva, such as a saltine cracker, graham cracker, or sugar cookie, between the child's upper and lower molars on the side of the mouth. Place two fingers or the thumb on the lower jaw directly

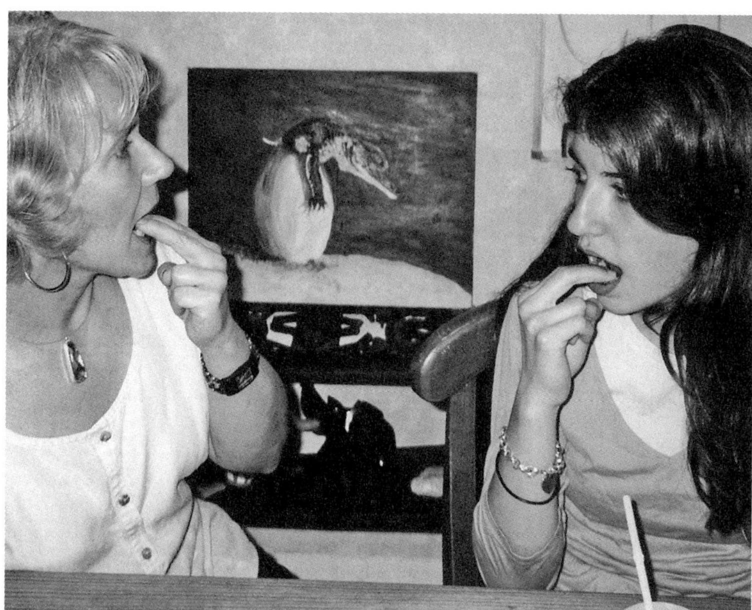

FIGURE 18-6 The child imitates the "jaw tug" by tugging downward 10 times on the lower teeth.

under the molars, and press straight up with firm, steady, sustained pressure (Figure 18-7). In theory the child will first respond to the sustained upward pressure by closing the molars on the food and then resist this pressure by opening the jaw. As the OT practitioner maintains upward pressure, rhythmic chewing often results.[10]

5. Put a tasty, juicy item like a piece of meat or fruit inside a piece of cheesecloth (available in kitchenware or houseware stores and some grocery stores). Place the wrapped food between the molars, and apply steady upward pressure to the lower jaw, as explained in strategy 4.[10]
6. Use a "bite and tug" game immediately before eating.[29] (**Precaution:** The practitioner needs to be careful to prevent the fingers from being bitten.) First, the practitioner wraps a clean, thick washcloth or dishrag around the fingers. Next, the cloth is dipped in a liquid the child likes, such as juice or broth. Then the cloth is inserted between the child's molars. A child who is ready for this strategy will then bite the cloth and suck out the juice. Finally, the therapist quickly and rhythmically tugs the cloth, allowing the child to simulate and feel a chewing motion with the molars. This technique is not used with children who have a tonic bite reflex (the involuntary forceful and prolonged clenching of jaws together, which is triggered by touch or light pressure to the gums or teeth).
7. With close supervision from the OTR or SLP and if the child tolerates vibration, place a small, vibrating rubber wand (available from equipment catalogs) on the cheek near the jaw or between the molars. Vibration, especially at a frequency of 60 Hz or higher (or 60 vibrations or more per second), facilitates muscle contraction (tightening). The teeth are excellent conductors of vibration. Therefore, when the vibrating wand touches the teeth, the vibration moves through the teeth to the jaw muscles and helps the child bite down on the wand. (**Contraindications:** (1) Do not use vibration with children who have a tonic bite reflex; their forceful biting reactions could hurt them. (2) Never place a vibrating item on the front of the neck or near the heart; the vibrations might interfere with the individual's natural heart rhythm.)

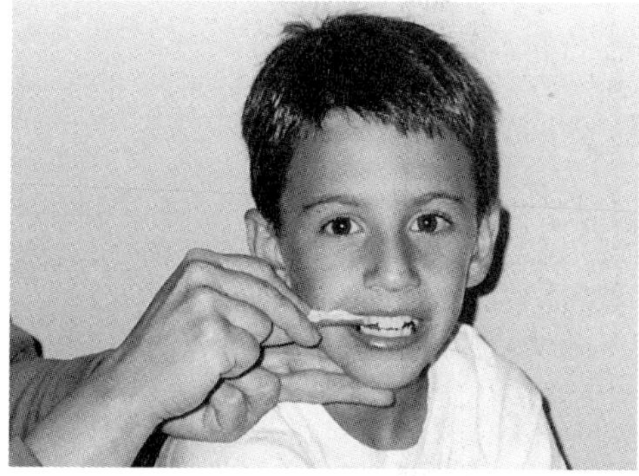

FIGURE 18-7 To facilitate chewing, a cracker is placed between the molars while applying steady upward pressure to the lower jaw.

Managing tongue thrust

Tongue control with rhythmic tongue retraction (pulling the tongue back into the mouth) is necessary to control both liquids and solids. Excessive tongue protrusion (sticking the tongue between the lips) and **tongue thrust** (extending the tongue outside the lips) are involuntary movements often seen in children with cerebral palsy, Down syndrome, and other disabilities interfering with muscle control. Tongue retraction, protrusion, and thrust all interfere with swallowing and can cause food to be pushed out of the mouth. Promoting mature tongue retraction can help the child with excessive tongue protrusion or thrust. Excessive tongue retraction can also be an obstacle to efficient feeding.[25]

Proper positioning is vital for tongue control. The trunk, head, neck, and shoulders need to be stable and aligned. Abnormal tongue movements tend to occur more frequently when the head is hyperextended. After the child is positioned, tongue retraction can sometimes be initiated by placing a thumb or two fingers on the soft part of the skin directly under the chin, behind the jaw, and in front of the neck. The practitioner presses upward, being careful to avoid touching the trachea. This facilitates contraction of the muscles at the base of the tongue, which pulls the tongue back into the mouth.

The OT practitioner can help a child retract the tongue several times before feeding. Tongue thrust can also be inhibited during feeding. Each time the child takes a bite, the practitioner presses the spoon down firmly on the center of the tongue and holds this pressure for about 3 seconds, after which the tongue usually relaxes and retracts.

Transition from fingers to utensils

Learning to feed with utensils instead of the fingers is a major developmental task for children. It requires visuomotor coordination, fine motor skills, motor planning, motor memory, and sensory processing. Lightweight plastic utensils commonly used in schools, hospitals, and even on family picnics can be especially problematic. Adapted holders and utensils may help children with special needs. See the following list for examples.

1. Attach a universal weighted handle to a plastic utensil. The term "universal" refers to the capacity to hold a variety of utensils, such as spoons, knives, toothbrushes, and pencils. Pediatric universal weighted grips and pediatric weighted spoons and forks are available from several equipment companies. Adding weight to the handle increases sensory feedback and stability for those children who have trouble feeling, handling, and steadying utensils.

CLINICAL 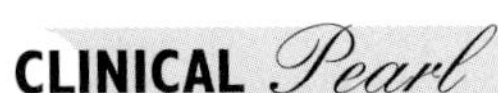

To inhibit tongue thrust, the spoon must be pressed downward in exactly the center of the tongue. If the spoon is too far forward, pressure on the tip of the tongue stimulates a stronger tongue thrust. If the spoon is too far back, a gag reflex may occur.

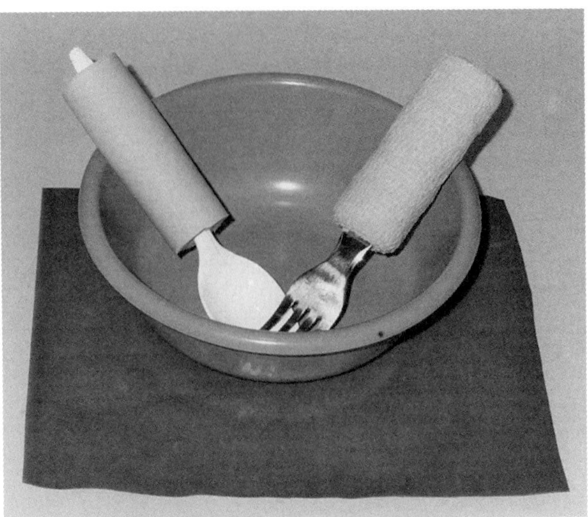

FIGURE 18-8 A spoon with a built-up foam handle, a fork with a built-up Coban handle, and a bowl stabilized with a Dycem nonslip mat.

(**Note:** These strategies may not work for a child with severe weakness.)

2. Slide foam tubing or foam from a new hair curler onto any utensil to make the handle larger and easier to grasp (Figure 18-8).
3. Wrap Coban (a textured elastic material similar to an Ace bandage that adheres to itself) around handles to increase their size and slightly increase the weight of the utensil (see Figure 18-8).
4. Curved utensils can help children who are able to bring their hands close to their mouths but cannot properly orient the utensils. Curved utensils are made for both right- and left-handed users.
5. Children who have a strong tonic bite reflex can use rubber-coated or plastic or rubber spoons.
6. Small, flat spoons can be used by children with a strong tongue thrust.
7. Children with tremors or incoordination can use swivel or weighted utensils.
8. Children who are unable to grasp utensils can use long-handled, bendable (wrap-around) spoons and forks that wrap around the hand, eliminating the need to grasp them.
9. Pediatric universal holders can be attached to a child's hands and a spoon or fork inserted into the sleeve.
10. Cutting play food, such as wooden and Velcro fruit and vegetables, is a fun way for children to learn how to hold a knife and cut safely with it (Figure 18-9).
11. Visual cues can be used to make spreading and cutting with a knife easier. A piece of tape or a red dot on the top edge of a knife shows proper placement for the index finger.

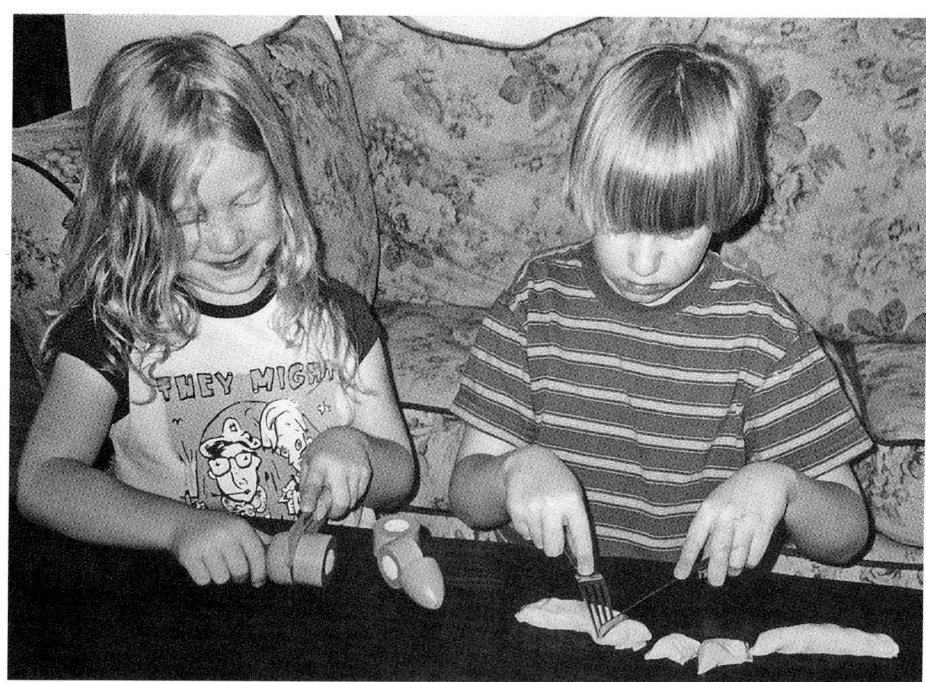

FIGURE 18-9 The girl learns to use a knife by cutting wooden and Velcro vegetables. The boy learns to use a knife and fork by cutting pieces of putty.

ALEX'S SPOON STORY. Alex is a nonverbal 5-year-old boy with pervasive developmental disorder, severe mental retardation, severely low muscle tone, severe sensory defensiveness, poor sensory discrimination, excessive self-stimulatory finger flicking, and severe delays in all areas of function. He actively resists holding any utensil, even after engaging in sensory modulation and resistive hand/arm activities. When encouraged to hold a spoon, he either pushes it away or flicks it back and forth while watching it from the corner of his eye.

The COTA worked hard to analyze his behavior and its possible causes, reasoning that if (1) his sensory defensiveness caused discomfort in holding the spoon and (2) his poor discrimination did not allow him to properly handle and adequately feel the spoon, then (3) maybe the use of a deep pressure technique would address both problems.

After consulting with the OTR, the COTA ordered pediatric weighted hand patches. The small fingerless neoprene gloves were placed on Alex's hands. Tiny 1-ounce weights slid into a pocket on the dorsum of the hand. After a short time of getting used to the new feeling, Alex stopped flicking his fingers and tolerated holding the spoon. He began bringing the spoon to his mouth (Box 18-5).

CLINICAL *Pearl*

Deep pressure techniques may be calming and can increase proprioceptive (deep pressure) awareness in muscles and joints. If people cannot feel things properly, they cannot handle things properly. Accurate interpretation of sensory feedback is necessary for body awareness, motor planning, and motor memory.

BOX 18-5

OT Supervision of Oral-Motor Intervention

- The registered occupational therapist recommends and specifically directs oral-motor intervention by the certified occupational therapy assistant.
- Medical personnel are consulted if the registered occupational therapist suspects that the child's oral-motor limitations are caused by physical problems. Specific tests or other interventions may be requested before oral-motor intervention begins.
- Certain techniques may be contraindicated for a child who is medically fragile or being fed through a tube.

Using tableware

The following list describes some of the many types of adapted plates and bowls available for children with special needs:

1. A bowl with a suction attachment on the bottom prevents the bowl from sliding.
2. Scoop plate, or a plate with a high rim around the edge, against which to push the spoon or fork makes food slide onto the utensil more easily and not spill onto the table.

3. For travel, a plastic or metal plate guard can be attached to most plates. Food is scooped against the plate guard, which helps push the food onto the spoon or fork.
4. Dycem, a type of nonslip material, prevents tableware from sliding (see Figure 18-8) and can be used as a place mat. It comes in a variety of forms, including thick precut rectangles and circles; long, thin rolls that can be cut into different sizes; and a lightweight mesh.
5. Holders for scoop bowls and plates can be created by carving out a block of firm foam.[33]

Managing special feeding and eating problems

Opening packages and containers

The ability to open packages and containers is a skill often overlooked in the development of independent feeding. The child may have mastered oral-motor skills and the use of tableware but still need help opening a juice carton, straw or ketchup package, plastic food container, or sandwich wrapped in plastic. The child can encounter these challenges at home, school, and in community settings.

The OT practitioner helps children develop the basic hand and finger skills needed to open packages (e.g., tactile discrimination, bilateral coordination, strength, and dexterity). In addition, the OT practitioner helps children, parents, and involved adults with problem-solving skills. For example, the practitioner may schedule a weekly treatment session at lunchtime to work with a child on opening packages or may ask the parents to wrap the child's sandwich in aluminum foil or put it in a plastic bag, which is easier to manage. Twist ties can be especially confusing and difficult to handle. The practitioner can work with teachers to design intervention strategies. The child may need adaptive equipment like a sandwich holder, which stabilizes the sandwich while freeing both hands for unwrapping. The child may need a small pair of scissors to use only on food packages or instructions to ask the teacher for help.

Gastrostomy tube

For medical conditions, some children must be fed through a gastrostomy tube, which is inserted directly into the stomach. If a child's tube feeding is temporary, the COTA may be asked to work on goals to help the child develop intraoral sensory awareness and motor control in preparation for future feeding by mouth. In some cases the COTA may be allowed to give the child a teaspoon of water or other liquid through the mouth. The previously described methods for reducing oral defensiveness can also help prepare a child who has a gastrostomy tube for feeding by mouth.

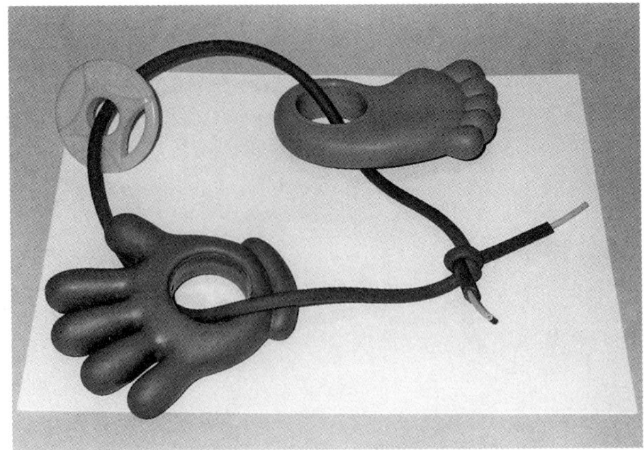

FIGURE 18-10 A chewy with toys safe for mouthing and biting. This chewy is designed for a child who bites people. Narrow tubing is threaded inside wider tubing to simulate the feeling of skin sliding over muscle.

Biting

Excessive biting of inedible objects is a problem occasionally encountered in children with developmental disabilities or other impairments. These children may bite things to calm themselves to reduce fear or anxiety or to explore the environment using the mouth because they are unable to perform tactile discrimination. They may also bite things because they have inadequate jaw stability or discomfort in the teeth or gums, or because they are trying to organize their bodies by giving pressure to the mouth and jaw, especially when learning new skills (e.g., children may bite their sleeves when struggling to learn handwriting in the first grade). Children may also bite to express anger or frustration or to attempt to communicate.

A "chewy" can be helpful for children who bite excessively (Figure 18-10). A chewy consists of chewable objects such as thick rubber toys, teethers, or oversized beads threaded onto a string or rubber or latex tubing.[27] The chewy can be worn as a necklace, attached to a belt, or even put in a pocket so it is always available. Adults use consistent teaching strategies to redirect the unsafe and improper biting of things and people to biting the chewy. The child is praised for biting the chewy each time s/he has the urge to

CLINICAL *Pearl*

Pen Suspenders (available from PDP Products) can be worn around the neck or fastened to clothing. The child slides a pen or pencil into the sleeve of the plastic holder, which is attached to a string. The holder is then readily available for biting, and it looks more mature and socially acceptable than a tubing necklace.

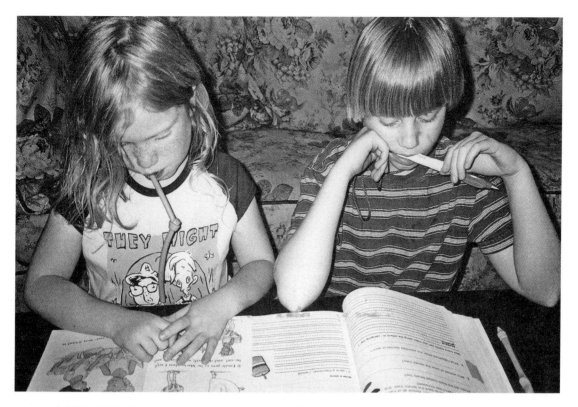

FIGURE 18-11 To help modulate, organize input, and increase focus on their work, the children mouth a "chewy" made from stretchy tubing and a "Pen Suspender" (from PDP Products).

bite. (**Precaution:** the chew toys need to be especially durable so that the child cannot bite through them. Chew toys made for animals are usually very durable.) School-age children may benefit from using a chewy that doubles as a pen or pencil holder (Figure 18-11).

The COTA may implement additional approaches for children who bite to explore objects. The child may be allowed to bite and explore safe objects with the mouth so that s/he can learn about shape, size, texture, and temperature. The child is taught which objects are not safe to put in the mouth. Simultaneously, the COTA addresses the use of the hands. The COTA can implement activities involving weight bearing on the hands, such as crawling over rugs, pillows, or other textured surfaces. Deep pressure applied to the hands can increase proprioceptive (muscle-joint input) awareness. Squeeze toys can be used to increase sensory awareness in the hands and the fine motor control needed for manipulating objects.

The sensation of biting the skin and muscle can feel very satisfying to some children. Once biting the skin becomes a habit, it can be dangerous and hard to stop. Children who persist in biting people can be given a special *chewy* made of two widths of Theratubing (see Figure 18-10). A piece of narrow, stretchy rubber or latex tubing is threaded inside a piece of wider tubing. The double layer, with one piece of tubing sliding over the other, simulates the feeling of the skin sliding over muscle and provides a safe alternative to biting people.[21]

Spitting

Some children spit excessively or play with their own saliva. In these cases the team and a doctor are consulted to determine the possible causes of the behavior. Some children may have problems with s-s-b synchrony such that saliva pools in their mouths. Others may produce excess saliva. Still others may be experimenting with cause/effect relationships, watching to see what happens when the saliva drips onto the table or floor, or exploring the texture of saliva by sliding their fingers or hands in it. Given a consistent team approach, many can be taught to handle saliva in an acceptable way.

RICKY'S SPITTING STORY. *Ricky, a nonverbal 4 year old, spits excessively on floors and tables. Consultation with his family revealed that he might be imitating his father, who sometimes spits in the sink or toilet at home. After ruling out medical and s-s-b problems, the team decided to show Ricky that spitting into a sink or wastebasket was an acceptable way to get rid of his excess saliva. He was encouraged to practice spitting in these places in school. When he spit on the table or floor, he was physically assisted in getting paper towels and cleaning it up. After Ricky learned the cleaning sequence, he was asked to clean up his spit independently when necessary. He was instructed in a matter-of-fact way and praised for every step toward managing his saliva. Even though Ricky could not ask for a place to spit, he soon learned to use only the sink or wastebasket for spitting at school.*

Ricky's spitting behavior was under control in the school environment. The team did not anticipate that he might have any problems outside of school. One day while on a field trip, the teachers noticed Ricky scanning an unfamiliar room and becoming increasingly agitated as he searched for a sink or wastebasket. He needed to spit and had learned not to do so on floors or tables. Ricky urgently darted to his teacher's large open pocketbook, the object looking most like a wastebasket to him, and spit into it. Ricky had solved his dilemma. The startled yet level-headed and wise teacher remained calm and praised him for not spitting on the floor. The staff regarded the incident with a good sense of humor but also learned an important lesson: when teaching a new behavior, all potential factors that could affect the behavior, like different settings, need to be considered.

Regurgitation and pica behavior

Certain children with special needs regurgitate food (return food to the mouth from the stomach) and display **pica behavior** (craving and eating inedible items such as plaster and dirt). Both behaviors are unsafe and socially unacceptable. Regurgitated stomach acid can destroy the teeth, and ingestion of dangerous substances like paint chips or pins can be physically harmful. In the following stories, the OT practitioner is instrumental in providing alternative activities for the adolescents involved. She chooses activities for their behavior plans that fit the adolescents' severe cognitive, social, and visual impairments.

ERNIE'S REGURGITATION STORY. *Ernie is a tall, lanky adolescent who lives in a residential institution. He is nonverbal and blind. He has severe mental retardation and few remaining teeth due to stomach acid from food regurgitated after every meal. After regurgitating, Ernie keeps the food in his mouth for some time before finally swallowing it. The treatment team determined that Ernie had developed this unhealthy habitual behavior because he was bored from the lack of stimulation in the institution and he was still hungry after eating his meals.*

To address his boredom, the team increased Ernie's activity program, emphasizing his favorite activities and social interactions with staff and peers. Physical activities were increased and included jumping on large and small trampolines as well as going through an obstacle course that the OT practitioner had designed for the residents with visual impairments.

To address his hunger, the nurse, psychologist, and SLP devised an unusual strategy that proved quite successful. After each meal, Ernie was allowed to eat as much bread as he wanted. At first he ate more than half a loaf. With so much food in his stomach, he felt satiated. The bread proved to be too bulky for Ernie to regurgitate. As his activity program continued, Ernie began to realize that he could eat as much as he wanted. Regurgitation stopped and smiling increased. After a few weeks, Ernie reduced the amount of bread he ate to two or three slices after each meal.

MELVIN'S PICA BEHAVIOR STORY. *Melvin is a large adolescent who weighs more than 250 pounds. He is nonverbal, blind, and profoundly retarded and lives in a residential home. Melvin plays with pieces of lint from the floor or tiny pieces of regurgitated food, alternately playing with them in his mouth and rolling and flicking them between his fingers. In addition, Melvin is self-abusive (banged his head on walls, furniture, or people) and becomes aggressive when frustrated or pressured to perform.*

While considering possible causes for his maladaptive pica behavior (craving and eating nonfood substances), the team determined that it had developed as a coping behavior. Pica behavior helped Melvin handle growing up blind in an institutional environment with inadequate social or environmental stimulation. He was bored and needed to play with something. Because Melvin was so emotionally fragile and dangerous to himself and others, his intervention was carried out slowly and cautiously in phases.

- *Melvin was first given one-to-one staffing with carefully chosen gentle primary caretakers who liked him and were successful at calming him.*
- *Melvin was given a variety of small tactile and auditory toys. He developed a strong attachment to one toy in particular, a small plastic cube with a tiny marble inside. When Melvin shook the cube, it rattled. He kept the cube and took it with him everywhere.*
- *Melvin was given additional nurturing social contacts.*
- *Melvin was engaged in an enhancing, calming activity program that the OT practitioner developed with input from primary caretakers and educational, recreational, psychological, and music therapy staff members. This program included rocking in a rocking chair, handling vibrating toys, listening to music, playing in water, and engaging in other activities that soothed Melvin.*
- *When Melvin displayed pica behavior, his primary caregiver gently redirected him into a calming, desirable activity like playing the plastic cube.*
- *When Melvin appeared agitated and resisted redirection, the caregiver avoided getting involved in dangerous power struggles. He was soothed until he was calm enough to give his primary caretaker the piece of lint or regurgitated food.*

After about 3 months of using this consistent nurturing and socially and environmentally enriched program, Melvin's pica behavior disappeared.

Bowel and Bladder Management

Bowel and bladder management refers to the capacity to control bowel movements and urination and the use of adaptive equipment or agents to aid regular bowel evacuation and bladder elimination.

Sensory awareness of pressure in the bladder (sack holding urine until its release) and urethra (tube carrying urine from the bladder to outside the body) develops before muscle control to release urine develops. Sensory awareness of pressure in the lower intestines near the anus (exit aperture for bowel movements) develops before the muscle control necessary to release a bowel movement develops. Daytime control develops before night-time bladder control. Some children sleep so soundly that they have trouble developing night-time bladder control. A variety of devices that help make the child aware of when s/he is wet are available from stores and supply catalogs.

Children with low muscle tone may develop both sensory awareness and control later than other children. Those with motor control problems such as cerebral palsy with spasticity may develop sensation long before they are able to control muscles. Other children, such as those with spinal cord injury or those born with severe cases of spina bifida (incomplete growth of spinal vertebrae), may be physically unable to develop sensation or control of the bladder or bowels. Because they cannot control the muscles used in bowel movements, these children may use suppositories regularly to assist them.

For any toileting program to work successfully, the child's diet must be considered. To ensure regular bowel movements, the child's diet should include enough fiber (contained in many vegetables and whole grains). With a physician's approval some children may take natural fiber supplements or use suppositories as part of their toileting program. To ensure regular urination, be sure the child drinks plenty of water and/or other liquids.

Resistance to toileting

Children may resist using a toilet for a number of reasons: (1) Diapers feel warm, snug, supportive, and comforting; (2) the feeling of underwear is unfamiliar and cool, and it does not provide the same support or comfort; (3) the toilet may appear too high and therefore frightening; (4) sitting on a toilet can feel cold and hard; (5) the sound or sight of the toilet flushing may be scary; and (6) depending on their level of cognitive and emotional development, some children may believe that part of the body is disappearing into the toilet.

Consider the following solutions:

1. Provide transition underwear that is extra thick and snug, similar to the feeling of the diapers. Some children may benefit from neoprene shorts, which are warm and provide external support (see Appendix C of this chapter). In contrast, some children need to wear underwear that feels completely different from diapers, so they will readily sense the difference. The realization that they are wearing different underwear can direct their attention to the new way of toileting: sitting on the potty.
2. Use a padded toilet seat or warm the seat with a hair dryer or heat lamp. Make the bathroom environment comfortable.
3. Use a "potty seat" that is close to the ground and has a wide, stable base. If this is not possible, provide a footrest and a potty insert to make the opening of the regular toilet smaller.
4. Temporarily omit flushing from treatment sessions to determine whether it helps the child tolerate the toilet better. Once the child masters eliminating in the toilet, develop strategies to address the fear of flushing (e.g., use a quieter toilet, let the child flush the toilet, or let the child go outside the bathroom door and then tell the OT practitioner when to flush).
5. Help young children deal with their fear of losing part of the body in the toilet by placing a diaper in the bottom of a potty seat. The child is reassured by seeing the urine or feces go into the diaper, just like it did before the potty was used.[37]

FEAR OF THE BATHROOM STORY. *In a special preschool setting, a team of teachers and a COTA became frustrated in their attempts to toilet train a classroom of children with severe developmental delays. When approaching or attempting to go into the bathroom, four of the six children cried, screamed, pulled away, threw tantrums, and refused to enter. The team identified both sensory defensive and fear reactions in the children, so they tried modifying numerous environmental factors to help them relax. The toilet seat was warmed to reduce the sudden feeling of the cold on their skin. Flushing the toilet was avoided so as to keep the loud noise from frightening them. The children still refused to enter the bathroom.*

The teacher and COTA eventually determined the cause of the children's fear. They could not tolerate the "sound of the lights" in the bathroom. The children tolerated the same level of fluorescent lighting in the classroom, so team members had assumed that the lights were not a problem. The difference was that every time the bathroom lights were turned on, a faint, high-pitched whine emanated from them and the children began to cry. The sound was barely audible to the team members. When the bathroom lights were turned off, the children calmed down and entered the bathroom without resistance.

The teacher's and COTA's careful and repeated observation and analysis, in context, and problem solving led to discovering the problem of the "sound of the lights" and an easy solution.

Schedule toilet training

Schedule toilet training programs are often effective in helping children learn to urinate in the toilet at regular intervals. These programs take place both at home and in the classroom. At home the parent and home care nurse or at school the teacher and OT practitioner usually coordinate this intervention. At school the teacher and OT practitioner work together on schedule toilet training. An adult takes the child to the bathroom every 30 to 60 minutes. Each time the child is taken to the bathroom, the toileting routine is repeated, including pulling the pants down, sitting on the toilet, wiping, pulling the pants up, and washing the hands. Drinking fluids 30 to 60 minutes before toileting may be part of the schedule training program. During the training, the children have so many opportunities to use the toilet that they begin to successfully use it for eliminating or having bowel movements.

It is important to make the toileting experience as comfortable and successful as possible. The following strategies may be helpful:

1. Buy a small toilet seat and place it next to the adult toilet seat. Some parents provide a picture book about toileting for the child to look at. The OT practitioner and parents can strategize to find the best approach for that child. At home, parents can encourage the child to use the potty seat at the same time that one of them uses the toilet. Children want to be like their parents, who can provide a model for them to imitate.
2. Simply turning on the water at the sink may facilitate urination. The running water sends an auditory message to the child, who unconsciously associates the sound with the feeling of urination.
3. Experiment with different potty seats. Some children prefer to start toileting on an adult-sized toilet to be "just like mommy and daddy." Some potty seats fit on top of a standard toilet seat with smaller openings to fit a child's small body.

CLINICAL *Pearl*

The Pediatric Toilet Safety Armrests (Achievement Products, Canton, Ohio; see Appendix C of this chapter) are relatively inexpensive, useful for most children and adults, and easy to attach. The armrests curve under the toilet seat, and the child's weight on the toilet keeps him or her from moving. The Pediatric Toilet Safety Armrests have two advantages: (1) the armrests are out of the way so that they cannot present obstacles to bump into or trip over, and (2) if a child accidentally pulls up instead of down on them, they tend to stay in place and provide support. However, the armrests themselves are at an adult height 7 to 8 inches above the seat.

Adapted equipment for toileting

A variety of adaptive equipment for toileting is available from equipment companies.

Children who have motor limitations often need adaptive equipment to facilitate independent toileting. Many factors need to be considered when choosing a toileting device. The caregivers' concerns are extremely important. If a device is too cumbersome to set up or clean, the caregivers may revert to putting their children in diapers.

Many children benefit from additional hand support beside the toilet to aid in sitting, staying on the toilet, and standing. Sometimes a grab bar beside the tub is close enough to the toilet to use. The OT practitioner may place a tension-operated floor-to-ceiling pole beside the toilet.

Some children need only a step stool or low toilet seat along with armrests to ensure their security.

Rolling toilet chairs may prove useful for some families. The toilet chair is rolled over the toilet when the child needs to use it. It can be rolled away when the parents or other family members use the toilet. Rolling toilet chairs can also serve as shower chairs.

Children with significant motor limitations might need a toilet seat with a backrest, lateral head support, lateral trunk support, seat belt, chest belt, footrests with straps to hold the feet in place, and armrests or grab bars.

Positioning for toileting

It is important for children sitting on a toilet to have their feet firmly on the ground for stability. Footrests may be necessary. To facilitate evacuation and elimination, the child can lean forward from a regular sitting position.

Balancing on an adult-sized toilet seat can be a challenge for any small child. Some children learn to support themselves with their hands placed beside them on the toilet seat. One toddler had her own idea of climbing onto the toilet seat backward. She straddled the toilet while holding onto the toilet tank to steady herself. She used this backward strategy without a potty seat and felt safe and secure until she was big enough to face forward.

Climbing onto an adult-sized toilet can also be a challenge. Step stools are available at children's stores and through equipment catalogs. Some children benefit from using the step stool as a footrest to promote stability and add a sense of security.

Little boys often first learn to urinate while sitting on a potty seat. The sitting posture reduces the need to balance, aim, and concentrate on releasing urine all at the same time. Little boys' potty seats usually come with a "splashguard," a high curved lip at the front of the seat. The splashguard prevents urine from accidentally spraying onto the floor. The splashguard also eliminates the need for little boys to aim accurately while concentrating on the release of urine on demand. Once postural control and urinary release have been mastered, some splashguards can be removed. Some boys may be ready to get rid of the potty seat and stand at the toilet.

To stand at a regular toilet and urinate, boys need to be tall enough and have adequate standing balance, a certain degree of spatial awareness and motor planning, and sufficient focus of attention. To help a boy learn to aim into the toilet while standing, small biodegradable foam donuts and other shapes can be obtained in children's stores and drugstores. The adult or little boy drops a foam shape into the toilet. Boys seem to love the "game" of aiming at the floating target, and it can increase their motor planning and attention while keeping the bathroom cleaner. For a less expensive method, simply drop a small piece of toilet paper into the water to serve as a target.

Children who have physical limitations may need more assistance for positioning when toileting. For those with spasticity, pediatric toilet seats often include a splashguard that also serves as a *pommel*, which is a device designed to keep the knees apart and reduce the spasticity that involuntarily pulls the knees tightly together. Sometimes the pommel can be detached when the child gets into or out of the chair.

Toilet Hygiene

Toilet hygiene is the ability to clean oneself after using the potty and includes knowing how to obtain and use the necessary supplies, managing clothing, holding oneself in the proper position, transferring to and from toilet facilities, managing menstruation, and managing incontinence (the inability to control the release of urine and feces). The management of catheters, colostomies, and suppositories is also part of toilet hygiene.

Except for medical procedures such as using a catheter or colostomy tube, COTAs might have the primary responsibility of training children in toilet hygiene, including how much wiping is necessary, how much toilet paper to use, and how to pull it off the roll and bunch it up. The COTA might also be responsible for reminding a child to wash his/her hands with soap every time he/she uses the toilet. Female COTAs might be responsible for helping girls learn how to manage menstruation and what to do with dirty underwear.

KENNY'S WIPING STORY. *Kenny had poor trunk rotation, weakness, distractibility, and insufficient knowledge about the need for cleaning after toileting. Because of his poor proprioceptive (muscle-joint input) discrimination, most of his actions were guided by vision. In other words, to control hand and foot movements, he needed to watch them closely. He was unable to successfully use feedback from the muscles and joints to plan his motor activities. The OT practitioner noticed that Kenny smelled after using the toilet for a bowel movement. His underwear was dirty. When Kenny showed the OT practitioner how he wiped, it was noted that he used almost no pressure and did not rotate his trunk or look at what he was doing. As a result, he did not get clean. Kenny's parents said that they were at a loss on how to teach him to wipe and asked for help.*

During OT sessions, Kenny was engaged in activities to achieve the following: discriminate different textures and shapes through touch; develop trunk rotation and reach behind his back; and strengthen the arms, hands, and trunk. He was given explanations and repeated requests to discuss why wiping is important. In addition, work took place in the bathroom. Whenever Kenny needed to use the toilet, the opportunity was taken to teach him. To show him the amount of pressure required, the OT practitioner wore plastic gloves and gave him hand-over-hand assistance in wiping. To make it easier, handi-wipes were used. Kenny was then asked to wipe himself from behind and look at the handi-wipe. He initially needed close supervision and much encouragement to continue wiping and checking until the handi-wipe was clean. Gradually Kenny moved to using toilet paper. With carryover from teachers and parents, he also began using more pressure, rotating more, and independently checking the toilet paper. In a few months his mother stated that he came home with his underwear clean.

Supplies

Toilet paper for wiping and water, soap, and towels for washing hands are the basic supplies needed for toileting. Children need to know how to get more supplies when the toilet paper roll is empty, the soap is gone, and the towel needs washing. Depending on the child's age and capabilities, this could involve getting and replacing it themselves or calling the caregiver's attention to the situation. The COTA may be responsible for training a child in what to do to get more supplies.

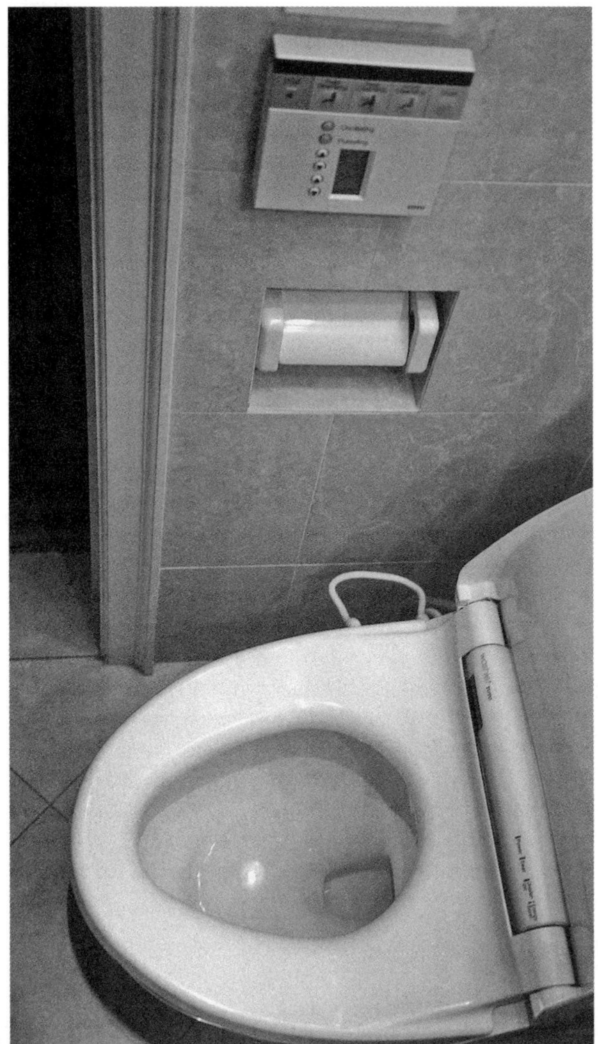

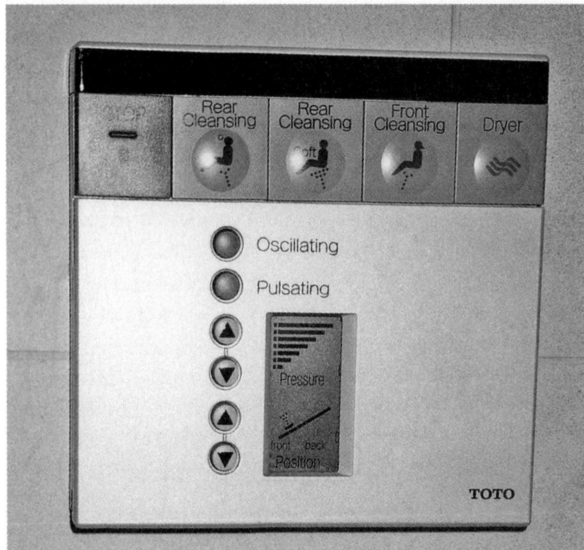

FIGURE 18-12 **A,** This electronic bidet toilet is operated by **B,** push buttons.

CLINICAL *Pearl*

Be sure that the wipes are alcohol free because alcohol can be irritating to the skin of some children. Also be sure that the wipes are not too cold. For children with extreme negative reactions to the cool sensation of wipes, it may help to place them in a microwave oven for a few seconds initially. Check to be sure that the wipes are warm and not hot.

Children who have sensory defensiveness may react negatively to the feeling of toilet paper. They may feel more comfortable using moist wipes until they become more familiar with wiping.

Children with significant physical limitations require special supplies. For example, a child with a spinal cord injury, who cannot reach behind the body or grasp toilet paper, might use tongs designed to hold it. A mirror might be used along with the tongs to check for cleanliness. Children who are unable to manage the tongs and mirror may need an electronic bidet with an automatic dryer. Bidets are large cleaning devices that look like toilets. When a person sits on one, it sends a spray of water that cleans the private parts. They can be separate pieces of equipment next to the toilet (Figure 18-12).

Managing clothing

Children need to independently operate the fasteners on their pants and pull regular pants and underwear down and then up over the hips. They usually learn to do this while standing in front of the toilet. Some children need to hold a grab bar or a solid chair with one hand and use the other hand to loosen the pants, pull them down, and later pull them up and fasten them. Children with hemiplegia (paralysis on one side of the body) might need to lean on the wall or first sit on the toilet to prevent falling while sliding clothing over the hips.

Menstrual care

Adolescence brings a new toileting challenge for all girls—menstruation. Menstrual care is even more challenging for girls with physical or cognitive disabilities. In their books and CD-ROMs called *Personal Success*, the Attainment Company (see Appendix C of this chapter) offers excellent picture guides for changing a sanitary napkin (pad) and tampon. These aids are oriented toward

CLINICAL *Pearl*

The most common type of glove is made of latex. If the child, nurse, OT practitioner or caregiver has latex sensitivity, then latex-free gloves must be used.

adolescents and young adults who have limited cognitive, learning, sequencing, body awareness, and social skills but may prove useful for other populations as well.

KELLY'S MENSTRUAL CARE STORY. Kelly was a 13-year-old girl with severe mental retardation, severe sensory defensiveness, a decreased ability to interpret touch-pressure feedback, weakness, incoordination, motor planning and motor memory problems, and limited range of motion, including decreased trunk rotation. She experienced difficulty in caring for menstrual needs in several ways. The OT practitioner helped her address these personal needs.

During OT sessions, Kelly regularly practiced trunk rotation activities to help her develop the skill of reaching behind her back during toileting. To increase her awareness of how much pressure to apply while wiping, she performed many resistive finger/hand activities. She performed weight bearing activities on her hands and wiped tables and blackboards. She also practiced regular toileting routines, including wiping in a front-to-back motion (to prevent urinary tract infections), adjusting clothing, and pressing hard enough during hand washing to wash and dry the hands thoroughly.

Kelly's parents provided large pads with adhesive tabs and side wings because they were the easiest for her to manage. When she was menstruating, Kelly brought her own pad to the OT sessions. She also brought picture cues of her bathroom sequence, which her COTA and speech therapist had created together. Combined with the COTA's verbal and demonstrative guidance, the picture cues reminded Kelly to (1) look and see whether her pad needed changing, (2) fold up the dirty pad, (3) wrap it in toilet paper, (4) discard it in a special container, (5) open a new package, and (6) stick a new pad to her underwear. Kelly could not estimate if there was only a little or a lot of blood on her pad. She was instructed to change the pad if there was any blood on it.

When Kelly's underwear had blood on it, the COTA used additional verbal and visual cues to help her change it. Wearing plastic gloves, the COTA assisted Kelly in washing the dirty underwear with cold water and soap. She then put the wet underwear in a plastic bag and brought them home for laundering.

Catheters

Children who cannot control the muscles for urination may be fitted with catheters. A catheter is a small tube inserted through the urethra into the bladder. The catheter allows urine to pass out of the body and into a bag attached to the child's leg, walker, or wheelchair. When the bag is full, the child or caregiver empties the urine from the bag into the toilet. The OT practitioner and nurse work closely together to make catheterization comfortable for the child. They also work together to teach catheter management if the child is cognitively and physically capable of learning it. When the catheter is inserted, cleanliness and comfort are most important. The hands are washed with antibacterial soap, and new plastic gloves are used.

BECKY'S CATHETER STORY. Becky is a 10-year-old girl who was born with spina bifida (for a discussion of spina bifida, see Chapter 15). She receives OT and nursing services at home. Becky does not have sensation below her waist and cannot control the muscles for urination. She has received help with catheterization from nurses and caregivers since she was a toddler. Now Becky has asked to learn to do this by herself. The OT practitioner and Becky's nurse arrange with her parents to meet for a joint session at home. Becky's mother helps during the session. The OT practitioner and Becky have been preparing for this session by using a catheter mirror. It is a 9-inch-wide round mirror attached to a flexible metal wire that Becky clips to her bed. She bends the wire so that when she is lying back and supported by pillows, she is able to push her legs open and see her urethra reflected in the mirror.

Before getting into bed, Becky empties the urine from her catheter bag into the toilet. When the nurse arrives, Becky is in position in bed and the OT practitioner and Becky's mother are ready. Everyone has prepared by washing the hands and putting on plastic gloves. The OT practitioner makes sure that Becky is comfortable. The nurse instructs Becky, the OT practitioner, and her mother in the following: cleansing the urethra with antibacterial soap; carefully removing the catheter she is wearing; looking for areas that have become red or irritated by the catheter; properly cleansing the skin again; applying cream or lotion for healing; and applying ointment for easy insertion as needed, preparing the urethra for the new catheter. The OT practitioner guides Becky in using the mirror and following the nurse's directions. Next, Becky must insert the new catheter tube. The package is opened and precautions are taken to keep the new catheter clean according to the nurse's directions. As the nurse instructs them, the OT practitioner guides Becky in using the mirror to gently insert the catheter into the urethra. The practitioner makes sure that Becky continues to be supported properly in bed and checks to be sure that her position will allow smooth insertion of the

CLINICAL *Pearl*

Children with spasticity may need pillows or pommels (firm supports between the knees) to keep the knees apart during catheterization. They may benefit from using a side-lying position, which can help inhibit spasticity.

catheter all the way into the bladder. The nurse tells Becky how to proceed and how to decide when she has inserted the catheter far enough. The nurse then instructs her and the OT practitioner in how to check the catheter's position using the mirror, how to be sure that it is connected securely to the bag, and how to prevent leakage. Becky attaches the catheter bag to her leg or wheelchair. Everyone removes their gloves and washes their hands again. Now Becky dresses herself and transfers out of bed, feeling satisfied that she has taken a big step forward toward independence.

Personal Hygiene and Grooming

Learning and remembering when and how often to perform personal hygiene may be a challenge for some chil-

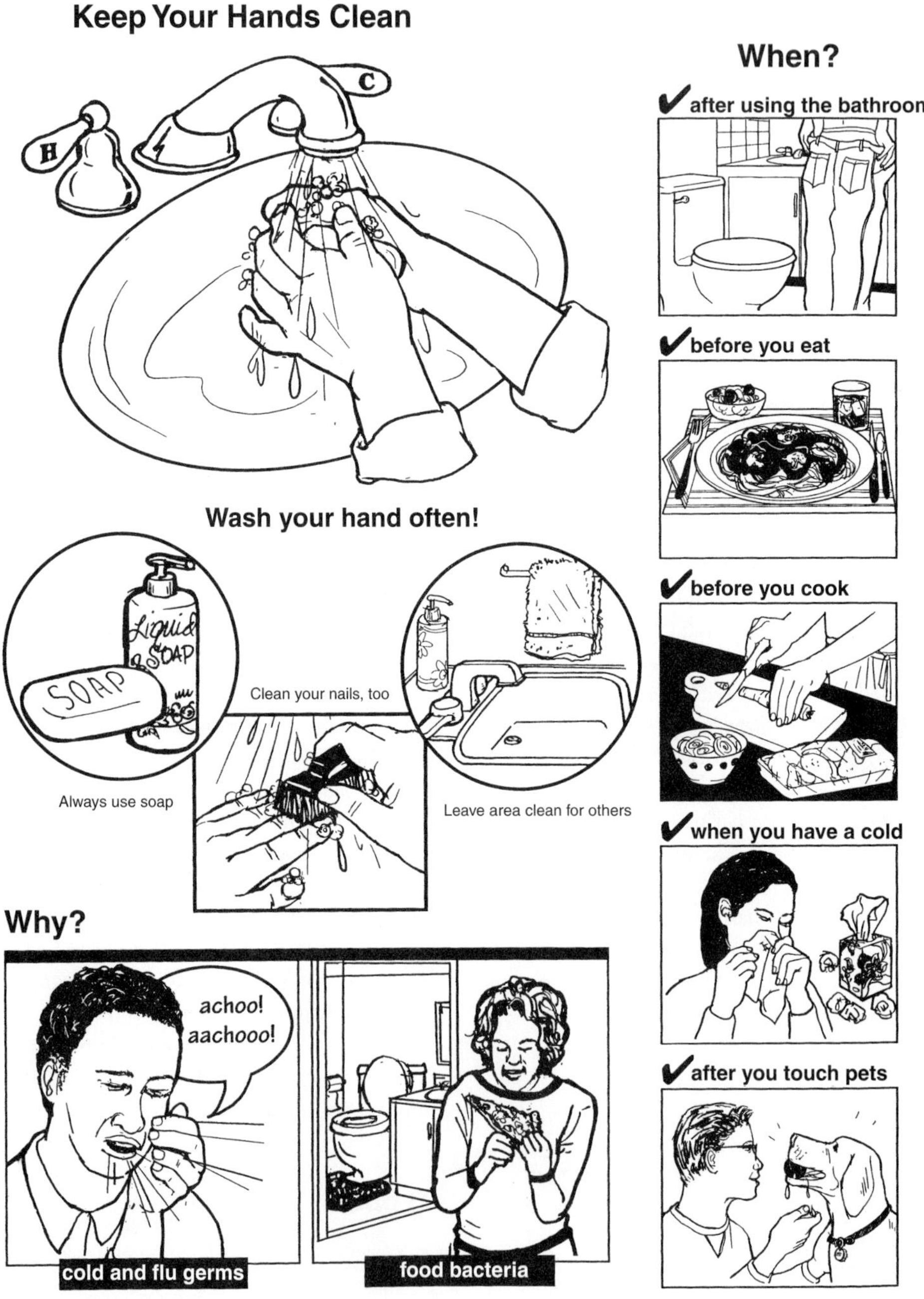

FIGURE 18-13 When this picture is posted in a bathroom, it can help children remember and follow the rules for hand washing. (From Reynolds J: *Attainment's personal success: an illustrated guide to personal needs,* Attainment Company Inc, 1999, Verona, Wis.)

dren with special needs. A primary role of OT practitioners is to help children learn the skills required to clean themselves adequately. COTAs may work on organizational skills related to hygiene and grooming. This requires reviewing bedtime and morning sequences and developing picture or written checklists with them. For example, a night-time checklist might include showering and shampooing hair, getting out clean clothes to wear the next day (that match in color and are appropriate for the predicted weather), and preparing their backpacks for school.[11]

Hand washing

Hand washing is performed every time an individual uses the toilet, comes inside from outdoors, and before and after eating. One of the most common causes of bacterial and viral transmission is insufficient hand washing.

The COTA may either assist with hand washing or ask the child if the hands were washed with soap and water.

Picture cues inside the bathroom can help children with special needs who have trouble remembering the sequence and physically performing the steps (Figure 18-13).[31] They sometimes wet only their fingertips, or they may get their arms, face, and shirt completely wet and become lost in playing with the soap bubbles. Some children do not know how to interlace their fingers to clean between them. Others do not know how to make lather with soap and do not realize that this is part of hand washing. Children with sensory defensiveness may ask to wash their hands more often than other children, or they may resist touching warm water, soap, and paper towels. Try to prevent potential outbursts by helping children push up long sleeves before turning on the water. Those with sensory defensiveness may pull off a shirt with wet sleeves or become so preoccupied with them that they cannot focus on anything else. Try to find comfortable ways for children to clean and dry their hands. Handi-wipes and liquid hand cleaner are alternatives to soap and water. Using a clean cloth towel and air drying are acceptable methods of drying hands.

Hair care

Having hair shampooed, cut, and groomed can be a trying experience for a child and caregiver. The child may scream and cry during shampooing no matter how gentle the process. Just one memory of getting soap in the eyes can cause a fear response in a toddler. During shampooing, the multiple texture and temperature changes (dry hair, wet hair, soapy hair, watery hair, warm air, cool air) and actions such as towel drying may cause the child to feel bombarded with attacks to the head.

When the hair is brushed, combed, braided, or put into hair bands or barrettes, the child receives multiple alternating sensations, from tickly to tugging and sometimes pinching, especially if the hair is tangled. These sensations may seem completely unpredictable and therefore more painful to a child with sensory defensiveness. The tickly vibration of an electric trimmer on the back of the head or neck, combined with intense buzzing beside the ears and prickly, newly cut hairs, may be more than the child can handle. Some of the following interventions for hair care may help.

1. Use a baby shampoo that causes little or no stinging when it gets in the eyes.
2. Rinse-free shampoos are now available from many equipment catalogs, pharmacies, and surgical supply companies.
3. A spray detangler works well on dry hair. Look for products that are alcohol free because alcohol dries out hair.
4. Even if the child does not yet understand language, each time the hair is shampooed and dried, use a soothing voice to repeat what will happen next. The rhythmic repetition of words can be calming. If the child understands the words, knowing what is going to happen can lessen anxiety.
5. Carry out each hair care step with a smooth, firm touch. Sometimes in their well-meaning attempts to be careful with a sensitive child, caregivers are too gentle, resulting in tickly sensations instead of firm, deep pressure. Light-moving touch is the most uncomfortable.
6. Be sure water and room temperatures are warm but not too hot. Keep a towel handy in case the face or eyes need to be wiped quickly.
7. Whenever possible, allow the child to control the hair care procedure. Even if attempts are unsuccessful and the caregiver must take over, the child may begin to get accustomed to the sensations by controlling part of the procedure.
8. Make the hair-cutting experience fun by providing special treats. Many barbers know that giving a child a lollipop during a haircut can be soothing and distracting. Some children need multiple distractions, such as a favorite story along with a toy and lollipop.
9. Use the Wilbarger Deep Pressure and Proprioceptive Technique (DPPT) two or three times before giving

CLINICAL *Pearl*

The Attainment Company (see Appendix C of this chapter) markets materials such as booklets, videos, games, and sequencing picture cards that teach independent living skills to children and adults with mild to severe cognitive and/or motor impairments. Their picture sequences use clear drawings of individuals performing the steps of bathing, showering, toileting, tooth brushing, and other daily living skills.

a child a haircut.[38] If possible, spend an hour in the park and sing songs or play with blowing toys right before the haircut. These activities help modulate the child's nervous system. Applying deep pressure to the head before the haircut, as with a head massage, may also help.
10. If an electric trimmer is not necessary, ask the barber not to use one.
11. Consider asking a trusted family member to cut a child's hair in the home. The secure feeling provided by a familiar relative and the home environment can help the child tolerate a haircut. A child who screams and throws a tantrum at a barbershop may sit quietly for an uncle who cuts the child's hair at home, even when an electric trimmer is used.

Independent hair care is taught on different levels, according to children's needs. Some need to gain knowledge about how often to wash and comb their hair and have it cut. Others need to learn step-by-step procedures for each skill. Still others need to have a positive attitude with regard to taking responsibility for hair care, checking themselves, and evaluating the outcome of their efforts.

Some children benefit from using a mirror during hair grooming, whereas others are confused by the backward mirror image. Adaptive devices such as a long- or bent-handled hairbrush may be helpful. A heavy hairbrush with a large handle and indented finger and thumb holds provides extra physical feedback for the child with limited sensory awareness.

MARY'S HAIR CARE STORY. *Mary is a 13-year-old girl with severe mental retardation, sensory defensiveness, a poor ability to reach across her midline, and an inability to accurately feel the hairbrush; she needs a special approach to hair care. Mary depended on visual feedback to guide her hand movements, so she practiced in front of a mirror. She used spray detangler and a large-handled hairbrush with a well defined handhold. The brush had bristles on all sides, so it was effective no matter which way Mary turned it.*

Although Mary was right handed, she brushed more thoroughly on the left side of her head using her left hand. By using each hand to brush each side of her head, Mary did not have to struggle to rotate her trunk and reach across her midline. Mary alternated using each hand to brush the back of her head. If Mary were younger or had fewer physical disabilities, it might have been possible for her to develop trunk rotation and spontaneous midline-crossing skills for more efficient hair brushing.

Shaving

Because of safety issues, make sure to obtain administrative approval, written permission from parents or guardians, and input from supervisors and team members when implementing a shaving program. Extra supervision is needed for girls and boys with emotional impairments; razors may need to be stored in a locked cabinet.

Shaving may not be necessary for girls unless a girl is highly invested in shaving her legs or underarms. For adolescent girls, shaving instructions should consist of how often to shave, the materials needed, how to obtain the materials, the cost of the materials, the motor sequence of shaving, safety precautions, positioning methods, self-evaluation, cleanup, and how to change the razor.

A group shaving program can be helpful for adolescent boys with limited coordination, cognition, sequencing abilities, sensory awareness, and strength. The camaraderie and pride associated with shaving independently can be shared.

EARL'S AND GREG'S SHAVING STORY. *At age 17, neither Earl nor Greg had the coordination to safely handle regular razors. Earl was diagnosed with fragile X syndrome (a genetic disorder, which can result in autism and intellectual disability, caused by a "fragile site" on the X chromosome), and attention deficit disorder. Greg had a history of lead poisoning, resulting in mental retardation. Both boys had emotional problems. Their COTA used activity analysis and knowledge of the boys' strengths and limitations to implement an effective training program for both of them.*

The COTA obtained permission from school administrators and the boys' parents. She searched in catalogs, local stores, and newspaper ads until she found a low-priced, good-quality, safe, wet-and-dry use electric razor.

Mirrors can help or hinder the shaving process, depending on the child. With Earl and Greg, tabletop mirrors proved helpful in carrying out the shaving sequence as well as checking their success. Because of Earl's severe sensory defensiveness, the COTA kept the water warm and allowed him to be in control of all contact with his face. The program included learning to clean the razors and change the blades. A pictorial guide showing the sequence provides visual cues for the boys to follow.

Nail care

Being given the opportunity to choose from a variety of trimming and cleaning tools may help a reluctant child participate in nail care tasks. Girls are often enticed by pretty nail polish and interested in keeping nails long.

Nail clippers can be dangerous or difficult to operate for children with limited coordination or weakness. A variety of adapted nail clippers are available. For example, some attach to a board that has suction cups on the bottom, eliminating the need to simultaneously hold, position, and pinch the clippers with one hand. Instead, the child positions the finger with the nail to be trimmed on the device and pushes down on the clippers. An oversized emery board may be easier and safer for other children. Some may prefer to use fingernail scissors. Scissors with a round tip are the safest, and they are often found in the baby section of the pharmacy. Children with limited motor planning skills, hand strength, and dexterity may benefit from preparatory resistive fingertip exercises, frequent and short practice sessions, and extra help in evaluating their performance by looking at and feeling their nails.

In addition to trimming nails, cleaning fingernails can be addressed in a nail care program.

Skin care

Children with spinal cord injuries, limited mobility, or limited sensory awareness must be taught to check their skin for bedsores, which are also called decubitus ulcers. They range from bruises to open red wounds and result from prolonged pressure to one area of the skin, depriving it of circulation and subsequently oxygen and nutrients. Bedsores are difficult to heal, so prevention is critical. Different sizes of mirrors with various bed or wall attachments can be angled to check the skin. After training by a doctor, nurse, or OTR, the COTA may teach children the procedures for the prevention and treatment of bedsores.

Many children have skin problems such as acne, eczema, psoriasis, scar tissue, and dry or oily skin. With advice from doctors and nurses, OT practitioners can help children learn what types of cream, lotion, or ointment need to be used and when and how to apply them; they need to watch children's responses carefully. Substances containing alcohol can irritate the skin and cause dryness. Children with sensory defensiveness may have a hard time tolerating substances for a variety of reasons: too cold, too slimy, too tickly, and/or too smelly. It is the OT practitioner's job to find reasons for children's resistance to any recommended substance and help find solutions. For example, the substance could be warmed in the practitioner's hands before application; excess moisturizer could be wiped off with soft tissues; it could be applied with firm pressure and long downward strokes; or a fragrance-free substance might be used.

Children with developmental delays, emotional impairments, or physical disabilities may need extra help in taking care of their skin. In dry or cold climates they may need to learn ways to check their skin to see whether it is rough, red, dry, or chapped and when and how to use skin lotion and lip moisturizer.

TERRI'S SKIN CARE STORY. Terri is a 7-year-old girl with Turner's syndrome (a genetic disorder in which the individual has only one X chromosome), attention deficit hyperactivity disorder, learning disabilities, and severe sensory defensiveness. She is extremely distracted by tactile, visual, and auditory input, so much so that she cannot screen out background stimulation without help. Every winter her lips become so chapped that she cannot stop touching and picking at them. This behavior not only causes her lips to bleed but also interferes with her focus on classroom activities.

Terri's intervention focused on three areas: (1) finding a tolerable lip moisturizer, (2) creating a schedule for its application, and (3) creating a plan to help Terri cope with her sensory defensiveness.

Finding a lip moisturizer that Terri would tolerate was not easy because her olfactory and oral sensory defensiveness were severe. Terri's mother and the OT practitioner found two kinds of lip balm that Terri tolerated. One day she would choose one kind, but the next day she would change her mind and choose the other one. Both were made available to her at all times.

Terri needed a schedule to apply the lip moisturizer frequently so that her lips would heal and stop distracting her. As a reminder to apply the moisturizer, a drawing of lip balm was taped to her school desk. School staff members also verbally reminded her to use the moisturizer.

Terri also benefited from the Wilbarger DPPT[38] to help her tolerate sensations. Terri stopped picking her lips during OT activities such as blowing bubbles and jumping on a trampoline. When the techniques were used consistently throughout the day and Terri used her lip balm frequently, she picked at her lips significantly less. She was able to pay attention more consistently in school.

Using deodorant

Children with special needs may find spray deodorants easier to use than roll-on deodorants. Adapters for spray cans may make it easier for children to use. Children with sensitive skin may be unable to use antiperspirants, but may be able to use a natural crystal deodorant.

COTAs can instruct children in deodorant use as well as practice the technique with them in a way so that children are not embarrassed.

EARL'S AND GREG'S DEODORANT STORY. Earl and Greg, the previously mentioned 17 year olds who had difficulty shaving, also had trouble using deodorant regularly. They

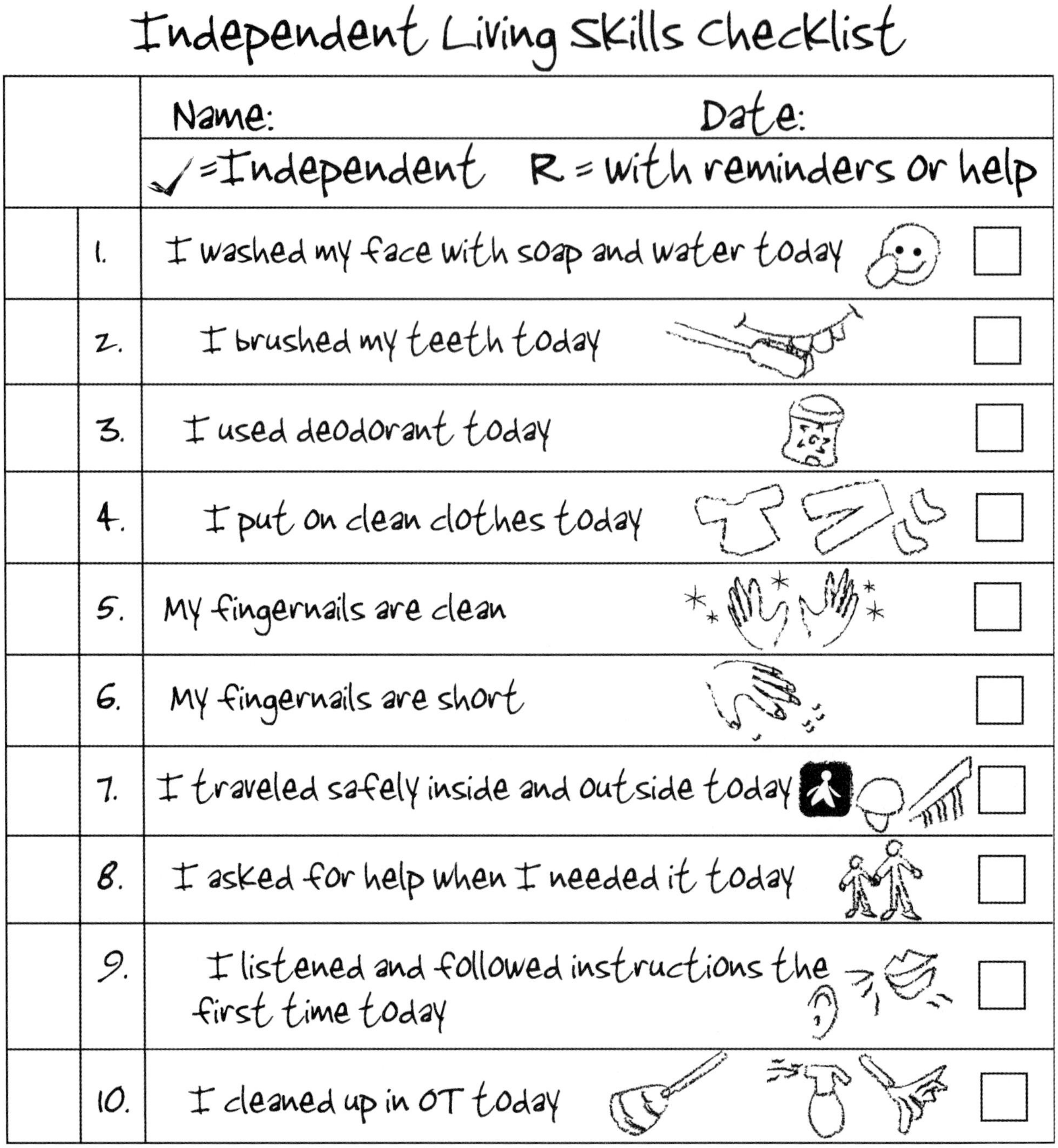

Independent Living Skills Checklist

		Name: Date:	
		✓ = Independent R = with reminders or help	
	1.	I washed my face with soap and water today	☐
	2.	I brushed my teeth today	☐
	3.	I used deodorant today	☐
	4.	I put on clean clothes today	☐
	5.	My fingernails are clean	☐
	6.	My fingernails are short	☐
	7.	I traveled safely inside and outside today	☐
	8.	I asked for help when I needed it today	☐
	9.	I listened and followed instructions the first time today	☐
	10.	I cleaned up in OT today	☐

FIGURE 18-14 Greg's and Earl's checklist for independent living skills.

had cognitive, sensory, motor planning, and emotional problems. Earl could not read, and Greg could read at only a third-grade level. At home they were given responsibility for their own daily hygiene and dressing tasks.

Figure 18-14 illustrates a checklist of daily living skills that can be used to help children take responsibility for their own hygiene, grooming, and functional interaction.

Earl and Greg completed their individual checklists daily to remind them to carry out their daily living skills. For

CLINICAL *Pearl*

Use caution when selecting an electric toothbrush. Some children are frightened by the vibrations, whereas others find the sound aversive, especially that of sonic electric toothbrushes.

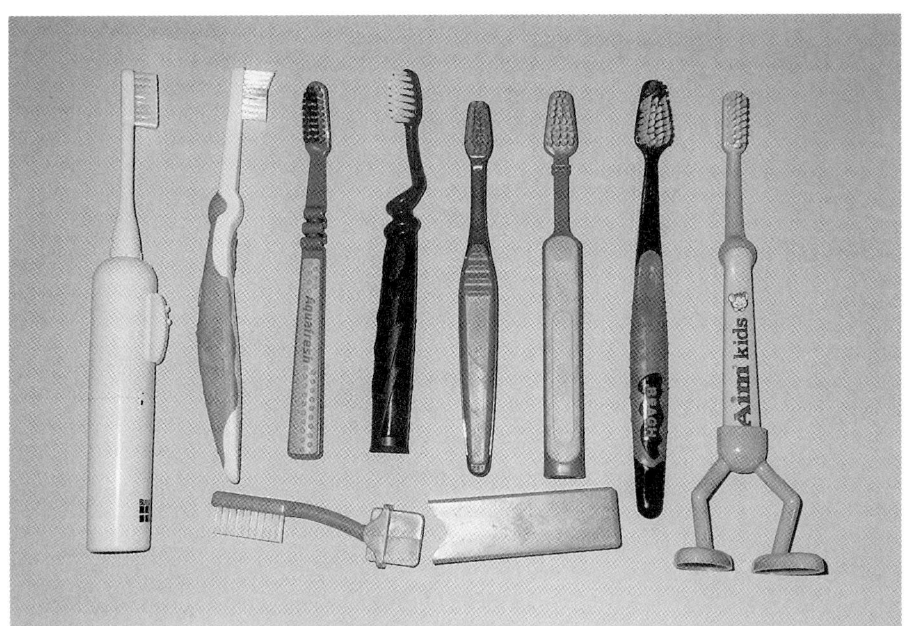

A

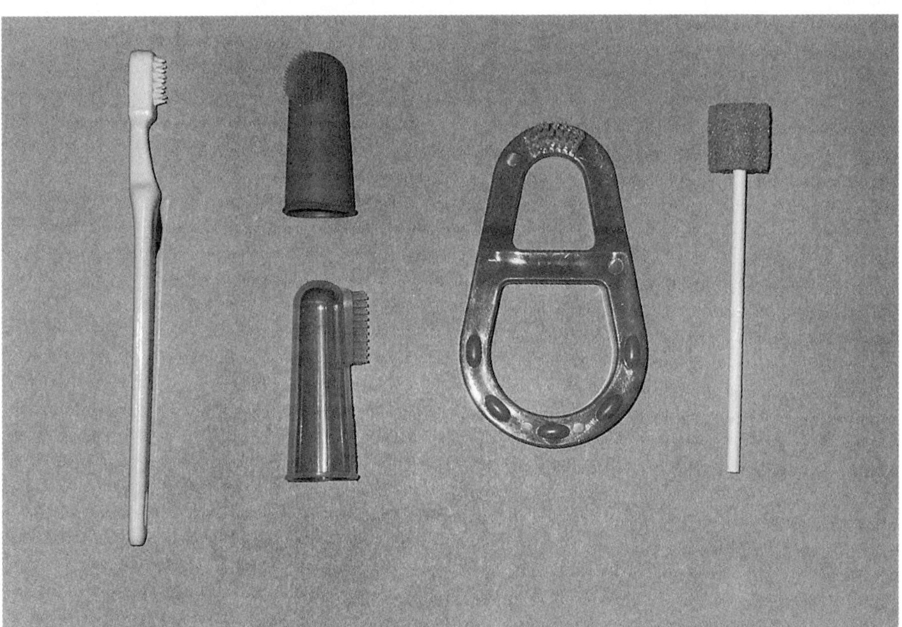

B

FIGURE 18-15 A, Different styles of large-handled toothbrushes, including an electric toothbrush, that can make tooth brushing easier. **B,** Modified toothbrushes *(left to right):* Nuk training brush; fingertip toothbrushes; rounded toothbrush, which is safe for infants; and toothette.

example, after reviewing his checklist, Greg often reported that he had forgotten to use deodorant. He was then given deodorant and asked to go to the men's room to put it on. His privacy was respected, and he was trusted to complete the job by himself.

Oral hygiene

A number of modified toothbrushes (e.g., large-handled toothbrushes, electronic toothbrushes) may ease the task of tooth brushing for children with limited coordination or motor planning (Figure 18-15, A). Small or precisely coordinated brushing actions are unnecessary when an electric toothbrush is used; the toothbrush is simply moved slowly across all tooth, gum, and tongue surfaces.

Before being introduced to actual tooth brushing, children can chew the pleasing textured surfaces of Nuk brushes, which have rubber nubs instead of bristles. Small, soft toothbrushes with oval handles can be independently grabbed and put in the mouth by children; the toothbrush's wide handles prevent the children from being gagged or poked (Figure 18-15, *B*). The fingertip training toothbrush (see Figure 18-15, *B*) has small, soft, molded plastic bristles and slides over the tip and first knuckle of a finger. The child or caregiver slips it on and uses it like a toothbrush to clean the teeth and gums. Children with severe motor impairments need hand-over-hand assistance to brush their own teeth or need their teeth cleaned for them. Toothettes, which are cardboard sticks with minty sponges on the end, can be used by some children (see Figure 18-15, *B*). Toothettes are not safe for children who have a strong tonic bite reflex or a tendency to chew or swallow inedible objects.

DARREN'S TOOTH BRUSHING STORY. *Eight-year-old Darren has resisted having his teeth cleaned since he was a baby. His mother says that he also refuses to attempt many other self-care tasks. He allows his mother or father to brush his teeth only once a day. His parents request the OT practitioner's assistance in school.*

In Darren's first OT tooth brushing session no toothpaste was used. He was told that it was more important to brush than use toothpaste. His parents found a type of toothpaste that he tolerated, the strawberry-flavored Tom's Toothpaste for Children, which was purchased for Darren's OT sessions.

Darren tolerated the feeling of water on his hands and learned the way to adjust the water temperature and rate of flow. Although he tolerated the sticky feeling of toothpaste in his mouth, he became agitated when he felt toothpaste and water dripping on his lips or chin. He showed a strong aversion to the smell of toothpaste.

Considering Darren's tactile aversions, a gentle approach was taken. He used his strawberry-flavored toothpaste, an appealing two-piece travel toothbrush, and the preparatory jaw tug technique.[26] *Practice sessions were short and included demonstrations, humor, and verbal prompting. Before starting a tooth brushing activity, Darren was given a paper towel to wipe the drips from his mouth and chin.*

Darren used a mirror and he was given slow, verbal instructions and repeated visual cues to remind him to reach all teeth on the inside and outside. Humor was easily incorporated into the session as the OT practitioner tried to give clear verbal instructions and demonstrate tooth brushing at the same time. To reinforce the skills Darren had learned, the practitioner periodically asked Darren to explain the sequence of tooth brushing and how often and why people need to brush their teeth. With his parents' gentle encouragement, Darren began brushing his teeth at home within several months.

Nose blowing

Limited facial sensory awareness can prevent a child from feeling the sensation of a runny nose. If the child already knows the sequence of nose blowing, the COTA may simply provide reminders about when it is necessary and instruction in how to check in a mirror to see if the nostrils are clean.

Other children with special needs have problems developing the skill of nose blowing. Limited respiratory control, motor planning, or touch-pressure discrimination may prevent them from sequencing or carrying out the task. Sensory defensiveness may cause aversive reactions to tissues. Caregivers and team members may need to work together to develop creative, individualized strategies for learning this difficult skill.

Demonstrating nose blowing is almost impossible because the tissue or handkerchief hides the nose during the task. Even when the tissue is removed and the practi-

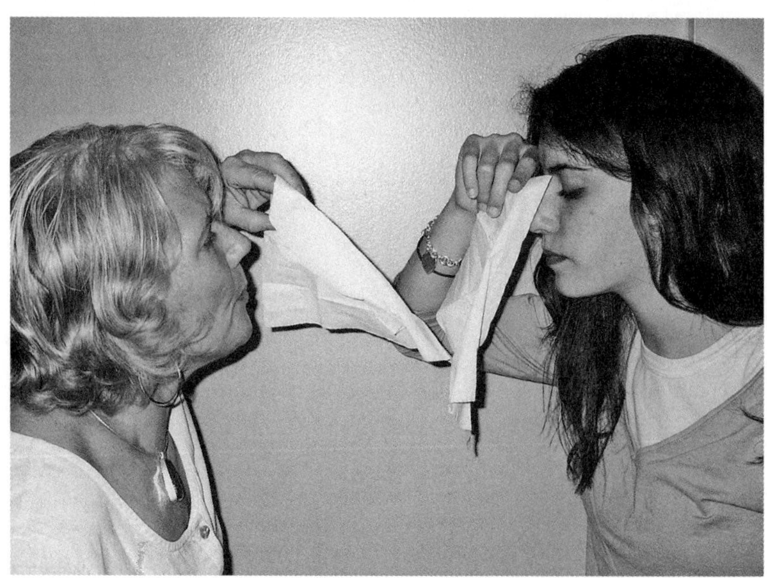

FIGURE 18-16 The girl learns how to blow out through the nose in preparation for nose blowing. When she sees the tissue flutter, she knows this is the right way to blow.

tioner forces air through the nostrils, the action can only be heard, not seen. Many children confuse breathing in through the nose with breathing out because they sound alike.

Several techniques may prove helpful. First, while demonstrating how to blow air through the nostrils while the lips are tightly closed, the OT practitioner places the child's hand under the practitioner's nose so that the child can feel the blowing air. Second, the practitioner shows the child how tissue flutters when it is held in front of the face and air is blown on it through the nostrils with the lips closed (Figure 18-16). Third, powder is sprinkled on a piece of dark paper or cardboard and placed under the practitioner's nose. A child who learns visually can benefit from seeing the powder fly away as the OT practitioner forcefully blows air through the nostrils. The powder-covered paper is then placed under the child's nose to encourage the same response. When the child is successful, s/he receives immediate visual feedback. The OT practitioner may need to spend extra time helping the child keep the lips closed while blowing out through the nose.

Extra care may be needed to help children with sensory defensiveness tolerate the sensation of tissues. Clean the nose gently and avoid vigorous wiping. A tissue dampened with warm water can make it feel less scratchy, and some children may tolerate a soft cloth handkerchief or a handi-wipe more easily than paper. Lotion (without alcohol) or petroleum jelly may be applied after wiping the nose to prevent the skin from becoming chapped. Some children with defensiveness choose to wipe their own noses, even if they are unable to blow them since control over the activity reduces aversive responses.

JAY'S NOSE BLOWING STORY. Jay, a 5-year-old boy with low muscle tone, poor sensory awareness, and learning disabilities, repeatedly confuses breathing in through the nose with breathing out. He asks for a tissue when his nose is runny but simply sniffs hard, imitating the sound of nose blowing. He is confused when no mucus appears on the tissue and his nose continues to run.

The OT practitioner worked hard with Jay, helping him hold a tissue in front of his nose and watch it flutter as he breathed out with his mouth closed. He easily mastered this preparatory technique but was completely unable to carry it over to actual nose blowing.

The OT practitioner helped Jay hold the tissue to his nose with the mouth closed. Then he imitated her slowly and rhythmically breathing in and out into the tissue, first gently and then gradually with greater force. She exaggerated the body movements associated with breathing in—straightening the back and pushing the chest out—and breathing out—bending forward to squeeze air out of the lungs. As Jay imitated her and increased the force of his breathing, mucus began to be blown onto the tissue. Jay was ecstatic because he had worked at this so hard for so long. The technique was also taught to his mother, so Jay could experience mastery at home as well. Training continued in OT until Jay developed adequate body awareness in his nose and trunk to successfully and consistently blow his own nose.

CLINICAL *Pearl*

Basis, Neutrogena, Ivory, and many types of glycerine (natural skin softener) soap are relatively gentle. Rinse-free body wash lotions and shampoos reduce the number of steps used to bathe, saving time and effort for caregivers and children. Rinse-free body washes and shampoos are available from some equipment catalogs, pharmacies, and surgical supply companies.

Bathing and Showering

The areas of bathing and showering include getting supplies as well as soaping, rinsing, drying, and getting into and out of a tub or shower. COTAs often help children and their families with bathing and showering needs.

Caregivers may need help in choosing the types of soap and body wash that fit children's special needs and skin types. For example, although they use soap to wash their bodies, children with dry skin probably need to use facial cleansers followed by moisturizers to wash the face. Advise these children and their caregivers to watch for red or irritated skin that can be related to a certain type of soap or cleanser.

Children with special needs may benefit from picture sequences about bathing and showering. COTAs assist children and their families in choosing adapted equipment and learning to use adapted methods of bathing and showering. Although many children can learn to get safely into the tub or shower and bathe themselves, other children with severe physical or cognitive disabilities may require physical assistance.

Transferring a child with severe disabilities into the tub or shower is demanding for caregivers. Lifting and lowering an adolescent or large child into a tub on a regular basis may easily injure the caregiver's back. The families of children with severe physical disabilities may consider the following modifications:

1. Create a roll-in shower, which is a large shower with a sloped floor entrance instead of a lip and is designed to allow a wheeled bath chair to roll inside and turn around. The child is transferred into the chair before entering the shower.

2. Adapted bath chairs may be equipped with seat belts, a chest harness, pommels (smooth wedges often made of plastic or foam that keep the knees apart and out of a reflexive, crossed position), and footrests or headrests. The chairs may feature netting that supports the child in a semireclined position. Some wheeled shower chairs can be rolled into a roll-in shower or over a toilet for dual use.
3. Create a raised tub in the home, which eliminates the need to lower the child into and lift him or her out of a deep tub and significantly reduces the strain on the caregiver's back.
4. A Hoyer or other hydraulic lift with a sling seat can be used to eliminate lifting for the caretaker.
5. Portable, inflatable tubs are also available. A common style is made by the EZ Bathe Company and marketed by Sammons-Preston (see Appendix C of this chapter).

Safety is the primary concern for the child with mild to moderate physical disabilities who is learning bathing and showering skills. The COTA teaches transferring and bathing skills to ensure that they are safely carried out in the home. Ideally, these skills are taught and refined with the caregiver in the child's home. Transferring into and out of a tub or shower requires the motor skills of weight shifting without losing balance, standing, turning, flexing (bending) the knees and hips, and weight bearing on the hands. Washing body parts requires all of these skills as well as reaching, grasping, manipulating faucets, and holding and using soap, a sponge, a washcloth, and often a handheld shower device.

Adapted equipment for bathing, showering, and transferring in and out of tubs and showers is available from equipment catalogs and companies, medical supply stores, and some pharmacies. Examples of adapted equipment and their uses include the following:

1. A nonslip mat in the bathtub or shower is essential to prevent slipping.
2. A bath mat with nonslip coating on the bottom, low pile, and no fringe is safest for outside the tub or shower.
3. The simplest bath chair is a stool that can be easily placed into and removed from the tub or shower. If the child is susceptible to skin problems, a padded chair may help. Children with poor balance may need a chair with a backrest.
4. Children that need extra help in transferring use a chair that extends over the side of the tub. To transfer from a wheelchair to a bath chair, transfer boards or pivot transfers may be used. Transferring from a wheelchair to a tub or shower is similar to that from a wheelchair to a bed.
5. A handheld shower device (a shower head on a long hose attached to the faucet) is useful for most children. Holders can be attached to the tub wall close to the dominant hand.
6. Tub-side grab bars that clamp onto the side of a tub are inexpensive, functional adaptations that do not require permanent installation. Permanently installed grab bars make bathing safer for everyone.
7. Many bathing aids are available, including the following: suction soap holders, which are attached to the wall; long-handled sponges and brushes; curve-handled sponges and brushes; small sponges on long handles to clean between the toes; terry cloth bath mitts; "soap on a rope"; and bath mitts with soap pockets, eliminating the need to hold soap or pick it up if dropped.

DONALD'S HYGIENE STORY. *Some children may not tolerate the slimy feeling of bar soap or the cold sensation of liquid soap. Paper towels may feel too scratchy or dry. This was the case for Donald, a 7 year old who told the OT practitioner that he never washed his hands. To determine the reason, the OT practitioner questioned Donald about his feelings on each aspect of hand washing. Fortunately, he was able to explain the ways in which the texture and temperature of the soap and temperature of the water bothered him.*

Several modifications were made for Donald. After reviewing the handwashing rules, such as when and why hand washing is done, Donald was given a choice of using bar or liquid soap. He chose liquid soap because the texture was slightly less aversive than that of bar soap. At first the OT practitioner warmed the liquid soap in her hands. She helped Donald rub it on his hands and then helped him rub his hands together under warm (not hot) water. Donald was then taught how to adjust the water temperature and warm up the soap in his own hands. Because he continued to resist using bar soap, liquid soap was always provided. He was given the option of air-drying his hands because he disliked the feeling of paper towels.

The OT staff and Donald's parents continued to reinforce the reasons why hand washing with soap was necessary after toileting and before and after eating. Soon Donald needed only periodic verbal cues to wash his hands and occasional reminders of how to regulate water and soap temperature.

Dressing

Learning to dress and undress is an important developmental achievement. The COTA can engage children in predressing games like pulling rings or hoops on and off the feet and hands or over the head or over the whole body. These games simulate pulling clothing on and off different parts of the body.[10] Adaptive techniques may help children with physical limitations, mental retardation, sensory or motor planning problems, attention deficit, learning disabilities, and in some cases, emotional problems. Two primary issues need to be addressed to help children achieve independence in dressing and undressing.

First, the OT practitioner chooses (with input from the parents and child) the type of clothing and fasteners best suited to the child's capabilities and living situation. Sleeve style, neck opening, fabric quality (i.e., stretchy, soft, nonslipping), fastener style, and placement are all addressed. Second, the practitioner decides on the teaching method that is most likely to lead the child to independent dressing.

Each step of dressing and undressing is analyzed according to its sensory, cognitive, spatial, postural, and fine and gross motor planning demands. The child's strengths are used, and limitations are accommodated. Forward or backward chaining methods are frequently used to teach dressing and undressing.

Because undressing is easier than dressing, it is generally taught first. In the following sections, the selection of adapted clothing and fasteners is addressed simultaneous with the methods of training.

Shirts and dresses

For children with weakness, abnormal movement patterns, or limited range of motion, loose, oversized shirts and dresses are the easiest to put on and take off. Use shirts or dresses with neck openings that are easy to

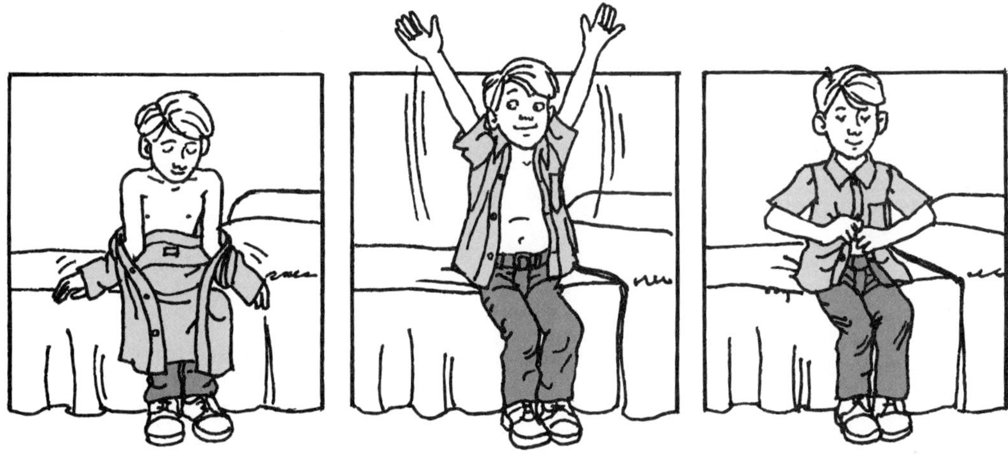

FIGURE 18-17 Adapted method of putting on a shirt: lap and over-the-head method.

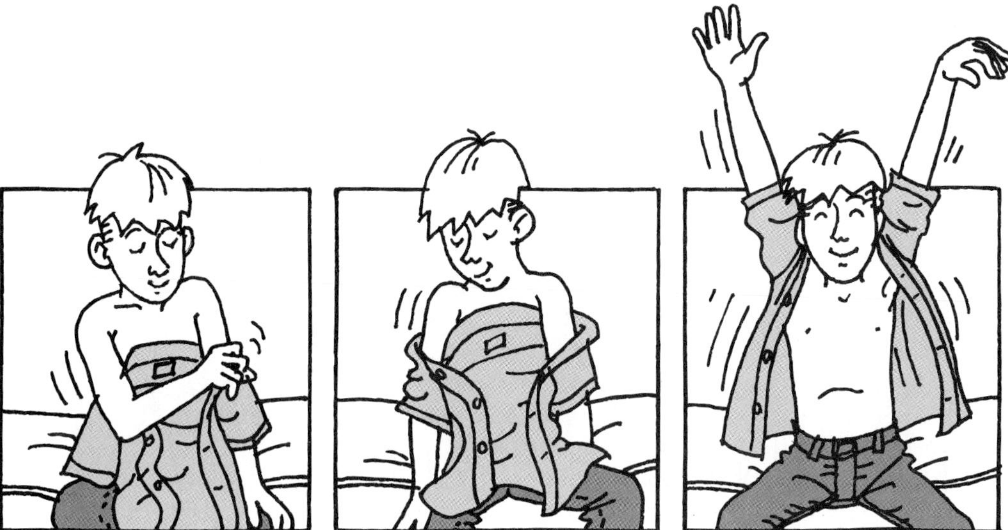

FIGURE 18-18 Adapted method of putting on a shirt: lap and over-the-head hemiplegic method.

handle, such as a horizontal crossover neck, V-neck, or boat neck opening.

To prevent a shirt from becoming untucked by an active child, try adding buttons to the waistband of the pants. The shirt can then be buttoned to the pants, as they are in some infant clothing. To prevent the fingers from getting caught while pushing the hands through the sleeves, have the child hold a small object or wear mittens while dressing.

Many adapted methods have been developed to put on and take off shirts (Figures 18-17 through 18-26). Adapted methods of removing shirts include the over-the-head method, the duck-the-head and sit-up methods, and the arms-in-front method.

Pants and skirts

Pants and skirts with elastic waistbands are usually easy to put on and take off. Waistbands need to be loose for children with severe weakness, abnormal movement patterns, or incoordination. Wrap-around skirts are easy to put on and take off.

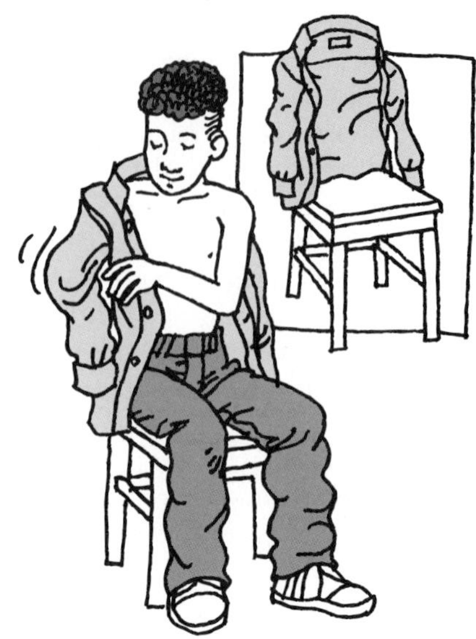

FIGURE 18-21 Adapted method of putting on a shirt: chair method.

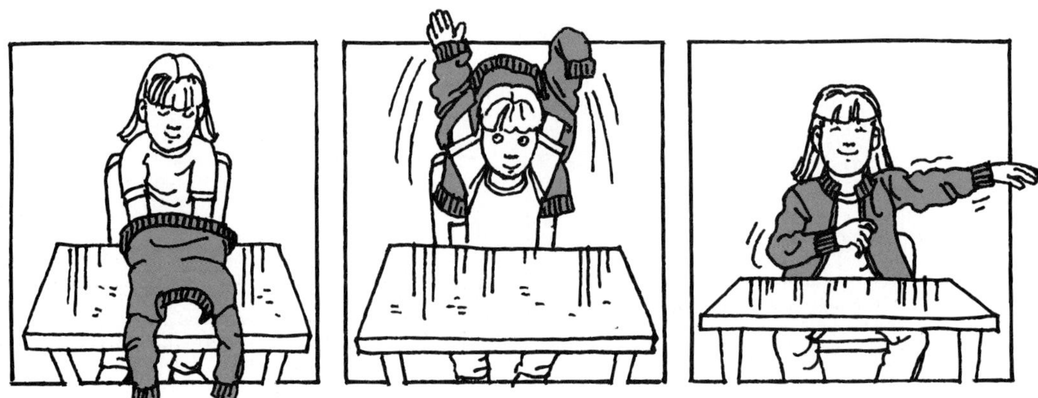

FIGURE 18-19 Adapted method of putting on a shirt: front lap and facing down method.

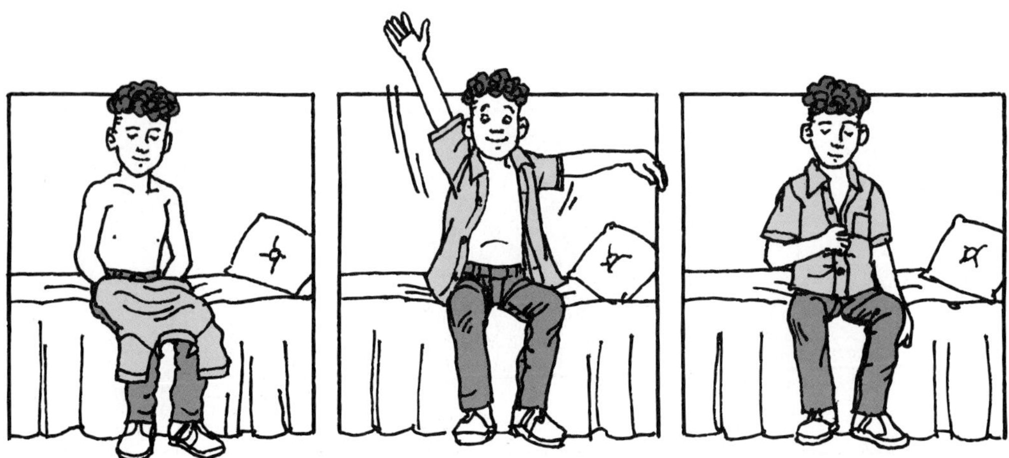

FIGURE 18-20 Adapted method of putting on a shirt: front lap and facing down hemiplegic method.

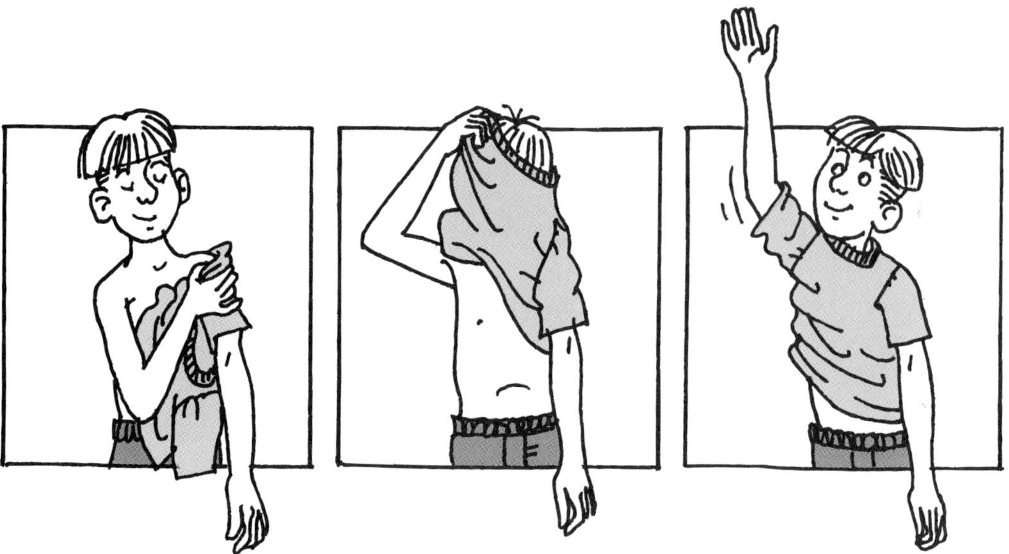

FIGURE 18-22 Adapted method of putting on a shirt: arm-head-arm method.

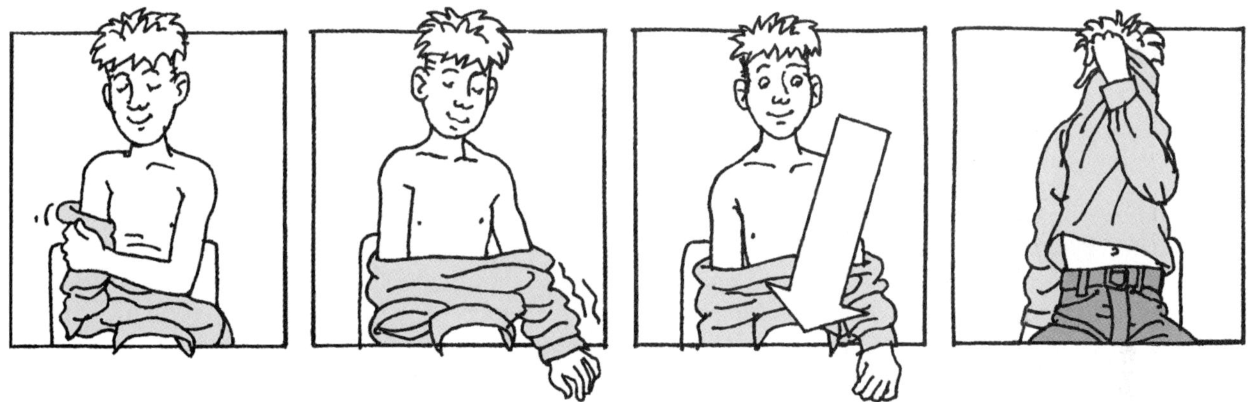

FIGURE 18-23 Adapted method of putting on a shirt: lap-arm-arm-neck method.

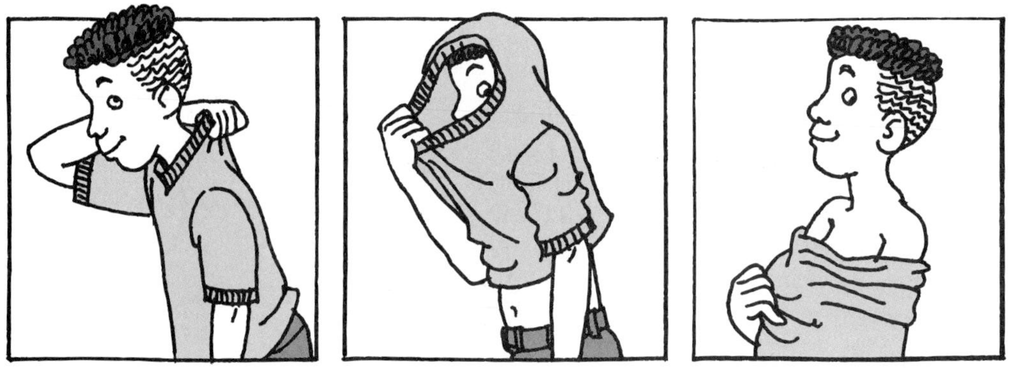

FIGURE 18-24 Adapted method of taking off a shirt: over-the-head method.

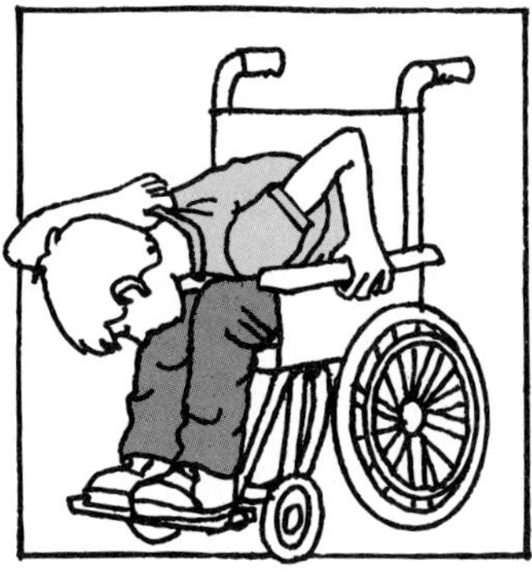
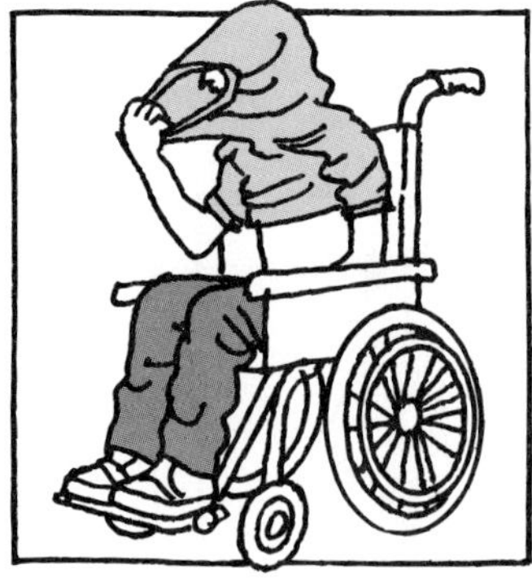

FIGURE 18-25 Adapted method of taking off a shirt: duck-the-head and sit up method.

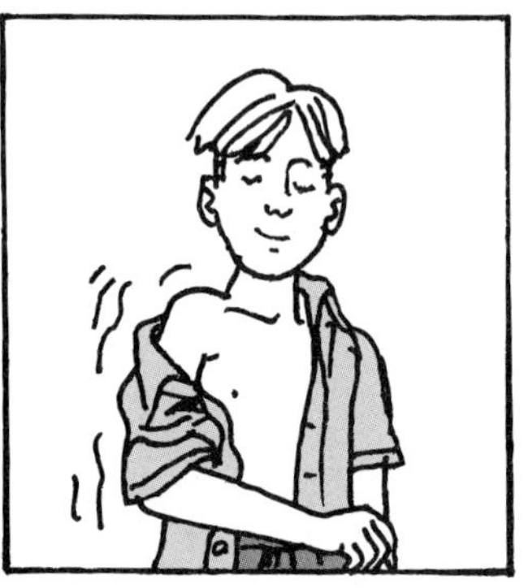
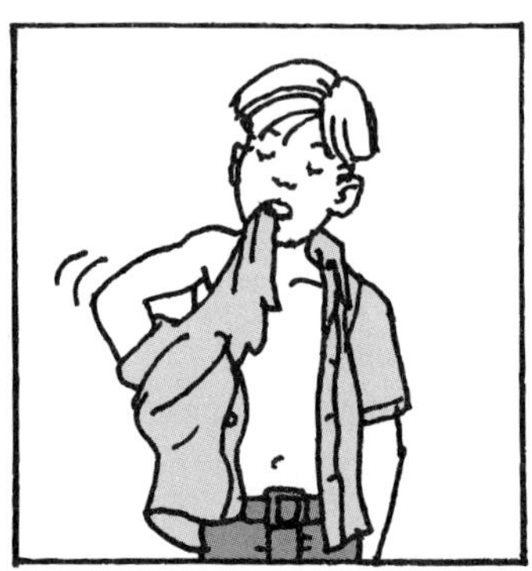
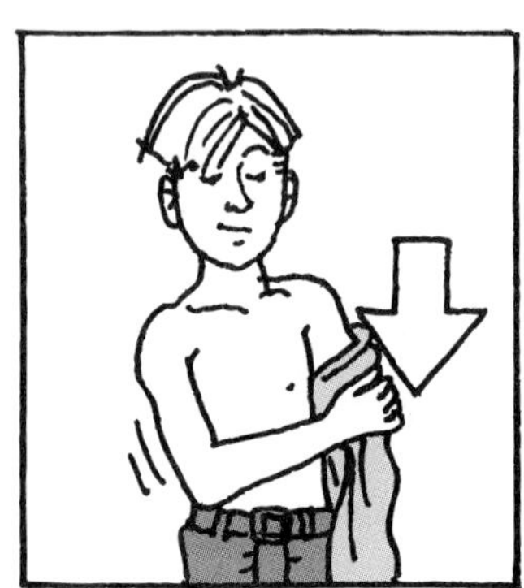

FIGURE 18-26 Adapted method of taking off a shirt: arms-in-front method.

Children who spend much of their time sitting in wheelchairs often feel more comfortable wearing pants with no back pockets because back pockets can potentially cause pressure sores. Many adapted clothing companies make pants with extra fabric in the back, allowing them to come up higher in the back than in the front. These are often more comfortable for children who use wheelchairs.[5]

To make dressing in pants easier for some children, clothing hooks can be used. Clothing hooks attached to a wall at various heights can help stabilize clothing while dressing or undressing. For example, before dressing in pants the child may sit in a chair next to the wall and hang one side of the waistband on a hook attached to the wall around ankle height. Then s/he uses one hand to hold the pants open while placing each foot in a pant leg. Next, the child may move the waistband to a higher hook to continue to hold the pants open and stable while pulling them over the knees with the other hand. To pull the pants over the hips, s/he moves them to a higher hook. The child may need to hold onto a grab bar attached to the wall to kneel or stand up. Finally, s/he uses the other hand to pull the pants over the hips.

There are many adapted methods of putting on pants (Figures 18-27 through 18-31). All of these steps can be reversed to take them off. Children with physical limitations on one side of the body need to dress and undress on the affected side first. Those with spinal cord injuries or limited grasping or reaching ability or hip flexion might benefit from using long-handled dressing hooks or the quad-quip trouser pull method (see Figure 18-31). The quad-quip trouser pull, a series of fabric loops with a clip for clothing on one end, is attached to the waist of the pants before the feet are placed in the pant legs.

Capes, jackets, and rain gear

Capes are usually easier to put on and take off than jackets. Certain adapted clothing companies make rain gear designed to fit over an individual in a wheelchair (see Appendix A of this chapter). An inexpensive, hooded, plastic rain poncho may prove equally functional.

CLINICAL *Pearl*

Children with spasticity, weakness, or limited balance may find the following positions useful to dress in pants: a high-kneel position (hips straight) while holding onto a grab bar, sitting in the corner of a room so there is support behind both arms, lying on the back on the floor while pushing the feet against the wall, and lying on the side in bed.[3]

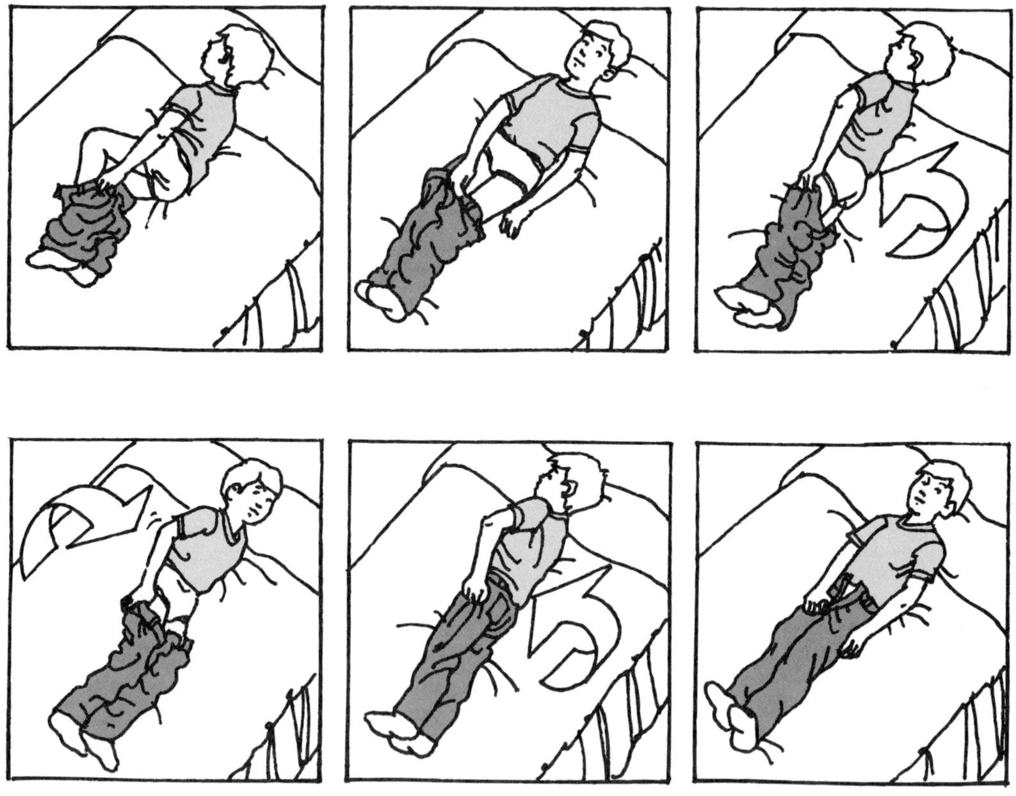

FIGURE 18-27 Adapted method of putting on pants: supine-roll method.

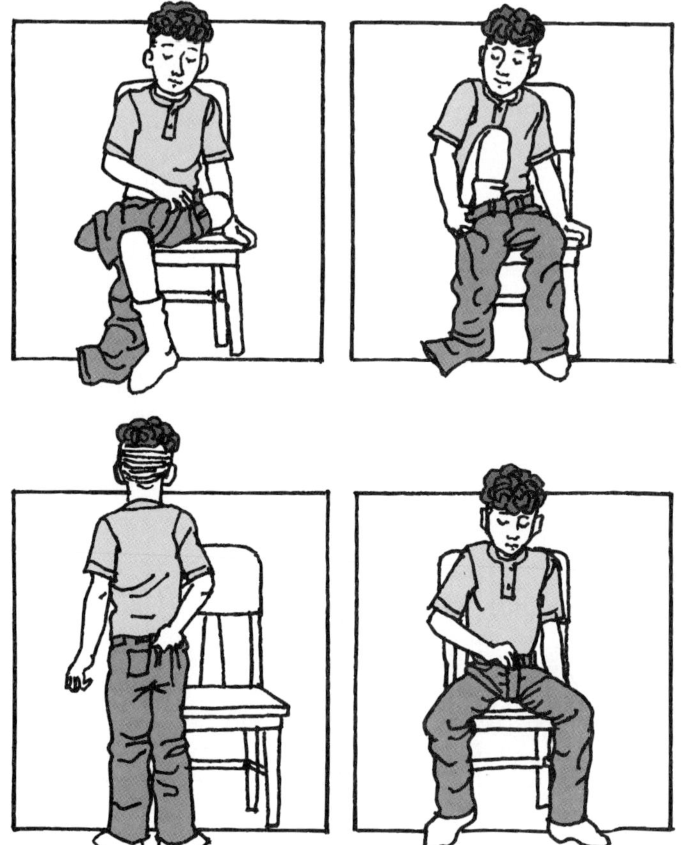

FIGURE 18-28 Adapted method of putting on pants: sit-stand-sit method.

Hooded rain jackets or ponchos are easier to use than umbrellas, which require the use of two hands to open and close them.

MARK'S COAT STORY. Mark is a 7-year-old boy born with several missing bones and tendons in his left arm and hand. Because his range of motion and coordination are moderately to severely limited in all left-sided shoulder, forearm, wrist, and finger movements, putting on a jacket was a problem. Mark has developed his own compensatory but inefficient method of putting on his jacket. First he puts his right arm into the sleeve. Then he twirls around quickly to the right so the jacket flies over toward his left arm. Occasionally, after only one or two twirls, the jacket comes close enough to the left arm for him to catch it and slide the left arm in. However, he usually twirls and twirls his jacket with it flying around him while the school bus, his classmates, or his family are waiting. Eventually Mark asks for help.

Because Mark was embarrassed by his limitations, the OT practitioner made sure to engage his curiosity and be respectful of his situation. She told him that she had a new idea for him and needed his opinion about it.

Mark was taught to put on his jacket more efficiently. The practitioner used a forward chaining method (teaching each step of an activity from beginning to end) accompanied by a demonstration and clear, slow verbal explanation to teach him to use the following sequence: (1) find the collar by looking for the label; (2) hold the collar in the right hand; (3) reach across the body to pull the left sleeve onto the left arm; (4) while still holding the collar, bring the right arm around the head, pulling the jacket around the right shoulder; and (5) keep the right hand loosely holding the jacket while sliding the hand toward the right sleeve and then down into it.

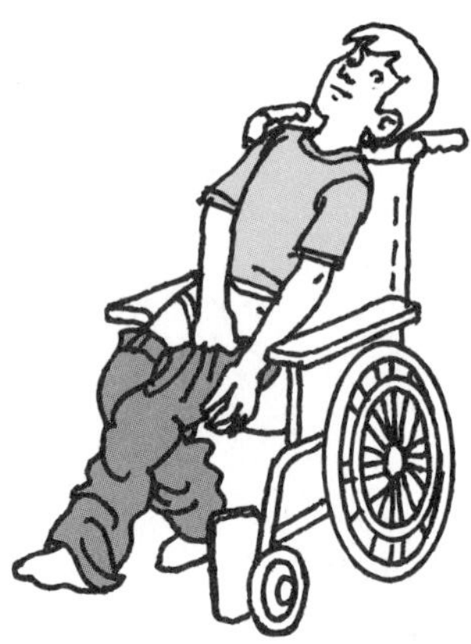

FIGURE 18-29 Adapted method of putting on pants: one-side bridge-sitting method.

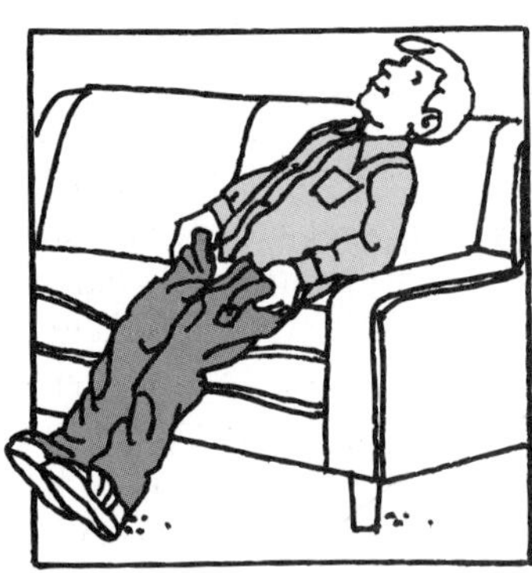

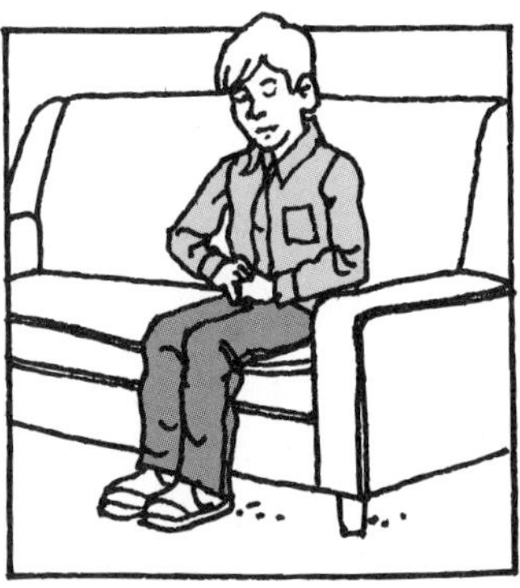

FIGURE 18-30 Adapted method of putting on pants: bridge-sitting method.

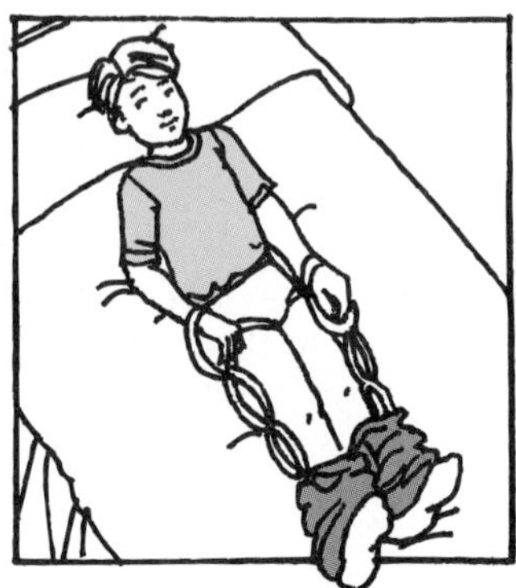

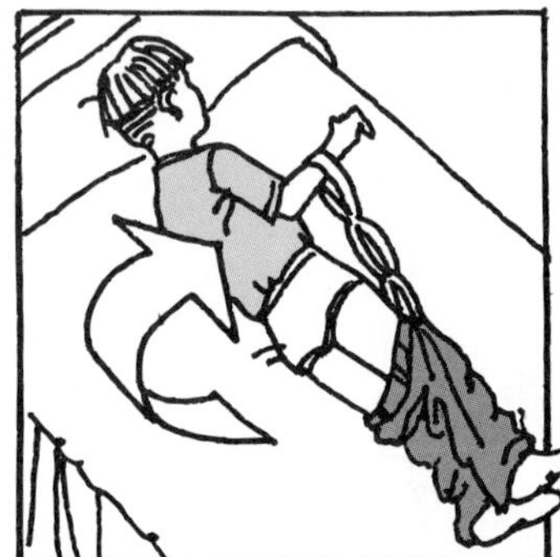

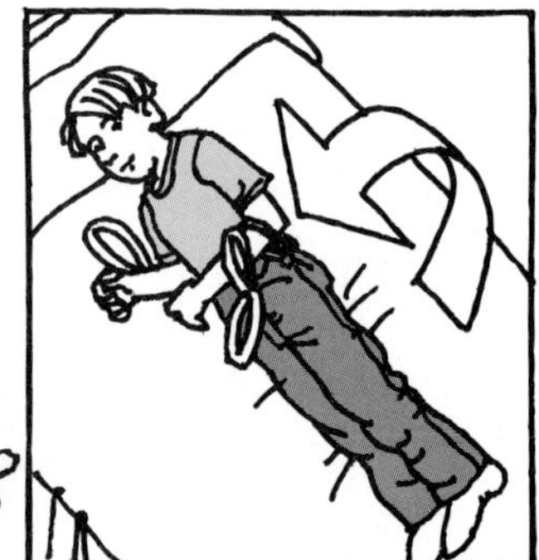

FIGURE 18-31 Adapted method of putting on pants: quad-quip trouser pull method.

It took Mark only a few attempts to succeed. Despite his problems with memory, attention, and sequencing, he never forgot this skill. He put on his jacket quickly and independently from that day on.

SUSAN'S JACKET STORY. *Susan is an 8-year-old girl with mild spasticity, severe mental retardation, severe sensory defensiveness, severely limited discrimination of touch-pressure feedback, severely limited motor planning, limited bimanual coordination, and autism (developmental disorder characterized by abnormal social interaction, sensory sensitivity, and a host of other behavioral manifestations). She does not understand verbal explanations. Visual demonstrations involving simple movements with heightened sensory feedback are the most effective ways to teach her to dress in her jacket.*

After using calming and focusing sensory activities, the clinician showed Susan the lap and over-the-head method (see Figure 18-17) to put on her jacket. The jacket was first placed upside down and spread open on the table in front of Susan, with the collar squarely in front of her. Demonstration and physical assistance were used to help her slap both hands onto the armholes. Then she was assisted in forcefully flinging both arms up and back over her head, sliding her arms through the sleeves at the same time. The heightened touch-pressure-kinesthetic feedback, from slapping the hands down and then flinging the arms overhead, provided meaningful information to Susan. She learned these two steps within a few months and was later taught to first place the jacket on her lap in the proper position.

Socks

Sitting with the back supported may be the best posture to use when learning to manage socks because this posture reduces the need to concentrate on balance while learning a new skill.

If one side of the body is different from the other (such as that with hemiplegia), the child may lift the affected leg onto a box or step to bring the foot closer to the preferred or unaffected hand. Sitting sideways on a bench can increase sitting balance by expanding the area of the child's body being supported. Removing socks is easier than putting them on, and it is often learned by 12 months of age, especially by those children who love to be barefoot. To remove socks, a child often uses the pull-the-toe method. First the child uses a thumb or one or two fingers to push the sock down around the heel. Then s/he grasps the toe of the sock and pulls it off.

Putting socks on can be challenging. Many of them have the toes and heels sewn in different colors than the other socks. These are the best for children who are able to use visual cues. The first step is to place the sock correctly before pulling it on. The visual cues of toe and heel in different colors helps them place the sock alongside the foot, with the toe pointing away from the body and the heel underneath. Those who cannot use color cues may benefit from socks in which the heel is stitched with thicker fabric or in a highly rounded fashion, providing extra tactile feedback. If these cues are inadequate, tube socks, in which the child's heel can fit on any side, may work. In addition, a wide sock opening can prevent frustration during the most difficult part of pulling socks on, which is inserting the toes.

Sock and stocking dressing aids are available through equipment catalogs. They help keep the sock or stocking openings wide while children slide their feet in. These aids may benefit children with limited reaching, coordination, and lower extremity function. Sock and stocking aids are usually inserted into and attached to the sock or stocking before the item is pulled on. While seated, children place their toes into the sock or stocking and then pull the straps or sticks on the dressing aid to pull them up completely. These aids can be difficult to use, so children need to try using several different types before purchasing one.

Putting on nylon stockings or tights can be challenging. They are difficult to grasp and provide little touch-pressure feedback for children and adolescents with coordination or sensory problems. Some dressing aids are designed specifically for stockings but can be difficult to use. If possible, try to use stockings made of thicker fabric, which provides more feedback. Choose a size that is one or two times larger than the child normally wears so that they will be easier to pull on and require less adjustment.

CLINICAL *Pearl*

Dress and undress on affected or weaker side first. Undressing is usually easier than dressing, and unfastening is usually easier than fastening.

Adjusting clothing

Adjusting clothing is sometimes problematic. A child may lack the tactile discrimination needed to determine whether the pants are on straight or a shirt is tucked in. Visual cues might help, such as lining up the top button or front seam of the pants with the child's belly button. Checking the appearance of the clothing in a mirror (front and back) before leaving the house and after using the toilet can be taught as part of the dressing and toileting routines.

Fastening

For individuals who have the use of only one hand or have limited strength, range of motion, or coordination, a variety of fastening aids may be helpful. These aids include such items as buttonhooks, bow ties, Velcro shoe closures, and zipper pulls. A dressing stick with a hook or clasp at the end can be used to reach the back fasteners. Velcro fasteners can make dressing and undressing easier and quicker; they can be sewn into clothing in place of buttons, snaps, zippers, or ties. Some clothing with Velcro closures, like shoes, are commonly sold in stores or through catalogs.

Fastening boards and cubes laid on a table or the floor provide stable surfaces for children who are developing beginning fastening skills. Playing "dress-up" is a valuable learning activity. Children can put on costumes with fasteners to act out scenes such as playing house or going shopping. Dress-up dolls, which come with a variety of fasteners, are also fun and useful learning tools. Some child-size pop-up tents are made with four entrances that are opened by four different fasteners and can also be used for fastening practice. However, practicing these skills during the actual occupation of dressing is always recommended.

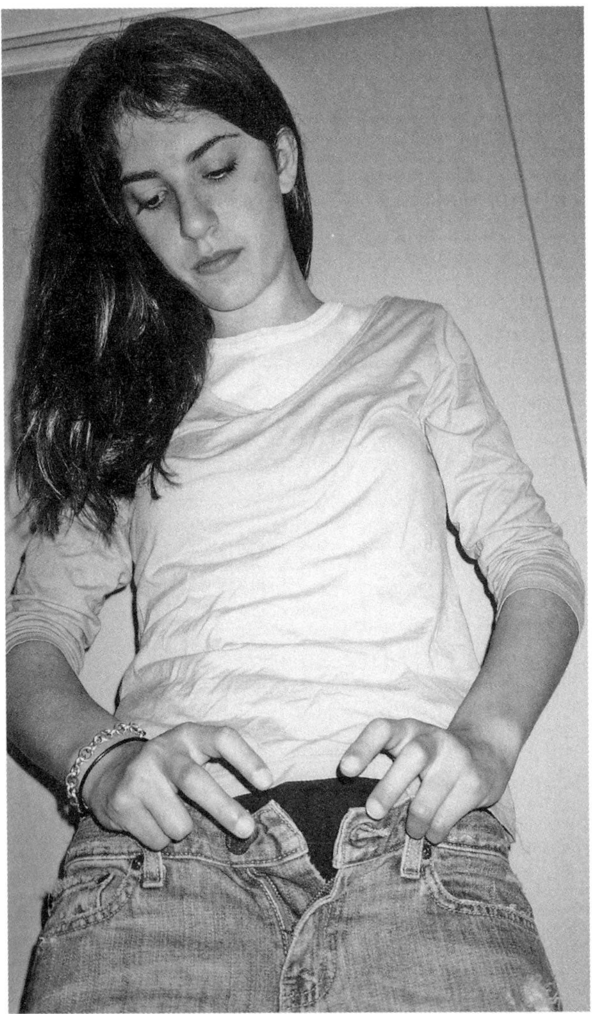

FIGURE 18-32 The girl shows how radial-ulnar separation makes dressing in pants easier. Using the strong, stable (ulnar) parts of the hands, she pulls and holds the two sides of the waistband together. She uses the skill (radial) parts of the hands to operate the fasteners.

Buttoning

Buttoning is a bimanual (two-handed) task that requires refined touch-pressure discrimination and fine motor skills. Also required for buttoning is an in-hand manipulation skill called *shift*, in which the thumb slides things across the fingers.

Another skill used in many dressing and fastening activities is separation of the two sides of the hand, also called dissociation of the ulnar and radial sides of the hands, or radial-ulnar dissociation. The ulnar (little finger) side of the hand is used to stabilize or hold something still, while the radial side (thumb and index and middle fingers) perform skilled actions or manipulate an item. Picture a child who is trying to fasten a pair of stiff blue jeans. The child grasps the waist on each side of the jeans, using the ulnar side of each hand to pull the button next to the hole for fastening. Holding the fabric in place with the ulnar sides of each hand frees the radial sides to fasten the button (Figure 18-32). Some children may never learn to effectively separate the two sides of the hands for dressing and fastening activities. Wearing especially loose clothing can reduce the need for this skill.

Some children learn to unbutton a practice vest with the following simple words sung in any tune, paired with graded physical assistance.

"Pinch the button and pinch the cloth. Pull the hole open and push the button through."

"Pinch the button and pinch the cloth. Pull the hole open and pull the button through."

With buttoning the same tune and almost the same wording are used. Singing simple instructions helps children attend to and remember motor sequences.

EVAN'S ADAPTED BUTTONING STORY. *Evan, a 19 year old with quadriplegia (paralysis in both arms and legs), struggled with learning to use a variety of buttoning aids. Although he eventually succeeded, the task required much time and energy. He asked the OT practitioner about adapted clothing (see Appendix A of this chapter) and eventually requested Velcro closures.*

Evan brought in several of his own shirts, and the OT practitioner sewed buttons over the buttonholes and Velcro closures inside the front opening. He could then fasten and unfasten his favorite shirts easily; they still appeared as if they were buttoned.

CARL'S BUTTONING STORY. *Carl is a 3½-year-old boy with severely low muscle tone, weakness, and limited body awareness, but he has excellent visual discrimination and average to above average intelligence. He cannot determine what sensations he feels while using his fingertips, which keeps him from establishing a motor plan for a sequence of actions. He has no idea of how to begin dressing or fastening tasks and actively avoids them. The flimsy texture of cloth feels confusing to him because he cannot properly interpret or respond to the sensation.*

The COTA graded (changed one or more aspects of a task to make it easier or harder for the child) the buttoning task for Carl to help him achieve success. He began each session by engaging in many resistive hand and finger activities to increase strength and discrimination. He then played a game designed to simulate buttoning, which provided firm touch-pressure feedback that allowed him to discriminate among sensations with his fingertips. The practitioner presented a plastic lid with a slot and held it vertically for Carl; he was shown the way to push a penny through the slot with one hand and remove it with the other (Figure 18-33). Because Carl tended to push the penny in but forget to pull it out, the COTA prompted him in a playful voice, saying, "Don't let the penny fall! Get the penny!" Carl laughed each time she repeated the cues. He repeated the activity in order to hear her say the words over again. The activity simulated the bimanual sequence of buttoning while giving Carl increased sensory feedback that he could interpret.

After a few weeks, the penny activity was followed immediately by a task that involved buttoning and unbuttoning large buttons on a vest that was on the floor. The floor provided a firm support, and the OT practitioner provided physical assistance. A backward chaining method was used to give Carl a feeling of immediate success. At first Carl was prompted to watch the practitioner push the button through the buttonhole. Carl was then asked to pull the button out, allowing him to feel that he successfully completed a buttoning or unbuttoning activity. Soon, with physical assistance, Carl began to (1) pinch the vest with the fingers of one hand, (2) pinch the button with the fingers of the other, (3) pull the buttonhole open, (4) push the button through the hole, (5) feel and pinch the button with the fingers of his opposite hand, and (6) pull it through.

Within 3 months Carl was holding the practice vest on his lap while buttoning and unbuttoning it himself. He was then able to button and unbutton the vest on his own body. Eventually Carl began practicing with his own clothing.

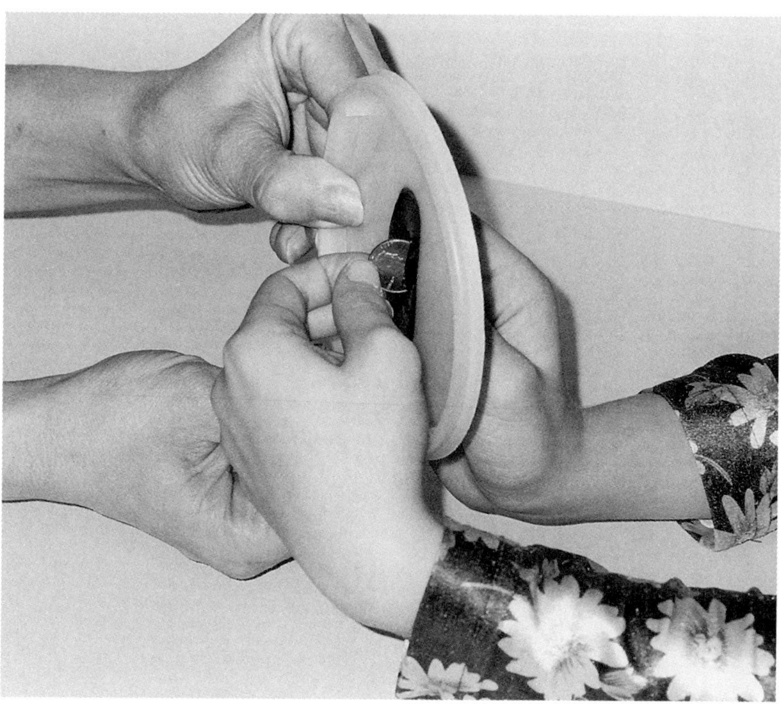

FIGURE 18-33 Penny-through-the-slot pre-buttoning activity.

Zipping

The OT practitioner generally teaches a child to unzip first and then zip (after the zipper has already been inserted for the child). The child is taught to insert a zipper only after learning to pull it up and down and usually after mastering buttoning and unbuttoning.

An oversized, easy-to-insert, smooth-sliding zipper is best for teaching zipping. It may be helpful to first insert the zipper in a garment, board, or dressing cube placed on a table in front of the child. Whether through verbal, physical, or visual means, the child must learn that the zipper has three parts that are tightly connected in a specific sequence. The three parts are labeled as follows for the purpose of explanation: (1) the puller, (2) the stopper, and (3) the post (Figure 18-34). Children with average verbal and cognitive skills can benefit from these concrete distinctions among the parts.

The zipper puller is a moving handle with an opening; it is grasped and pulled up and down. The following sequence is used for zipping. (1) The puller is pulled down tightly against the stopper (the tiny bar that stops the puller from sliding off). (2) The puller and stopper are pinched and held snugly together. (3) While one hand is used to pinch the puller and stopper tightly together, the other one takes the post and guides it down all the way through the puller and stopper. (4) The puller is zipped up.

The bimanual coordination demands of zipping prove especially difficult for some children to master. Many need extra training to properly orient the post to the opening in the puller and hold the puller and stopper together during insertion. Strategies of jiggling the closure, pinching, pulling tight, and starting over can be taught.

Children need to practice zipping and unzipping vests, shirts, or jackets on their own bodies. New demands like reaching, getting extra fabric out of the way, and accommodating visual focus increase the challenge. Children tend to become frustrated when fabric bunches up or gets caught in the teeth of the zipper. Watch for faulty zippers that are too stiff and difficult for adults to operate so that children do have to struggle with them unnecessarily.

Snapping

Oversized fasteners are useful tools for teaching the task of snapping. Because of the increased **proprioceptive feedback** (muscle-joint input) provided by snapping, many children learn to snap before inserting a zipper and sometimes before buttoning. However, if a child has weakness or poor discrimination of touch-pressure feedback or relies primarily on visual guidance to learn (as many children with low muscle tone do), snapping may prove challenging.

To teach children to snap, start with practice clothing or snapping toys that rest on a table or the floor. Have them look carefully and feel carefully with their fingertips to line up the top half of the snap over the bottom half. When the top is placed over the bottom, the children again need to feel carefully with the fingertips and rely on touch-pressure feedback to be sure that the parts stay together and do not slide apart. They then feel and press carefully, using both tactile and proprioceptive feedback to gauge the amount of strength needed to push the two parts together.

Buckling

The motor skills needed for buckling include the ability to pinch with two or three fingers and separation of two sides of the hand.

Buckling can be broken down into a five-step sequence. (1) With a long belt, use the ulnar and radial sides of the hands to straighten both sides of the belt and orient the ends to face each other. (2) Slide the end of the belt under the first bar of the buckle. (3) Use both

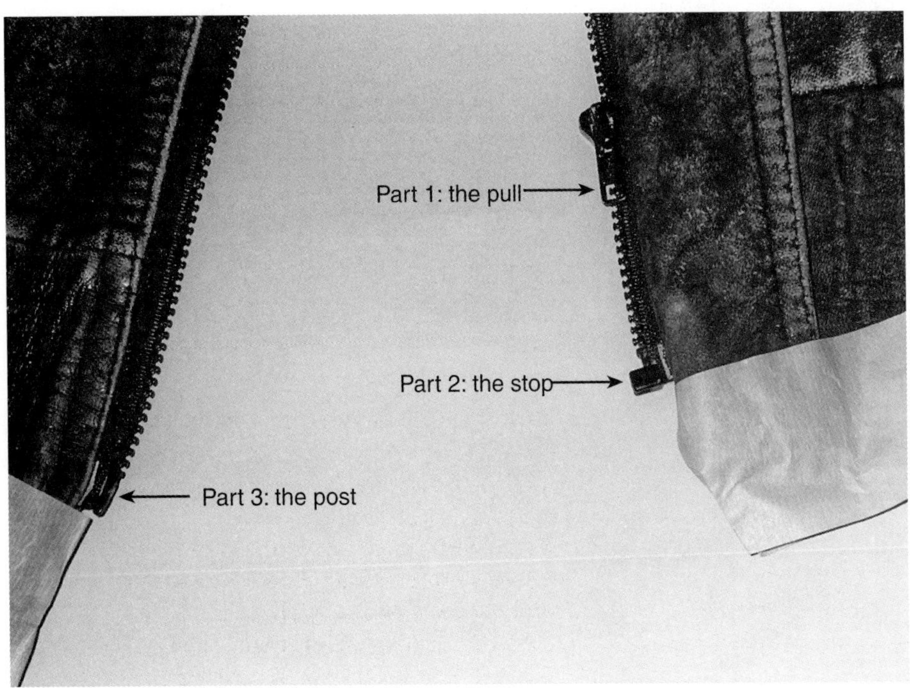

FIGURE 18-34 Three parts of a zipper.

hands to pull the belt tight so it is snug yet comfortable. (4) Insert the prong into the closest hole. (5) Slide the end of the belt under the second bar.

Buckling can sometimes be accomplished with only one hand. It becomes more challenging if the buckle is small or located on a shoe or sandal. Once buckling is mastered on a practice item (e.g., doll, dressing cube) the child can put on and buckle clothing that has a wide, easy closure. When buckling belted pants, skirts, or dresses, the most efficient method is to thread the belt through the belt loops before pulling on the clothing.

Shoe tying

Grading activities involves changing one or more aspects of a task to make it easier or harder for the child. This is of particular importance in shoe tying. Each child's abilities and needs dictate the type and amount of grading to use for shoe tying. A seemingly small change in an activity can significantly increase the chance for success.

One way to grade shoe tying is to sequence the steps. **Forward chaining** (teaching each step of shoe tying from beginning to end), **backward chaining** (teaching the last step of shoe tying first, then the next-to-last step, and so on), or both can be used. During forward chaining, the child starts shoe tying and the OT practitioner finishes the steps the child has not yet learned. During backward chaining, the practitioner starts shoe tying and the child performs the last step. By executing the last step and seeing the finished outcome, the child feels an immediate sense of accomplishment and mastery. Eventually the child learns and performs the last two steps independently and so on.

The OT practitioner may choose to use both forward and backward chaining. The child initially learns only the first and last steps of the sequence. The practitioner performs the steps in the middle. The child feels early success by knowing how to both start and finish the task. The child gradually performs more steps until the entire sequence is learned.

Fading assistance is another means of grading an activity. As the child gains proficiency and confidence in carrying out each step in a skill sequence, the practitioner progressively decreases the amount of help. For example, the practitioner may initially use hand-over-hand or maximum physical assistance. The assistance is gradually reduced from maximum to moderate to minimum physical, then to tactile, then to verbal, and finally to visual or gestural cuing only.

Shoelaces provide little sensory feedback to a child with poor sensory discrimination. The child may be completely unable to manipulate the laces and consequently simply twist them around. Use wide, thick, stiff laces to provide increased touch-pressure feedback, which facilitates a calmer response and an improved ability to interpret touch-pressure feedback, subsequently improving motor planning.

Using extra-long laces can also reduce frustration. Children often tie loose bows at first. Long laces prevent them from pulling out during the last step of tightening. Black laces on a black shoe can be confusing for the child with learning disabilities or perceptual problems. To increase visual cues, two laces of different colors are tied together before lacing the shoe, so each side of the bow is a different color. The shoe is a third color, increasing visual contrast.

Before working on bow tying, prepare the child's hand muscles and improve sensory discrimination by performing resistive finger activities. A few examples are using squeeze toys, pulling pennies or pegs out of putty, picking up small items with tweezers or small tongs, playing miniature travel games like mini-Perfection, and pulling ropes. *Bunny Bow Tie* (from OT Ideas; see Appendix C of this chapter) is a popular beginning bow tie device. The book *Shoe-Tying Made Simple*[39] comes with a long, wide, and stiff lace in blue and yellow. The book has clear picture cues, which provide important additions to demonstration. The child can check each picture in the book to see if the laces and hands in the picture look exactly the same as the child's laces and hands.

Repeat the same motor sequence and use the same cuing phrases during each trial to aid a child's memory. Sing the phrases or use a voice with a sing-song pattern to further enhance the child's memory. Remember that some children cannot listen and watch at the same time; the OT practitioner needs to decide whether the child learns better by hearing instructions and watching a demonstration at the same time or by performing the steps in silence with only the picture cues (Box 18-6).

Adjusting laces is best taught as part of the initial bow tie sequence, as described above. Some children master the steps of lacing a shoe and tying a bow but continue to have problems adjusting, checking for tightness, retightening, and untying knots. The laces may come untied repeatedly throughout the day, and children may still need adult assistance to keep the shoes tied. Some children need to work on adjusting and tightening for several years before they are mastered.

CHUCK'S SHOE-TYING STORY. *Chuck is an 11-year-old overweight boy with poor abdominal muscle strength and limited hip flexion (bending ability). He cannot balance to squat or kneel on one knee. Even when sitting in a chair with his foot on a step stool, he needs to rotate his hip internally and stretch with effort to reach the side of his shoe. His strength and range of motion are so limited that he cannot reach the middle of his shoe, where the bow is typically tied.*

Using the OT tools of activity analysis and grading and adapting activities, the OT practitioner devised a way for

BOX 18-6

Bow-Tying Steps

Typical Bow Tying: A shoe is laced with stiff red and blue laces, one on each side of the shoe, and prepared for a right-handed child. When laced and with the toe of the shoe pointing toward you, the blue part will be on the left and the red on the right. In addition, because children have trouble estimating how big to make the loops, mark visual cues on the red part of the lace as follows: draw black dots at the points where you want children to pinch the loop together.[5] Place the shoe in front of the child with the toe pointing toward him or her.

Note: For the left-handed child, prepare a different shoe with other thick, stiff, bicolored laces. Lace the shoe in such a way that the red part is on the left and the blue on the right. Then reverse the instructions for "the left hand" and "the right hand" below.

Note: For children who are unable to distinguish right from left, show them the sequence below and substitute words such as "this side," "that side," and "the other side" as needed.

The guidelines below are designed to make the sequence as easy as possible and facilitate success. During a training session, the certified occupational therapy assistant might say the following.

1. Do you see the red and blue laces? Stretch the red lace out to the right and put it on the table. Stretch the blue lace out to the left and put it on the table.
2. Now take the red lace with your right hand; cross it over the shoe and put it on the table. Take the blue lace with your left hand; cross it over the shoe and put it on the table. Do you see the "X" you made?

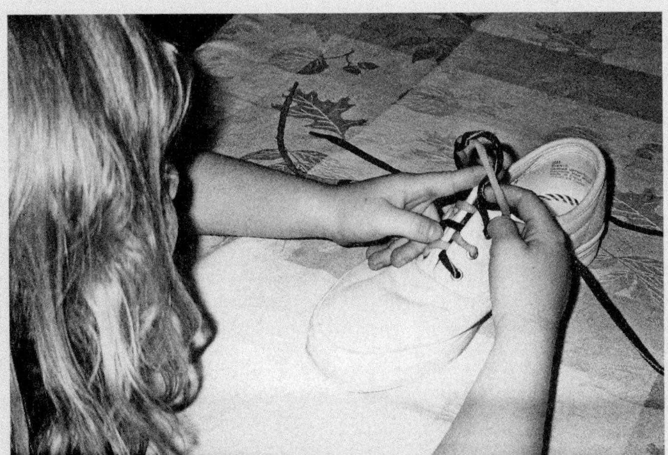

A

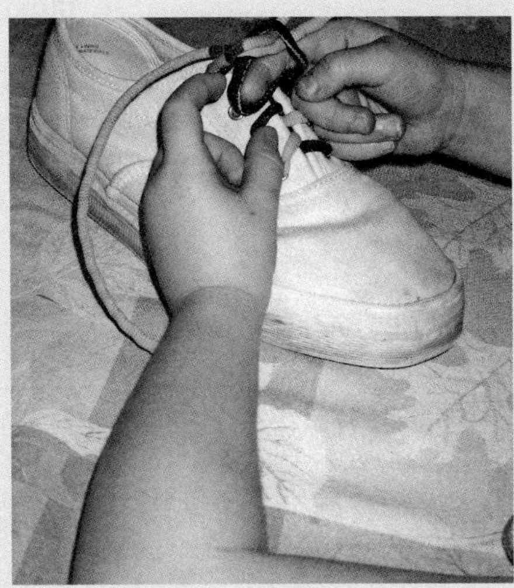

B

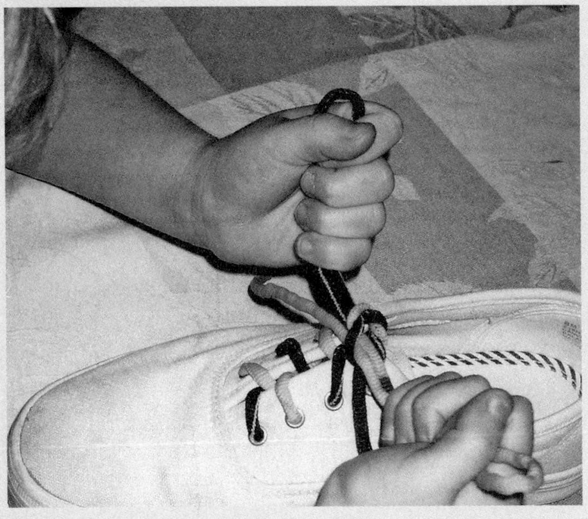

C

FIGURE 18-35 A child with right-hand preference performs a few tricky steps in shoe tying. **A,** Pull the blue lace through the first "tunnel" 2 times to help keep the bow snug. **B,** Switch hands when the second loop is pushed through the second tunnel. **C,** Turn the hands palms up and use their strong ulnar sides to pull the loop "super-duper" tight.

BOX 18-6

Bow-Tying Steps—cont'd

3. With your left hand, show me how you can put your pointer finger and thumb together to pinch. Now pinch the middle of the X where the blue lace crosses the red lace. Pinch the red and blue laces together hard so that they will stay together. Look for the big "tunnel" below your fingers. Where is it?
4. For the rest of this step, keep using your left hand to pinch the red and blue laces against each other where they make an X. Now use your right hand to fold the blue lace over and behind the red lace. Take your right pointer finger and push the blue lace through the tunnel and out the front. Pull it all the way out. Now fold the blue lace over and pull it through the tunnel again (Figure 18-35). Pulling the blue lace through the tunnel two times will help keep the laces tight.[5] (**Note**: This technique of pulling the blue lace through the tunnel twice can help children compensate for poor radial-ulnar separation during shoe tying.)
5. Now use both hands to pull the laces tight. Pull sideways, not down against the shoe and not up but straight out to the sides, as tight as you can.
6. Get ready to make a loop with the red lace. Do you see the two black dots? Can you fold the red lace over so that the two black dots will be touching each other?[39] Pinch the black dots together with your left hand. You made a big red loop!
7. Keep pinching the red loop at the bottom with your left hand. Use your right hand to carefully wind the blue lace around the red loop one time. Gently make the blue lace snug around the bottom of the red loop. Do you see the new little blue tunnel that you made?
8. Continue pinching the bottom of the red loop with the left hand. Take your right pointer finger and push a small fold of the blue lace through the little blue tunnel. It is a tiny blue loop!
9. Now it is time to switch your hands. Take your left hand off the red loop and switch it to pinch the tiny new blue loop. Switch your right hand over to pinch the red loop.
10. Make the tiny blue loop as big as the red loop; slide the blue loop until it is bigger.
11. "Pinch tightening" is next. Move your fingers close to the middle of the bow. Pinch each loop. Keep your fingers outside the loops. If you put your fingers inside the loops, they will come untied. Pinch and pull the loops out to the sides. You made a bow!
12. Now comes adjusting. Look at my mouth and say "adjusting." Do you know what it means? (Take a minute to explain it to the child as needed.) Is any part of the bow touching the table? The blue lace is touching the table. Pull the blue loop on the other side gently and watch the lace come off the table. The red loop looks so big. It is touching the table. Can you slowly pull the red lace on the other side to make the loop just the way you want it?
13. Every time we adjust, we do pinch tightening again. Can you show me?
14. Now it is time for "super-duper tightening"! Make your hands do this. (As you demonstrate turning both hands from palms down to palms up, make a sound like "Woop!") Grab each loop in a fist and pull the loops out to the sides three times as tight as you can (see Figure 18-35). Keep your fingers on the outside of each loop. (**Note**: This step engages the stronger ulnar side of each hand in tightening.) Pull tight and then relax, pull tight again and then relax again, and pull very tight again.
15. Let's do "checking." Pinch the middle of the bow. If the middle of the bow feels hard, it is very tight. If it feels soft then it is only a little tight, so we do super duper tightening again. Do you think your bow is very, medium, or only a little tight?

Symmetrical Bow Tying: Some children become too frustrated with the method of Typical Bow Tying because of its greater demands for bimanual coordination and visual perception. These children may be more successful using a symmetrical method, which is described in the following sequence. Prepare the shoe in the same way as above, starting out by following steps 1 through 6.

1. Use your right hand to fold the blue lace over and turn it into a loop just like the red loop. Take your right hand and pinch the bottom of the blue loop just like the left hand pinches the bottom of the red loop.
2. Carefully slide your fingers up each loop so you have a fist around each one.
3. Cross the middle of the red loop over the middle of the blue loop, making another X (Figure 18-36).
4. Use your left hand to pinch the blue and red loops together at the point where they cross, leaving a new tunnel below your fingers.
5. Keep your left hand pinching the two loops together in an X, and use your right hand to fold the red loop over and behind the blue loop and pull it through the new tunnel (see Figure 18-36).

BOX 18-6

Bow-Tying Steps—cont'd

6. Still using your right hand, pull the red loop all the way out of the tunnel.
7. It is time to switch hands. Put the red loop in your left hand between your pointer finger and thumb, and then switch the blue loop to your right hand between your pointer finger and thumb.
8. Pull the loops out to the sides, doing pinch tightening. (just like Step 10 in Typical Bow Tying).
9. Then follow Steps 11, 12, and 13 of Typical Bow Tying so that the laces will be very tight and adjusted evenly.

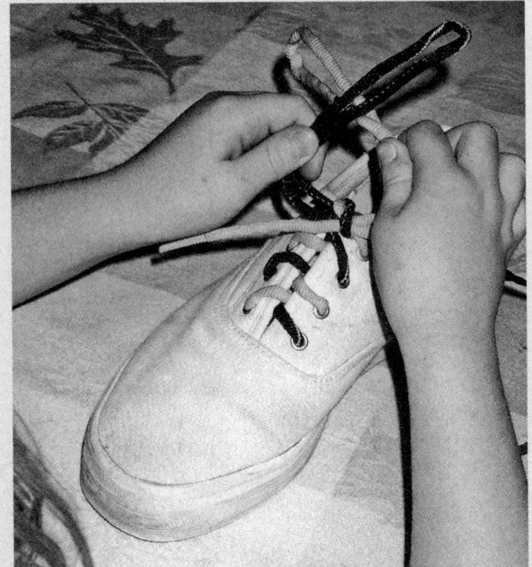

A

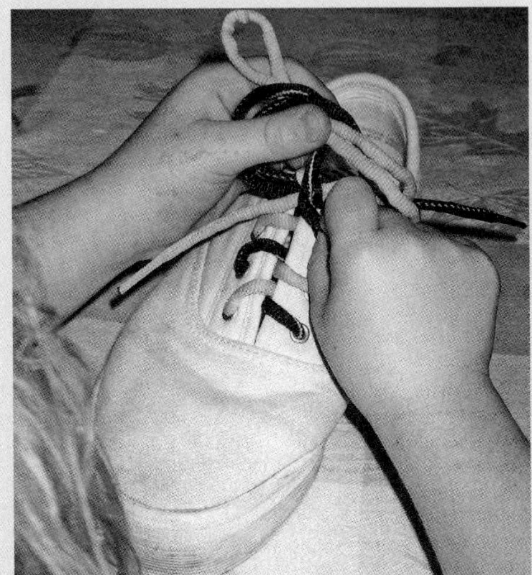

B

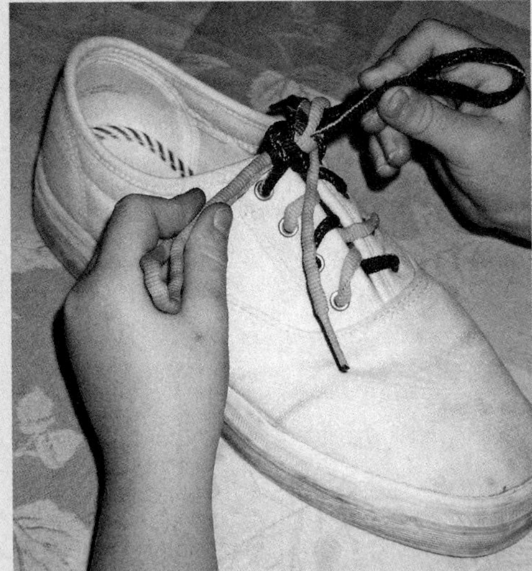

C

FIGURE 18-36 A child with right-hand preference ties a double knot. **A,** Cross the blue loop over the red loop to make a big "X". **B,** The left hand pinches the middle of the "X," and the right hand folds the blue loop behind the red loop and brings it through the "tunnel." **C,** Pull a little tight; make it snug.

CLINICAL *Pearl*

While teaching shoe tying or any challenging activity, use positive words. For example, instead of saying "The bow is not tight," say "Well, that seems medium tight to me" or "Wow, that is pretty tight, but I bet you could make it *super* tight." By phrasing it in this way, the child may feel successful and motivated to try for "very tight" instead of giving up.

CLINICAL *Pearl*

Numerous shoe-tying aids are available from equipment catalogs. For example, after a child ties elastic shoelaces once, they can be slipped on and off without tying or untying them again. Many shoe-tying aids are designed for one-handed manipulation.

Chuck to become independent in shoe tying. The key questions addressed were (1) how much postural strength, flexibility, balance, and control were needed for Chuck to tie his own shoes and (2) how the task could be modified so that Chuck could succeed.

The postural demands of shoe tying were more problematic for Chuck than the bow-tying sequence. The OT practitioner adjusted the length of his laces so that a bow tied on the side of his shoe would hang evenly. His mother was notified of the new strategy so she could help reinforce the procedure. Because Chuck was self-conscious about his weight, care was taken to reinforce his self-esteem by praising his bow-tying progress and using an accepting, matter-of-fact tone to address his postural problems.

ALISON'S SHOE-TYING STORY. *Alison was a 15-year-old girl with moderate mental retardation, visuomotor problems, sensory defensiveness, extreme distractibility,impulsivity, poor sitting tolerance, and poor judgment. She attended a special school that provided extra structure and emphasized functional and prevocational skills. Because Alison could not tie her shoes properly, they came untied repeatedly every day. A staff person always had to take time away from teaching to retie her shoes.*

To address this problem, Alison's COTA began each session with intensive sensory modulation activities to increase sitting tolerance, focus of attention, and tolerance for physical cuing and the tickly feeling of shoelaces. Frequent but short practice sessions involved forward and backward chaining with color-coded laces. Alison first practiced bow tying on a board, then on an oversized wooden shoe, then on a real oversized shoe placed on a table, and eventually on her own sneakers. Despite her lower developmental level, Alison learned the higher-level splinter skill of tying her own shoes, thereby increasing her independence and self-esteem at home and school. A **splinter skill** *is a specific, often complex task that is mastered by a child who lacks the underlying developmental capabilities. It is accomplished through compensatory methods and practice rather than the remediation of underlying developmental components.*

Personal Device Care

Personal devices include hearing aids, glasses, splints, orthotics, braces, prosthetic limbs, artificial eyes, and aids to mobility. An OTR, nurse, hearing specialist, physical therapist, or other professional initially gives the COTA all pertinent information about the device and trains him or her in why, when, where, and how the device is used.

After learning the way to apply and remove the device, the COTA may then be responsible for teaching the child to apply and remove it as well as for routinely reinforcing the child's performance. In some cases, such as one involving a child who uses a hand splint, the COTA may be in charge of instructing parents, teachers, or other involved persons. Drawing pictures or writing down the sequence of putting on the device, its proper fit, the frequency and duration of its use, and precautions to take with it can be helpful.

The COTA's role may include instructing the child and caregivers in the following: cleaning personal devices (especially glasses) (Figure 18-37),[29] storing them when they are not in use, replacing parts, and scheduling a doctor's appointment for a new one. Once trained, the COTA may also instruct caregivers or other staff about the issues. Hearing aids need periodic adjustment and battery replacement. An SLP or audiologist can instruct the COTA in adjusting the level of the hearing aid and recognizing when the batteries need replacement.

Depending on the level of expertise, the COTA may create splints for a child with a doctor's prescription and OTR supervision. S/he may design a variety of accessories for personal devices, making them more attractive to the child. When children participate in the process, they will be more invested in using personal devices. For example, the COTA can help a child create a beaded strap to hold glasses or a zipper bag to store a hearing aid and battery. Some devices can be personalized by letting a child add stickers or drawings.

The COTA can be instrumental in identifying problems and developing creative solutions associated with personal devices. For example, an observation of the child's appearance and behavior may reveal skin irritation or an asymmetrical fit. A simple solution would be to ask the parent or family worker to help get the item refitted. Many children resist wearing their devices. They may repeatedly lose or break their glasses, hearing aids, or other personal devices so that they do not have to wear them. The COTA might request team meetings to explore the causes of and solutions for personal device problems. The team may recommend reducing the amount of time the device is worn. For example, a child who wears glasses may need to wear them only at school or while doing homework.

FORGETTING TO BRING GLASSES STORY. *After gently questioning an adolescent, the OT practitioner discovered that the boy did not bring his glasses to school because he did not have an eyeglass case. This was remedied by asking a staff member to donate an old eyeglass case.*

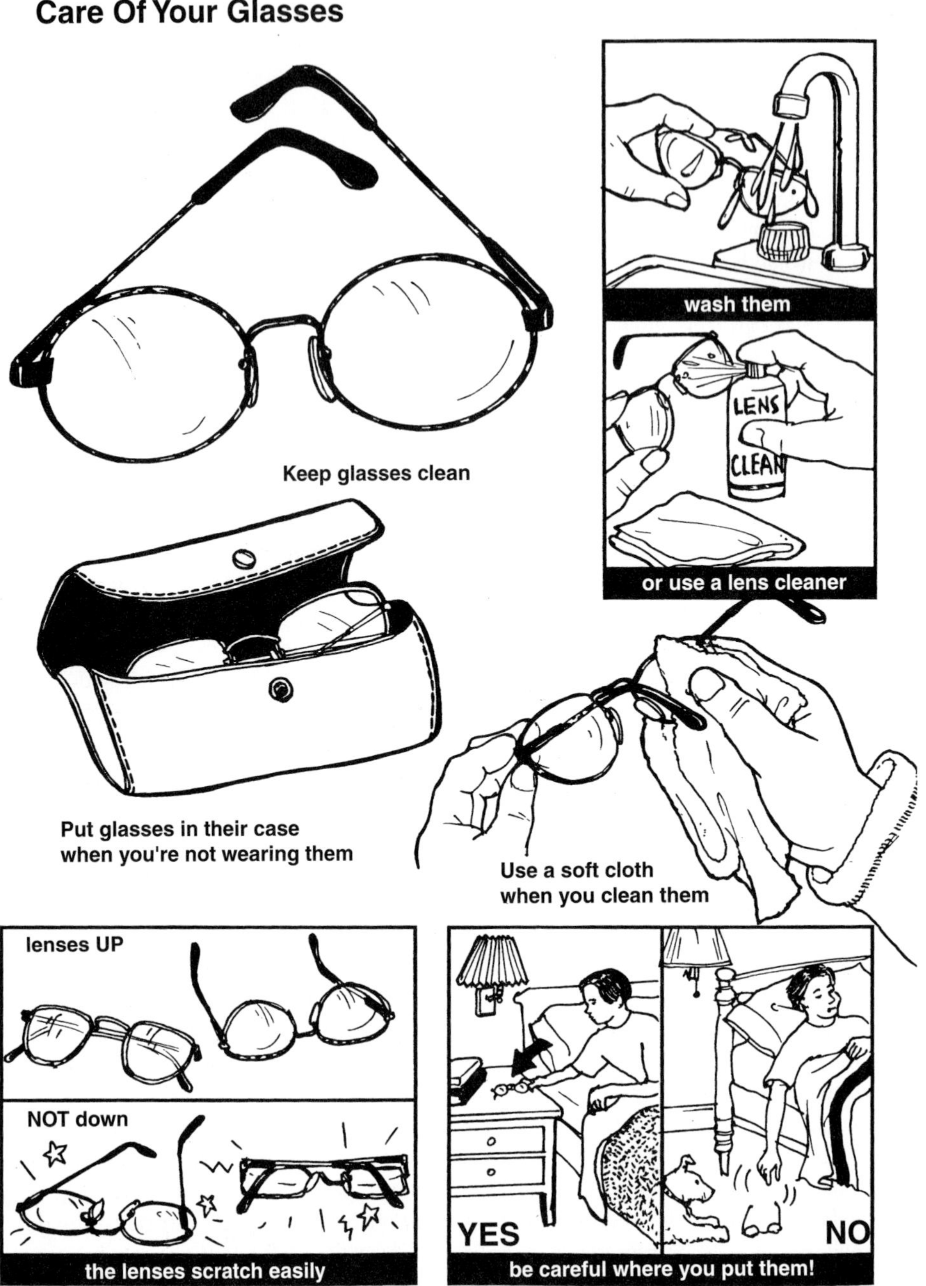
Care Of Your Glasses
Keep glasses clean
wash them
LENS
CLEAN
or use a lens cleaner
Put glasses in their case
when you're not wearing them
Use a soft cloth
when you clean them
lenses UP
NOT down
the lenses scratch easily
YES
NO
be careful where you put them!

FIGURE 18-37 "Care for your glasses" picture sequence. (From Reynolds J: *Attainment's personal success: an illustrated guide to personal needs,* Attainment Company Inc, 1999, Verona, Wis.)

CLINICAL *Pearl*

Some children benefit from wearing snug eyeglass straps to prevent the glasses from falling off the head and breaking. There are a variety of eyeglass straps on the market. One unique style consists of a soft, stretchy, coiled band that attaches to the earpieces of the glasses and goes around the back of the head.

REFUSING TO WEAR GLASSES STORY. Another child refused to wear his glasses because he did not like the way they looked or felt; fortunately, he also needed a new prescription. His parents were able to afford a new pair of glasses that fit him better. All the staff members complimented him on his new glasses, which seemed to help his self-esteem. Combined with the improved fit and prescription, the praise increased his tolerance for wearing glasses.

Sexual Activity

Sexual activity refers to engaging in activities that result in sexual satisfaction. Teenagers may struggle with how to properly express themselves sexually and knowing when it is okay to do it. For older, married teenagers, exual activity can involve how to make love. For married clients, team members may ask the COTA to address issues such as positioning, adaptive equipment, and techniques related to sexual activity.

Sexual expression includes the self-identity of boys and girls and their social interaction. It can be extremely important to adolescents. The COTA needs to consider adolescents' unique issues so as to develop possible intervention strategies. A dyadic treatment session involving a boy and girl could help them learn to interact respectfully with the opposite sex. Team members can help adolescents set up lunch dates or attend dances or social events with their peers.

COTAs need to prepare themselves for potential encounters involving boys and girls who are exploring their own sexuality. Adolescents with mental retardation or other developmental delays, head injuries, or emotional problems may flirt with or make sexual remarks to COTAs. Immediately report any incident of this nature to the OTR, family worker, psychologist, parents or caregiver, or on-site supervisor. Being matter of fact and setting firm limits against touching are often the best approaches. Some adolescents will need to meet with counselors to discuss why their behavior is unacceptable and explore avenues for developing a romantic relationship with a peer.

Some children and adolescents may touch their genitals excessively. Very young children tend to do this when they need to use the bathroom, and the COTA can help them learn what to do. This socially unacceptable behavior can elicit negative reactions from peers and people in the community. Many children need to be reminded repeatedly about when it is and is not okay to touch their genitals. For children with limited cognitive skills, establish concrete rules such as "It is okay to touch your private parts in the bathroom or bedroom when no one else is there."

When this technique is not enough, use a team approach. Some children may need a medical evaluation to rule out infections. Anxiety may be a factor, so fidget toys such as squeeze toys or even handheld video games can positively redirect the child. Reward children who behave in a socially acceptable way for short periods by offering them their choice of toys.

BOB'S SEXUAL APPROACH STORY. *Bob was a 17 year old with fragile X syndrome (a type of autism caused by an abnormality in the X chromosome), mental retardation, and poor judgment. He frightened several young female staff members by lunging at them and trying to touch their legs when they wore skirts. A COTA reported this behavior to the OTR, who then consulted with the family worker. The family worker discussed the issue with Bob's mother, who greatly appreciated the feedback. She had never witnessed this behavior and was unaware that it was happening. She and her husband had always taught Bob to interact respectfully with everyone.*

Bob's parents said that even though he often talked about imaginary girlfriends, they did not think that he was ready to handle intimacy. His mother stated that he was capable of satisfying himself at home by masturbating in his bedroom. She and her husband said that they would address the problem at home. They asked school personnel to continue to gently but firmly enforce limits with Bob. During supervision sessions the OTR and COTA discussed ways in which the COTA could redirect Bob's behavior in a matter-of-fact way and help him learn how to interact more positively with females.

TEDDY'S MASTURBATION STORY. *Teddy was a 16 year old with severe mental retardation and autism. Sometimes in school he touched his genitals continuously. When encouraged to stop, he became agitated and aggressive. The parents and multidisciplinary team determined that Teddy's behavior could be caused by frustration resulting from being asked to stop what he was doing. Because the parents and team knew he was capable of satisfying himself through masturbation, a behavior plan was devised that incorporated this behavior. When Teddy became so agitated by the need to touch his genitals that he could not participate in class work, he was asked to go to the bathroom. A male staff person respectfully monitored him until he was finished and then assisted him in refocusing on his class work.*

Sleep and Rest

Sleep and rest refer to times when an individual is inactive and may or may not be conscious (aware of self, others, and surroundings). Sleep and rest allow the brain to absorb new information and allow the body and brain to recuperate from work and/or play or heal from stress, injury, or illness. The COTA can be instrumental in helping a family with adaptive equipment for and furniture arrangement in the bedroom.

Bed safety railings provide protection and support when getting in and out of bed.

The following are some potential problems for children related to sleep and rest:

1. They may have trouble with self-regulation or modulation of their own level of arousal (alertness and readiness to perform the activity at hand). It may be hard for them to stop playing or stop thinking or talking about an exciting idea as a result of overarousal, with limited inhibitory (slowing or stopping) control. They could be overexcited about special events such as birthdays, vacations, movies they hope to see, and relatives coming to visit.
2. Sensory defensiveness can cause self-regulation problems. These children react negatively to harmless events and are often unable to inhibit these feelings. For example, the sensation of sheets or blankets can be too scratchy or tickly. Background noises such as family members walking outside the bedroom might keep them awake, while other children would not notice the noises.
3. They might have eaten too much or eaten something that does not agree with them. They might have unknown food sensitivities that cause them to feel uncomfortable hours after the food was eaten (e.g., the caffeine in some foods could cause sleeplessness).
4. Unfamiliar surroundings, such as those found when staying in a motel or trying to nap at the babysitter's house, can cause restlessness.
5. Parents may be inconsistent in maintaining a calming bedtime routine.
6. Children may be unable to calm unreasonable fears (e.g., monsters under the bed, thunder, space alien attacks).

Some possible solutions include the following:

1. Be sure the child is getting enough exercise every day. If his or her muscles are tired, sleep may come more easily.
2. It is important to establish a bedtime routine that helps a child calm down and go to bed at the same time every night. While many children need about 30 to 45 minutes to slow down and get ready for bed, others might need 1 or 2 hours. Let the child know what time to start getting ready for bed. The repetition of familiar sequences, like reading the same bedtime book every night, can be calming. Baths tend to be more calming than showers, but this is not true for all children. Take time for quiet play during the bath. Engage the child in blowing soap bubbles if possible. This activity requires slow, deep breathing, which is relaxing. Dry the child using firm, slow, and rhythmic drying movements. If the child has sensory defensiveness, using DPPT both before and after the bath may help the child get to sleep more easily. Read bedtime stories. Turn the lights off. Complete darkness (without even a night light) promotes deep sleep.[4]
3. Carbohydrate foods (e.g., potatoes, rice, bread) may promote sleep. In their SANE workshop, Anne Buckley-Reen, an OTR, and Debra Dickson, a physical therapist, recommend that children eat breakfasts and lunches that are high in protein and dinners that are high in carbohydrates so as to promote a good night's sleep.[4]
4. A number of sleep and relaxation CDs are now available (e.g., Mealtimes/New Visions; see Appendix C of this chapter). Some replicate the rhythms of a mother's heartbeat. Others have the soothing sounds of waves on a beach or rain in a forest. Try them out yourself and carefully follow all instructions for their use. The major emphasis in using these CDs is to promote the soft sounds. Check the volume on the headphones frequently to be sure that it is not accidentally increased.

Functional Mobility

Bed mobility

Mobility in bed is needed to get in and out of bed, protect the skin and joints, and find a comfortable sleeping position. The COTA may be responsible for teaching bed mobility to children who are unable to stand independently or are bedridden due to illness or injury. Bed mobility skills include scooting or sliding, bridging, rolling, and sitting from the supine position.

Scooting or sliding is necessary to get in and out of bed. Sliding toward the head of the bed and propping the head on pillows are necessary for eating in bed. To slide or scoot from side to side on the bed, the child can use a hand to pull on the bed rail or the edge of the mattress. S/he may use the opposite hand or foot to push to the side.

Rolling to the side and holding the body in a side-lying position are necessary for dressing. Rolling from side to side for dressing may be the easiest bed mobility skill to learn. Use caution with these movements so as to protect unstable or painful joints. When teaching a child with hemiplegia (paralysis or weakness on one side of the body) or a stroke, first relax the shoulder blade on the affected side. It is easier to roll to the affected side first because the stronger muscles can perform all the work (Figure 18-38). In general encourage the child to use the muscles in the arms, trunk, and legs that will help in rolling and dressing.[28]

Bridging involves lifting the hips off the bed from a supine position and is always helpful for dressing and scooting to different positions (Figure 18-39). It demands more muscle strength and control than rolling. The hips can be bridged during dressing in order to pull the pants up.

Pulling from a supine to a sitting position is helpful for getting in and out of bed. The child first rolls to a side-

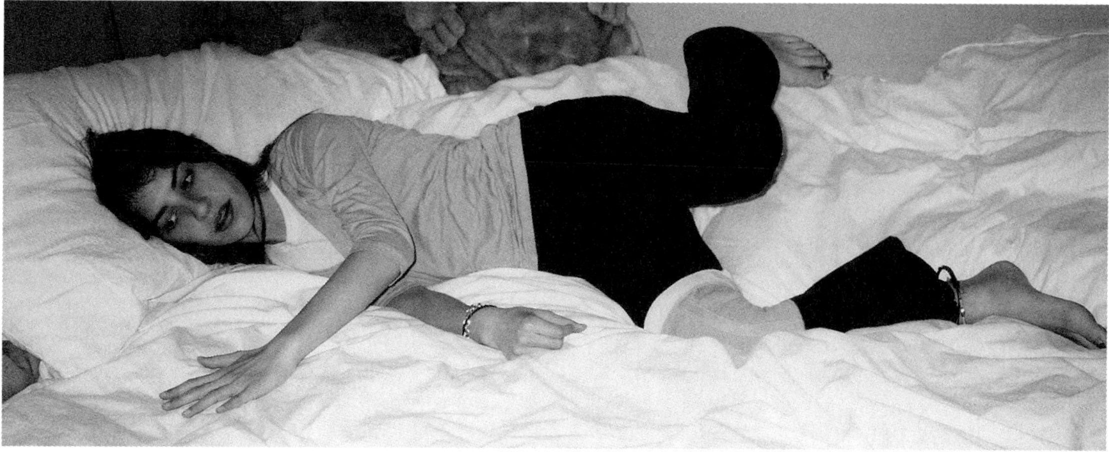

FIGURE 18-38 When moving in bed, it is easier to roll toward the affected side.

lying position. Next, s/he swings the lower legs off the bed. Then s/he rolls a little more to place the hands flat on the bed. Finally, s/he pushes the body up to a sitting position.

Adaptive equipment such as overhead trapezes (Figure 18-40) can be especially useful for children with paraplegia (weakness in the legs), hemiplegia, or lower extremity amputations. To use an overhead trapeze successfully, the child needs adequate neck, upper back, and chest strength along with hand and arm strength on one side. The trapeze is suspended over the bed in such a manner that the child can reach it easily from the supine position. S/he can grasp the trapeze to pull toward the head or side of the bed or into a sitting position. S/he can also pull on the trapeze to lift the hips off the bed during dressing, while using a bedpan, or for other ADLs. For children who lack the hand strength to grip the trapeze, like those with quadriplegia (weakness or paralysis in the arms and legs), a bed hoist or quad-quip pull might work. A bed hoist is a series of five or six rungs connected with rope, similar to a small ladder. A quad-quip pull is a series of five or six connected loops of sturdy fabric webbing. The bed hoist or quad-quip pull can be secured firmly to the foot of the bed. A child can insert the arms alternately into successive rungs or loops to pull themselves up to a sitting position.

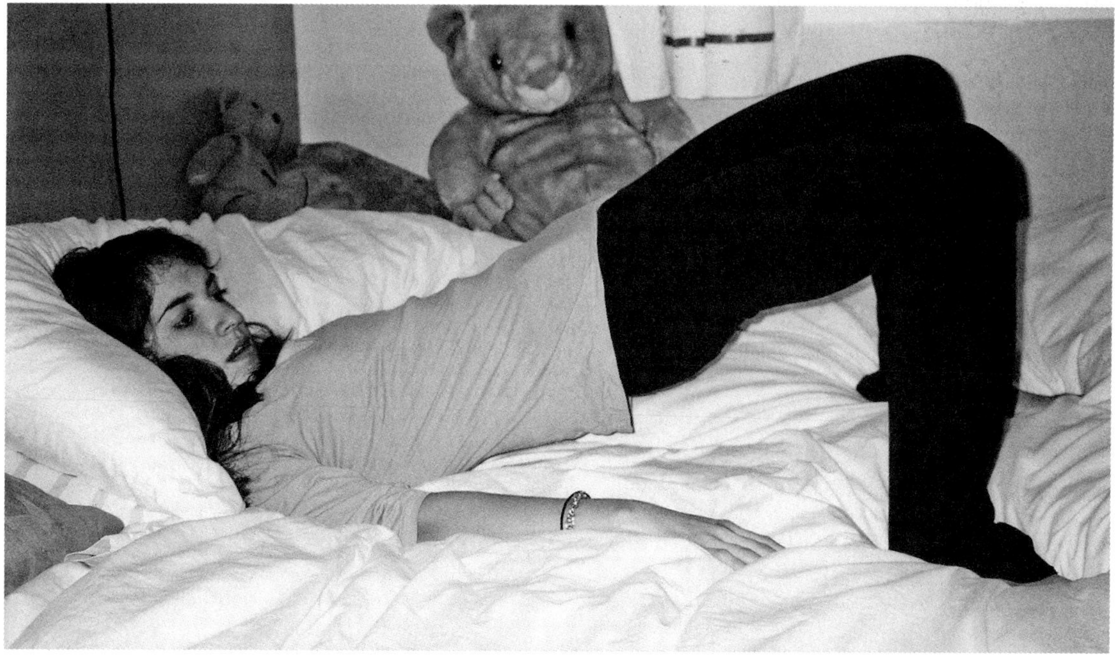

FIGURE 18-39 Bridging the hips is a useful skill in bed mobility.

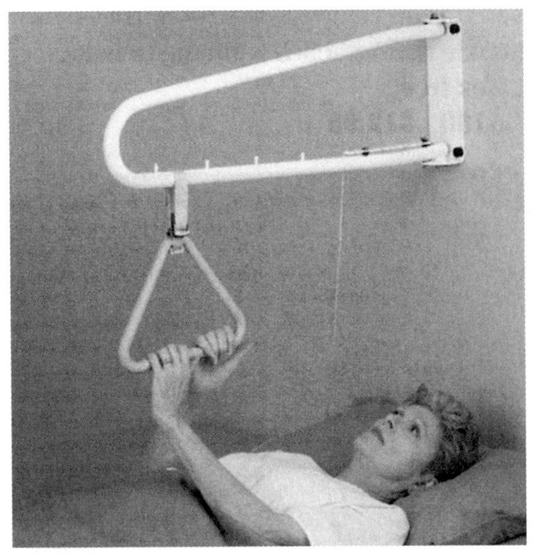

A

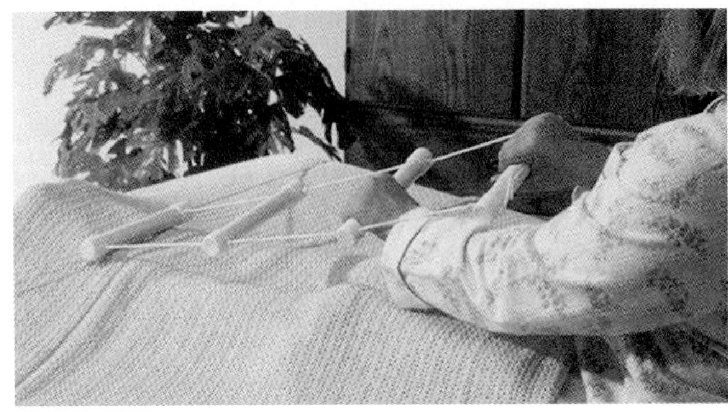

B

FIGURE 18-40 **A,** An overhead trapeze or **B,** bed hoist can help individuals pull up to the sitting position in bed. (Courtesy Sammons Preston Rolyan, Bolingbrook, Ill.)

Wheelchair transfers

Wheelchair transfers refer to getting in and out of a wheelchair. The sections below address wheelchair transfers for children who are ready for training by the OT practitioner. To learn independent transfers a child needs safety awareness, motor planning skills, and some upper extremity strength.

Transfers between wheelchair and bed

A transfer board, sometimes called a sliding board, is a piece of wood, plastic, or metal used by a child who is unable to stand to move from one surface to another. A wide variety of transfer boards are available. Be sure to practice with the desired transfer board before purchasing one for the child.

It is easiest to use a transfer board between a wheelchair and bed when they are close to the same height. If the bed is lower than the wheelchair, leg extenders (available from equipment catalogs) can raise the bed a few inches to make the transfer easier. When using a transfer board to move from a wheelchair to a bed, first position the wheelchair so that the child's stronger side can be next to the bed. Second, lock the wheels and remove the armrest that is closer to the bed. Next, release the seat belt and slide one end of the transfer board under the thigh, resting the other end on the bed. Then lean forward for balance, place the hands on the transfer board, and slide little by little onto the bed. Finally, when securely seated on the bed, remove the transfer board. Bed-to-wheelchair transfers are performed in a reverse sequence, with the wheelchair turned so it is beside the bed on the stronger side of the child's body.

If the child can bear some weight on the legs but is unable to use a transfer board, a *standing pivot transfer* may work. In a standing pivot transfer the OT practitioner helps the child stand, turn, and sit down. As with any handling, care is taken to protect unstable or painful joints. In a wheelchair-to-bed transfer, the wheelchair is first positioned as described above, with the wheels locked and the armrest on the side next to the bed removed. Second, the OT practitioner places her own feet against the outside of the child's feet her knees against the outside of the child's knees. In this way the OT practitioner can control the child's feet and knees throughout the transfer. The practitioner bends her knees and reaches under the child's arms, locking the hands together around the child's back. Next, the clinician pulls the child up and close to her body. The child supports his or her own weight on the feet. Then the OT practitioner takes small steps, turning his/her own feet and body in such a way that the child turns along with him/her. When the child is positioned with the back of the knees against the bed, he/she slowly bends his/her knees, lowering the child onto the bed.

If the child's joints are unstable or s/he is too weak to stand reliably, the OT practitioner may lift the child by grasping the pants or using a transfer belt (Figure 18-41). Transfer belts are usually made of strong fabric webbing about three inches wide, with secure closures. To provide extra support and prevent falling during transfers and ambulation training, caregivers and OT practitioners hold onto the transfer belts. During wheelchair-to-bed transfers, the transfer belt is first placed securely around the child's belly. After stabilizing the feet and knees and reaching around the child's back, the OT practitioner grasps the transfer belt to help lift and move the child. Some transfer belts are made to fit around the hips; these are more comfortable for the child and offer more control to the caregiver or practitioner.

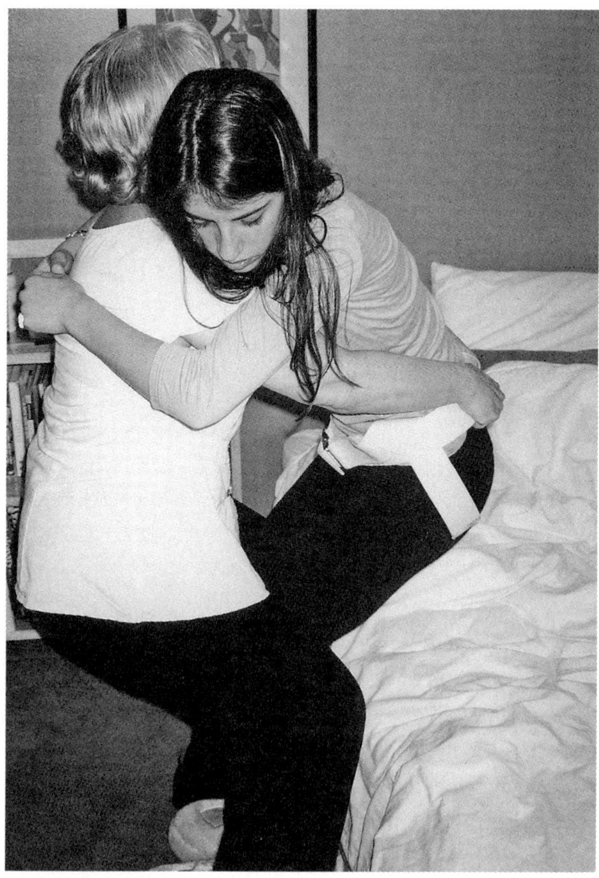

FIGURE 18-41 The occupational therapy practitioner uses a transfer or gait belt to increase safety when helping a child get out of bed.

Transfers between wheelchair and toilet

COTAs can help children learn transfers between the wheelchair and toilet. These transfers are similar to those between the wheelchair and bed, with some differences. Limited bathroom space can interfere with the optimum positioning of the wheelchair beside the toilet. The wheelchair may be positioned at a right angle (90 degrees) or opposite the toilet. Wall-mounted grab bars are sturdier than tension-operated floor-to-ceiling poles, but both can provide hand support during transfers. Toilet armrests might help during a standing pivot transfer, described above in the section on transfers between the wheelchair and bed. However, armrests would prevent a sliding board transfer.

If the bathroom doorway is too narrow for the wheelchair to pass through, the child may use a toilet chair in the bedroom. The toilet chair has a regular toilet seat with a bucket below it. The bucket slides out easily for emptying and cleaning by the caregiver. Transfers between the wheelchair and toilet chair are also similar to those between the wheelchair and bed.

Transfers between wheelchair and tub or shower

COTAs may have the responsibility of training children and/or caregivers to transfer between a wheelchair and tub or shower. Tub transfers are similar to but more difficult than bed transfers. Bathroom space may be limited, and extra strength is required from both the child and caregiver to lower the body down into the tub and later lift the body up and over the side. Many individuals prefer to use bath chairs as a quicker and less strenuous way to transfer into the tub. These chairs allow children to sit and use handheld shower devices to bathe themselves. Children transfer between wheelchairs and bath chairs using a transfer board, standing pivot, or other style of transfer. When the body is wet, it may not slide as easily on a transfer board. Try placing a dry towel on it to make sliding easier.

Another option is an electric bath chair lift, which some children learn to operate independently. An electric bath chair is permanently installed in a bathtub. The cushioned chair swivels in and out of the tub and is lowered and raised when electric buttons are pushed. The child first transfers from the wheelchair to bath chair by means of a sliding board or pivot transfer. Next s/he swivels the chair into the tub, carefully lifting the legs over the side. Then s/he operates the lift to lower them into the tub. The child can fill the tub with water and bathe using adaptive bathing aids like long-handled sponges and soap held in the pocket of a wash cloth mit. Finally, s/he gets out of the tub by following the sequence in reverse.

Children who lack the strength to perform either board or pivot transfers may need to use manual or electric lifts. A lift consists of a large metal frame suspending a detachable canvas sling that can be lowered and raised. The lift frame often has lockable wheels so that the child can be transferred from the wheelchair to the lift in one room and then rolled into the bathroom before being transferred into the tub. To do this, the sling is first detached from the lift. Next, as the child sits in the locked wheelchair, the caregiver or OT or physical therapy practitioner carefully rocks the child's hips from side to side while gradually sliding the sling underneath. The ends of the sling are kept free and ready for attachment to the chains or ropes of the lift. The lift is moved close to the wheelchair, and the wheels are locked. Then the canvas sling is attached to fasteners on the chains or ropes of the lift. With manual lifts a crank is turned to raise and lower the child in the sling. With electric lifts the buttons are pushed for raising and lowering. Once the child has been safely raised, the wheels are unlocked and the lift is carefully rolled to a position next to the tub. The wheels are again locked and the suspension arm over the sling is swiveled into position, with the child over the tub. The sling is then lowered until the child is securely in place in the bath chair. The sling is removed in the same way that it was initially positioned. Finally, the child can be bathed.

Transfers between a wheelchair and shower can be tricky because of the 2- to 4-inch-high lip, also called a threshold, at the shower door. With physical assistance, children who are able to bear some weight on their legs and shift weight from side to side may negotiate this obstacle. The following are other means of transfer between a wheelchair and a shower that involve either bath/shower chairs or structural modifications. (1) A bath chair that straddles the lip may be the most economical solution. When the wheelchair is positioned as close as possible to the bath chair, the child can transfer onto the shower chair using a sliding board or pivot transfer and then scoot across the chair into the shower, avoiding the lip. (2) A contractor or plumber can modify the entrance to the shower by sloping it. Plaster or tile can be slanted upward before the lip and slanted downward after the lip, making it easier to negotiate.

Transfers between wheelchair and floor

Transfers between a wheelchair and the floor are not essential for most ADLs, but they can increase safety, freedom, joint flexibility, muscle strength, self-esteem, and opportunities to play and learn. In an emergency like a fire, a transfer from a wheelchair to the floor or vice versa can be lifesaving.

To transfer between a wheelchair and the floor, children need sufficient strength to move on the floor. They can creep on their hands and knees, belly crawl, scoot on their seats, or pull and push themselves with the arms and legs. They need to be able to judge which environmental supports, like a heavy sofa, will be secure enough to hold their body weight without slipping. To transfer from a wheelchair to the floor, the child carries out the following sequence: (1) positions the wheelchair with the stronger side of the body beside a support like a sofa or next to floor pillows; (2) locks the wheels, lifts the footrests, and removes the armrests; (3) slides forward toward the front edge of the seat and twists the body toward the stronger side, placing the hands on the seat of the wheelchair or on a stable support like the sofa; (4) leans forward for balance and carefully slides off the edge of the wheelchair, lowering the body to the knees or to a sitting position on the floor or pillows; (5) if lowering to a high kneeling position (resting on knees with hips straight), continues lowering to a low kneeling position (resting on knees with bent hips); and (6) moves the hands to the floor and proceeds to a side-sitting position, creeping on the hands and knees or crawling on the belly to a desired location. An alternative method of lowering to the floor, which requires more arm and shoulder strength, is as follows: After sliding forward to the edge of the chair, place the hands on each side of the body on the seat of the wheelchair and then slowly slide the body forward off the edge of the wheelchair and lower the body onto the floor or pillows.

Transferring from the floor to a wheelchair requires enough strength to lift the body against gravity. The child might use the following sequence: (1) Get into a low kneeling position facing the locked wheelchair, with the armrests removed and footrests raised. (2) Using a stable support like a heavy sofa or the wheelchair itself, pull up into a high kneeling position. (3) Place the hands on the seat of the wheelchair on the child's stronger side. (4) Keeping the body as close as possible to the wheelchair, lean forward and hoist the body off the floor, rotating slightly to lift one hip onto the seat of the wheelchair. (5) Push the hips all the way back in the wheelchair to get the body into a stable position. (6) Lower footrests, fasten seat belt, and replace armrests.

A child who is not strong enough to lift the whole body into the wheelchair at once might try lifting the body up in stages. For example, first the body can be lifted onto pillows or an ottoman, then onto a sofa, and then into the wheelchair.

Transfers between wheelchair and chair or sofa

It is important for children who use wheelchairs to sometimes sit on other surfaces. Changing their seating can increase circulation, help prevent pressure sores, and increase opportunities for peer and family interaction. Transfers between a wheelchair and a chair or sofa are performed in a manner similar to those between a wheelchair and bed. If the seat heights of the wheelchair and chair or sofa are significantly different, the child may need additional training or physical assistance. The child may also need extra help getting in and out of the corner of a soft sofa.

Car transfers

Car transfers with vans or SUVs that have sliding doors are easiest. These vehicles allow plenty of space to position mobility devices. Transfers through other car doors are more difficult due to the small transfer space in the angle of the open door.

From crutches or a walker, children carefully back up to the car seat. When the backs of the legs touch the seat, they slowly lower themselves into a sitting position. Next they move one hand to a stable support inside the car, possibly the console, back of the front seat, or seat itself. The other hand might remain on the walker or one crutch or the armrest of the door if it is stable enough. Using hand support, children then lift and turn until their hips are facing forward. Then they lift the legs into the car one by one. They may need to use the hands to pick up each leg. Finally, they fasten their seat belts.

Swivel seats are round cushions that require minimum effort to turn. They can ease many transfers by eliminating the need to lift up the body when turning to the proper position.

To get out of the car, children position the crutches or walker as close to a right angle to the car as possible. They follow the above sequence in reverse and use extra care to bear weight on stable supports when pulling up to stand.

Transfers between a wheelchair and car may require additional maneuvering to get the seat of the wheelchair as close as possible to the car. The wheelchair is positioned almost parallel to the car seat, especially when a transfer board is used. The sequence described above in the section on transfers between a wheelchair and bed is followed.

Survey of wheelchair and eye contact

Well-meaning adults often make the mistake of not speaking at eye level to children who use wheelchairs. In a survey of five group homes for children in wheelchairs, only 3 of the 12 observed were spoken to at eye level.[20] Verbal interaction at eye level helps them feel respected and safe, whereas that above eye level can cause children to feel controlled, intimidated, and unimportant.

In the same survey, two types of social interaction were observed: (1) the staff giving physical assistance or verbal instructions to children and (2) the children conveying their needs to the staff through speech, gestures, and facial expressions. A study of the children's interaction with each other revealed a pronounced deficiency in peer interaction.

This survey illustrates the importance of enhancing social interaction. Simple solutions may facilitate socialization, such as moving two children so that they can sit side by side or face to face.

Transporting objects

Children with mild physical limitations and/or problems with sensory processing, motor planning, and motor memory often need assistance when transporting or carrying objects. COTAs may instruct children in how to carry clothing by looping it over one arm or how to carry a few folders or books by tucking them under an elbow. Some children benefit from wearing a shoulder bag with a wide opening for school notebooks. A bag that has a soft strap crossing the body is best. One drawback is that shoulder bags can pull children off balance. Backpacks are practical and popular for all children. They can give additional proprioceptive feedback and promote stability when walking. Rolling backpacks are also useful, but children using them might need training on how to manage curbs and steps. To carry drinks, it is best for children to carry unbreakable items with lids, such as plastic sports bottles and straw cups with lids.

Children with moderate physical limitations who use walkers might carry items in a homemade cloth bag with strong Velcro loops attached to the walker. Some pediatric walkers have optional baskets or trays that can be purchased. Check the measurements to be sure that the basket or tray will fit your client's walker.

Children with more severe physical limitations who use wheelchairs often carry items on their lap boards, which are wide trays that attach to wheelchair armrests. They are often created for specific wheelchairs and children. A lapboard is used for eating and schoolwork as well as for transporting objects. The COTA may give input about the child's capabilities and needs when choosing a lapboard.

Safe mobility

The COTA's responsibilities may include teaching safe mobility skills to children who use wheelchairs or are unable to walk. Those who use manual or electric wheelchairs need to learn the following safe mobility skills: (1) locking and unlocking the wheelchair; (2) starting or stopping for obstacles such as walls or people; (3) going straight; (4) slowing or stopping on request; (5) timing, sequencing, and gauging the force and direction of movement; (6) negotiating around corners and furniture; (7) moving through tight spaces such as doorways, bathrooms, and elevators; (8) moving over different surfaces, such as ramps and carpets; and (9) refining actions such as opening and closing doors or going over thresholds. For children with manual wheelchairs, gloves may be used to increase friction on the wheels while protecting the hands.

Children who are able to walk may have problems moving safely for several reasons. Limited head or eye control can interfere with environmental awareness. Limited postural control, body awareness, or motor planning can impair children's ability to control their bodies. Those with mobility problems may tend to run instead of walk and may bang into walls or doors, letting obstacles stop them instead of slowing down and stopping on their own. They may have trouble estimating distance and knowing where to move. An inability to anticipate potential accidents and time their actions accordingly can result in collisions with people or furniture. The following strategies may help children improve safety while being mobile:

1. To increase environmental awareness, improve eye control as needed.
2. To improve body awareness, move under, between, or through small spaces (e.g., between two chairs, under heavy pillows, or through tunnels or makeshift tents).
3. To improve body awareness, make a "mat sandwich." Have the child lie down between two mats or

cushions. Press down firmly on the upper mat and child and pretend to put on sandwich toppings.
4. To improve motor planning, use obstacle courses or relay races in which children must avoid touching certain items.
5. To learn what a normal moving speed is (not too slow or too fast), move the wheelchair in rhythm or march in rhythm to music.
6. To increase awareness of the environment, play a game in which the child moves onto visually located targets such as shapes, letters, or numbers on the floor.
7. To improve attention to visual cues, play a game in which the child stops moving when the OT practitioner holds up a red sign, moves slowly in response to a yellow sign, and moves quickly in response to a green sign.
8. To increase attention to auditory cues and enhance postural and impulse control, play games in which the child "freezes" in place when music that is playing is turned off. The child may also be told to move very slowly, very quickly, or in a different direction on command.
9. To increase postural control, especially in a child who is able to walk but tends to run or bang into walls or people, have the child carry a weighted object such as a bucket of sand while moving from one room to another.
10. To help the child remember safe mobility skills, review rules for safe mobility before each session. For example, have the child describe the proper speed for walking in the halls or up steps and what to do if a person is in the way.

SAFE HALLWAY TRANSITION STORY. *In a special school for children with pervasive developmental disorder and emotional impairments, classroom transition (moving from classroom to classroom) was problematic. The children had poor body and environmental awareness, sensory defensiveness, and limited motor planning skills. During transition from one room to another, they swayed and repeatedly bumped into furniture or each other and then overreacted by pushing or hitting, stumbling, running, or grabbing artwork from the walls. They were unable to coordinate their bodies long enough to follow the frequent clear verbal directions from the teachers.*

To address the transition problems, the OT practitioner utilized the theory that deep-pressure (proprioceptive) feedback to the joints and muscles could enhance body awareness and initiate a calming response. S/he hypothesized that the children might improve body control if they carried weighted objects during transition from one room to another.

The practitioner purchased pumpkin-shaped plastic pails (the ones commonly used for trick-or-treating on Halloween) for each child. A volunteer sewed about 2 pounds of rice into terry cloth hand towels to make weights. The weighted towels were then placed in the pumpkin pails, and each child carried one during room transition.

The results were amazing. The children stopped swaying and bumping into furniture and each other during room transition. They stopped grabbing artwork from the walls, walked using a steady pace with little stumbling, and were even able to follow verbal directions.[3]

INSTRUMENTAL ACTIVITIES OF DAILY LIVING

IADLs are more complex than ADLs (i.e., they require more cognitive skill, problem solving, and judgment) and include more interaction with the environment.

Communication Device Use

Communication device use refers to managing the equipment used for sending and receiving information. These devices include writing equipment, telephones, keyboards, computers, communication boards, telecommunication devices for the deaf, Braille writers, emergency call systems, and environmental control systems. If trained by the OTR, COTAs can help children with communication devices in a number of ways: assessing their ability to use these devices, choosing or adapting the devices to fit special needs and capabilities, helping them develop the foundation skills necessary to operate the devices, training them to operate the devices, and helping them use the devices during daily functions.

Postural control and positioning

Postural control in sitting provides the foundation that supports the eye and limb movements necessary for children to operate most communication devices. Upright sitting frees the arms and hands for pointing, writing, and

CLINICAL *Pearl*

Simply practicing sitting in a chair does not increase postural control. To develop and maintain the muscle control needed to sit in a chair for extended periods, children of all ages need to perform regular exercises and activities designed to activate and strengthen the muscles in the trunk, back, stomach, hips, shoulders, and neck. Proper positioning benefits all children.

typing. COTAs assess postural control to help children use communication devices. Proper positioning is also addressed and is a basic component affecting the ability to focus on and succeed in most activities.

Determining seat height

Children must be seated at the correct height to use a communication device. If only the sole of the foot is on the ground, lower body stability is insufficient to support upper body mobility, and the seat is too high. If a child's feet dangle or if scooting forward is necessary to get the feet flat on the ground, the seat is too high. When children must slide forward to get the feet on the ground, the hips begin to straighten. In children with spasticity this leads to hyperextension (excessive straightening) of the hips and abnormal posturing of the upper body as well.[2] High seats can prevent them from using their hands functionally.

It is often necessary for the OT practitioner to measure the distance between the bottom of the child's shoe to the crease behind the child's knee. The proper seat height is 1 to 2 inches less than this distance. The feet need to be flat on the floor or footrest, with the child's weight solidly on the heel and the sole but slightly more on the heel.

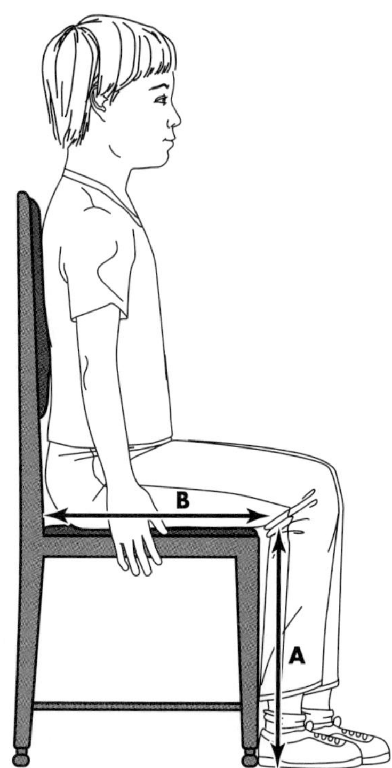

FIGURE 18-42 Positioning for instruction. Seat height *(A)*: 1 to 2 inches less than the distance between the heel (with shoes on) and the crease behind the knee. Seat depth *(B)*: 1 to 2 inches less than the distance between the back of the hip and the crease behind the knee.

Determining seat depth

The OT practitioner measures the distance between the back of a seated child's hips and the crease behind the child's knees. The proper seat depth is 1 to 2 inches less than this distance, which allows the child's hips and back to rest firmly against the back of the chair, promoting hip and trunk stability (Figure 18-42).

Determining tabletop height

The OT practitioner measures the distance between the floor and the child's elbows while the arms are hanging at the child's side; the most functional tabletop height is about 2 inches higher than this distance. When working at a table the shoulders tend to *flex* forward, raising the elbows slightly.

Positioning problems and simple solutions

When seated, many children with special needs have trouble maintaining the hip and trunk stability required to support hand, head, and eye mobility. Signs that the child needs more stability or that the seat may need an adjustment include the following: straddling the seat, wrapping the feet around chair legs, sitting with a wide base of support, putting the feet up on the seat of the chair, sliding to the side or front edge of the chair, sitting or kneeling on the feet, slouching, banging the chair legs, and rocking.

Consider using the following inexpensive methods for footrests and backrests:

1. Telephone books covered with duct tape make fairly sturdy and cost-effective footrests.
2. Detachable footrests or backrests for small children can be made out of cardboard blocks that look like bricks.[22] Add weight as needed to the cardboard footrests by filling them with sand. Cover them with contact paper so that they can be cleaned with a wet sponge. Attach them to the chair legs with sticky Velcro or tubing.
3. Footrests can be created with sturdy, closed-cell foam for children weighing up to about 100 pounds.[22] Cut the foam into blocks with a bread knife. Foam footrests take little time to make and can be wiped clean easily.
4. Pieces of corrugated cardboard glued together to the desired width can make firm, portable backrests. Cover them with contact paper so that they will look more attractive and can be cleaned. Children can carry them to different classes as needed.
5. Rectangular boxes 2 to 3 inches deep filled with newspaper and covered with contact paper can make portable backrests.[41]

Children may need seating alternatives; consider using the following:

1. A child who rocks continuously may be more attentive when sitting in a child-size rocking chair.
2. A child who fidgets or squirms around too much despite proper positioning can try an air-filled moving seat cushion to increase comfort and ease postural adjustments (Figure 18-43).
3. A child who leans heavily on a desk or has trouble staying seated despite proper positioning may benefit from sitting on a therapy ball in class. Keep the ball in a stabilizer ring. The bouncy feedback from the ball may facilitate trunk and head control as well as increase alertness. Using the stabilizer ring is important to prevent the child from straining postural muscles. In addition, to prevent straining the muscles, the child needs to change to a different seating option with back support after 20 to 30 minutes. Chairs with backrests that hold therapy balls are now available. Children may sit in these chairs as long as they stay comfortable and focused.
4. A child who is unable to stay seated for more than a few minutes may be able to stand near the desk for schoolwork. Standing next to a desk does not necessarily interfere with writing or using other devices. Place colored tape on the floor to designate the child's workspace. Consider allowing the child to work at a podium, countertop, or other raised surface to promote a straight back and reduce postural demands.
5. A child who is unable to sit safely because of physical limitations may benefit from using a seat belt to aid hip stability. This might apply to a child with low or high muscle tone who tends to fall out of the chair

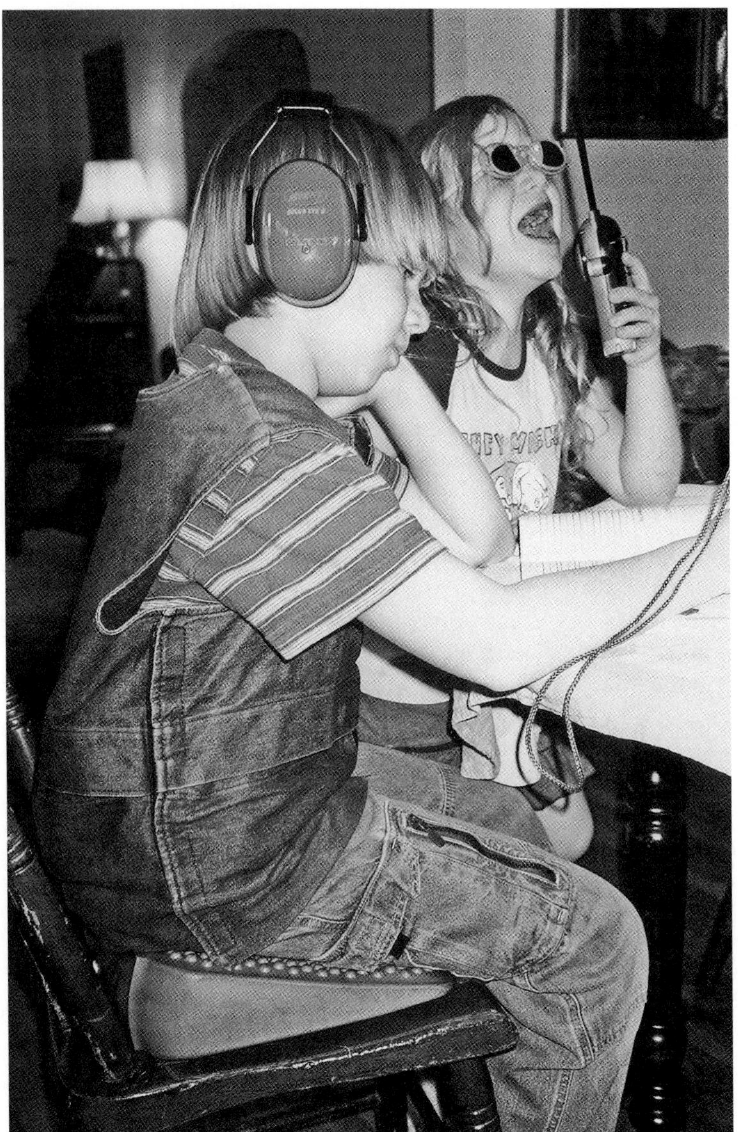

FIGURE 18-43 The boy uses three assistive devices to help him complete his work: (1) a weighted vest to increase proprioceptive feedback for postural control and provide a calm, secure feeling; (2) an air-filled seat cushion to allow for easier postural adjustments and increased comfort; and (3) noise reduction headphones to decrease background auditory distractions.

but is able to sit briefly. Seat belts are not used with children for the simple reason that they frequently get out of their chairs.

6. Chairs with wooden armrests and side supports afford a little extra stability for children who tend to slide around due to physical limitations.

Those with typical development use a wide variety of postures during the day. Preschoolers use the floor; they crawl with trains and cars or sit on their sides to complete puzzles. They use numerous different positions on the floor, with frequent postural transitions to play with dolls or action figures. During all this floor play, children develop the strength and postural control they will eventually need to sit in chairs. Even children in elementary, junior high, and high schools need to use various positions and participate regularly in strengthening activities to maintain comfortable postures for writing or using communication boards or computers.

Visual function

The OT practitioner often addresses visual function as a foundation skill to help children improve handwriting, communication board use, computer use, and other communication device use. Visual function involves visual acuity, oculomotor (eye movement) skills, and visual perception. Children who have severe visual impairments need specialized intervention. They may need referral to a developmental optometrist.

The development of any visual skill requires careful grading of activities. The OT practitioner begins with simple activities and gradually increases their complexity.[2,36] Because of the intricacy of visual function, the OTR gives precise directions for intervention. The COTA may intervene at different levels during the same session. Teachers and SLPs also address various visual perceptual and visuomotor skills. Whenever possible, coordinate treatment efforts with these professionals.

Visual acuity

Visual acuity is the "capacity to discriminate the fine details of objects in the visual field"[32] or "a descriptive means of expressing the sharpness, clearness, and distinctness of vision."[6] Ophthalmologists and optometrists assess acuity. A referral is recommended if the COTA notices that a child brings objects very close to the eyes; squints; or appears unable to see obstacles, people, or writing on the blackboard.

CLINICAL *Pearl*

Seat belts are considered restraints and are *not* used on children who are capable of sitting independently. Many agencies require a physician's prescription in order for seat belts to be used with children.

Oculomotor skills

Oculomotor skills are multiple coordinated eye movements produced by the eye muscles.[6] These skills are also known as ocular control or oculomotor skills. Eye muscles pull the eyes in horizontal, vertical, and oblique (diagonal) directions. Combinations of eye muscle actions move the eyes in a circle. Children need oculomotor skills for communication activities like writing, eye gaze during conversation, and finding the keys on a keyboard or symbols on a communication board. Any problem in this area can significantly interfere with communication device use.

Difficulty in finding and holding the correct head position interferes with maintaining a stable visual field, which provides the base of support for the eye movements involved in activities such as reading, writing, and finding symbols on a communication board or keys on a keyboard. The visual field is "the entire area that can be seen while the eye is fixing or gazing steadily at a target in the direct line of vision."[6] Strong neck muscles, which position and steady the head, are needed for a stable visual field.

Visual fixation, or a sustained eye gaze, in the direction of a target is necessary for ADLs or IADLs.[6] Children who have limited convergence, the "simultaneous turning of the eyes inward,"[6] are unable to bring their eyes together well enough to see objects close to their faces (i.e., within a 12-inch distance).

Head-eye dissociation refers to the ability to move the eyes independently without moving the head. The inability to separate head and eye movements interferes with writing or finding symbols on a communication board.

Poor head-eye dissociation makes visual tracking (following moving targets with smooth eye movements) difficult.[6] Children who have poor visual tracking skills often lose focus while trying to follow or find an object. Their eyes may also stop or jump when crossing the midline of the body. They often have problems reading and writing and finding keys on a keyboard and may skip letters or words without an awareness of doing so.

Gaze shift (accurately moving the eyes from one target to another) and quick localization (pinpointing items with the eyes) are required to find the next line of text while reading, find symbols on a communication board, or copy from the blackboard.

Oculomotor difficulties can be detected by the observant COTA. Watch for asymmetry in the eyes (e.g., they do not seem to point in the same direction or one eye wanders in or out); how the eyes and head move when the child visually follows moving objects or switches focus from paper to the blackboard; skipping words or lines when reading or copying; or difficulty in finding symbols or pictures on a communication board. When noticing or suspecting oculomotor problems, the COTA alerts the OTR and checks the child's medical record for past eye examinations. After the OTR further screens the child, the parents may be given information about getting a developmental optometry evaluation and subsequent vision therapy.

Several factors interfere with oculomotor control, including weakness of the neck and eye muscles, poor discrimination or interpretation of proprioceptive feedback (from muscles and/or joints) in the neck and eyes, and nystagmus (involuntary jerking of the eyes). The OTR may request that the COTA carry out the following specific activities to help a child improve oculomotor skills:

1. To help a child maintain a stable visual field, use strengthening exercises for neck flexion (bending) and extension (straightening).
2. To increase convergence, encourage the child to watch an appealing object move slowly toward the nose. Watch each eye to be sure that both are equally directed at the target to within about 4 inches from the face.
3. To help the child synchronize eye, neck, and head control, use specific movement activities like riding on a scooter board in a prone (face down) position while reaching for toys positioned on the floor.
4. To improve gaze shift and quick localization, the child can aim at stationary or moving targets such as a ball or balloon suspended from the ceiling while riding on moving equipment. In a dark room, the practitioner can shine a flashlight on objects and the child can then point to or identify them. Visual games like dot-to-dot and mazes also require gaze shift and quick localization. Play board or card games or try shape-matching activities. Choose those activities that require moving the eyes quickly between targets like the card game Memory and the shape-matching game Perfection.
5. To improve head-eye dissociation and tracking skills, move a toy in vertical, horizontal, and circular patterns as the child watches. If s/he does not automatically keep the head still, use gentle physical manipulation of the chin to stabilize the head. Playing with toy cars, marbles, balloons, and bubbles can also help. Watch carefully to see if the child always moves the head along with the eyes or the eyes move independently.

Visual perception

Visual perception refers to "the ability to interpret and use what is seen"[35] or "the capacity to interpret sensory input, recognize similarities and differences, and assign meaning to what is seen."[6] It includes the ability to discern edges, shapes, light and dark, figure-ground discrimination, visual closure, and spatial orientation and relations. Visual perception increases with maturity and "occurs through an active process between the child and his environment."[35] It requires cognitive (thinking) analysis as well as perception (receiving information) through sight.

Object perception refers to the "visual identification of objects by color, texture, shape, and size: what things are."[32] An important area of object perception for reading, writing, and using communication devices is *form constancy*, or "the recognition of forms and objects as the same in various environments, positions, and sizes."[32] Form constancy is the skill that allows children to recognize a letter as the same whether it is lowercase, uppercase, cursive, or italic. To help improve form constancy, a child can compare the details of various pictures or shapes to determine whether the forms are the same. The child can examine worksheets, looking for two shapes that are the same, with one being smaller, larger, darker, or lighter than the other, turned on its side, or inside another shape.

Figure-ground discrimination refers to the ability to distinguish important foreground features from background objects. For example, figure-ground discrimination is required to find a pencil on a cluttered desk; the child must be able to pick out the pencil (which is in the foreground) while distinguishing it from the desk and other items on the desk. Many activities that help develop visual figure-ground discrimination can be found in bookstores and equipment catalogs. The *Where's Waldo?*[15-18] book series, "Find What's Different" worksheets, "Find the Hidden Figures" pictures, and "What's Wrong with This Picture" worksheets all involve figure-ground discrimination.

Spatial perception refers to the "visual location of objects in space: where things are."[32] An area of spatial perception commonly addressed by clinicians is position in space, which "provides the awareness of an object's position in relation to the observer or the perception of the direction in which it is turned."[32] The perception of position in space provides the basis for the development of directional concepts such as "in," "out," "beside," and "behind." The spatial perception of position also allows the child to decipher one word as separate from another while reading and to space letters evenly while writing.[32]

Children's ability to use spatial and directional concepts such as "in" and "off" usually develops by about 30 months of age. By about 36 months, children usually begin to understand the concepts of "on," "under," "out of," "together," and "away." By about 5½ years of age, children are able to use basic spatial concepts such as "behind," "ahead of," "first," and "last"[35] (Box 18-7).

BOX 18-7

Activities to Improve Awareness of Position in Space and Spatial and Directionality Concepts

1. When children are first learning directional concepts, use directional terms to describe their actions. For example, as the child places a toy train on the tracks, say "On," or as the child removes a jacket, say "Off." Ask children later to describe the actions themselves.
2. To learn about body position in relation to objects in the environment, set up equipment so that children can play at squeezing through small spaces. Provide obstacle courses or playground activities in which children must use spatial concepts (e.g., going up, on top of, and over a giant pillow or slide).
3. To teach children how far to stand from a person during conversation, ask them to extend an arm and stand at a distance of an arm's length for social interaction. On an elevator or in other crowded situations, ask children to check on all sides to be sure that they are not touching anyone.
4. To teach children where to start reading and writing, emphasize a starting point. For example, place a sticker at the top left corner of a page.[35]

Visuomotor skills

Visuomotor skills are sometimes referred to as visuomotor integration skills or eye-hand/eye-foot skills. They require coordination of the eyes with the hands or feet such that the eyes guide complex, precise limb movements. A few examples of visuomotor activities are (1) following dot-to-dot patterns or mazes, (2) drawing, (3) handwriting, (4) copying designs with pegs or beads, (5) using a computer, (6) cutting with scissors, and (7) moving through obstacle courses.

Pointing

Pointing is used with communication boards and computer keyboards. Caregivers and team members rely on the OT practitioner to inform them about the child's fine motor capabilities and any obstacles to pointing, such as being unable to isolate the index finger and use it separate from the other fingers. During intervention, the practitioner helps the child develop underlying hand skills or adapted techniques. The following strategies may be helpful:

1. To isolate the index finger for pointing, the child uses the middle, ring, and little fingers to hold a pencil.
2. To facilitate extensor (straightening) muscles, the OT practitioner strokes the back of the index finger.
3. To help develop isolated index finger movements, the child handles tiny objects such as pieces of cereal, raisins, or small beads.

CLINICAL *Pearl*

Use a developmental approach to address visual problems. Higher-level visual-motor and visual-perception skills cannot develop properly unless lower-level skills of oculomotor control, visual acuity, and maintenance of full visual fields are adequate.[36]

If the child is completely unable to point with a finger, then consider having the child use the following alternative techniques:

1. Use the fist.
2. Use a universal art holder that has a pointer.
3. Use a pediatric weighted utensil holder that has a pointer.
4. Use a universal cuff that has a pointer.
5. Use a head pointer.
6. Attach a pointer to another part of the body that has more precise control.
7. Children with severe incoordination or spasticity can direct their eye gaze to objects, words, or widely spaced pictures to communicate their needs or thoughts.

RUSTY'S COMMUNICATION DEVICE USE STORY. Rusty is a bright 10-year-old boy with learning disabilities, self-regulation problems, and distractibility. He has trouble with handwriting, keyboarding, and checking for errors in his written work both in handwriting and on the computer. Rusty has problems with head-eye separation. When he is overexcited and distractible, he tends to quickly move his whole head from side to side when writing or keyboarding such that he often loses his place. Problems with visuomotor function further interfere with handwriting. Rusty is motivated to work on cursive handwriting. However, he has trouble forming certain letters correctly, spacing letters and words evenly, and keeping them on a line. When Rusty is overexcited and distractible, his writing deteriorates even more such that letters are oversized and placed all over the page. He is unable to follow visual demonstration. He repeatedly makes the same errors in formation and spatial orientation. Because of Rusty's spatial issues and problems identifying written errors, the OTR and COTA wonder if he has visual perception problems. When overstimulated, he is completely unable to focus on visual search activities. At best, after much repetition of the instructions, Rusty may be able to say that his letters are all over the page, but he is unable to find a detail like the letter "t" that is not crossed.

Visual acuity problems are first ruled out. According to Rusty's recent eye exam, visual acuity is 20/20. The COTA is careful to help Rusty calm down and maintain a low state of arousal (alertness and readiness to learn) during OT sessions. Then the COTA works with him on neck-strengthening activities like riding the scooter board in both the prone and supine positions, and playing games in a side-lying position while propping himself on one elbow or the other. The COTA also works on eye muscle activation (starting or increasing eye muscle exercises). Spinning activates eye muscles, and Rusty craves the spinning motion.[21] *Deep breathing activities like blowing soap bubbles, blowing bubbles with sugarless gum, and sucking on a straw to lift feathers or cotton balls are also used to activate his eye muscles.*[26]

The COTA then helps Rusty synchronize head and eye control. Over a number of sessions she may ask him to keep his head still while watching a favorite toy move in circular motions (tracking). She also asks him to switch his gaze back and forth from one visual target to another while keeping his head still. Furthermore, he is asked to switch his gaze from distant to nearby targets and back again without moving his head (gaze shift). The COTA then uses alphabet blocks and numbered beanbags during eye control games. The beanbags are spread out randomly in front of Rusty so that he can see all the letter on the blocks and numbers on the beanbags. Rusty must turn over each block or beanbag in the proper order. The COTA watches to see how long he can automatically (without reminders) keep his head still and accurately move his eyes from target to target. Gradually he develops functional head-eye separation during tracking and gaze shift.

Visuomotor function improves along with Rusty's oculomotor control. In addition to the activities mentioned above, the COTA has him work on a variety of fine motor games and exercises to enhance the finger coordination needed for handwriting and keyboarding. After engaging in calming and therapeutic activities, Rusty is now able to imitate the COTA's visual demonstration of how to form and space letters and keep them on a line. He also improves in keyboarding accuracy.

The OTR and COTA wondered whether Rusty had real visual perception problems or his oculomotor, visuomotor, and distractibility problems were preventing the development of visual perception. The COTA first addressed the early developmental skills of oculomotor control. When hand skills were also addressed, Rusty's visuomotor skills increased. With the aid of the COTA's calming techniques, he began following directions to visually search for handwriting and keyboarding errors in a systematic way, starting at the top of the page and moving from left to right one line at a time. He easily found spatial errors and omissions as his visual perception skills quickly improved.

What had initially appeared to be a visual perception problem was actually problems with oculomotor control and visuomotor skills, which were exacerbated by limited self-regulation. The COTA learned some critical information: if lower-level or early developmental skills are first resolved, they may reveal that higher-level skills like visual perception easily improve and fall in place. Always work on the most basic level of visual function first.

Computers

Computers are now used in schools as instructional tools and for recreation. Children who have significant problems with handwriting may find a computer or word processor to be the pathway to successful written communication. Numerous keyboard options are available, such as alphabetically arranged, one-handed, and pointer (one-finger) keyboards. Word prediction computer programs help children transmit their ideas into writing more quickly. As the child starts typing a word, the program anticipates what the word might be and finishes typing it. Word prediction programs can reduce oculomotor demands and frustration for individuals who use them. Some computers are equipped with programs that allow operation through voice recognition or by pointing to the monitor (see Chapter 22).

Communication boards

Children who are unable to speak might point to pictures, symbols, or words on communication boards. A beginning communication board might have only two or three items. Children who have a large vocabulary might need a communication book with pages of words or symbols. OT practitioners often work with SLPs to identify problems such as how many pictures a child can scan on one page; how large the pictures need to be for the child to perceive them; whether problems with figure-ground discrimination necessitate dark, wide borders between pictures; and whether fine motor skills are adequate for pointing to small symbols.

Sign and reduced language

Although OT practitioners do not usually teach sign language, some settings require them to use it. Children can have a variety of issues, such as hearing impairment, delayed or limited speech development, or combined limitations in both vision and hearing. When both vision and hearing are impaired, children learn to interpret signs through touch. The OT practitioner would make a sign and then physically cup the child's hand over the sign (Figure 18-44). The OT practitioner might physically assist the child in pressing and moving the fingers over the sign to gain more information through touch-pressure feedback. The OT practitioner would also physically assist the child in making signs with his or her own hands.

During treatment sessions, the practitioner would help him or her improve the foundation skills of fine tactile discrimination like **stereognosis** (the ability to identify objects through touch).

Sign language is often used along with other methods of communication. For example, children may communicate by (1) pointing to pictures on a communication board and (2) using sign language at the same time they are (3) learning to speak. Some parents teach their babies with typical needs to use sign language in addition to spoken words. Because communication with gestures and facial expressions naturally develops earlier than speech, these children may begin expressing themselves with sign language before they are capable of speaking.

The OT practitioner may use reduced language with a child if the team determines it could help. Reduced language omits articles, adjectives, prepositions, and extra phrases. It is used when a child has some verbal skills but becomes easily confused by rapid or verbose speech. For example, instead of saying "Excuse me, Timmy. Would you mind putting the spider plant on the windowsill for me? My hands are full," the adult would say, "Timmy, take plant window, please." Although reduced language is often effective, all team members and caregivers need to use the same system so that the child does not become confused. To prepare the child for community interaction that does not involve reduced language, gradually increase the language complexity in communicating with the child.

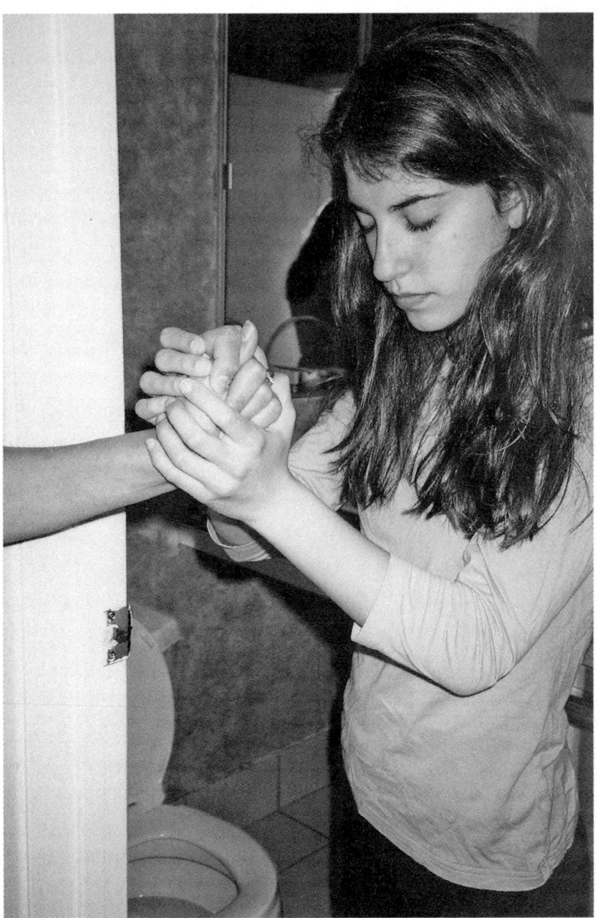

FIGURE 18-44 A child with visual and hearing impairments is assisted to feel and form her hand around the occupational therapy practitioner's sign for "toilet."

Telephones, telecommunication devices for the deaf, Braille writers, call lights, emergency systems, and environmental control systems

Technology has expanded the range of communication systems available for children with disabilities. COTAs can be involved in helping to obtain the devices, placing them in the best locations for children, and teaching the children and caregivers how to use them. They may help devise ways for children to press buttons by enlarging them, sticking tactile cues to them, or finding head, mouth, or finger pointers. COTAs also help children develop the foundational skills needed to operate these devices. For example, to feel and operate the devices with their hands, children might need to improve finger dexterity, pointing skills, and discrimination of touch-pressure feedback in the hands and fingertips. To operate mouth sticks or head pointers effectively, they might need to increase neck strength and control.

Telephones can be adapted in numerous ways. It may be the COTA's responsibility to find a suitable adapted phone system or teach children or adolescents the proper social skills for the phone. Phone companies offer adapted phone systems for children and adults who have various limitations. Some phones have extra-large push buttons and enlarged print for those with incoordination or visual impairments. Phones can be hooked up to computers for those with hearing impairments. Children or adults with limited hand use may benefit from using speakerphones, hand-free phones with headsets, or holders for phone receivers.

Children may need instruction in what to say and not to say on the phone. For those who can read, use written scripts for them to follow when answering, starting a conversation, or making an inquiry over the phone. They can practice their phone skills using disconnected phones. Children need to be taught not to give personal information to strangers, tell strangers who is home, or tell strangers when the family will be on vacation.

Braille writers look similar to keyboards, and the keys are imprinted with Braille letters and numbers so that individuals with limited vision can type. Special paper is used that prints in Braille. Braille writers can be important for children with visual impairments who are in school, especially for those who also have limited hearing, and for those attending college. COTAs require special training to work with children who are learning to use Braille writers.

Call lights can be used for different purposes. They may be used to alert caregivers when bedridden clients need help. These clients press a button that switches on a light in a different location, like the nurses' station or the kitchen, wherever the caregiver might be. Call lights are used for a different purpose with people who have hearing impairments. The lights are attached to doorbells or phones in such a way that ringing causes the lights to blink. A blinking light over the front door indicates that someone is ringing the doorbell, and a blinking light on the phone indicates that someone is calling.

Emergency systems are used to alert emergency medical technicians or the fire department to come to the aid of the clients. In case of an emergency, clients press a button that might be worn on a strap around the neck like a necklace. COTAs might be involved in working with older adolescents on judgment skills (e.g., learning what constitutes a true emergency).

Environmental control systems are useful. The remote control device for a television is an example of an environmental control. More complex environmental control systems are individualized for clients who may need help operating common household appliances such as the lights in different rooms, CD or DVD players, heaters or air conditioners regulating room temperature, and fans and security features such as door locks.

Safety Procedures and Emergency Responses

Safety

Safety skills can be the most serious factor interfering with progress toward independence. They can lead to injury of the child or others, prevent movement to a less restrictive environment, and block improvements in areas such as social interaction and self-esteem. Some children play with peers by hitting them, while others bite their own hands when frustrated. Whatever the cause, safety issues need to be addressed immediately.

While planning and implementing treatment for safety problems, the practitioner needs to use methods that quickly resolve the issues. Self-injury and aggressive behaviors can be prevented by reducing overstimulating sensory input and increasing pleasing sensory input. Methods such as using a helmet, using a consistent behavior management plan, reducing demands, and providing one-on-one supervision may help ensure the safety of the child and others. The clinician also addresses underlying developmental factors and coping skills. With the help of caregivers and other team members, the child may eventually be able to function without modified sensory input, adaptive equipment, strict limits, or constant supervision.

Emergency response

OT practitioners, caregivers, and teachers may be involved in teaching children how to take care of themselves in an emergency. The first skill that children often need is being able to say, write, or otherwise indicate their names, addresses, and phone numbers. If they are unable to speak or write but able to understand the question, they can use printed cards with their names, addresses, and phone numbers to show to the proper individuals when they are lost.

Emergency responses may be different for children in wheelchairs. In case they ever fall out of their chairs, the practitioner should make sure that children know how to pull themselves to a phone, pull themselves back into their chairs from the floor, or operate an emergency call system.

In preparation for a fire emergency, practice the "stop, drop, and roll" sequence with children. In institutions such as schools, fire drills with full evacuations are practiced regularly. The staff should maintain a calm atmosphere while quickly and quietly helping children get out of the building and move to a safe location. Fire alarms frighten some children, causing them to cry, scream, or become aggressive. OT practitioners provide assistance as needed and arrange in advance the assistance of children with special needs.

In settings in which children are in wheelchairs, a supply of evacuation chairs may be needed for evacuating the building in case of a fire or other disaster. Evacuation chairs are lightweight, small, and designed to go down steps more easily than standard or electric wheelchairs (Electric wheelchairs are extremely heavy because of the battery.) In many facilities, the nursing staff is responsible for acquiring evacuation chairs and training other personnel in their use. In other facilities, OT practitioners may have this responsibility.

Some children may not know what constitutes an actual emergency. One mother reported that her son was so excited to know how to dial 9-1-1 in school that he came home and tried it out. Of course, police cars swarmed the house and the parents needed to apologize and provide a lengthy explanation to the boy so that he would understand that he could dial 9-1-1 only in a real emergency. In an OT session it can be revealing, fun, and useful to work on solving problems that are related to emergencies. The practitioner asks a child to choose a card that describes or depicts an emergency, and s/he explains or acts out what s/he might do in the situation. Have the child practice dialing, reporting the emergency, and stating his or her name and address on an unplugged or toy phone.

Children with special needs often need additional instruction to be wary of strangers. Children need concrete definitions of who is actually a stranger, such as "a stranger is someone who does not work at or go to your school." They also need specific strategies to use when approached by strangers, such as going to their teachers.

ANNIE'S SAFETY SIGN STORY. *A COTA who was working in a special school setting with an adolescent girl named Annie, who had pervasive developmental disorder, mental retardation, and emotional impairment, became concerned about her ability to respond to an emergency. She could not read and depended on adults to tell her what to do.*

After discussing Annie's plan with the OTR, the COTA ordered safety signs that included clear pictures and words such as STOP, EXIT, FIRE, POISON, and DANGER. For a few minutes of each OT session, Annie was quizzed on the meaning of each sign. At first she had the goal of distinguishing between or among two or three signs. As her skills improved, she began to differentiate among eight or more signs. Safety procedures were reviewed for various emergency situations, and she was asked to explain them. She eventually used role playing to act out emergency situations with the COTA. While walking in the halls and during field trips, she practiced looking for and identifying safety signs. Annie seemed to enjoy these activities and felt proud that she had learned this important information.

Health Management and Maintenance

Nutrition

Nutrition is an area that OT practitioners are incorporating into their work more often. It makes sense that children will improve the thinking skills needed for daily living and school success when they have optimum nutrition. This means eating enough protein and vegetables and having a sufficient vitamin intake every day and minimizing their intake of processed foods, sugar, food colorings, artificial preservatives, and food additives.

Childhood obesity is a problem in the United States. Obesity may occur more often in the special populations with whom OT practitioners work. Children with special needs often have limited opportunities to exercise because they require one-to-one attention for safety reasons. Some children may resist exercising because of limitations such as low muscle tone, which make physical activity more tiring than it is for those with typical muscle tone.

Some caregivers use food to manage children's behaviors, but this technique can result in overfeeding. Childhood obesity coupled with inactivity can lead to joint problems and an impaired social life. In these cases, family workers and other team members, including the COTA, help caregivers learn alternative behavior management techniques.

CLINICAL *Pearl*

Avoid foods with added sugar and "empty calories" (food that has no nutritional value). Encourage parents and children to do the same. Based on current research in the field of nutrition, additives such as artificial preservatives, taste enhancers, texture enhancers, and artificial colors may negatively affect children's behavior, ability to learn, and attend school. Persistent diarrhea or constipation is a common indicator of either an unbalanced diet or food sensitivities.[4,31]

In their attempt to be the best possible caregivers, some parents become overly concerned with feeding their child. They may believe that their picky child is not receiving proper nutrition. In some cases making a list of all the food that the child eats reveals that s/he is actually eating a balanced diet, which reassures the parents.[15] In other cases, the list reveals that the child does have limited food preferences.

Factors such as poor oral-motor skills, oral defensiveness, limited access to nutritious food, limited knowledge of nutrition, food allergies or sensitivity, gastrointestinal problems, and limited food preferences present obstacles to proper nutrition. The following techniques may encourage positive habits for nutrition:

1. *When is the right time to eat?* Try to pay attention to children's requests for food. If they say they are hungry, take the opportunity to give them nutritious food. If requests for food are repeatedly ignored or if required to eat when not hungry, they may become unable to recognize their own bodily needs. Poor eating habits can result, such as gorging at every opportunity. Children with poor sensory awareness in the mouth or stomach may not sense when their mouths or stomachs are full. These children and those who frequently use food to calm themselves need assistance to distinguish hunger from their desire for oral stimulation. They need help in choosing oral activities that do not involve food, like blowing bubbles or whistles.
2. *Create a calm, accepting, positive social atmosphere during the meal.* A quiet place to eat can help children with sensory defensiveness. They can concentrate on eating instead of being distracted by background noise or activity. If necessary, they can begin their meals before or after others. Noisy dishes or utensils can be overstimulating and disturbing. Plastic dishes make less noise than metal or ceramic dishes when utensils knock against them. Children who are relaxed and content will be able to enjoy their food.

3. *Creative and personal touches make children feel happy about eating.* Provide children's favorite utensils, special cups with straws, or painted character bowls. Caregivers can create designs with food. Take a bowl of tuna salad and surround it with carrot sticks to look like the rays of the sun. Make food more interesting. Dip raw vegetables into dressing or spread celery with peanut butter. Melt cheese or pour tasty sauces over cooked vegetables. Place frozen peas or blueberries in a Dixie cup. Cut broiled chicken into strips for dipping. Form lean hamburger or turkey burgers into shapes with cookie cutters. Substitute brown rice and vegetables for buns. Wrap deli meat slices around long pieces of red pepper or cooked green beans. Even teenagers appreciate these personal touches.
4. *Talk about the food.* One way to facilitate eating is to direct everyone's attention to the look, smell, and taste of the food. Talk about how good it is or how it is made. The discussion can lead to eating.[23]
5. *What do you say about eating to children who cannot speak?* Communication board symbols are helpful and can be attached to place mats. Children use the place mat symbols to request things by pointing to pictures of juice, utensils, a sandwich, carrots, dessert, an apple, or a napkin. Caregivers can point to place mat symbols that demonstrate wiping the mouth with a napkin, scooping food with a spoon rather than the fingers, chewing completely, or swallowing. Communication place mats are easy to make out of stiff paper or cardboard covered with clear contact paper.
6. *Give children extra time to eat.* Although children with cerebral palsy or other motor problems may be difficult to feed, patience and nurturing are key aspects of the process.
7. *Offer food in the order of nutritional priority.* Mealtime may seem like one big struggle to get children to eat nutritious food. The plate contains all the food groups, but this may be too tempting or confusing for children. Many will fill up on carbohydrates and avoid proteins and vegetables. These children may benefit by having food offered in the order of the highest nutritional value. Begin by making a list of all the proteins that the child will eat. Begin meals by putting food containing only one of these proteins on the plate. After that food is consumed, offer the next food in order of nutritional value (e.g., vegetables second and whole grain carbohydrates or fruit third).[4]

Food allergies and sensitivity

Many children with special needs, such as those with autism, attention deficit hyperactivity disorder, learning disabilities, or minimum brain dysfunction, can have food allergies or sensitivity. Nutritional programs may be necessary. With the consent of the administration and the OTR, the COTA may explore the possibility of food ensitivity with the parents.

Food allergies are often accompanied by rashes or red patches on the skin or ear lobes; itching; swelling; and, in their most severe form, difficulty breathing. In extreme cases, food allergies can shut down the respiratory system and require emergency medical attention. In highly allergic individuals, simply smelling the food can set off a severe allergic reaction.

Food sensitivity or intolerance is harder to observe and diagnose. Behavioral, cognitive, and muscular deficits may indicate sensitivity to particular foods or additives.[7,8] Nutrition experts or physicians specializing in the relationship between food and behavior can help determine which types of food contribute to a child's problems.

Food allergies or sensitivity may occur as a result of eating some of the following types of food or the chemicals or ingredients in the food:

- Gluten and wheat products
- Casein, milk, and lactose products
- Products containing excess yeast, such as bread, vinegar, and pickles
- Excess amounts of sugar, sugar substitutes, or carbohydrates
- Nuts
- Natural salicylates, which are found in apples, all berries, cucumbers, tomatoes, raisins, oranges, plums, and peaches
- Synthetic salicylates, which are found in aspirin and medications that contain aspirin
- Synthetic or artificial colors that are listed as "U.S. certified color" or in a numerical form such FD&C yellow No. 5 or FD&C red No. 40
- Synthetic or artificial flavors that are listed as "flavoring" or "artificial flavoring"; additives and salicylates that are found in the child's daily diet
- Antioxidant preservatives

When certain foods and synthetic chemicals are eliminated from the diets of food-sensitive children with various diagnoses, dramatic improvement can be seen.[7,8] COTAs who are interested in learning more about their role in nutritional intervention with children are encouraged to attend workshops (see Appendix D of this chapter).

Yeast sensitivity has received attention in recent years. Yeast is a substance found in normal digestive systems, primarily the intestines. However, yeast overgrowth can damage the walls of the digestive tract by creating tiny holes. It then passes through these holes and into the bloodstream and travels across the blood-brain barrier to the brain. There it interferes with the functioning of neurotransmitters, the chemicals that carry messages from one neuron (nerve cell) to another.[30,31]

Yeast overgrowth is believed to cause a wide range of symptoms, from headache, fatigue, and confusion to frequent ear or sinus infections to diarrhea or constipation. Yeast feeds on sugar. Consuming excessive amounts of sugar and carbohydrates promotes yeast overgrowth. It is especially hard to manage because it is part of a vicious cycle. It causes sugar and carbohydrate cravings, so you consume more sugar to feed the growing yeast. The yeast continues to grow and needs more sugar to keep growing.[30,31]

The treatment and control of yeast overgrowth is difficult. Unfortunately, antibiotics promote the unchecked growth of yeast. Most cattle and chickens are fed antibiotics to increase their size. Today's diets expose people to unnecessary antibiotics through the meat and poultry they eat. It seems that the best approach to this problem is dietary intervention.[4,30,31]

Food reinforcers

Food rewards are sometimes given after children perform an activity; these are called primary reinforcers. Food rewards given too often can decrease the child's interest in participation and can interfere with the ability to recognize hunger sensations. Before giving food or drink rewards, carefully consider why a small food item is necessary. Is it to reward children for their behavior or performance, help them focus on challenging work, modulate their level of arousal, or satisfy their hunger or thirst? Instead of relying on the rewards of primary reinforcers, try substituting rewards of "choice time" or "free time" using therapeutic equipment. In addition to helping children feel "rewarded," the opportunity to play freely with therapeutic materials promotes creativity, cognitive problem solving, spatial and motor planning, and environmental interaction.

JERRY'S FOOD REINFORCER STORY. *Jerry is an 18-year-old boy living in a residential institution. He has normal intelligence but is totally deaf and blind. Jerry has severe behavior problems that are partially due to the overuse of primary food reinforcers. He has been taught that he will receive a piece of candy each time he performs a requested activity. Jerry learned to expect the reward, so when he is not given a piece of candy after performing a requested activity, he becomes enraged, destructive, and aggressive, throwing furniture and attacking people. The overuse of primary reinforcers limited his curiosity and exploration of the environment and restricted his development.*

Jerry needed activity rewards that were suited to his normal level of intelligence and would stimulate further environmental exploration and social interaction. His OT practitioner introduced him to assembly activities such as the use of screws, nuts, and bolts to put together a stationary bicycle for the wing where he slept. Jerry was also taken more frequently on walks outside the residence with staff members and peers. With the help of all involved staff members, Jerry's insistence on primary reinforcers gradually decreased.

Physical fitness

COTAs are often involved in helping children with disabilities engage in fun and realistic activities that include swimming, playing in a park, roller skating or riding a bike with assistance, dancing or exercising to music, playing catch, horseback riding, and modified sports activities. The goal of the intervention is for the child to be able to participate in activities.

The COTA may have to improve the underlying skills required for participation, such as muscle tone, range of motion, strength, and gross and fine motor functions. However, the goal is to perform the activity to promote physical fitness. Some activities may be used as preparation to help the child be ready for the actual physical activity. The following is a list of sample preparatory activities.

- *Muscle tone:* In general, activities are used to either increase hypotonicity (low muscle tone, or loose muscles and joints) or decrease hypertonicity (high muscle tone, or unusually tight muscles and joints). Repeated activities can gradually increase muscle tone. Engaging children in trunk activities such as riding a scooter board in the prone and supine positions; wrist and hand activities including hanging from a trapeze, working with theraputty, using a variety of squeeze toys, and weight bearing on the hands; and climbing a jungle gym and doing modified pushups against a wall or desk strengthen trunk, shoulder, arm, and wrist muscles.
- *Range of motion:* Intervention may increase joint mobility and/or stability. The COTA engages a child in stretching and imitation games such as "Simon Says" as well as activities performed seated on the floor in order to help increase hip flexion. Work on trunk strengthening, including the stomach and back muscles, will provide better postural support for a child.
- *Strength and gross motor function:* Activities to increase strength and gross motor (large muscle) coordination may benefit children. Given safety rules at the beginning, the COTA may have a child engage in activities such as crawling over or under obstacles with a weighted toy on his back, hopping up and down the hall on a hoppity-hop ball, pulling himself

with a rope while riding the scooter board, and performing "Egg rolls" for stomach strength and "Airplanes" for back strength. In these gross motor coordination activities, the motor planning and timing demands are gradually increased.

- *Fine motor function:* Therapeutic activities to increase fine motor (small muscle) function are beneficial to children. The COTA may initially engage a child in games of catch using large balls when the activity requires using both hands together. Over the next several therapy sessions, s/he may ask the child to string tiny beads or snip paper to make fringes. These activities require each hand to perform a different job. The left hand stabilizes and positions items like paper, while the right hand carries out skilled actions like cutting with scissors. Bimanual coordination will eventually become natural and engrained into the child's motor memory for life.

To maintain cardiovascular fitness, children need to engage in a physical activity at least three times a week for 20 minutes each. In a school, hospital, or clinic setting, the COTA could lead a movement group for children with special needs. A variety of books, videos, CDs, DVDs, and cassette tapes contain practical and fun physical activities for children with disabilities (see Appendix C of this chapter). Yoga, which promotes flexibility and postural and respiratory control, can also be adapted for children with special needs.[24]

Too few physical fitness and after-school programs exist for children with special needs in both rural and urban settings. COTAs can help alleviate this deficit significantly by developing and managing fitness programs for children with special needs. Many community sports or after-school programs now enroll children who have mild to moderate disabilities. Some parents are able to hire an adolescent or young adult to assist the child during class.

Although children may express interest in karate or lifting weights, carefully consider all factors before enrolling them in a class. Adolescents who have mild or moderate mental retardation, head injury, or emotional impairment might not have the judgment to safely use the abilities required for these activities.

PETER'S WEIGHTLIFTING STORY. *Peter is an overweight 15 year old with mild mental retardation due to lead poisoning. As part of his OT sessions he engaged in strengthening activities and began learning to use small dumbbells. He expressed great interest in this and worked hard on increasing his strength. During OT sessions, Peter also told his COTA about seeing a woman on the street being bothered by a man. Of course she took the opportunity to problem-solve with Peter about what to do if he saw an incident such as that again: Tell his father, an adult at school, or a policeman. However, the topic surfaced again, and this time Peter told her that he wanted to help the lady by beating up the man who had been bothering her.*

The COTA immediately told her supervising OT, and together they consulted with Peter's counselor. His counselor provided additional information that Peter imagined himself to be a superhero and thought that he could right injustices wherever they occurred. He believed that lifting dumbbells made him extremely strong and powerful. The OTR helped the team come up with a plan for Peter. It was decided that weightlifting would stop in OT and that other areas of intervention, like safety awareness, would be emphasized. Peter did not have the judgment skills necessary to determine whether an injustice was occurring, and he definitely did not have the skills needed to correct it. The staff members were concerned that he might confront someone on the street and, as a result, get beaten up himself.

Someone like Peter may try to protect a person who is being mugged and get seriously hurt or may hurt someone else. However, learning one of the martial arts or how to use weight machines in a gym could perfectly fit other adolescents' needs. Martial arts such as Karate or Judo help students develop strength, flexibility, and deep breathing. With proper supervision for safety, using weight machines in a gym can help adolescents develop strength, joint stability, body awareness, and motor planning skills. (**Note:** Weightlifting is contraindicated for children who have not reached their full height. It can potentially damage the joints where growth occurs.)

In hippotherapy, an OT practitioner, physical therapist, or speech therapist trained in hippotherapy uses a horse's movement to promote therapeutic goals.[19] Children are placed on a horse's back in a variety of positions that facilitate postural control, speech, breathing, and other functional skills. An aide walks on one side of the horse, with the therapist on the other side. The therapist directs a horse trainer to lead the horse in different movements.

The wide base of support provided by the horse's back increases the child's balance while sitting. The vestibular (i.e., movement) input helps coordinate postural and head control with visual focus and hand movements. Feeling the strong rhythm of the horse's gait may help improve a child's unsteady gait. Leg, trunk, and neck strength may be increased for a child with muscle weakness. High muscle tone may be reduced through gentle stretching of the hips and legs.

Numerous benefits can result from hippotherapy and therapeutic riding, which teaches horseback riding to children with special needs. Sitting high up on a horse increases the child's sense of well-being and self-esteem.

Learning to care for and guide a horse can help an adolescent who has behavioral problems. Even a child who is unable to walk may learn to ride a horse. A child who learns to control the reins gains a functional recreational and physical fitness skill that can be used throughout life.

Principles of joint protection

In all areas of ADLs and IADLs, be sure to follow the principles of joint protection with those children who have unstable joints, especially those with juvenile rheumatoid arthritis, which is a degenerative disease characterized by swollen and painful joints. Several examples of the principles of joint protection are as follows. (1) Always use the strongest joint possible for the task. (2) Avoid forces that push the wrist toward the ulnar (little finger) side of the hand, as when lifting a pitcher of water by the handle. (3) Bear weight on the whole palm instead of the knuckles because the finger joints can be easily injured.

Medication routine

Caregivers, nurses, teachers, or other team members collaborate to give children their medication according to a prescribed schedule. Through team meetings and chart reviews, COTAs learn the type of medication prescribed and its purpose. If asked to do so, they will take children to the nurse to receive scheduled medication.

Unusual sleepiness, silliness, inattention, crying, complaints of stomachache or headache, tics (i.e., repetitive involuntary movements), and other atypical behaviors may be related to increases, decreases, or changes in medication. The COTA reports significant behavioral changes to the child's OTR as well as his or her doctor, nurse, team, and/or caregivers as needed. This type of information can be invaluable to doctors, who may use team members' anecdotal observations to modify the child's prescriptions.

Home Establishment and Management

Home establishment and management refer to obtaining and maintaining a dwelling and the things in and around it, including indoor and outdoor space, furnishings, and personal belongings. COTAs working in pediatric OT usually have clients who already live in established homes. They live with their parents or possibly in foster or group homes.

COTAs might occasionally work with teenagers who are planning to establish new homes. They might provide them with information or teach them the homemaking skills needed for new settings. For example, teenagers with physical limitations, learning disabilities, or emotional impairment might need preparation to move into a group home, an apartment with a relative, a dormitory, or their own apartments with hired home health aides. More often, COTAs teach children to participate in home management by cleaning their rooms, making their beds, setting and clearing the table, washing and drying the dishes, and helping with the laundry.

Cleaning up

Cleaning up one's personal items and putting them back where they belong are skills taught in early childhood. COTAs who work in preschools will soon learn one or more "Cleanup" songs that help children know what to do at the end of any activity. One example is sung to the tune of "Do you know the muffin man?" It goes as follows.

"Do you know what time it is?
It's cleanup time, it's cleanup time.
Everybody helps at cleanup time.
Playtime (or OT, painting, Legos, etc.) is finished.
It's time for *lunch* (or Speech, bath, bed, etc.)."

During and after the singing, adults help children clean up by modeling, instructing, and assisting. Singing a "cleanup" song helps children at home as well as school. OT practitioners working in home care or group homes can teach the song to caregivers, who often need guidance to have the expectation that children clean up. If we pick up after them, we only teach them dependence and helplessness. It is better to teach them how to clean up so that they can become capable and independent. Picking up one's personal belongings and putting them away is just the beginning.

COTAs can help children learn to clean up the bedroom. A model known as "the sweep" can be used as a method. Think of your arm sweeping everything off a tabletop so that it can be completely clear. Of course the method does not entail sweeping everything onto the floor. Instead, the image of the sweeping arm represents thoroughly clearing and cleaning one space before moving on.

Children follow a set of rules for "the sweep." Clean in small sections. Start in one small area of the bedroom, such as the desktop, and completely clean it. Keep your eyes focused on that area without being distracted. Do not begin to clean a new area until the desktop is finished. Nothing goes back on it. Once the desktop is finished, move to another small area, such as the bookshelf, and organize it. Then move to one small section of the floor and clean it, and so on. By "sweeping" through a small area first and cleaning it thoroughly, children quickly achieve a sense of accomplishment. They gain a sense of mastery by experiencing one section of the room as organized and clean. This can motivate them to continue "the sweep" until the whole room is clean.

Along with "the sweep" as the organizational method, children also need to learn when to clean up, what supplies they need, where to get them, and how they are used. COTAs may teach children any or all of these aspects. In addition, they may consider the following:

- Put items in logical places where it makes sense to use them. For example, books go on bookshelves, not in desk drawers. Hairbrushes go next to a mirror, on a dresser, or in a basket in the closet. CDs go in CD boxes or storage containers next to the CD player, not on the desk. Dirty clothes go in a hamper or dirty clothes bag, not on the floor.
- Find containers that fit the size and purpose of the items. Find pencil cases or cups for pencils. Find small baskets, plastic containers, or large cups for crayons and markers. Find narrow horizontal shelves for paper (e.g., one shelf each for lined paper, blank construction paper, and graph paper if needed). Find big bins or wall nets for balls. Other types of ball holders can be found in equipment catalogs and sporting goods stores. Put small stuffed animals in baskets, bins, or boxes.
- Be sure children can reach all the materials. Place the objects used the most often at the level of the child's chest. Children who use wheelchairs need items placed on the lower shelves. Reachers, which are found in equipment catalogs or surgical supply stores, can help them obtain items from very low or very high places.
- Put away materials from one activity before starting another.
- Throw away or give away everything you haven't used in the last year.
- If you drop something, pick it up right away. If you spill something, wipe it up right away. It's OK to drop or spill things; everyone does. We just clean it up.
- Children with special needs may not know how to perform routine cleanup. A few examples are keeping a shirt from falling off a hanger, operating a spray bottle of cleaning solution, cleaning the whole mirror, using a feather duster gently on breakable objects, and managing a broom and dustpan at the same time.

Making the bed

Part of cleaning the bedroom is making the bed every morning Figure 18-45. COTAs can teach making the bed in home care, day care, group homes, or other settings. It can be taught at a young age (e.g., 4 to 6 years), depending on the child's cognitive and motor skills.

Children can begin making the bed by pulling the sheet and then blanket or bedspread to the head of the bed. To prevent stress to the back, they can try kneeling or sitting on the bed when pulling up the sheet and spread. The pillows can be placed on top or under the bedspread, depending on family style and individual capabilities. Sheets and blankets are spread smooth by sliding flat hands (palms down) over them. Move the hands toward the ulnar side to prevent stress to the radial (thumb) side of the hand and protect wrist joints. It is critical for children with unstable joints, such as those with juvenile rheumatoid arthritis, to move the hands toward the stronger ulnar side.

Another important skill for teenagers to learn is changing their own sheets. COTAs can train them to remove the sheets and bedspread, sort them into piles, and decide whether the bedspread needs to be washed along with the sheets. Children who wet their beds can benefit from learning these skills.

When changing sheets, shake out the bottom sheet so it lands open on the bed. Line up the corners and edges of the sheet with the corners and edges of the mattress. Tuck in fitted or unfitted corners, starting with the hardest corner to reach. Fitted sheets with extra-deep pockets are easier to tuck in and are available in department stores. Reaching across the bed causes stress to the lower back and can aggravate back problems. To protect the back, OT practitioners can show children how to walk around the bed or kneel or lie on the bed while tucking the sheets and blankets under the mattress. Details that add to an attractive, neat appearance are folding the edge of the top sheet over the blanket and arranging colorful pillows at the head of the bed.

Maintaining clothing

Taking care of clothing is part of the occupation of home management. Some categories of clothing maintenance are cleaning clothes, folding and storing them, polishing shoes, and managing minor repairs such as sewing on buttons.

Laundry

Some teenagers do their own laundry; many of them help their parents or caregivers with the laundry for the entire family. When older teenagers prepare for transition into the community, it is important for them to be able to do the laundry independently. COTAs can train children in laundry skills in home, school, day care, hospital, or group home settings.

Start by gathering supplies. Prepare laundry detergent, chlorine or nonchlorine bleach, stain remover, and fabric softener. Sort clothing by color and fabric. Read the washing instructions on clothing tags. Pretreat stains. Read the directions for operating the washing machine. Use mesh laundry bags (available in most supermarkets) for delicate items. Set the washer on the regular or delicate cycle. Put the detergent in either before or after turning on the water according to the directions. Front-loading washing machines work best for children in wheelchairs. Avoid letting wet clothes stay in the washing machine for longer than 30 minutes because they can

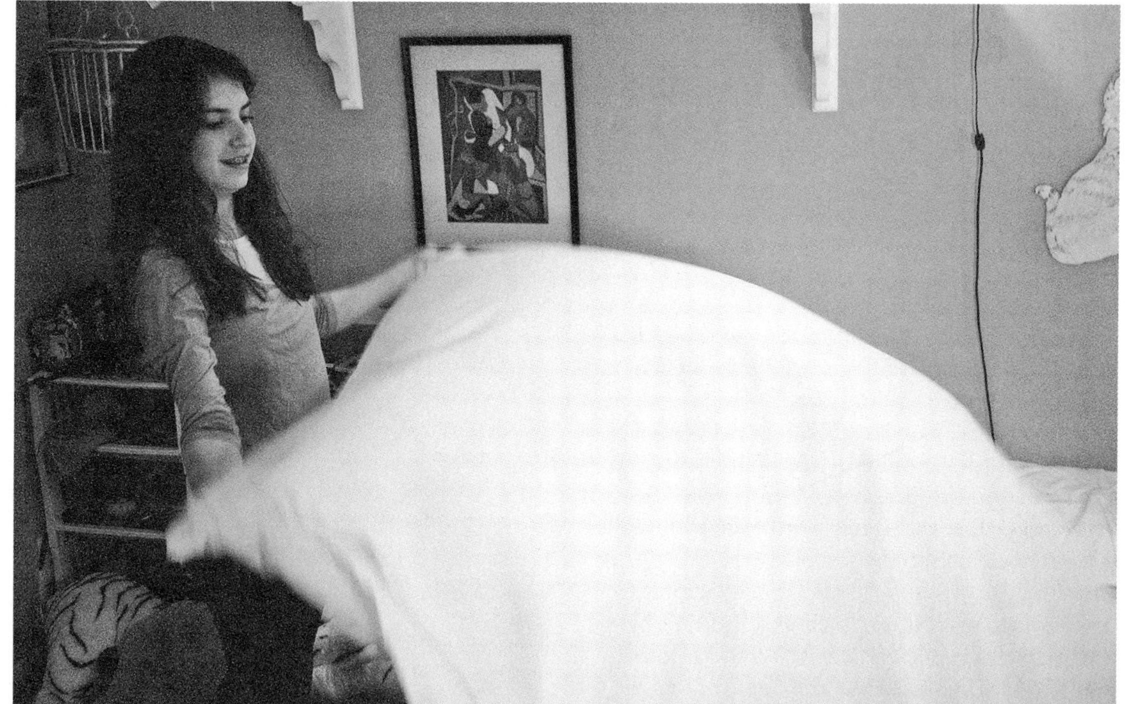

A

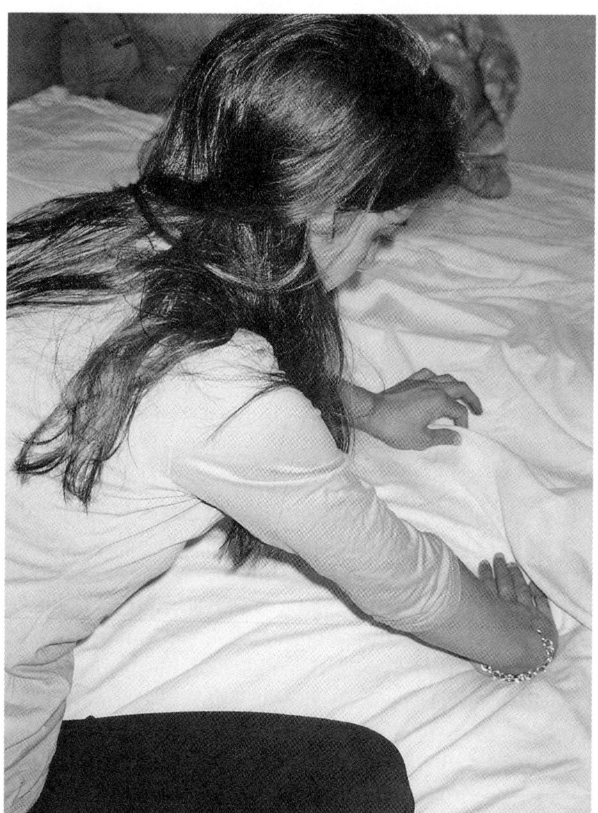

B

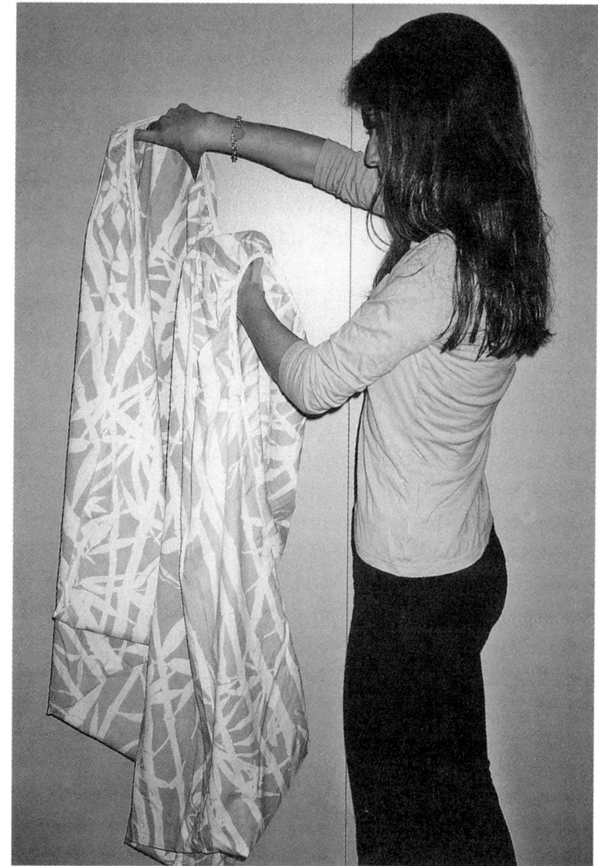

C

FIGURE 18-45 Bed-making techniques. **A,** The teenager learns to shake a sheet in the air so that it will land spread out on the bed. **B,** She uses joint protection for her wrists, smoothing out wrinkles by sliding her hand in an ulnar direction, toward the little finger side of her hand. **C,** Before folding and putting away her clean fitted sheet, the teenager pockets each corner into the corners of other fitted sheets.

mildew, which causes an unpleasant smell that is hard to eliminate.

Shake out clothing before placing it in the dryer so that it will dry more quickly. Remove clothing from the dryer as soon as it stops to minimize wrinkling. Hang or fold clothes quickly. Children who are not yet ready to use the washer and dryer can participate in laundry preparation by putting their own clothes away.

Folding

Folding and hanging clothes are difficult for children with special needs. The necessary skills for these tasks are functional tactile discrimination, fine motor planning, and visual perception. Fabric provides only light tactile feedback, which is hard for children with limited sensory awareness to interpret; they also need to rely on visual cues. On the other hand, children with limited visual skills need to rely on tactile cues for folding.

When folding sheets and blankets, it is helpful to have a large surface to work on, such as a bed or table. COTAs can help children learn to match corners exactly and smooth wrinkles out by sliding the hands across the sheets. Children need to think ahead and visualize what size they want the folded sheet to be. To fold bottom-fitted sheets, simply match corners and stuff each corner pocket into the other pockets (Figure 18-45, C). Then fold the sheet to the desired size.

To fold T-shirts and sweaters, a cardboard guide can be used (Figure 18-46). Cut a piece of cardboard to about 6 × 8 inches, depending on the finished size desired. The guide will last longer if laminated or covered with contact paper.

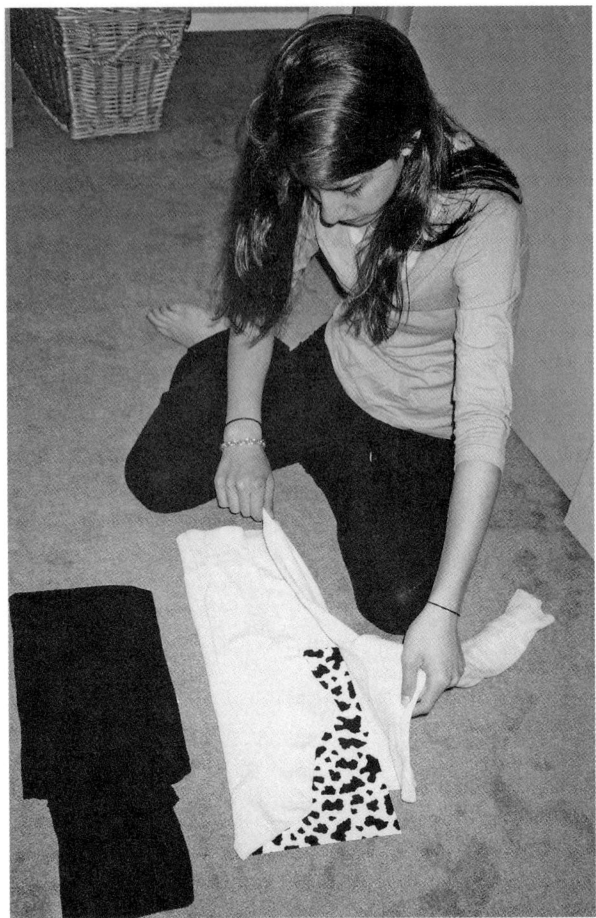

FIGURE 18-46 A teenage girl folds shirts and sweaters neatly using a cardboard guide covered with contact paper.

Storing clothes

Children may need to learn how to properly store clothing and keep their dressers and closets organized. Put similar items together. For example, put T-shirts in one drawer and pajamas in another. Store socks and underwear in smaller drawers. Hang pants on one side of the closet and shirts on the other. Put clothes away exactly where you found them. Put them in the same place every time. Dirty clothes go in a hamper or dirty clothes bag, not on the floor.

Shoe care

COTAs can help children learn to care for their shoes. Sneakers require little care. Canvas sneakers can be washed in a washing machine when dirty. Remove the laces first and place them in the washer along with the shoes. Dry canvas sneakers in the sunlight outside because drying them in a dryer may shrink. Sneakers made of leather or other materials can be wiped clean with soap and water.

Some sneakers and other shoes can be polished with shoe polish. An easy and quick way to shine shoes is to use shining sponges, which are available in different colors in many drug stores in the shoe care section. Simply remove the top and brush the sponge over the shoe (Figure 18-47). Children may need help in recognizing when shoes need to be polished, repaired, or replaced.

Sewing

COTAs may have the responsibility of teaching children who live in group homes or attend daycare centers how to mend clothing by sewing. Sewing on a button or mending a small tear can provide a quick sense of mastery. The finished product can be seen, felt, and used right away. As always, safety is the most important part of sewing. Children need to be able to demonstrate and/or describe how to handle a needle safely. Two safety rules for needles and pins are as follows. (1) Keep needles and pins in a pincushion whenever they are not in use. (2) When a needle or pin is lost, it is essential to find it immediately to prevent possible injury. Threading a needle is made easier with the help of needle threaders, which are found in most mending kits available from fabric stores. If children have sufficient sensory awareness

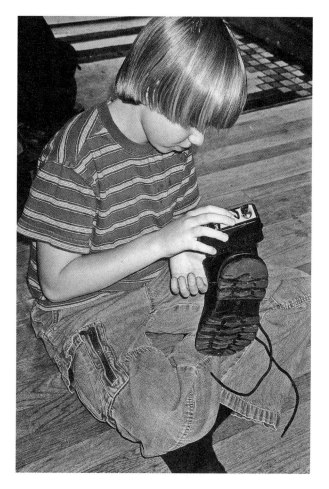

FIGURE 18-47 The boy shines his shoes in one step using a shoe-shining sponge.

and fine motor and cognitive skills, it is helpful for them to learn the different stitches used to repair a hem and sew on a button.

If children have insufficient fine motor control or touch-pressure discrimination, they will need other options for mending. Caregivers often perform mending for them. One teenager with learning disabilities and fine motor and sensory limitations learned how to take her clothes to the tailor. While using a tailor is an expensive option, this girl was fortunate that her parents paid for the service, and she increased her self-confidence by handling the mending herself.

Handling unexpected problems

COTAs who work with children in group homes or daycare centers or in transition to a home setting could help them learn what to do if there are problems with appliances or other items. The following are examples of dilemmas that children might encounter: changing a light bulb; dealing with a toilet that clogs up or overflows; recognizing when the refrigerator or air conditioner leaks or stops working and knowing who to call; staying safe when a window breaks; and problem solving about what to do when the keys stick in lock on the front door.

Meal Preparation and Cleanup

Meal preparation and cleanup refer to "planning, preparing, and serving well balanced, nutritious meals and cleaning up food and utensils after meals."[28] COTAs could work with children on setting and clearing the table, washing and drying the dishes, or preparing food. Skills could be as simple as passing out cups or as complex as preparing a meal for the family.

Setting and clearing the table

Children begin learning to set the table as early as preschool. Younger children usually set the table with paper or plastic plates, plastic cups, and plastic or metal utensils. Older children may use ceramic or glass plates and cups. They will need to learn how to position the knife with the blade facing toward the plate.

Preschool-aged children also help clear the table. The use of trays may help make carrying the items easier. Children need to be aware of how objects balance in space so that trays or plates will not tip over. Children need adequate memory and visual scanning or tactile search skills to check the table and remove serving items, like pitcher of water or salt and pepper shakers. The hands are always washed after clearing the table. The demands of the tasks are gradually increased as children mature.

Washing and drying dishes

COTAs can help children wash and dry the dishes more easily by following these strategies:

1. Use scrub brushes that are attached to the insides of sinks with suction cups. Children apply soap to the brush and then wash the plates and utensils by sliding

CLINICAL *Pearl*

Place mat guides can be used to show children where to put tableware. Teachers, caregivers, speech therapists, OT practitioners, or the children themselves can create them. Cut out paper shapes of a plate, cup, napkin, spoon, and fork and attach them to a larger rectangular sheet of paper in a contrasting color. Then laminate or cover the place mat in clear contact paper so that it can be cleaned after each use. One modification for children with visual impairment is to cut the tableware shapes out of cardboard. The raised edges of cardboard will provide tactile cues for placement of the plate, cup, napkin, and utensils.

them over the brush. Tall scrub brushes with suction cup attachments are made for washing cups and glasses and can also be found in equipment catalogs.
2. Use rubber gloves to help grip items more securely or reduce discomfort from the sensation of running water or soap.
3. Many grocery stores sell plastic squeeze bottles with brushes on top for easier dishwashing. Bottles are filled with water and liquid dish detergent. Scrubbing dishes with the brush requires less time, effort, and range of motion than using a sponge.
4. To save effort, consider air drying the dishes in a dish rack.
5. When drying dishes by hand, stabilize them on a piece of Dycem or a damp dishcloth. This reduces bimanual and finger coordination demands.

Food preparation

Most children in the United States, including those with special needs, learn to prepare basic breakfast, lunch, and snack food. They usually learn to prepare a bowl of cereal, make cold sandwiches, spread bread or toast with peanut butter and jelly, make toasted or grilled cheese sandwiches, boil hot dogs, scramble eggs, heat up canned soup, and microwave potatoes or popcorn. COTAs could teach children to do the following:

1. Pour slowly while estimating the needed amount of water, juice, milk, or other liquid. Be sure to use joint protection methods with children who have unstable wrist or finger joints.
2. Follow a series of steps in preparing food, as in making a cold sandwich with turkey slices, lettuce, and tomato.
3. Spread butter, mustard, mayonnaise, peanut butter, cream cheese, or jelly with a knife. When performing this type of food preparation, people usually hold the knife handle with the index finger extended on top, which helps guide the knife. One way to help the child remember where to put the index finger is to place a red dot or a piece of tape at that point on the knife. Figure 18-9 provides an example of knife positioning. Spreading requires the ability to grade pressure according to the texture of the bread, toast, or cracker, and it requires considerable wrist rotation.
4. Before heating or cooking anything, safety knowledge for the stove, toaster, and standard and/or microwave oven needs to be developed. Children need to know how to operate the appliance, how to protect themselves from getting burned by wearing oven mitts and keeping the arms and body away from heating elements, how to handle hot pans and food, and what to do in case of emergency.
5. Depending on what is being cooked or heated, children need to learn how to manipulate utensils like tongs for hot dogs and spatulas for turning grilled cheese sandwiches, how to time and check on the process so foods are not overcooked, and how to prepare food such as piercing potatoes to keep them from exploding in the microwave.

COTAs might be responsible for adapting food preparation to children's specific capabilities and limitations. A number of picture cookbooks for nonreaders are available from equipment catalogs. Those with limited fine motor skills could use a cutting board to stabilize food for spreading and cutting. They might use a rocker knife or a knife with a cuff to aid the grip. The handles of pans on the stove can be stabilized with a pan holder attached to the stove with suction cups.

Children who use wheelchairs need accessible surfaces on which to work. This could be their wheelchair lapboard or a leaf table that can be folded out from the wall. Children with limited balance while standing might sit or use a locked walker for support when standing. Grab bars can be attached to the walls of the kitchen if needed.

Community Mobility

Community mobility refers to the ability to move around the community or neighborhood, including using public transportation, taxis, and driving.

Travel training in the community

Children who use wheelchairs benefit from OT intervention in travel skills. Those with vision impairments are trained to travel by an orientation and mobility teacher. Children who are able to see are taught ways to travel in the community by a travel trainer, OT practitioner, or special educator trained in this area.

Propelling a manual wheelchair down a sidewalk is not a simple task. Sidewalks are generally sloped toward the street for water drainage. To keep the wheelchair going straight, the child must push almost twice as hard on the street side of the chair. Children with electric wheelchairs also need to learn to adjust their steering to accommodate the slope of the sidewalk.

Moving around corners, people, and obstacles outdoors is similar to moving indoors; however, more vigilance and caution are required outdoors because of increased variability in terrain, high-speed automobiles, and unpredictable obstacles. Regardless of whether they use a wheelchair, children may encounter problems negotiating cracks or bumps in the sidewalk, gravel, hills, and grassy or rocky surfaces. Those who are able to walk are often referred to a physical therapist for help with their gait and negotiating different types of surfaces. Children who have problems with sensory processing, body awareness, coordination, and/or motor planning have particular difficulty accommodating the changes in terrain.

Crossing the street

Numerous individuals, including parents and older relatives, OT practitioners, and other adults involved with children, can teach children to cross the street. Young children may benefit from learning rules involving little or no problem-solving tasks, such as the following:

1. Cross the street only with an adult present.
2. Always cross at an intersection.
3. Even when you are with an adult, look both ways before stepping off the curb.
4. If you see a car coming toward you, wait until it passes no matter how far away it is.
5. Watch for cars turning into your path from side streets.
6. Talk only about the current traffic situation when crossing a street.
7. Listen to the traffic noises around you; if you hear a siren, watch out for it.

Children who are attempting to become independent in the community need to practice crossing the street at different types of intersections—with traffic lights and stop signs and without any traffic signals and stop signs at all. They need to learn to estimate the speed of traffic that is far away so as to assess their ability to cross the street in a safe amount of time.

FEAR OF THE CURB STORY. *Sherry is a 14-year-old girl with incoordination, mental retardation, severe sensory defensiveness, and problems with environmental awareness. Her teachers report that she was afraid to step off the curb, and her COTA was asked to help. Sherry's parents report that as an infant she refused to walk on grass and became frightened when encouraged to walk on different surfaces.*

The COTA first ruled out the possibility that Sherry needed glasses. According to her eye doctor, she did not have any problems with visual acuity (i.e., clarity or distinction). To address Sherry's problem with curbs, the COTA started therapy sessions with techniques designed to reduce sensory defensiveness. These techniques calmed Sherry and also decreased her anxiety and distractibility. The COTA then worked with her on indoor and outdoor mobility skills.

In Sherry's school, the COTA assisted her with moving through obstacle courses involving numerous surface changes. To increase her environmental awareness, Sherry played with a ball and performed tasks that involved reaching for targets, especially with her feet. These activities were often combined with vestibular (movement-gravity) tasks to help her time and coordinate her actions while moving. Sherry was sent on errands, such as delivering messages to classrooms on different floors, so that she could practice going up and down the stairs.

The COTA also took Sherry outside regularly. After using calming techniques, the COTA and she went behind the school to a safe, relatively private curb. The two of them practiced stepping up onto and down from the curb numerous times. Sherry was unable to look both ways for cars and step off the curb at the same time, so the task was broken down into smaller steps. She learned to (1) stop at the curb, (2) look both ways for cars, (3) look down at the street, (4) step down from the curb, and (5) look both ways again before (6) walking across. The COTA accompanied Sherry on weekly class trips to the grocery store to help her master the curb task and learn other community travel skills.

Public transportation

Adolescents often begin travel training for a specific purpose, such as going to and from school, the store, or a prevocational program. They may be preparing to travel to a vocational program that does not provide transportation, which usually means that they must learn to use public transportation.

To help children and teenagers become familiar with travel routes, COTAs may incorporate subway, bus, or street maps into therapy sessions. Map activities may also be used to help children improve their environmental awareness, sense of direction, eye movement, sequencing, and problem-solving skills.

Children who use wheelchairs need to learn and practice the way to enter adapted buses and wheelchair-accessible commuter train stations. This task is commonly an OT practitioner's responsibility. Regardless of whether children have physical disabilities, they need to learn how to buy tickets, tokens, or transit cards and deposit change on a bus. They need to learn how to determine when their stop is approaching and how to prepare to exit. They need to learn when and how to signal a bus driver to stop a bus. As children become more proficient at performing the sequence of actions, the OT practitioner reduces the level of assistance given to them and presents problems for them to solve. For example, the OT practitioner could allow children to miss a bus stop to see how they handle the situation and allow them to think of solutions.

Role of the shadow

Most community travel training programs designed for children who are able to walk use a "shadow" person. The shadow is usually someone from the program who is unknown to the child. Once s/he is able to carry out a travel sequence consistently in the presence of a trainer, the child is allowed to travel semi-independently. The shadow follows the child at a distance, getting on and off buses and/or subways at the same stop as the child and observing the situation for any problems that could arise. While using public transportation, some children engage in excessive self-stimulation, unknowingly push people, or talk to strangers. The shadow does not intervene unless a dangerous situation develops or the child has trouble solving a problem.[13]

Public phones

Using public phones is an essential tool for independent community travel. This skill may be taught by an OT practitioner, special education teacher, caregiver, travel trainer, prevocational teacher, or a combination of these individuals. Even if they have cell phones, children need to always carry extra change for a phone call because the charge on the cell phone battery might run out. The following techniques may be helpful in teaching children to use public phones:

1. Identify all the public phones along the children's travel routes.
2. Have children practice using pay phones on the street to call their schools, homes, or vocational centers.
3. Have children think of solutions to possible phone predicaments, such as encountering a phone that is out of order or having no money.
4. Have children handle coins and practice translation skills (moving coins between the palm and fingertips), which are required to remove coins from a wallet and insert them into a public phone.

Community interaction

Again, depending on the setting and the funding and purpose of the agency, the COTA may be responsible for teaching children to use community services such as a library, bank, post office, or grocery store. Learning these community skills may involve the assistance of several disciplines, such as OT, special education, social work, and speech therapy. Whenever possible, the OT practitioner participates with the child in community interaction. During outings identify and address complex problems, such as being too friendly to strangers or unable to count change correctly under pressure.

Social conduct

Basic social interaction includes using polite greetings, responding when spoken to, and saying "good-bye," "thank you," or "excuse me" when necessary. Caregivers and team members need to model polite interaction and provide opportunities for children to use them in different contexts.

Many polite phrases that are needed for proper social conduct can be inculcated through the rote method of learning. *Rote learning* refers to the acquisition of routine behaviors that may not be completely understood or performed with sincerity by the individual using them. It is usually acquired through memorization and repetition. If social phrases are used correctly, the child may be treated more kindly in the community. If they are not used, the child may be considered rude. Whether they are used in a rote manner or as the result of genuine understanding, basic social conduct interaction eases the child's ability to move in and out of different social contexts.

Financial Management

Financial management refers to the use of funds for purchases; planning and using money in different forms, such as checks and cash; and creating short- and long-term goals related to money. Financial management can be taught at home, in school, and/or in OT.

Children may become aware of financial management issues on trips to the grocery store with caregivers. Other ways to enhance awareness might include playing with pennies, putting coins in a bank, counting pennies, and getting an allowance. Children love imaginary play, and playing "store" is a fun way to help children understand some of the things that money pays for. Many games, play cash registers, and play automatic teller machines are available.

More formal training in financial management often begins in school by learning the names and values of different coins. Under the supervision of staff members, students could run a school store where both the children and staff purchase small items. The students are responsible for telling the customers the prices, taking and sorting money, and making the correct change.

OT practitioners may provide more individualized training of money skills for children who have perceptual or motor problems. Those who have visual impairments learn to distinguish coins by tactile discrimination, using the fingertips to feel the size and texture along the edges of each coin. Although pennies and dimes are a similar size, pennies have smooth edges and dimes have ridges. Likewise, nickels have smooth edges and quarters have ridges. To distinguish among bills, an individual with a visual impairment asks a trusted friend to fold one of them for him or her before putting it in a wallet or purse. Different values of paper money are folded in different ways, so the individual uses the fingertips to perceive how a certain bill is folded and identify its value before paying for things.

Coin carriers with slots for each type of coin may help children with tactile discrimination problems because only one type of coin fits in each slot. The individual memorizes the sequence of the slots so as to choose the right coin. Paper money needs to be stored in different ways. For example, all one-dollar bills can be kept in the right pocket, five-dollar bills in a back pocket, ten-dollar bills in the coin section of a wallet, and twenty-dollar bills in the paper section.

Whenever possible, have children use money skills during real community outings. For example, during OT sessions children can work toward earning an outing to buy a pack of sugarless gum.

In junior high or high school, students often learn how to keep checking and savings accounts and how to write checks. Students may begin having their own savings accounts very early if caregivers set it up for them. When teenagers begin working, sometimes at age 16, it is important for them to have checking or savings accounts. Some teachers or OT practitioners teach children how to write out deposit and withdrawal slips. Guides for check writing and deposit/withdrawal slips are sold at educational stores and equipment companies. Grids or templates are used for students with limited vision or poor coordination. Templates are simple pieces of cardboard or plastic with rectangles cutout where the number amounts and signature belong. The individual uses the fingers to feel the openings and writes inside them. The pen hits the edges of the openings on the template and keeps the writing within their boundaries.

Budgeting refers to making a plan for spending and saving money. COTAs may be instrumental in teaching adolescents budgeting skills. Many children are surprisingly naïve about how much a salary will allow them to buy. Teenagers with jobs need to use math skills to figure out the difference between their income and expenses. It is important for them to understand what things they need to buy to live on as opposed to what they want to buy for pleasure.

EARL'S FINANCIAL MANAGEMENT STORY. *Earl is a 17-year-old student at a school for children with special needs. He has intellectual disability resulting from mild lead poisoning. He also comes from a family with little income. Earl is proud to have an after-school supported job with a job coach. He is earning minimum wage for about 4 hours a week. Although Earl now has income to buy new clothes, he still wears the same sweatshirt to school every day and does not wear a belt. Earl's COTA has been helping him with rules for wearing fresh clothes every day, developing checklists with him, and reviewing with him how to get new clothes, but these changes are not occurring. When questioned, Earl said he did not have the money because he spent it on comic books.*

Coordinating a plan with Earl's school counselor and his father, his COTA helped Earl understand what he needed to survive in contrast with what he wanted for pleasure. Together they looked at clothing ads in the newspaper. They wrote lists of how much shirts and belts cost at different stores. Earl knew of a clothing store near his house. After cashing his next paycheck, the COTA and Earl went to the store, where he tried on a number of shirts and belts. He selected and bought two shirts and a belt. Wearing a new shirt and belt the next day, Earl's smile told everyone how proud he felt about his new budgeting and shopping skills.

Shopping

Shopping includes preparing lists for groceries and other purchases, finding and choosing the items needed, choosing a way to pay for them, and completing the purchase. COTAs might work on different levels of shopping, depending on the children's needs and the focus of therapy. Older children may need to develop independent shopping skills for settings such as group homes, daycare centers, and high schools. Younger children may work on beginning shopping skills as part of their community mobility. Some very young children may need help in the area of self-regulation in order to manage their behavior during shopping trips with caregivers.

Lists are useful when teaching most shopping skills. To prepare for grocery shopping, older children first make lists of food they will need during the next few days. They omit items from the list that they already have. Shopping lists should be arranged by grouping related items. For example, dairy items would be listed together, as would fruit and vegetables.

It is important for children with limited mobility to prepare for shopping trips. Call the stores in advance to be sure that they are accessible. Find out which entrance is best, the location of elevators, and when the store is the least crowded. For children with limited vision or hearing, ask whether a salesperson could be available to help on the chosen shopping day. To learn where merchandise is located and practice asking for assistance, it may help some children to visit the store with the COTA first before actually going shopping.

During a shopping trip, some children have trouble reading and following grocery lists. It may be helpful for COTAs or speech therapists to develop portable picture cards for supplies such as detergent, toilet paper, hand soap, canned beans, apples, meat, and bread. Next to the picture on each card, include the approximate price of the item. Laminate cards or cover them with clear contact paper and punch a hole in one corner. The picture cards are kept in a notebook during the week. Before a shopping trip, children choose the cards picturing the supplies they need. They place these cards on a large key ring so that they can flip through them in the store as they choose each item. They need only the abilities of matching pictures with items and reading and comparing prices.[13]

Children who are trying to stay within a budget need to keep track of how much money they are spending. They need to know how to quickly estimate the cost and add and check their change, either in their heads or with a calculator. It is helpful for children to use calculators when shopping. COTAs can teach them an easy way to estimate how much money to give the sales clerk. They simply round up the total amount due and offer the next higher dollar amount. For example, if a can of tuna fish costs $1.59, the child gives the clerk $2.00.[24]

Many foundational skills for shopping can be addressed during OT sessions, but actual shopping experiences often reveal unusual problems. Social skills may turn out to be more problematic than any other aspect of shopping.

JOHN'S SHOPPING STORY. *John, a 15 year old with fragile X syndrome, has sensory defensiveness with gaze avoidance as well as mild intellectual disability. His mother asked his school COTA to work on buying simple things like a soda because she was having trouble teaching him how to do it. The COTA worked on every aspect of the sequence: finding the soda, placing it on the counter, looking at the clerk, paying, and taking and counting the change. John liked to wear sunglasses to relieve the stress of looking into people's eyes due to his sensory defensiveness. During the actual shopping trip to the deli on the corner, everything went as planned until it came time to pay. John put the money on the counter and the sales clerk took it. When the clerk tried to hand him the change, he cringed and backed away from the counter. Despite the COTA's encouragement, John could not take the change, so she helped him complete the transaction.*

Back at school John felt more comfortable in a one-on-one situation with the COTA, and he told her of his feelings. He said that he hated how the clerk's hand might feel when giving him the change. John's sensory defensiveness caused withdrawal reactions when faced with the possibility of a stranger touching his palm.

During mock shopping transactions in school, John easily tolerated the COTA handing him change. Although she and his parents had been treating his defensiveness, it remained severe. He needed a compensatory strategy when shopping to reduce his overwhelming fear of touch from a stranger. John figured out that he could tolerate picking up change from the counter, and the COTA role-played with him how to ask the clerk to put down the change. During his next visit to the deli, with encouragement from the COTA, John carried out the plan and the clerk placed the change on the counter. John was greatly relieved and pleased with his success. The COTA informed his parents of the new strategy.

CLINICAL *Pearl*

Some problems can be discovered only during real outings. Completely unexpected issues often arise, which can then be addressed in therapy.

Care of Others

Care of others can be direct or indirect. It includes arranging for and supervising people who provide care. Pediatric clients may be asked to help care for a parent with a disability.

Sometimes pediatric clients participate in choosing their own caretaker or babysitter for after-school hours or weekends. Their input can be quite helpful. It is important for parents and other involved adults to carefully watch a child's reactions and listen to reports about caretakers. Occasionally an unqualified caretaker is inadvertently hired. A situation may occur in which the caretaker behaves in a deceitful or puni tive manner. The child's behavior may be the only way for parents to determine if the arrangement is working.

Other pediatric clients are asked to care for family members who have physical or emotional problems. It is natural for family members to help one another, but some families impose adult responsibilities on children. The following account illustrates this situation.

JUNE'S CARE OF OTHERS STORY. *June is an 11-year-old girl with learning disabilities, mild hearing impairment in both ears, decreased oculomotor control, problems with motor planning and motor memory, and limited handwriting skills. She is enrolled in a school for children with learning disabilities and mandated to receive counseling, OT, and additional help from a reading specialist. June's father works full time. Her mother has a seizure disorder, depression, and anxiety. The mother is unable to work because of her disabilities. June rarely goes to school, and when she does, she usually arrives unprepared and without her homework. She appears happy and unconcerned about school requirements.*

Because of June's poor attendance, she makes little progress in reading and writing. She is unable to complete projects with her classmates because she is always behind in her work and understanding. When the staff gently discussed her difficulties with her, June often complained that the school was "bad" because she was "not learning anything." Her counselor called the family numerous times, asking them to help June get to school more frequently. The family always responded in an agreeable way, assuring the counselor that she would attend regularly. But after 3 or 4 days of regular attendance, June's old pattern would return.

During their infrequent OT sessions, June told the OT practitioner that she spent most of her time at home taking care of responsibilities for her mother. She went to medical appointments with and for her. She helped her mother with shopping, going to the laundromat, and cooking and cleaning. Some days her mother stayed in bed all day. June also talked about how she liked to cook. When questioned about career interests, she said that she did not need a career because she would get married. By listening to her and consulting with team members, the pieces of the puzzle began to fall into place. June performed much of the care for her mother and family. The family placed little importance on school, and June readily accepted this way of thinking. Because of her problems with reading and writing, thinking that school was unnecessary helped June "save face," and retain her self-esteem.

June's counselor then tried a different approach. She helped June's mother get a home attendant 4 hours a day to accompany her to medical appointments and help her clean and cook. A family therapist began working with all the family members to get them to focus more on June's issues. In addition, the counselor elicited assistance from the family's church, which provided a tutor to come to her house and help her with homework after school. June's attendance, interest in school, and progress in class and OT slowly began to increase.

Child Rearing

Child rearing is the provision of care and supervision to support the development of children. Although we do not readily think of child rearing as a pediatric IADLs, it can be an important activity in some cases. Teenagers with typical cognitive function who have physical limitations such as cerebral palsy, amputation, visual or hearing impairments, hemiparesis (weakness on one side of the body), and muscular dystrophy may be asked to babysit for younger siblings, or they may choose babysitting as a means of earning extra money. As with any teenager, they need to be instructed in safety procedures and emergency responses specifically for their charges and fitting their own limitations and strengths. For example, they need to know the addresses and phone numbers of the caregivers, the young children's doctors, the police and fire departments, and the neighbors. They need to be comfortable and mobile in the babysitting setting. This may be easier in the teenager's own home, where it is assumed that suitable environmental modifications are already in place.

Sometimes children with or without disabilities are given too many child-rearing responsibilities. Parents who themselves have physical or emotional problems may depend on one child to care for his or her siblings. These children may lose out on necessary play and the development of social skills. They may feel responsible for their siblings' well-being or their parents' difficulties, thereby becoming resentful or depressed. If the COTA suspects that a pediatric client is being given overwhelming child-care work, it is best to consult with the OTR and the client's social worker or counselor to determine a course of action. A social worker or counselor might be able to explain the situation to the parents and smoothly resolve the problem. Team members can also work to strengthen the client's coping skills, which can make the demanding home situation easier to handle.

Another example of pediatric child rearing occurs with teenage parents. Some older teenagers with disabilities have children. To raise a child, any teenager needs additional help and a strong support system. Teenage parents with disabilities require assistance specifically suited to their individual needs and abilities. OT practitioners can be asked to provide intervention for teenage parents with disabilities. Given this complex scenario, a COTA would request guidance from the supervising OTR and multidisciplinary team.

Care of Pets

The care of pets may involve directly feeding, cleaning up after, and providing shelter and health care for house pets. It may also involve arranging for and supervising the maintenance of house pets, farm animals, and/or service animals. With the increased use of service animals such as dogs and monkeys for individuals with visual or hearing impairments and/or physical disabilities, the care of pets can be an important IADL for COTAs to address with certain pediatric clients. The care of pets is discussed in Chapter 24.

MANAGING ACTIVITIES OF DAILY LIVING AND INSTRUMENTAL ACTIVITIES OF DAILY LIVING

Knowing how to independently manage ADLs and IADLs such as dressing, bathing, school assignments, household chores, and financial management can help prepare children for adult life. The practitioner can provide them and their caregivers with useful strategies and assistance. It is not surprising that attention to instruction is a common problem for all populations. Children need to develop the ability to attend when learning new skills and sustain attention when using them. An optimum **level of arousal** (i.e., alertness and readiness for the job at hand) is required for learning.[38] Children with attention deficit disorder, hyperactivity, sensory processing problems, anxiety, low frustration tolerance, impulsivity, sequencing or motor memory problems, or auditory processing problems have even more trouble attending and sustaining attention when learning and performing.

Regulating levels of arousal can improve attention. Many OT practitioners and some teachers use sensory input for the mouth, ears, eyes, muscles, and vestibular (movement-gravity) system to help children regulate levels of arousal.[38,40] These sensory methods include allowing children to suck from a sports bottle or water bottle with a straw at their desks, asking fidgety children to run errands or help with jobs like sharpening pencils, asking anxious children to pass out heavy books or reposition chairs and tables for class activities, allowing children to move around and talk during group activities, lowering bright lights to change the mood, and incorporating stretch breaks into learning activities.

Strategies such as the following can be incorporated into routines at home during self-care, dressing, and cleaning bedrooms or into the classroom with challenging academic exercises, keyboarding, handwriting, and other routines.

- Before children begin challenging work, try table or chair pushups, leg lifts, trunk and head twists, or other exercises requiring muscle work or movement. These actions increase body awareness and can help individuals regulate their arousal for increased attention.
- Deep breathing is a powerful way to focus attention and relax the brain and body. Before challenging work, have children use straws to blow cotton balls into a make-believe corral created by their hands or a piece of paper.[40] Have children take a deep breath and then quietly recite the alphabet or count to 30 without taking another breath. Children could also slowly count to 10 or produce a rhyme in one breath.
- Oral activities are useful during challenging work. OT practitioners frequently use resistive oral-motor treats to provide deep-pressure sensations inside the mouth. The treats can promote an *optimum level of arousal* and increase the focus of attention and concentration. Small resistive oral-motor treats are best used before or during a challenging activity such as keyboarding or before a transition between activities, rooms, or buildings. A few examples of resistive oral-motor treats are popcorn, pretzels, carrot sticks dipped in salad dressing, dried fruit, baked potato chips, baked corn chips, nuts, and water or juice from a straw cup. Add water to juice because juice tends to have too much sugar. Organic snacks are always the best but not always cost effective. Avoid snacks with food coloring and food additives because they may cause unusual behavioral reactions. Children often chew on pieces of tubing or pencil holders (see Figure 18-11) instead of eating food.
- Children with sensory defensiveness may benefit from using the Wilbarger Deep Pressure and Proprioceptive Technique every hour or two throughout the day to reduce anxiety and defensive reactions (per clinical observations as opposed to research-based evidence).
- Children who are distractible and unable to screen out background visual input, such as bright bulletin boards or people walking by, may benefit from using study carrels (partitions or cubicles). They block out visual stimulation from the front and sides.
- Children who are unable to screen out background noise, such as chairs sliding or footsteps outside the room, may be able to work independently when wearing headphones with or without music (see Figure 18-43). They can still hear the instructor while wearing noise reduction headphones.
- Children can be given the option of completing work in a quiet area such as an alcove, sitting in a beanbag chair in a corner of the room, or in the hallway just outside the room.
- Attempts to maintain upright sitting can cause discomfort or distract children with poor postural control. Because they must concentrate on trying to stay upright, they cannot focus sufficient attention to instruction. Using a seat cushion (see Figure 18-43) or adaptive seating may increase comfort and decrease the effort required to sit up, allowing them to attend to the job at hand.

ERIC'S LEVEL OF AROUSAL FOR ADLS AND IADLS STORY. *Eric, a bright 8 year old, has the following issues: poor regulation of his level of arousal, sensory defensiveness, distractibility, poor environmental and body awareness, limited postural control, limited ADLs in the area of shoe tying, and decreased IADLs in the area of safety.*

Eric's extreme overarousal, distractibility in response internal and external stimuli, and decreased safety awareness are the primary obstacles to school participation. He constantly fidgets with his feet, slides his body around his chair, and inadvertently pushes the chair away from his desk and into other people. At times he even falls out of his chair. He taps out rhythms on his desk and hums and acts out scenes from Sponge Bob cartoons. Eric's fidgeting and noises tend to block out important information from his teacher.

He becomes distracted and unable to focus on instructions. He has trouble moving safely around his class and the school. On the other hand, he is verbal, curious, friendly, and motivated to try new activities.

Eric has trouble with shoe tying for many reasons, among them sensory defensiveness, frequent overarousal, limited postural strength, and control. He becomes immediately overstimulated by the tickly shoelaces and breaks into hysterical laughter. Of course, he is unable to focus on instructions and soon exhibits unsafe behavior. He may even fall out of his chair because of limited body and safety awareness. At this point it is hard for the COTA to help Eric recover a state of equilibrium. He could lose a whole day of learning if he returns to class in this state of unsafe, unfocused, and uncontrolled silliness.

Eric's treatment was multilayered. His most critical problem was determined to be in the IADL area of safety. However, his level of arousal, sensory defensiveness, and distractibility, resulting in unsafe and disruptive behaviors, had to be dealt with. The following describes his intervention:

- *Eric first engaged in listening to classical music.*
- *Eric is given noise reduction headphones (see Figure 18-43). He could still hear the teacher's voice but not distracting background sounds such as footsteps, classmates whispering, and the clock ticking.*
- *The COTA asked Eric's parents to send in a sports bottle with a straw top every day. He filled it with water and kept it on his desk, taking sips throughout the day.*
- *The COTA replaced Eric's hard finger tapping with a different form of fingertip pressure—the COTA slowly and rhythmically squeezes his hands.*
- *Eric received extra proprioceptive feedback to calm his body and increase body awareness, control, and safety. The COTA met with Eric's teacher to discuss adaptive equipment that could help him in the classroom and also brought a weighted vest and an air-filled seat cushion to the class (see Figure 18-43). The vest contained 3 pounds of weight. The teacher was given written instructions for when and where Eric is to use the weighted vest.*
- *Eric received a seat cushion that enables him to move around in his seat without slipping off the edge.*
- *Eric received a sturdy wooden chair. It did not move easily when he fidgeted with his feet, so he could not accidentally push his chair into other people. The COTA double-checked to be sure that his feet were flat on the floor in order to provide maximum stability.*
- *Eric's desk was moved to the front of the room next to the teacher's desk. His desk no longer faced his classmates, so distractibility was reduced. His close proximity to the teacher's desk provided a calming and organizing influence.*

The effectiveness of these techniques was dramatic for Eric. His humming and finger tapping stopped. The IADL area of safety improved. He was calm and focused. He followed demonstrations and verbal instructions. Finally, the COTA worked on the ADL area of shoe tying. He steadily progressed in acquiring independent shoe tying. His transition back into the classroom is now safer.

ORGANIZING ACTIVITIES OF DAILY LIVING AND INSTRUMENTAL ACTIVITIES OF DAILY LIVING

One of the first parts of organizing activities involves making a list of steps or assigned jobs. As each step is completed, children cross it off the list. The physical act of crossing a step off the list is rewarding in itself. For an ADL routine such as morning hygiene, caregivers or COTAs can make a written or picture list, cover it with clear contact paper, and place it on the wall or mirror in the bathroom. Children can keep a homework list in the front of a notebook or folder so that it will be the first page seen when the notebook is opened. Home chores can be listed on a chart designating each day of the week and placed on the refrigerator, kitchen table, or corkboard in the kitchen.

For young children and those who do not read, COTAs can create lists using symbols, photographs, or objects attached to a Velcro board. For example, a toothbrush could represent tooth brushing and a mini-washcloth a bath. The practitioner attaches the symbols, photos, or objects to the board in the desired order. As each job is completed, children pull the related item off the board. They receive gratification from mastering each job as well as removing Velcro items from the board. They also have a visual representation of activities that they have accomplished. For some activities the sequence can be varied. For example, children could choose the order of home chores and attach symbols, photos, or objects to the board before starting.

Timing is important when scheduling activities. Ask children to get schoolwork or chores done before dinner because they may be too tired to concentrate afterward. Make sure that there is enough time to complete the activities. Some children need the times to be specified on the assignment list. Others need the sequence specified. For example, "After your snack, take the water bottle, gum, and swivel chair to your room." Still others benefit from timers, which encourage them to stay focused until the timer rings, take a break at a certain time, or stop for dinner. Try using kitchen or liquid timers, but carefully observe the responses. They help many children but cause others to become distracted or anxious and then work more slowly.

To help children focus on a school assignment, include only those items on the table or easel that are needed for that assignment or support the focus of attention and an optimum *level of arousal*. Keep other materials in the book bag or desk. Once each assignment is finished, it is stored back in the book bag or desk.

SHAPING POSITIVE ATTITUDES FOR ACTIVITIES OF DAILY LIVING AND INSTRUMENTAL ACTIVITIES OF DAILY LIVING

Learning skills are often the focus of treatment, but clients may also need gentle shaping of their attitudes. Low self-esteem, hopelessness, boredom, expectations of failure, anger, frustration, anxiety, and a need to be nurtured and dependent are just some of the feelings that can interfere with performance. An adolescent may know exactly how to accomplish hygiene tasks, but negative feelings prevent the daily completion of the steps.[5]

Eliciting children's positive feelings and their desire to learn a skill or carry it out at specific times can be difficult. The COTA can use the following techniques to shape positive attitudes and increase self-esteem:

- Frequently praise the child's attempts to learn a particular skill.[9,33]
- Use a "matter-of-fact" approach when needed; this method may be especially helpful when treating adolescents.
- A positive, concrete description of children's behaviors tells them exactly what they are doing correctly, even if their performance is not perfect.[9,34] For example, even if a child's shoe tying is not completely successful, the practitioner can still say "You're working so hard," "I really like how you concentrated on that job," or "Wow, you finished getting the laces into an 'X' shape!" Many children who have high cognitive skills but also have learning disabilities or motor impairments are painfully aware of their inability to perform like other children. Therefore, be honest in your descriptions and comments; they will know if you are not.
- Avoid using the words "bad" or "good." Even the experienced practitioner works at choosing the most effective words to use with each child. Although it is easy to understand why the word "bad" needs to be avoided, it may seem strange that the word "good" should also be avoided. Using the word "good" implies that if performance is not "good," the child or performance is "bad."[34]
- Never tell children to "be good" or ask them "Were you good today?" All children want to be good, and they can always be considered to be inherently good. Only their behaviors may need to change. Children need to know what is expected of them. Give concrete instructions or make specific comments about exactly what positive behaviors are needed.[33] For example, say "We're walking slowly to stay safe" or "Remember to follow directions and use nice words on the bus." Avoid using words like "no" and "don't," saving them instead for dangerous situations when you must yell "No!" or "Don't do that!" to prevent physical injury. If used sparingly, children will heed these negative warnings more readily than if they are frequently heard.
- Make sure the last words heard by the child explain the desired behavior. For example, "Yelling is finished. It's time to talk in a quiet indoor voice." The last words in the statement describe the desired behavior—to talk in a quiet indoor voice.[9] If you say "Don't yell!" the last word that is heard is "yell." Without hearing a description of a positive replacement behavior for yelling, the child may continue behaving in a manner that is consistent with the last word that is heard: yell.
- Being genuinely caring and having a sense of humor can really help at times. A positive social environment that includes opportunities to develop friendships, learn constructive ways of expressing anger and frustration, and experience even small successes may motivate a child to perform independently. When you hear the child say "Don't help me; I want to do it myself," you know you are on the right track.
- The OT practitioner's self-awareness is one of the keys to successful treatment. The ability to understand one's own feelings, behaviors, and beliefs improves his or her interaction with a child. For example, awareness of how the OT practitioner's behavior, such as a loud or quiet voice, affects the client can lead to more effective communication. Likewise, awareness of how a child affects the practitioner's own feelings and behaviors, both positively and negatively, enhances the therapeutic process. Finally, the OT practitioner needs to believe in his or her own effectiveness as a practitioner and believe that the child is capable of improving.[9]
- If a child responds in an avoiding, negative, or oppositional way, it is important not to take it personally but consider the underlying factors. Children may resist participation as an attempt to cope with feelings of confusion, anxiety, or fear of failure. As OT practitioners, it is our job to try to understand the sources of their feelings and help them express negative feelings in productive ways. It is also our job to give clear, understandable instructions in verbal, visual, physical, and/or multisensory ways. If we ensure that children experience frequent small suc-

cesses, their attitudes toward activities and learning, as well as their self-esteem, will increase.

Children with severe handicaps receive much attention because they are assisted in accomplishing daily activities. They may learn that one way to obtain more attention is to ask for more help or behave in a needy and dependent manner. In their attempts to be the best caregivers possible, some adults do everything for their children except encourage or expect them to perform independently. This relationship may produce learned helplessness. Even though the caregiver's aim is to help the child as effectively as possible, s/he does not learn to perform ADLs independently or accept responsibility for taking care of oneself.

The OT practitioner's role is to facilitate children's independence. Part of this role is to help caregivers understand how important it is to encourage independence. Mastery of any daily living skill enhances a child's self-esteem and allows freer movement in various environments.

INTERVENTION FOR ACTIVITIES OF DAILY LIVING AND INSTRUMENTAL ACTIVITIES OF DAILY LIVING

A common mistake made by OT practitioners is to practice an activity as a primary intervention. Although repetition and additional practice are especially important for many children with disabilities, repetitive practice may not lead to the desired outcome. The results can be quicker and more permanent when combined treatment approaches are used. A child with oral defensiveness may resist tooth brushing. Practice alone, even with one-to-one supervision, may not necessarily lead to independent tooth brushing. The practitioner needs to first reduce the child's defensiveness. As s/he becomes less defensive and more comfortable with tooth brushing, it will be more likely to grow into an independent activity or whole skill.

"Reading the child in context" focuses attention on the relationship between the child and the current situation. It is a moment-by-moment observation and analysis of the child's relation to the social and physical environments and his or her responses to the therapeutic process. The best practitioners continuously read children in context and modify their intervention plans accordingly.

To read a child in context, the practitioner monitors numerous factors before and during intervention. The following are some samples of questions that a practitioner tries to answer during a session with a child. Does the child perform best in a quiet individual setting or with peer models nearby? Are competing background noises or tactile sensations (like scratchy clothing) interfering with the child's concentration? What happened to cause the child to suddenly switch from laughing to screaming or from singing to hitting? If the child becomes more oppositional than usual, would it help to increase calming activities (such as listening to soothing music), reduce the task demands, or both? Is the child oppositional because of a factor such as sickness, thirst, lack of sleep, a long bus ride to school, or a family argument or an unexpected sensory event like getting the sleeves wet at the sink? Does the child's current facial expression show a fear or pain response? Would it help to use slower handling movements or change the child's head position? What are all of the possible causes of the current change in behavior, and what can be done to improve it? If the child is fully engaged in a purposeful, meaningful activity, how long do I allow it to continue? When do I intervene again to keep the activity going or change it? The number of possible questions is endless. Carefully adjusting therapy by reading the child ensures the therapeutic nature of the intervention.

SUMMARY

The occupations of ADLs and IADLs are occupational performance areas in which COTAs play broad and important roles with children. The role of COTAs involves analyzing, grading, and adapting activities; reading the child in context; consulting and collaborating with OTRs, caregivers, team members, agency administrators, and other professionals; utilizing combined treatment approaches; matching adaptive devices with an individual child's capabilities and caregiver preferences; and utilizing the numerous literary, media, and workshop resources available in OT and other disciplines. COTAs use their personalities, creativity, and sincerity to connect with children and help them feel safe and cared for. They can help children participate in ADLs and IADLs, thereby playing a vital role in helping children achieve maximum independence in life.

References

1. American Occupational Therapy Association: Occupational Therapy Practice Framework: domain and process, *Am J Occup Ther* 56:609, 2002.
2. Bergen A, Colangelo C: *Positioning the client with CNS deficit: the wheelchair and other adapted equipment*, Valhalla, NY, 1982, Valhalla Rehabilitation Publications.
3. Burton L: *Concept and design for weights used during hallway transitions*, Brooklyn, NY, 1996, The League School.
4. Dickson D, Buckley-Reen A: *The whole child: the S.A.N.E. system of pediatric assessment and treatment*, Professional Conference, New York, 2002.
5. Early MB: *Mental health concepts and techniques for the occupational therapy assistant*, New York, 1987, Raven Press.

6. Erhardt R: *Developmental visual dysfunction: models for assessment and management*, Tucson, 1993, Therapy Skill Builders.
7. Feingold B: *The Feingold handbook*, Alexandria, Va, 1982, Feingold Association of the United States.
8. Feingold B: *Why your child is hyperactive*, New York, 1974, Random House.
9. Filemyr J, Spears A: *Techniques for dealing with oppositional behaviors*, Presentation, Brooklyn, NY, 1994, League Treatment Center.
10. Finnie N: *Handling the young cerebral palsy child at home*, ed 3, Boston, 1997, Butterworth-Heinemann.
11. Fletcher P: COTA, Interview, Brooklyn, NY, 2004.
12. Frick R, Frick SM, Oetter P, et al: *Out of the mouths of babes: discovering the developmental significance of the mouth*, Hugo, Minn, 1996, PDP Press.
13. McCarthy K: *Activities of daily living: a manual of group activities and written exercises*, Framingham, Mass, 1993, Therapro, Inc.
14. Goldsmith MC: *Expanding children's diets: ketchup isn't the only vegetable*, Presentation, Kennebunkport, Me, 1996, Avanti Summit.
15. Handford M: *Find Waldo now*, Boston, 1988, Little, Brown.
16. Handford M: *The great Waldo search*, Boston, 1989, Little, Brown.
17. Handford M: *Where's Waldo?* Boston, 1987, Little, Brown.
18. Handford M: *Where's Waldo in Hollywood?* Cambridge, Mass, 1993, Candlewick Press.
19. Heine B: An introduction to hippotherapy, *J Strides* pp. 10–13, 1997.
20. Jones L: *Survey of accessibility in group homes for pediatric clients in wheelchairs*, New York, 1982, New York University and United Cerebral Palsy of New York State.
21. Koomar J, Masur S: *Sensory integration treatment*, Workshop, Boston, 1990, Sensory Integration International.
22. Liszkay E: *Closed cell foam foot rests*, Brooklyn, NY, 1998, The Joan Fenichel Therapeutic Nursery, The League Treatment Center.
23. Machover PZ: Consultation on promoting positive feelings around eating using social-environmental intervention, New York, 1990.
24. McCarthy K: *Activities of daily living: a manual of group activities and written exercises*, Framingham, Mass, 1993, Therapro, Inc.
25. Morris S, Klein M: *Prefeeding skills: A comprehensive resource for feeding development*, Tucson, 1987, Therapy Skill Builders.
26. Oetter P, Richter E, Frick S: *MORE: Integrating the mouth with sensory and postural functions*, Hugo, Minn, 1993, PDP Press.
27. Oetter P, Richter E, Frick S: *On MORE: Integrating the mouth with sensory and postural functions*, Workshop, Greenwich, Conn, 1995, Professional Development Programs.
28. Pedretti L, Early MB: *Occupational therapy skills for physical dysfunction*, ed 5, St Louis, 2001, Mosby.
29. Reynolds J: *Attainment's personal success: an illustrated guide to personal needs*, Verona, Wis, 1999, Attainment Co, Inc.
30. Rossi L: *Nutrition as cause and cure of systemic candidiasis*, unpublished master's thesis, Bridgeport, Conn, 2004, The University of Bridgeport.
31. Rossi L: Consultation, New York, 2005.
32. Schneck C: Visual perception. In Case-Smith J, editor: *Occupational therapy for children*, ed 5, St Louis, 2005, Mosby.
33. Stoller L: *Low tech assistive devices: a handbook for the school setting*, Framingham, Mass, 1998, Therapro, Inc.
34. Stringer K: *Staff behavior management guidelines*, New York, 1996, The Reece School.
35. Todd V: Visual perceptual frame of reference: an information processing approach. In Kramer P, Hinojosa J, editors: *Frames of reference for pediatric occupational therapy*, Baltimore, Md, 1993, Williams & Wilkins.
36. Warren M: Evaluation and treatment of visual deficits. In Pedretti LW, editor: *Occupational therapy practice skills for physical dysfunction*, ed 4, St Louis, 1996, Mosby.
37. Wilbarger P, Becker-Lewin M: *Sensory defensiveness and related social/emotional and neurological problems*, Workshop, Long Island, NY, 1998, Professional Development Programs.
38. Wilbarger P, Wilbarger J: *Intervention for persons with moderate to severe dysfunction*, Workshop, Brooklyn, NY, 1992, Comprehensive Network.
39. Wilk K: *Shoe-tying made simple*, Boston, 2002, Therapro.
40. Williams M, Shellenberger S: *How does your engine run?: A leader's guide to the Alert Program for Self-Regulation*, Albuquerque, 1994, Therapy Works.
41. Zielig S: *Inexpensive backrest*, Brooklyn, NY, 1998, The League School.

Recommended Reading

Amundson SJ: Prewriting and handwriting skills. In Case-Smith J, editor: *Occupational therapy for children*, ed 5, St Louis, 2005, Mosby.

Ball D: *Handwriting issues in school system practice*, Lecture, Charleston, SC, 1998, Trident Technical College.

Beauchamp R: *Fine motor activities*, Parent Workshop, New York, 1998, Reece School.

Benbow M: *Loops and other groups: a kinesthetic writing system*, Tucson, 1988, Therapy Skill Builders.

Berry J: *Give yourself a hand: an integrated hand skills program*, Framingham, Mass, 1993, Therapro.

Bissell J: *Coping in the classroom: sensory integration special interest section newsletter*, 1991, Bethesda, Md, American Occupational Therapy Association.

Bissell J, Fisher J, Owens C, et al: *Sensory motor handbook: a guide for implementing and modifying activities in the classroom*, ed 2, Tucson, 1998, Therapy Skill Builders.

Bissell J, et al: *Trouble-shooting pads: (a) Producing organized written work. (b) Beginning and completing tasks. (c) Sportsmanship and cooperation. (d) Organizing behavior during motor time. (e) Performing tasks while seated. (f) Copying from the blackboard. (g) Cutting with scissors. (h) Writing with pencils. (i) Maintaining order in line. (j) Organizing personal belongings*, Handouts, Tucson, 1998, Therapy Skill Builders.

Boehme R: *Improving upper body control: an approach to assessment and treatment of tonal dysfunction*, Tucson, 1988, Therapy Skill Builders.

Bortz S: *Improving classroom behavior with modified use of the Alert Program for Self-Regulation*, Master's thesis, Brooklyn, NY, 1997, The League School.

Bryte K: *Classroom intervention for the school-based therapist*, San Antonio, Texas, 1996, Therapy Skill Builders.

Burton GU: Sexuality: an activity of daily living. In Early MB, editor: *Physical dysfunction practice skills for the occupational therapy assistant*, St Louis, 1998, Mosby.

Case-Smith J, editor: *Occupational therapy for children*, ed 5, St Louis, 2005, Mosby.

Case-Smith J, Pehoski C: *Development of hand skills in the child*, Bethesda, Md, 1992, American Occupational Therapy Association.

Christiansen CH, Baum CM: *Occupational therapy: enabling function and well-being*, ed 2, Thorofare, NJ, 1997, Slack.

Crepeau EB, Cohn ES, Schell BAB: *Willard and Spackman's occupational therapy*, ed 10, Philadelphia, 2003, Lippincott Williams & Wilkins.

Duran GA, Klenke-Ormiston S: *Multi-play, sensory activities for school readiness*, Tucson, 1994, Therapy Skill Builders.

Early MB: *Physical dysfunction practice skills for the occupational therapy assistant*, St Louis, 1998, Mosby.

Exner C: In-hand manipulation. In Case-Smith J, Pehoski C, editors: *Development of hand skills in the child*, Bethesda, Md, 1992, American Occupational Therapy Association.

Exner C: Development of hand skills. In Case-Smith J, editor: *Occupational therapy for children*, ed 5, St Louis, 2005, Mosby.

Faustin D: *Cardboard brick block footrests*, Brooklyn, NY, 1995, The Joan Fenichel Therapeutic Nursery, The League Treatment Center.

Fink B: *Sensory-motor integration activities*, Tucson, 1989, Therapy Skill Builders.

Folio MR, Fewell RR: *Peabody developmental motor scales*, Chicago, 1983, Riverside.

Gans JS: *Including SI: a guide to using sensory integration concepts in the school environment*, Bohemia, NY, 1998, Kapable Kids.

Goldstein AP, McGinnis E: *Skillstreaming the adolescent: a structured learning approach to teaching prosocial skills*, Champaign, Ill, 1980, Research Press.

Haldy M, Haack L: *Making it easy: sensorimotor activities at home and school*, Tucson, 1995, Therapy Skill Builders.

Henderson A, Pehoski C: *Hand function in the child: foundations for remediation*, St Louis, 1995, Mosby.

Henry D: *Tools for teachers*, Glendale, Ariz, 1998, Henry Occupational Therapy Services.

Herring KL, Wilkinson S: *Action alphabet: sensorimotor activities for groups*, San Antonio, Texas, 1995, Therapy Skill Builders.

Huss AJ: *A neurophysiological approach to central nervous system dysfunction*, Workshop, Ann Arbor, Mich, 1981, Continuing Education Programs of America.

Jones L: *Survey of accessibility in group homes for pediatric clients in wheelchairs*, New York, 1982, New York University and United Cerebral Palsy of New York State.

Keplinger L: *Movement is fun: a preschool movement program*, Torrance, Calif, 1988, Sensory Integration International.

Levine K: *Fine motor dysfunction: therapeutic strategies in the classroom*, Tucson, 1991, Therapy Skill Builders.

Loiselle L, Shea S: *Curriculum-based activities in occupational therapy: an inclusion resource*, Framingham, Mass, 1995, Therapro.

McCarty H: *Energy and stress in the learning process: a neurophysiological approach to learning at any age*, Workshop, Phoenix, 1998, Sensory Integration International.

McGinnis E, Goldstein A: *Skillstreaming in early childhood: teaching prosocial skills to the preschool and kindergarten child*, Champaign, Ill, 1990, Research Press.

McGinnis E, Goldstein A: *Skillstreaming the elementary school child: a guide for teaching prosocial skills*, Champaign, Ill, 1984, Research Press.

Norton K: *Design of prevocational program*, Brooklyn, NY, 1984, The League School.

Okoye R, Malden J: Use of neurotransmitter modulation to facilitate sensory integration, *Neurol Rep* 10(4):67–72, 1986, Neurology Section of the American Physical Therapy Association.

Olsen J: *Handwriting without tears*, Potomac, Md, 1994, Janice Z Olsen.

Quirk N, DiMatties M: *The relationship of learning problems and classroom performance to sensory integration*, Haddonfield, NJ, 1990, Quirk and DiMatties.

Richardson BG, Shupe MJ: Management of disruptive behavior: the importance of teacher self-awareness in working with students with emotional and behavioral disorders, *Teach Exceptional Childr* 36:8, 2003.

Rubell B: *Big strokes for little folks*, San Antonio, Texas, 1995, Therapy Skill Builders.

Seroussi K: *Unraveling the mysteries of autism: a mother's story of research and recovery*, New York, 2002, Broadway Books, a division of Random House.

Sher B: *Different drummers—same song*, San Antonio, Texas, 1996, Therapy Skill Builders.

Sher B: *Moving right along*, Hugo, Minn, 1997, PDP Press.

Stackhouse T, Wilbarger J, Trunnell S: *Treating sensory modulation disorders: the STEPSI: a tool for effective critical reasoning*, Workshop, Boston, 1998, Professional Development Programs.

Sumar S: *Yoga for the special child*, Buckingham, Va, 1996, Special Yoga Publications.

Trombly CA, Radomski MV: *Occupational therapy for physical dysfunction*, ed 5, Baltimore, 2002, Williams & Wilkins.

Trott M, Laurel M, Windeck S: *Sensibilities: understanding sensory integration*, Tucson, 1993, Therapy Skill Builders.

Tupper LC, Miesner KK: *School hardening: sensory integration strategies for class and home*, San Antonio, Texas, 1995, Therapy Skill Builders.

Wilbarger P: The sensory diet: activity programs based on sensory processing theory, AOTA *Sensory Integration Special Interest Section Newsletter*, 18(2):1-3, 1995.

Wilbarger P, Wilbarger J: *Sensory defensiveness in children aged 2–12: an intervention guide for parents and other caregivers*, Santa Barbara, Calif, 1991, Avanti Educational Programs.

Wolf L, Glass R: *Feeding and swallowing disorders in infancy: assessment and management*, Tucson, 1992, Therapy Skill Builders.

Young S, Keplinger L: *Movement is fun: a preschool movement program*, Torrance, Calif, 1988, Sensory Integration International.

REVIEW *Questions*

1. Define ADLs and give examples of the problems that children might have and the intervention a COTA might provide in four ADL areas.
2. Define IADLs and give examples of the problems that children might have and the intervention a COTA might provide in four IADL areas.
3. Why is s-s-b synchrony important, and how would the COTA proceed if the OTR, SLP, and/or parents requested intervention for a child in this area?
4. Describe some common problems that children with disabilities have in toileting, hygiene, and grooming. In what ways can the COTA help address these issues?
5. What are five adapted dressing techniques or devices, and what types of children might benefit from using each of them?
6. How could a COTA help a teenager with paraplegia increase independence in wheelchair transfers and community mobility?
7. Describe a variety of ways in which a COTA might intervene with a 6 year old who has sleep problems.
8. How might a COTA intervene to improve room cleaning and cleanup after meals with a bright 12-year-old girl who uses a wheelchair?
9. When learning to use communication devices like a simple communication board or standard keyboard, how could a COTA address a teenager's mild to moderate limitations in the following foundational skills: trunk and neck strength, oculomotor control, and finger isolation? How can this intervention improve the use of communication devices?
10. In the categories of (a) Health Management and Maintenance and (b) Safety Procedures and Emergency Responses and based on your knowledge and opinions, describe the ways in which COTAs can help children with special needs. In which areas do you believe that children who are developing typically need help?
11. In what ways might a COTA help the following children improve financial management and shopping skills: (a) a bright 12 year old with visual impairment, sensory defensiveness, and anxiety and (b) a 19-year-old resident of a group home with moderate mental retardation and mild to moderate spasticity who uses a walker for mobility?
12. Give five examples of ways in which a COTA might help children with poor discrimination of tactile-proprioceptive feedback when they are learning and performing various ADLs and IADLs.
13. Describe five ways in which sensory defensiveness can interfere with children's success in different ADL and IADL areas. Explain how a COTA might intervene.
14. In what ways does the COTA work with the OTR, caregivers, other professionals, and administrators to promote children's independence in ADLs and IADLs?

SUGGESTED *Activities*

1. For 2 to 3 minutes, watch a child with typical development perform an ADL or IADL. Describe in detail the child's postures, sequence of movements, facial expressions, social interaction, responses to sensory or environmental input, eye-hand skills, and any other pertinent observations. How many different actions or behaviors did the child coordinate at one time? Using the same activity, observe a child of about the same age who has disabilities. Describe and compare the two children's results.
2. Using a watch with a second hand, document how often you swallow during a 3-minute period. Then see how long you can go without swallowing and describe what happens.
3. Try holding your nose while eating and describe what happens. Also try eating without closing your lips and describe what happens.
4. Wearing a thick pair of gloves or mittens, try zipping, buttoning, snapping, buckling, tying a bow, cutting with a knife and fork, grooming your hair, and keyboarding. What happens to your motor planning accuracy? Explain the ways in which you compensate for the decreased touch-pressure feedback in your hands.
5. Practice teaching shoe tying or other multistep ADLs to a classmate without using spoken language. Use only visual, tactile, and physical cues. Then describe what happens and ask your classmate for feedback.
6. Using only one hand, perform your typical bathroom routine, including toileting, showering or bathing, applying deodorant, brushing your teeth, and shaving. Which adaptations would make these activities easier?

7. Imagine that you are a child who is able to use only one arm and one leg. Try to dress yourself in clothing with fasteners. Which techniques help you accomplish this? What are the most difficult parts of the activity and why?
8. Following the sequences in the section on Wheelchair Transfers in this chapter, experiment with a classmate in assisting with transfers to and from a real or make-believe wheelchair. Which strategies might work with a teenager and which might not? What adapted techniques or devices would help?
9. Sit on a hard high stool or chair. Do not lean back. Let your arms hang to your sides and let your feet dangle. Try to stay perfectly still, keeping your head upright. Look forward at a visual target. How long are you able to stay comfortable and attentive? List the sensory input or postural changes that might help you. Why do you think these changes would help?
10. Try this activity with a classmate and then ask for feedback. Think of teaching an ADL or IADL activity to a child. List 8 to 10 directions that an adult might give to the child and incorporate negative words such as "no,'" don't" or "never." Then change the directions to use only positive phrases that describe desired actions or behaviors. For example, instead of saying "Don't put them there," try 'Can you show me how to put your socks side by side in the top drawer?"
11. During a class lecture, look around the room to find out what strategies other students use to regulate their own levels of arousal. What are they doing with their hands, hair, mouths, eyes, noses, feet, and the rest of their bodies? What do you do to stay focused during a dull ADL or IADL like balancing your checkbook? What do you do to calm yourself down before or during a challenging ADL or IADL like going to the dentist?
12. Create an assistive device to help train a child in an ADL or IADL. Try one described in this chapter, one from your other studies, or one of your own invention.
13. Think of a simple song to help children remember the steps and increase their enjoyment of ADLs or IADLs.

CHAPTER 18 APPENDIX A

Adapted Clothing Companies

Adrian's Closet
PO Box 9930
Rancho Santa Fe, CA 92067
(800) 831-2577
Fax: (619) 759-0578
http://www.adrianscloset.com/

Aviano USA
1199-K Avenue
Acaso Camarillo, CA 93012
(805) 484-8138
Fax: (805) 484-9789

Kotton Koala
908 West Moffet Creek Road
Fort Jones, CA 96032
(916) 468-5475
Fax: (916) 468-5492

Laurel Designs
5 Laurel Avenue
Belvedere, CA 94920
(415) 435-1891
Fax: (415) 435-1451

Marshons Fashions
PO Box 1848
Calumet City, IL 60409-7848
(708) 849-4610
Fax: (800) 850-4610

MJ Markell Shoe Company
PO Box 246, Main Station
Yonkers, NY 10702-0246
(914) 963-2258
Fax: (914) 963-9293
http://www.markellshoe.com/

Plum Enterprises
PO Box 85
500 Freedom View Lane
Valley Forge, PA 19481-0085
(610) 783-7377
Fax: (610) 783-7577
http://www.plument.com/

CHAPTER 18 APPENDIX B

Computer Teaching Resources

AccuCorp, Inc
PO Box 66
Christiansburg, VA 24073
(703) 961-2001

Aurora Systems
Box 43005
Burnaby, British Columbia V5G-4S2, Canada
(604) 291-6310
(888) 290-1133
Fax: (604) 291-6310
http://www.aurora-systems.com/

Brown Bag Software
2155 South Bascom, Suite 114
Campbell, CA 95008
(408) 559-4545

Bytes of Learning
(800) 465-6428

The Darci Institute of Rehabilitation Engineering
810 West Shepard Lane
Farmington, UT 84025
(801) 451-9191
Fax: (801) 451-9393
http://www.westest.com/darci/index.html

Don Johnston Developmental Equipment
26799 West Commerce Drive
Volo, IL 60073
(800) 999-4660
http://www.donjohnston.com/

Herzog Keyboarding
1433 East Broadway
Tucson, AZ 85719
(520) 792-2550
Fax: (520) 792-2551
http://www.herzogkeyboarding.com/

Infogrip, Inc
1141 East Main Street
Ventura, CA 93001
(800) 397-0921
http://www.infogrip.com/

Intelligent Peripheral Devices, Inc
20380 Town Center Lane, Suite 270
Cupertino, CA 95014
(408) 252-9400

Intellitools, Inc
1720 Corporate Circle
Petaluma, CA 94954
(800) 899-6687
http://www.intellitools.com/

Interplay/Brainstorm
(800) 428-8200

Keytime
5508A Roosevelt Way Northeast
Seattle, WA 98105-3631
(206) 522-TYPE
Fax: (206) 524-2238
http://www.keytime.com/

Knowledge Adventure
2377 Crenshaw Boulevard, Suite 302
Torrance, CA 90501
(310) 533-3400
Fax: (310) 533-3700
http://www.adventure.com/

Macintosh/Apple Computer Systems
PO Box 4040
Cupertino, CA 95014-4040
(800) SOS-APPL
http://www.apple.com/

Madenta Communications, Inc
9411A-20 Avenue
Edmonton, Alberta T6N 1E5, Canada
(800) 661-8406

Microsoft Corporation
One Microsoft Way
Redmond, WA 98052
(800) 876-4726
http://www.microsoft.com/

CHAPTER 18 APPENDIX B—cont'd

Computer Teaching Resources

Perfect Solutions
15950 Schweizer Court
West Palm Beach, FL 33414-7128
(800) 726-7086
Fax: (561) 790-0108
http://www.perfectsolutions.com/

Prentke Romich
1022 Heyl Road
Wooster, OH 44691
(800) 262-1984
http://www.prentrom.com/

Sierra Entertainment, Inc {AU: Street address or PO Box or phone number?}
Bellevue, WA 98007
http://www.sierra.com/corporate_overview.do

Sunburst Communications, Inc
US Payments & Mail Orders, Sunburst Technology
1550 Executive Drive
Elgin, IL 60123
(800) 786-3155
(800) 321-7511
http://store.sunburst.com/

Toolworks
25 Kearny Street, Suite 400
San Francisco, CA 94108
Voice: (415) 733-0990
TTY: (415) 733-0992
Fax: (415) 733-0991
http://www.toolworks.org/pages/home.htm

Words+ Inc
1220 West Avenue J
Lancaster, CA 93534-2902
(800) 869-8521
http://words-plus.com/

CHAPTER 18 APPENDIX C

Adapted Equipment Companies

ABC School Supply, Inc
3312 North Berkeley Lake Road
Box 100019
Duluth, GA 30096-9419
(800) 669-4222

Achievement Products
PO Box 9033
Canton, OH 44711
(800) 373-4699
Fax: (800) 766-4303
http://www.specialkidszone.com/

All the Write News Dixon Ticonderoga Co
PO Box 67096
Los Angeles, CA 90067
(888) 736-4747
Fax: (888) 329-4747

Attainment Company for Children and Adults with Special Needs
PO Box 930160
Verona, WI 53593-0160
(800) 327-4269
http://www.attainmentcompany.com/

Benik Corporation
11871 Silverdale Way Northwest #107
Silverdale, WA 98383
(800) 442-8910
Fax: (360) 692-5600
http://www.benik.com/index.html

Best Priced Products, Inc
PO Box 1174
White Plains, NY 10602
(800) 824-2939
http://www.bpp2.com/Merchant2/merchant.mvc?Screen=SFNT

Callirobics
PO Box 6634
Charlottesville, VA 22906
(800) 769-2891
Fax: (804) 293-9008
http://www.callirobics.com/

Different Roads to Learning, LLC
12 West 18th Street, Suite 3 East
New York, NY 10011
(800) 853-1057
Fax: (800) 317-9146
http://www.difflearn.com/www/index.cfm?action=article.show&id_article=4

Early-Learning Materials
ABC School Supply, Inc
6500 Peachtree Industrial Boulevard
PO Box 4750
Norcross, GA 30091
(800) 247-6623

Equipment Shop
34 Hartford Street
Bedford, MA 01730
(800) 525-7681
http://www.equipmentshop.com/

Free Spirit Publishing, Inc
217 Fifth Avenue North, Suite 200
Minneapolis, MN 55401-1299
(866) 703-7322
Fax: (612) 337-5050
http://www.freespirit.com/

Handwriting without Tears
8001 MacArthur Boulevard
Cabin John, MD 20818
(301) 263-2700
Fax: (301) 263-2707
http://www.hwtears.com/

Imaginart
307 Arizona Street
Bisbee, AZ 85603
(800) 737-1376

Jump-In
1035 Moon Lake Court
Pinckney, MI 48169
(734) 878-0166
Fax: (734) 878-0169

CHAPTER 18 APPENDIX C—cont'd

Adapted Equipment Companies

Kapable Kids
PO Box 250
Bohemia, NY 11716
(800) 356-1564
Fax: (516) 563-7179

The Lockfast Co
10904 Deerfield Road
Cincinnati, OH 45242
(800) 543-7157
Fax: (513) 891-5836

MADDAK, Ableware
661 Route 23 South
Wayne, NJ 07470
(973) 628-7600
Fax: (973) 305-0841
http://service.maddak.com/index.asp

Mealtimes/New Visions
Route 1, Box 175-S
Farber, VA 22938
(804) 361-2285

Milani Foods
2525 West Armitage Avenue
Melrose Park, IL 60160
(708) 450-3354

North Coast Medical
18305 Sutter Boulevard
Morgan Hill, CA 95037-9946
(800) 821-9319
Fax: (877) 213-9300
http://www.ncmedical.com/

OT Ideas
124 Morris Turnpike
Randolph, NJ 07869
(877) 768-4332
Fax: (973) 895-4204
http://www.otideas.com/

Oriental Trading Company, Inc
PO Box 2308
Omaha, NE 68103-2308
(800) 228-2269
Fax: (800) 327-8904

Orvis Fly Fishing Outfitters
PO Box 2861
Vail, CO 81658
(970) 476-3474
http://www.flyfishingoutfitters.net/

PDP Products
14524 61st Street Court North
Stillwater, MN 55082
Fax: (651) 439-0421
http://www.pdppro.com/product.htm

The Pencil Grip
PO Box 67096
Los Angeles, CA 90067
(888) PEN-GRIP
Fax: (310) 315-0607
http://www.thepencilgrip.com/contact.htm

Pocket Full of Therapy
PO Box 174
Morganville, NJ 07751
(800) PFOT-124
http://www.pfot.com/

Pro Ed
8700 Shoal Creek Boulevard
Austin, TX 78757-6897
(800) 897-3202
Fax: (800) 397-7633
http://www.proedinc.com/

Rifton
359 Gibson Hill Road
Chester, NY 10918-2321
(800) 777-4244
Fax: 800-336-5948
http://www.rifton.com/

Sammons Preston/Tumble Forms
PO Box 5071
Bolingbrook, IL 60440-5071
(800) 323-5547

CHAPTER 18 APPENDIX C—cont'd

Adapted Equipment Companies

Slosson Educational Publications, Inc
538 Buffalo Road
East Aurora, NY 14052
(716) 652-0930
Fax: (800) 655-3840
http://www.slosson.com/

Smith & Nephew, Inc
1 Quality Drive
PO Box 1005
Germantown, WI 53022-8205
(800) 558-7681

Southpaw Enterprises
PO Box 1047
Dayton, OH 45401-1047
(800) 228-1698
Fax: (937) 252-8502
http://www.southpawenterprises.com/

Sportime Abilitations
1 Sportime Way
Atlanta, GA 30340
(800) 850-8602
Fax: (800) 845-1535

Stanfield Publishing Co
PO Box 41058
Santa Barbara, CA 93140
(800) 421-6534
http://www.stanfield.com/index2.html

TFH (USA) Ltd
4537 Gibsonia Road
Gibsonia, PA 15044
(800) 467-6222
Fax: (724) 444-6411
http://www.tfhusa.com/

TherAdapt Products, Inc
11431 North Port Washington Road, Suite 105-5
Mequon, WI 53092
(800) 261-4919
Fax: (866) 892-2478
http://www.theradapt.com/theradapt/files/products/index.html

Therapro
225 Arlington Street
Framingham, MA 01702-8723
(800) 257-5376
Fax: (888) 860-6624
http://www.theraproducts.com/

Therapy Skill Builders
(A division of the Psychological Corporation)
355 Academic Court
San Antonio, TX 78204-2498
(800) 211-8378
Fax: (800) 232-1223

Therapy Shoppe
PO Box 8875
Grand Rapids, MI 49518
(800) 261-5590
http://www.therapyshoppe.com/

Toys to Grow On
Lakeshore Curriculum Materials
2695 East Dominguez Street
Carson, CA 90895
(800) 987-4454
Fax: (310) 537-5403
http://www.toystogrowon.com/

Velvasoft
MW Sales and Service, Inc
2549 O'Daniel Road
Seguin, TX 78155
(877) 656-5228
Fax: (830) 379-5411
http://www.world-net.net/home/mwsales/index.html

CHAPTER 18 APPENDIX D

Workshop Sponsors for Continuing Education

If parents are interested in pursuing nutrition as an area of intervention, consider referring them to the following books: *Special Diets for Special Kids*, by Lisa Lewis, PhD, and *Unraveling the Mysteries of Autism and Pervasive Developmental Disorder*, by Karyn Seroussi. Both have helpful recommendations and references for individuals interested in learning more about casein-free, gluten-free, and yeast-free diets. You can also contact The Autism Network for Dietary Intervention, PO Box 17711, Rochester, NY 14617-0711.

AOTA
4720 Montgomery Lane
PO Box 31220
Bethesda, MD 20824-1220
(800) 729-2682

Boehme Workshops
8642 North 66th Street
Milwaukee, WI 53223
(414) 355-8744
Fax: (414) 355-6837
http://boehmeworkshops.com/Default.asp

Clinical Developmental Seminars
6407 Overbrook Avenue
Philadelphia, PA 19151
(215) 879-2929
Fax: (215) 879-9979

Continuing Education Programs of America
PO Box 52
Peoria, IL 61650
(309) 263-0310
http://www.cgiworker.com/cepa/courses.html

Dove Rehabilitation Services
3305 Jerusalem Avenue
Wantagh, NY 11793
(516) 679-3683
http://www.iser.com/dove-NY.html

Education Resources
266 Main Street, Suite 12
Medfield, MA 02052
(800) 487-6530

North American Riding for the Handicapped Association
PO Box 33150
Denver, CO 80234
(303) 452-1212
http://www.narha.org/

Occupational Therapy Associates
124 Watertown Street
Watertown, MA 02472
(617) 923-4410
http://www.otawatertown.com/

OT Kids, Inc
PO Box 1118
Homer, AK 99603
(907) 235-0688
Fax: (907) 235-0688
http://www.alaska.net/~otkids/Webspecials.html

Professional Development Programs
14524 61st Street Court North
Stillwater, MN 55082
(651) 439-8865
Fax: (651) 439-0421
http://www.pdppro.com/

Sensory Integration International
PO Box 5339
Torrance, CA 90510-5339
(310) 787-8805
Fax: (310) 787-8130
http://www.sensoryint.com/

Vital Sounds
PO Box 46344
Madison, WI 53744
(608) 278-9330
Fax: (608) 278-9363
http://www.vitalsounds.com/

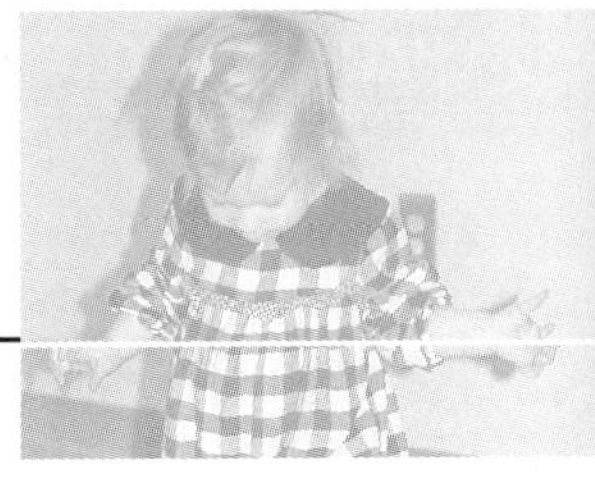

19

Occupation of School: Handwriting

DIANA BAL

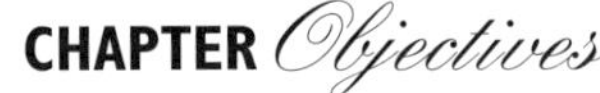

CHAPTER Objectives

After studying this chapter, the reader will be able to accomplish the following:

- After studying this chapter, the reader will be able to accomplish the following:
- Explain how handwriting skills affect the ability of children to perform written assignments in the school setting
- Recognize the client factors required for handwriting
- Identify the reasons handwriting difficulties occur
- Be able to suggest or provide intervention to improve handwriting and written expression

KEY TERMS

Handwriting
Visual perception
Prewriting
Grasping patterns
In-hand manipulation
Proprioception

CHAPTER OUTLINE

The most frequent referral for occupational therapy (OT) in schools is for problems with handwriting abilities.[6] **Handwriting** is an important aspect of a child's educational process because it is the primary way children share and express their academic knowledge. Children who are able to write and express themselves have better academic success and improved self-esteem and show more written creativity.[5]

In kindergarten the child is expected to be able to form letters, write his or her name, and copy words from a vertical surface. In first grade, the child sits at a desk and writes words on lined paper. In elementary school 30% to 60% of the school day is dedicated to the completion of fine motor tasks such as writing, using scissors, and keyboarding.[15]

Difficulties with handwriting may interfere with taking tests and completing written assignments. Such difficulties as poor letter formation, spacing, and organization of words on a page may interfere with learning. The teaching of letter formation is frequently discontinued after the third grade. Fifth graders are expected to complete written assignments in cursive formation spontaneously, without struggling with letter formation or organization of the letters on the page.

Handwriting is the tool teachers use to measure a child's academic abilities. It allows children to express themselves, learn information, organize their work, and communicate with others. Therefore, OT practitioners working in schools must address handwriting difficulties in order to improve the child's performance.

EVALUATION AND ASSESSMENT OF HANDWRITING SKILLS

Dominick attends the third grade. His parents have provided him with a day planner to write all his assignments down so that he can complete his homework. However, he frequently forgets to write this down, and when he does the letters are often illegible. As a result, his parents are not able to help him with his homework. The teacher reminds the class to write the assignments down; she sees Dominick writing.

During language tasks Dominick struggles to write about what he did over the weekend. Other children write paragraphs, smiling as they reminisce about such activities as playing with friends, going to the movies, and sliding. Dominick looks concerned and stressed. His hand hurts, and he feels inferior to the others in the class. He completes one illegible sentence, hands the paper to his teacher, and slowly walks back to his desk. Other students are frantically writing. Dominick starts to tell others about his weekend. The teacher reprimands him for being "off task." An OT consultation is scheduled to address Dominick's handwriting difficulties.

This case depicts the multilayered aspects involved in handwriting. OT practitioners are trained to evaluate, intervene, and provide classroom strategies to help children succeed in academic occupations.

Handwriting requires an evaluation of developmental, motor, sensory, and perceptual functioning. Observation and analysis of the child's hand skills allow the OT practitioner to ascertain the cause of the handwriting problem as it relates to occupational performance within the school context. Formal and informal assessments of the ability to imitate and copy lines and shapes, hold a pencil or tool, and complete perceptual motor and sensory modulation tasks help to identify the factors for intervention. Figures 19-1 and 19-2 are examples of checklists to identify whether a child has the prerequisites for handwriting.

The OT practitioner is responsible for evaluating all aspects of handwriting; designing intervention or compensatory strategies; and consulting with children, teachers, and parents. The goal of OT in the school is to promote participation in the general educational curriculum. As such, teachers and parents benefit from recommendations to enhance handwriting skills. Compensations and accommodations allow the student to be successful in the classroom or home (refer to the section on classroom accommodations later in this chapter).

Standardized Assessments

Standardized assessments are used to determine the factors interfering with handwriting skills. A variety of them are available to provide objective data on the aspects of handwriting.

Developmental Assessments

These tests examine the developmental level of a child's handwriting abilities. For example, in the case of Dominick, the assessment can answer the following question: Does Dominick have the handwriting abilities required of a third grader?

The Peabody Developmental Motor Scale–2 evaluates copying and writing readiness skills and provides an age-equivalent score on grasp development, manual dexterity, and developmental writing skills. The *Hawaii Early Learning Profile* (HELP) can be used to examine pre-handwriting skills for children 0 to 3 years of age. This developmental checklist is helpful in tracking the development of hand skills. *The Bayley Scale of Infant Development* assesses the motor development of children from 1 to 42 months of age. *The Erhardt Prehension Assessment* measures the components of arm and hand development in children. The *Bruininks-Oseretsky Test of*

Name : ______________________________ Date: ______________

1. Describe class work compared with the other students in class

2. Describe posture at the desk

Desk height 2" above bent elbow ____ Feet on floor ____ Wrist stable ____

Body symmetrical ____ Head aligned ____ Trunk upright ____

3. Imitation of whole body motions in a timely manner without touching:

Straighten arms over head ____

Stretch arms out to side ____

Cross arms in front of body ____

Right arm straight, bend left elbow ____ Left arm straight, bend right elbow ____

Shift arms and hands from one side of the body to the other ____

X midline of body with arms/hands ____

4. Imitation of hand and finger motions in a timely manner without prompts:

Rotate wrist ____

Open and shut fingers/thumb ____

Touch thumb to fingers ____ when told which finger to touch ____

Move each finger separately imitatively ____ when told which finger to move ____

Routine finger songs (Thumbkin, Itsy Spider) ____

5. Grasp on pencil: Static ____ Dynamic ____

fingers on pencil ____ Distal thumb ____ Pressure on paper ____

FIGURE 19-1 Handwriting checklist—manuscript.

Open web space ____ Distal control ____ Wrist stable ____

6. Hold down paper ____

7. Reversals ____

list

8. Hand dominance ____

R L

9. Write the following sentence on paper with lines and evaluate the following:

"The dirty plane flies up high into the sky"

Curved lines	Rounded	Straight
Sentence begins with capital		Ends with punctuation
All other letters lower case		Start “d” with a “c”
% letters initiated at top		% letters and words going left to right
% letters on the line		% spaces between words

10. Visual perceptual test results:

FIGURE 19-1, cont'd. Handwriting checklist—manuscript.

Name: ____ Date: _____________

1. Describe class work compared with the other students in class.

2. Describe posture at the desk.

Desk height 2" above bent elbow ____ Feet on floor ____ Wrist stable ____

Body symmetrical ____ Head aligned ____ Trunk upright ____

3. Imitation of whole body motions in a timely manner without touching:

Straighten arms over head ____

Stretch arms out to side ____

Cross arms in front of body ____

Right arm straight, bend left elbow ____ Left arm straight, bend right elbow ____

Shift arms and hands from one side of the body to the other ____

X midline of body with arms/hands ____

4. Imitation of hand and finger motions in a timely manner without prompts:

Rotate wrist ____

Open and shut fingers/thumb ____

Touch thumb to fingers ____ when told which finger to touch ____

Move each finger separately imitatively ____ when told which finger to move ____

Routine finger songs (Thumbkin, Itsy Spider) ____

5. Write the following sentence on paper with lines and evaluate the following:

"The brown dog wags his fat tail"

FIGURE 19-2 Handwriting checklist—cursive.

Curved lines	Smooth	On same slant	Rounded
Sentence begins with capital		End with punctuation	
All other letters lower case		All letters in word connect	
% letters starting at line		% letters and words going left to right	
% letters on the line		% spaces between words	

6. Grasp on pencil: Static ____ Dynamic ____

fingers on pencil ____ Distal thumb ____ Pressure on paper ____

Open web space ____ Distal control ____ Wrist stable ____

7. Hold down paper ____

8. Reversals ____

list:

9. Hand dominance ____

R L

10. Visual perceptual test results:

FIGURE 19-2, cont'd. Handwriting checklist—cursive.

Motor Proficiency measures the gross and fine motor proficiencies of children $4^1/_2$ to $14^1/_2$, testing such areas as response speed, upper limb speed, and visual motor control.

Visual perception assessments

Visual perception is the ability to organize and interpret what is seen. Handwriting requires children to visually perceive the organization of letters and spacing between words. They must also determine the direction of letters (e.g., *b* compared with *d*). Visual perception is required to know where to start writing on the page and how to sequence letters and space words. During handwriting, children must recognize that the size of a letter does not change its meaning. Dominick may be experiencing poor visual perception. In this scenario he is unable to make sense of how letters are formed. Dominick may not recognize the differences among *b*, *p*, and *d*.

The *Test of Visual Motor Integration–Revised* combines both the developmental sequencing of the geometric shapes and visual motor integration. The *Motor-Free Visual Perception Test–Revised* and the *Test of Visual Perceptual Skills* (nonmotor) (TVPS) measure nonmotor visual perception in children by testing visual perception without requiring a motor response. These tests examine the following perceptual skills.

- *Discrimination*: The ability to detect a difference or distinction between one item or picture and another
- *Visual Memory*: The ability to remember a shape or word and recall the information when necessary. In handwriting children must remember how to form letters, string them together, and develop paragraphs.
- *Form Constancy*: The ability to realize and recognize that forms, letters, and numbers are the same or constant whether they are moved, turned, or changed to a different size. This means that a square is always a square no matter what size or color.
- *Sequential Memory*: The ability to remember a sequence or chain of letters to form a word. For handwriting, children need motor as well as cognitive sequencing. Therefore, they need the ability to remember how letters make words and sequence them according to their motor capacities to make those words.
- *Figure Ground*: The ability to identify foreground from the background. When looking at pictures, people, or items, it is essential to separate the important visual aspects from the background. During handwriting, children identify written words on lined paper.
- *Visual Closure*: The ability to identify forms or objects when given an incomplete appearance. This enables a child to figure out objects, shapes, and forms by finishing the image mentally, such as finding a jacket when it is partially covered by others. This is required in cases in which the letter may not be completely formed.

Handwriting assessments

The *Children's Handwriting Evaluation Scales* (CHES-S and CHES) measure the speed and quality of the child's handwriting skills.[16] *The Evaluation Tool of Children's Handwriting* (ETCH) evaluates legibility and speed in six areas of handwriting: alphabet production of lower and uppercase letters from memory, numeral writing of 1 to 12 from memory, near- and far-point copying, speed, and sentence composition in both manuscript and cursive formation.[15] The ETCH provides legibility scores compared with the child's age level.

CLASSROOM OBSERVATIONS

Classroom observations allow OT practitioners to see children work, organize their work/desk surface, and use their time. When evaluating a child's handwriting, observation of the child's performance in the classroom is beneficial.

Classroom observation allows the OT practitioner to view the occupation (e.g., handwriting) in the context in which it occurs. Understanding the child's performance within the context of the classroom guides the intervention plan. For example, examination of the *physical* context provides information on such things as classroom space, seating arrangements, the height of the desk, visual stimuli, and environmental supports. Dominick may be sitting in a chair that is too high, and the classroom space may not be conducive to writing. In terms of *personal* context, classroom observation may reveal information about Dominick's needs. Perhaps he is easily distracted by the noise outside the door. OT practitioners will want to consider the writing demands of a third grade classroom as well as Dominick's temperament and attitude toward the writing task. From the case study we know that Dominick looks concerned and stressed during writing assignments, providing the clinician with a window into his feelings. *Temporal* context refers to the time of day in which the handwriting is performed. Classroom observation may provide insight into how Dominick is managing his time as well. *Cultural* context refers to classroom expectations. How organized is the teacher? Are accommodations a natural part of the classroom? Is the environment conducive to working on handwriting? *Virtual* context, or the use of computers in the classroom, may be beneficial to children with handwriting difficulties. *Social* context refers to the child's ability to interact with others in the classroom.

OT practitioners are interested in learning whether the child is able to participate in social interaction and whether the environment supports the child. Is the classroom too busy for a child who requires quiet writing time? Is the child able to interact easily with his or her peers? Does the family support the child's ability to write?

Classroom observations provide valuable information on what may be interfering with function in the classroom. Teachers are able to provide OT practitioners with information concerning the child's performance in the classroom, classroom expectations, and possible solutions.

CLINICAL *Pearl*

Visual or auditory distractions in the classroom may interfere with visual attention to handwriting tasks.

CLINICAL *Pearl*

Asking teachers and families what strategies they have used in the past saves time. Matching strategies to the classroom is effective.

DEVELOPMENTAL SEQUENCE

Referrals for handwriting are made based on children not performing at age-appropriate standards. Teachers notice that the child is not as fluent, clear, or legible as his or her classmates. OT practitioners are called in to determine the developmental level the child is functioning at and the cause(s) for the handwriting difficulties so that they can design appropriate intervention. Development occurs through the learning, experiencing, and acquisiion of the skills. The rate of development and the progression of skills vary in children but usually follow sequential patterns.

Prewriting

As the name suggests, **prewriting** skills (also known as writing readiness skills) are prerequisites for handwriting. Prewriting depends on the development of sensory, cognitive, and motor systems. It helps children develop the strength, in-hand manipulation skills, and coordination required for handwriting. Prewriting skills begin with children scribbling with their hands in their food, using a spoon as a tool, and leads to holding a crayon and making unrefined strokes and marks on the paper. This progresses to the imitation and copying of specific lines and shapes. Mastery of basic figures (e.g., circle, square, triangle, cross) is essential for manuscript and cursive handwriting.[1] Table 19-1 outlines the developmental sequencing of prewriting and handwriting skills.

TABLE 19-1

Developmental Sequencing of Prewriting and Handwriting Skills According to the Peabody Developmental Motor Scale–2

ITEM NAME	AGE (MONTHS)
Stirring spoon	12
Scribbling—1 scribble 1 inch long	14
Imitating vertical line 2 inches long	23-24
Imitating horizontal line 2 inches long	27-28
Copying circle—end points within 1/2 inch of each other	33-34
Copying cross—intersecting lines within 20° of perpendicular	39-40
Tracing line—deviates <2 times	41-42

Grasping Patterns

Children with handwriting difficulties show a less mature grasp, immature pencil grip, and inconsistent hand preference.[5] The most mature grasps are the dynamic tripod (Figure 19-3, *A*) and lateral tripod. The lateral quadrupod and four-finger grip can be as functional as the dynamic tripod, lateral tripod, and dynamic quadrupod pencil grips in fourth graders.[11]

Dynamic tripod grasps use finger movements rather than the whole hand or arm. When forming a letter, dynamic movement of the fingers creates smooth curves. Awkward grasping patterns result in poor letter formation, fatigue, and poor handwriting. Hank holds the pencil tightly with minimum web space and a cross thumb grasp (Figure 19-3, *B*). The resulting strain and contraction of the wrist and finger muscles may cause pain, fatigue, and discomfort.

Knowledge of the progression of **grasping patterns** is useful to the practitioner evaluating handwriting. Cross thumb or static tripod grasps can be fatiguing or painful and yet offer more stability and power. Tight grasps limit the variety of movements and make smooth, flowing motions difficult. Writers using tight grasps often press hard on the paper, resulting in dark, sometimes smeared letters.

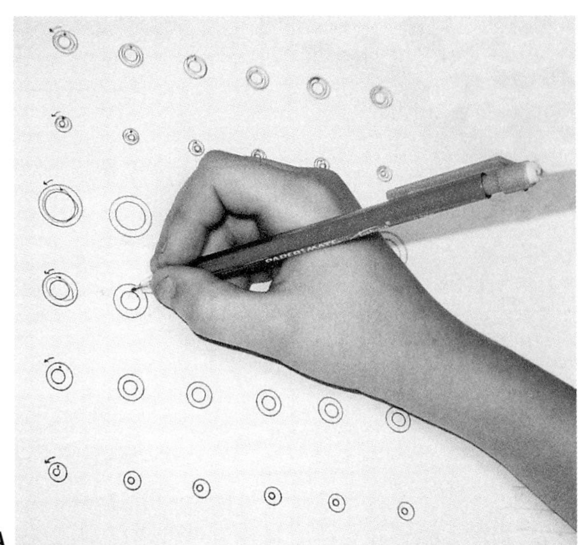

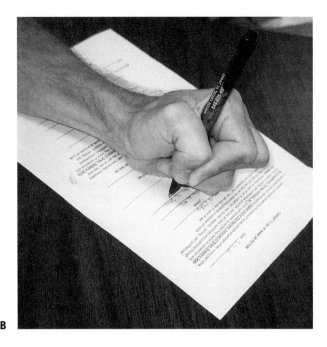

FIGURE 19-3 **A,** Dynamic tripod grasp. **B,** Cross thumb grasp.

CLINICAL *Pearl*

Many adults use a variety of pencil grasps with minimum web space and a very tight grasping pattern. Look around and observe the variety of grasping patterns that are used.

In-Hand Manipulation

In-hand manipulation refers to the precise and skilled finger movements made during fine motor tasks. To perform in-hand manipulation, the child needs to be able to adjust objects within the hand while maintaining the grasp of the object. In-hand manipulation skills during handwriting are observed when a child rotates the pencil to use the eraser. Another example is manipulating the pencil to write dynamically with a tripod grasp while the ring and little fingers remain still to stabilize the hand. In-hand manipulation requires strength, timing, and coordination.

CLINICAL *Pearl*

Children with Down syndrome tend to use their third finger and thumb to pick up small objects because their thumb does not curve, or oppose, enough to reach the index finger.[4]

CLINICAL *Pearl*

Look at how the tool, spoon, or pencil is given to a child. The child's handedness can be influenced by offering him or her the item consistently on one side of the body or to one hand. Frequently, when a right-handed parent sits opposite a child to feed him or her, s/he will tend to use the left hand for self-feeding. It is important to present items in the middle of the child's body.

INTERVENTION USING A DEVELOPMENTAL FRAME OF REFERENCE

A developmental frame of reference suggests starting at the level at which the child is comfortable and providing opportunities to develop the next level of skills. For example, a typical handwriting session, in which a developmental frame of reference is used, may include the following scenario.

The OT practitioner used the HELP to determine the most advanced skill that Trey accomplished. The practitioner determined that Trey was able to imitate a circle but unable to imitate a vertical stroke. In therapy, the practitioner played maze games with Trey. They had to move their fingers "down the winding road" in the sand and follow the snake by moving a piece of yarn through a trough; finally, they played a paper and pencil game of drawing lines. The

OT practitioner provided the teacher and parents with activities to promote this skill at home. (See Chapter 20 for a description of the normal sequence of hand skills.)

Developmental Activities

- Follow the developmental sequence as outlined in the Peabody Developmental Motor Scale–2 or HELP. Perform the listed developmental visual motor tasks, such as cutting with scissors.
- Trace simple line drawings, such as beginning shape designs. The lines of the shapes can be emphasized by highlighting them with a magic marker and then outlining with white glue. The glue will dry clear, making a raised border highlighted to call attention to the lines.
- Draw a line between two horizontal lines, two stickers, or two matching pictures.
- Tap a ball that is suspended on a string from a stick, moving the hands rhythmically.
- Using water, rice, beans, or bingo magnetic chips as the contents, pour those contents from one container into another.
- Use special handwriting paper to emphasize and highlight the lines with embossed, raised lines. The top line could be green and the bottom line red to indicate the boundaries.
- Color within a designated area; use a template to cover the area not to be colored, and put emphasis on that area.
- Have the child copy and imitate designs and body motions. S/he can imitate body motions as s/he moves from one location to another.
- Work with a variety of tools, such as screwdrivers, hammers, and tongs, encouraging one-handed working with the other hand stabilizing the object.
- Cut putty and paper with scissors to work on a one-handed task designed to strengthen the intrinsic muscles of the hand and further develop tool usage.

Named Activities

- Clip it up: Place paper clips on cardboard or paper. This can be a difficult task because of the need to motor-plan how to place the clip on the paper and then coordinate the two hands to secure the paper clip. A prerequisite for this task should be to clip a clothespin to secure the paper because clothespins are larger and the end can be colored or highlighted for finger placement.
- Feed me: Place coins in a narrow vertical slot, encouraging finger/thumb prehension and wrist rotation. Initially the placement of a coin in a horizontal slot is easier, so rotate the container slightly until the vertical slot is achieved.
- Manipulate me: Dump out the contents of the container on the table. Pick up a penny, button, and paper clip. Place them in a pan and then sort out one item at a time. Do this with vision occluded and using only one hand.
- Scarf throw: Throw scarves up in the air and catch them with both hands and then with one hand or turn and catch. Attach various weighted objects to increase the rate of fall.
- Toss it up: Toss a beanbag or ball from one hand to the other while holding the head still and watching the beanbag.

EVALUATION AND INTERVENTION OF MOTOR SKILLS

Motor skills play an important role in handwriting. Poor grip strength, contractions, and other factors may interfere with a child's handwriting.

For example, consider Brittany, who sits slumped in her chair and leaning to the right with her shoulders elevated and retracted. She holds the pencil tightly and is unable to use her left arm to stabilize her paper; instead, she is holding onto her chair seat. Brittany expends her energy staying upright, making smooth, fine motor movements (such as those needed for handwriting) difficult.

This case illustrates the importance of examining the motor skills required for handwriting.

Range of Motion

The OT practitioner evaluates the range of motion (ROM) available for the trunk, elbows, shoulders, wrist, and fingers. Contractures or limitations in ROM may interfere with the smooth, coordinated movements required for handwriting.

Integrity of arm, hand, and fingers

OT practitioners examine the integrity of the arm, hand, and fingers to determine whether deformities, edema, or open wounds are interfering with handwriting. For example, children with juvenile rheumatoid arthritis may experience periods of pain and edema in the joints that will interfere with writing.

Shoulder, wrist, and finger stability

Children must be able to hold the shoulder steady to use the wrist and fingers for writing. Sometimes children retract or "fix" their shoulders to keep them steady. This makes it difficult to write effectively. Wrist stability refers to the ability of the child to keep the wrist in one position. Wrist stability is important for the child to perform precise hand skills. A stable wrist position allows the child to move the fingers more efficiently. The wrist should be straight or slightly extended while writing. Using a vertical surface rather than a horizontal one promotes the development of wrist extension and strengthens arm and shoulder muscles.[21]

For example, try to use a hammer with a flexed wrist. The hammer cannot be securely held or controlled because the hand is not in a power-grasping pattern. The wrist, in a slightly extended posture, stabilizes the hand while using a tool.

CLINICAL *Pearl*

The sequence of the typical development of tool usage is provided below.

Initially children move the whole arm with shoulder movements while holding the utensil in a grasping pattern with the thumb and index finger toward the paper.
Movement occurs at the forearm, with the shoulder more stable.
The upper arm and forearm are more stable as movement occurs primarily at the wrist and with the whole hand.
Movement occurs at the metacarpal joints of all the fingers or with a static tripod grasp.
Finally, dynamic movement occurs at the thumb and index finger, with the middle finger stabilizing the writing utensil and the ring and little fingers stabilizing and maintaining the wrist angle.

Children must be able to hold the finger joints steady when writing. OT practitioners must examine how much control the child has in keeping his or her fingers in position. Children who cannot stabilize their joints will have difficulty with fine motor movements.

Posture

Children must be able to sustain an upright seating posture during writing. This requires strength and stability of the trunk. Leaning on the forearms for trunk stability impedes the ability to write effectively and may cause difficulty when using the nondominant hand to secure the paper.

Posture can be easily influenced by the height of the desk and chair. Although some teachers want classroom desks to be the same height, students are not the same size and require different-sized desks. The best sitting position is with the hips and knees at 90 degrees, the feet flat on the floor with the ankles at 90 degrees, and the desk at a height of 2 inches above the flexed elbow.[2]

Children must make postural adjustments during writing. If Brittany cannot automatically adjust to subtle changes while writing, she may have poor penmanship.

CLINICAL *Pearl*

Because children flex forward slightly while writing, those with poor trunk control may benefit from sitting at an angle of less than 90 degrees.

Strength and Endurance

Hand strength and endurance are required for performing the complex tasks of handwriting. Children must move their hands and bodies automatically. Students must be able to sustain motor movements over time to complete the required assignments. By the fifth grade, handwriting should be so automatic that the child is able to concentrate on written expression and not the mechanics of writing.

The *arches* of the hand are formed as the hand muscles develop. They shape the hand for grasping different-sized objects, allow for skilled movements of the fingers, and control the power and force of prehension. This force is modulated to pick up fragile items without breaking them, such as a pencil. Children with poorly developed hand arches have flat, underdeveloped, weak hands. The lack of hand arching interferes with the strength and development of the hand because the intrinsic muscles are not adequately developed.

When the arches are well developed, the hand is able to form a bowl in the palm and the creases in the palm are distinctly observed. Children with poorly developed arches may compensate by holding the pencil tightly against the palm, showing no web space.

Hand strength that is adequate to hold objects and the endurance to repeat motor patterns without fatiguing are important for writing tasks. The process of writing is continuous. Therefore, promoting optimum muscle strength and endurance for the task is an excellent initiation for the treatment of handwriting.

CLINICAL *Pearl*

To work at a table with a writing tool, the child's posture must be prepared and ready to work. Abnormal muscle tone interferes with body symmetry and positioning. Low muscle tone leads to fatigue and a lack of endurance for the task. Children may exhibit hand tremors, and children with low muscle tone may have hand tremors and lack the endurance for the task.

INTERVENTION USING A BIOMECHANICAL FRAME OF REFERENCE

Children with ROM limitations, poor hand strength, and poor endurance benefit from a biomechanical approach. The following is an example of an intervention session to increase handwriting skills by using a biomechanical approach.

The OT practitioner performs an ROM assessment (manual muscle strength) and determines how long the child is able to perform handwriting tasks without fatiguing. S/he examines the child's posture and makes the necessary adaptations to seating so that the child can sit in an upright position for handwriting. Next the OT practitioner addresses the ROM limitations through gentle stretching techniques, splinting, or serial casting if necessary. The session begins with a warm-up and then strengthening activities and ends with a "cool-down" period consisting of functional handwriting. Strengthening activities are designed to be fun for the child (see the following intervention activities) and are graded to challenge him or her. The OT practitioner works with the child to improve his or her handwriting endurance by increasing the writing time and decreasing the breaks. The length of endurance to be reached is dependent on the child's grade level and teacher expectations. Generally, children in the fifth grade write for 20 minutes continuously. However, children write throughout the day with frequent breaks. The practitioner may decide to emphasize the speed of the child's writing as well. In this scenario the child would work to write a certain amount of words in an allotted time period. This may in fact help the child function best in the classroom.

Motor Activities

- Have the child lie on his or her stomach to strengthen the back and upper trunk. Mike has low muscle tone in the trunk (Figure 19-4, *A*). He also has very poor ability to sustain trunk and neck extension. Working on the ball in a prone position optimizes body alignment and trunk extension. Facilitated handling to provide support to the elbows and co-contraction to the shoulders strengthens Mike's upper trunk and shoulders (Figure 19-4, *B*).
- Bounce the child on the ball to provide vestibular stimulation and joint proprioception to increase muscle tone throughout and to make the body ready for the occupational performance of sitting and writing (Figure 19-5, *A*).
- Swing the child on a suspended piece of equipment to provide vestibular stimulation and promote muscle tone. Using a bolster swing encourages Mike to hold on tight, strengthening his upper trunk and shoulder muscles (Figure 19-5, *B*). Mike loves swinging, which makes it an excellent tool to start the session and a wonderful reinforcement when he has completed working.
- Have the child pick up items with gentle hand-over-hand assistance to promote a thumb–index finger grasping pattern and flexing of the ring and little fingers. Provide hand over hand assistance to place the pencil in the optimum and most dynamic position in the child's hand.
- Have the child pinch a zip lock bag with the thumb and fingertips to promote finger strength and fingertip control. Put therapy activities in these bags to promote opening and closing with each task.

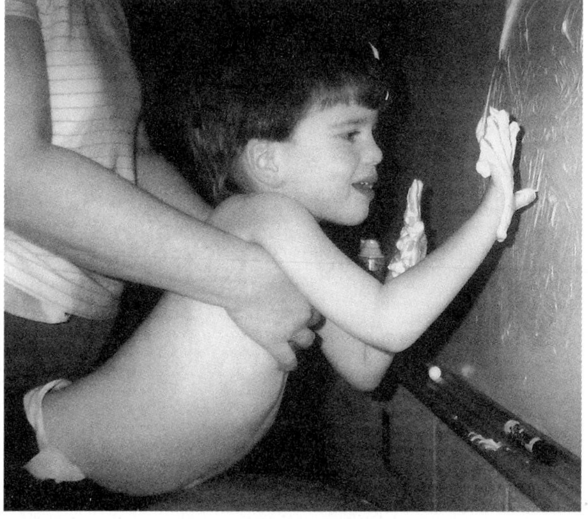

A

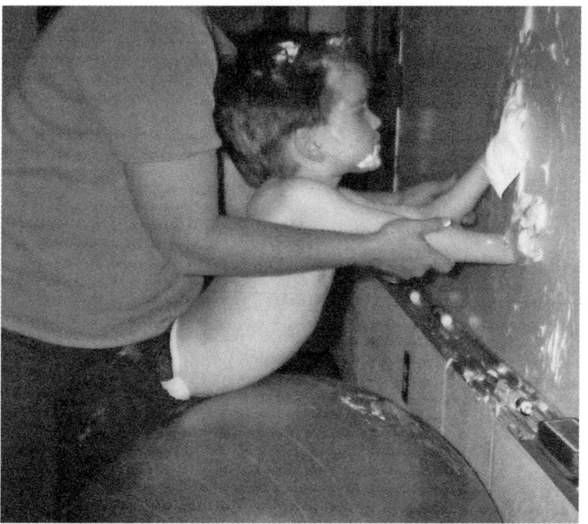

B

FIGURE 19-4 **A,** Low muscle tone in the trunk. **B,** Working on the ball in a prone position optimizes body alignment and trunk extension.

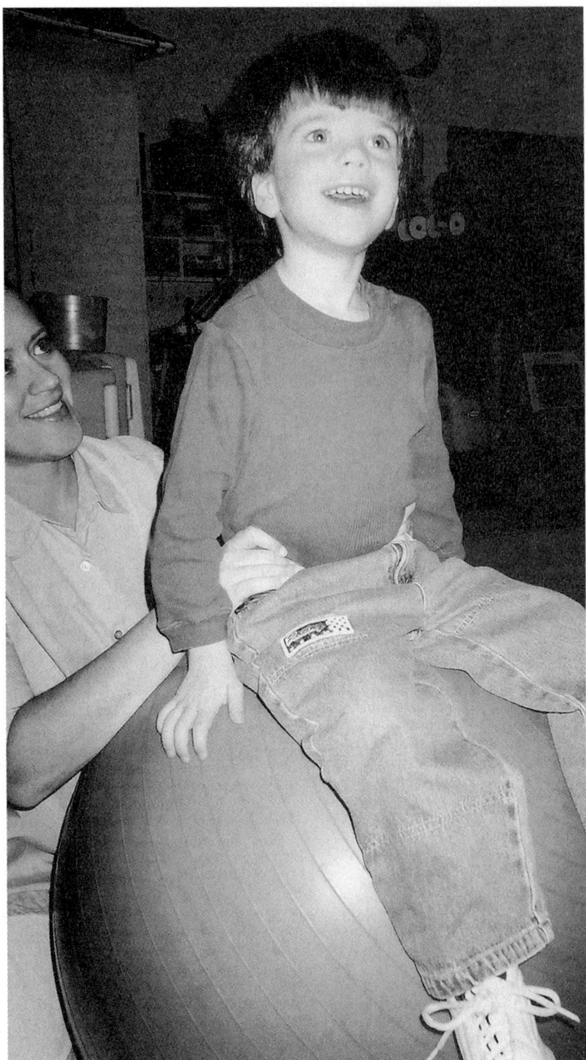
A

B

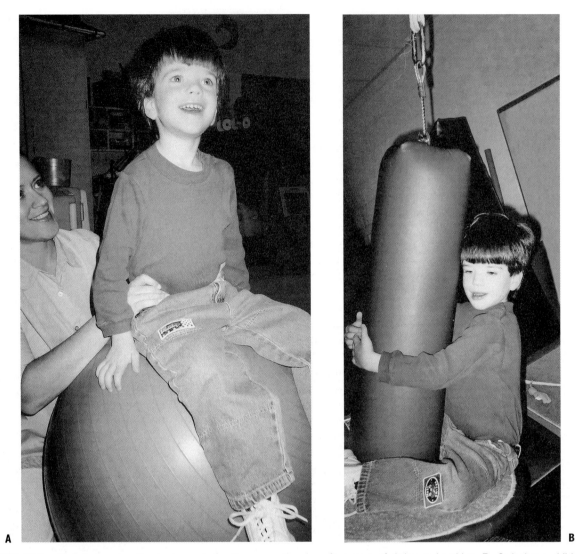

FIGURE 19-5 A, A ball makes the body ready for the occupational performance of sitting and writing. **B,** Swinging a child on a suspended piece of equipment provides vestibular stimulation to promote muscle tone.

- Have the child crumple and throw away trash. This activity works on hand movements and coordination.
- Commercially available programs have been developed to promote handwriting readiness. Diana Henry's *Tool Chest: For Teachers, Parent's, Students, and Teens* provides activities to promote a child's sensory needs and alertness in the classroom.[11] *Brain Gym* provides techniques that encourage movement and the integration of both sides of the body and crossing the midline.[8]
- Thread pegs or string beads on small eyehooks to encourage thumb and index finger prehension. Attaching the pegboard to the wall and vertically orienting it promote grasping and upper trunk strengthening (Figure 19-6).
- Arm strengthening and prone activities decrease arm tremors. Use wrist weights of varying heaviness, removing them when writing is finished so that accommodation cannot occur. These can also be made with fishing weights sewn onto neoprene. Another option is to glue magnets onto a wristband and place paper on a metal sheet (e.g., cookie sheet) to stabilize the wrist or use a commercially weighted pencil. (Commercially weighted pencils may be too large and often difficult for children to grasp.)
- A pencil gripper (Box 19-1) or a small pencil encourages a tripod grasp.[15] Large bulb-shaped grippers facilitate open web space. This may also be accomplished by wrapping a rubber band around the pencil at the grip site.[7] Many classrooms have a generic pencil basket, so the child does not have his or her own storage place. Providing a bag that attaches to the back of the child's chair frequently

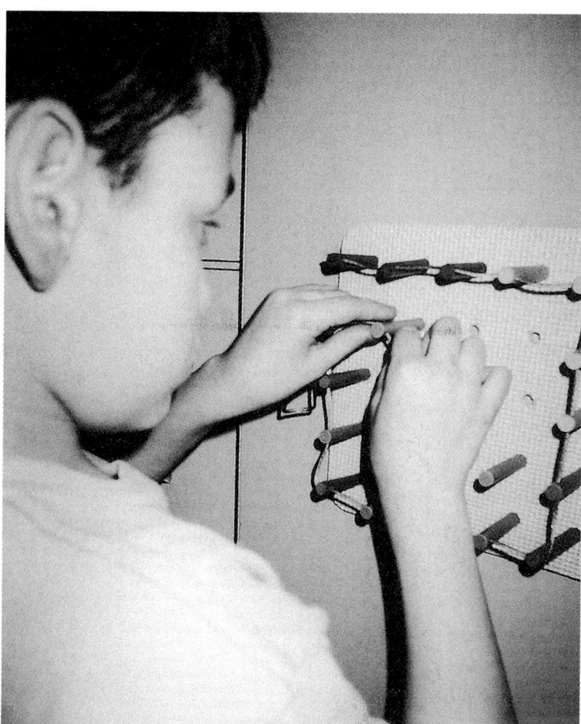

FIGURE 19-6 Grasping and upper trunk strengthening is promoted with the use of a pegboard.

helps with organization and keeping track of purchased pencil grippers.

Named Activities

Naming the activity so that it can be a routine in the child's daily occupational performance is both beneficial and fun. These activities may be organized as centers in a classroom and wonderfully fun home programs.

- *Squirrel Away.* Put objects into the child's hand. Have him or her try to keep the fingers closed while another child or adult tries to pry the fingers open to get the item out of the hand.
- *Pick a Hand.* Have the child hide an object in one hand and try to get another child to decide which hand the object is in.
- *Clip Away.* Clip clothespins onto a clothespin tree made of an old coffee cup holder. This activity encourages an open thumb, web space, and finger strengthening. Clip cards onto the clothesline in numerical order or flash cards in alphabetical order. Paint the clothespins with different colors to promote sorting by color. Clip together clothespins and small tiles that have the letters of the alphabet written on them in order to promote matching.

BOX 19-1

Companies That Have Pencil Grips and Handwriting Supplies

OT IDEAS, INC
124 Morris Turnpike
Randolph, NJ 07868
973-895-3622
www.otideas.com

POCKET FULL OF THERAPY
PO Box 174
Morganville, NJ 07751
723-441-0404
www.pfot.com/

SAMMONS PRESTON, AN ABILITYONE COMPANY
PO Box 5071
Bolingbrook, IL 60440-5071
800-323-5547
www.sammonspreston.com

THERAPRO PRODUCTS
225 Arlington St
Framingham, MA 01702
800-257-5376
www.theraproducts.com

THERAPY SHOPPE, INC
PO Box 8875
Grand Rapids, MI 49518
800-261-5590
www.therapyshoppe.com

LOCAL WAL-MART, K-MART, OR OFFICE SUPPLY COMPANY

- *Snakes and Snails.* Use putty to roll out 10 1-inch snakes and then place a penny in each snake. The snakes and penny then become a snail. When all the snails are made, hold the penny with the ring and little fingers against palm of the hand and roll a round ball with the putty into a ball with the thumb, index, and middle finger.
- *Tongs to You.* Use vegetable tongs or tweezers with scissor handles to pick up a variety of objects. Use the tongs to sort the items or objects by color or classification, such as cotton balls, blocks, or toys. Tongs that are commercially made to color Easter eggs can be purchased.
- *Hammer Down.* Use the dominant hand to hold on to a hammer to push golf tees into Styrofoam, balls into a cylinder, or pegs into a pegboard.

- *Open Me Up.* Open and close tubes or jar lids and turn knobs or turn over objects (pennies or cards) to encourage precision rotation skills. This task can be graded and made harder or easier with different-sized jars and lids or by loosening and tightening the lid. Placing items in these jars for the task that the child is going to work on makes the task functional and meaningful.
- *Take Me Off.* Put a variety of refrigerator magnets on a metal sheet. This task can be graded for difficulty by using stronger magnets to promote thumb-finger grasping patterns in picking or pulling the magnets off. Use magnets that are commercially made and have kitchen items on them to encourage language and functional skills.
- *Cut Me Up.* Use a pizza cutter or plastic knife to cut Play Doh or cut apart Velcro fruit or Velcro checkers that can be purchased or made.
- *Wrap Me.* Wrap masking tape around one hand and use the other hand to remove the tape.

EVALUATION AND INTERVENTION OF SENSORY PROCESSING SKILLS

Midline Crossing

Fluent handwriting requires that one cross the midline of the body without hesitation. Failure to cross the midline is a sign that the nervous system is not mature and the child is experiencing difficulties. Indications that a student is avoiding crossing the midline of the body include starting to write in the center of the paper, switching hands while writing, and poorly established hand dominance. Children may scoot over to one side of the seat or shift the paper over to the side of the table rather than cross the midline of the body.

Eye-Hand Coordination

Eye-hand coordination or visual-motor integration requires the child to visually observe his hand as it moves in a controlled fashion. Children with poor handwriting skills score lower on eye-hand coordination tasks than those with adequate handwriting skills.[5]

Visual Perception Skills

Many of the difficulties in learning letters or word recognition skills are due to a lack of understanding of the relationship between the perceptual elements presented and the other letters or words. In order to write, children need to recognize and perceive the letter forms and understand their differences and similarities. Children who do not perform well on the visual perception tests in the areas of visual memory and visual-motor integration typically have poor handwriting skills.[20]

Directionality

Directionality, or the understanding of which way to go or move the pencil, is essential for handwriting because writing is performed left to right and top to bottom, with some letters placed on the line and some under the line. Forming letters in the correct direction, orienting them on the page, and starting or stopping letters at the right location are essential for handwriting.

Motor Planning

Children with poor handwriting skills may have deficits in motor planning (i.e., figuring out how to move their bodies and then actually doing it) or motor memory (i.e., remembering the motor patterns and being able to repeat them).

Motor planning problems may be due to **proprioception** (awareness of muscle and joint positions). Children with motor planning difficulties are unable to maneuver around their school environment without bumping into other people or knocking things down. Sometimes walking in line or not running into other children or the wall can be a challenge. If walking down the hall in a smooth, coordinated manner is difficult, then doing a refined task such as moving a pencil around a piece of paper and creating letters is also. Smooth writing requires the ability to motor-plan the separation and isolation of finger movements for dynamic grasping patterns.

A well organized proprioceptive system provides an unconscious awareness of where our bodies are in space. It helps the child understand the touch and movement that they are experiencing. Therefore, the difficulties observed with poor proprioception consist in not knowing where ones arms or hands are positioned in space with the eyes open or closed, finger identification, and finger isolation. Children with poor proprioceptive abilities do not "feel" how much pressure to put on the pencil to hold it; how much pressure to put on the paper can also be the result of proprioceptive difficulties. These children may need to visually monitor or observe where their hands are positioned on the paper.

The *tactile* system plays a key role in handwriting. This important skill requires the ability to feel the pencil and manipulate it without the aid of vision. Some children with handwriting deficits do not feel objects adequately. For example, try writing while wearing mittens. The lack of tactile sensation interferes with one's ability to manipulate the pencil. To feel the pencil, you may have to hold it more tightly. Refined movements are impaired and the writing is messy.

INTERVENTION USING A SENSORY APPROACH

Providing tactile, visual, and auditory stimulation and combining them into handwriting tasks often help children remember the activity. Practitioners evaluate the sensory needs of children with the understanding that an inability to process sensory input may interfere with learning. Some children may benefit from a sensory integration approach to remediate their handwriting difficulties, while others require sensory activities.

The following is a sample session in which a sensory integrative frame of reference is used to improve handwriting abilities. The OT practitioner sets up the clinical environment so that the child can choose activities that will help him or her modulate attention (e.g., vestibular and movement activities) and prepare for postural control. This could include fast-moving vestibular activities such as swinging in a net or tire swing and wheelbarrow races.

Once the child is prepared, the practitioner engages in a variety of activities to improve the child's motor planning abilities (e.g., obstacle course, climbing a rope swing). Next, s/he engages in activities to promote hand strength, coordination, and tactile discrimination. Finally, s/he participates in writing tasks. The OT practitioner provides the child with opportunities for success throughout. (See Chapter 21 for more explanation of sensory integration intervention.)

Some handwriting sessions focus on the sensory aspects. In this case, the session may include preparatory tactile activity such as games in which the child has to find hidden objects in rice, water, or sand. These activities may be followed by in-hand manipulation activities using tactile media such as Play-Doh or Theraputty. The child may use a brushing technique to desensitize the hand. Other sensory activities may include participating in finger painting or writing over sandpaper for proprioceptive input. The *Brain Gym* program may provide activities to enhance the child's handwriting through sensory experiences. Finally, the child participates in handwriting activities.

Sensory Motor Activities

- Play common children's games for coordination and leisure, such as hopscotch or Simon Says. These may need to be done at a slower pace and rhythmically so that the child can perform the movement.
- Squat to pick up small objects on the floor and place them in a container with a small opening. This is an excellent activity for sorting objects, and the squatting will strengthen the trunk and lower extremities as well as challenge motor planning.
- Create an obstacle course out of the classroom furniture. Children will learn important directional language skills such as in/out, over/under, and top/bottom.
- Give the child a job or task in the classroom, such as handing out papers. Let him or her figure out how to accomplish it with a minimum of prompts.
- Imitate body motions by symmetrically following one another in a mirror image. Vary the difficulty by going faster or slower or having the child perform the exact body movements while facing each other.
- Imitate isolated finger patterns in different spatial orientations. Do the finger movements above the head to eliminate visual input. To make the finger patterns easier, doing them to a song or rhythmic chant (e.g., singing the ABCs) frequently assists with more automatic motions.
- Trace letters that have been drawn with a marker and highlighted with dried glue.
- Write or draw on a vertical surface with different media, such as shaving cream or pudding. Write letters or designs in zip lock bags filled with hair gel. Form letters on a tray in water mixed with cornstarch.
- Change the standard writing tool or surface by using magic markers, slanted writing surfaces, or vibrating pens.
- Practice handwriting using handwriting sheets or commercially available programs to facilitate fluid and automatic movements. Practice and hand-over-hand assistance promote directionality and correct letter configuration (Box 19-2).

Named Activities

- *Draw for Me.* Draw in dried Tang, sand, shaving cream, or pudding mix.
- *Paint the World.* Paint on chalkboards or an outside surface with brushes dipped in water or paint.
- *Animal Walks.* Activities such as Rabbit Hop, Crab Walk, Elephant Walk, and Duck Walk encourage imitation, motor planning, strengthening, laterality, and directionality as well as body position in space.
- *I Got Rhythm.* Encourage rhythmic patterning and flow to promote tactile and kinesthetic awareness. Perform the rhythms with both extremities together, either moving them against gravity or beating on the table or knees. Handwriting has rhythmic movements, whether forming the letters or connecting them together. Use beginning patterns such as R-L-R-L and then R-R-L-L-R-R-L-L and then with each

BOX 19-2

Commercially Available Handwriting Programs

This list provides a brief overview of some commonly used handwriting programs.

1. A Reason for Handwriting

A Reason For
700 E Granite
Siloam Springs, AR 72761
800-447-4332
www.areasonfor.com
This program uses a simplified version of Zaner Bloser's handwriting program and is based on Scripture verses and Christian content. It gives students a practical reason for using their very best handwriting and can be highly motivating.

2. Callirobics

Laufer
PO Box 6634
Charlottesville, VA 22906
800-769-2891
www.callirobics.com
This program consists of exercises that are repetitive, simple writing patterns done to music. Callirobics can be beneficial to students who are auditory rather than visual learners.

3. D'Nealian Handwriting

Thurber DN: *D'Nealian handwriting*, 1 Jacob Way, Reading, MA 01867, www.dnealian.com
This program is developed to ease the transition from manuscript to cursive writing because most of the manuscript letters are the basis forms of the corresponding cursive letters. These letters are formed with one continuous stroke rather than the "ball and stick" method. In addition, many of the letters have a "monkey tail," so the letters are easily converted to cursive formation. The program can be confusing to children who have directionality and orientation difficulties because they don't know in which direction to put the monkey tail.

4. First Strokes Multisensory Print Program

The Handwriting Clinic
3314 N Central Expressway, Suite A
Plano, TX 75074
972-412-4119
www.firststrokeshandwriting.com
This program was designed by an occupational therapist and provides a multisensory approach to teaching printing.

5. Getty-Dubay Handwriting

Continuing Education Press
Portland State University
http://www.cep.pdx.edu/
This program, developed by Barbara Getty and Inga Dubay, is an italicized handwriting program that promotes efficient, simple movements. Exercises to strengthen hand muscles and improve coordination are provided in the book *Write Now: The Comprehensive Guide to Better Handwriting.*

6. GUIDE-write Raised Line Paper

601 SW 13th Terrace, Suite G
Pompano Beach, FL 33069
954-946-5756
www.guide-write.com
GUIDE–write provides products such as raised-line letters and raised-line paper that can be helpful when teaching a student to form letters.

BOX 19-2

Commercially Available Handwriting Programs—cont'd

7. Handwriting Without Tears

Jan Olsen, 1990, 2000

8801 MacArthur Blvd
Cabin John, MD 20818
301-263-2700
www.hwtears.com

This handwriting program uses a developmental approach toward prewriting through cursive writing. The letters are grouped by difficulty in formation of the letter. In addition, the letters are formed with a simple vertical rather than a slanted line. In this program there are only two writing lines, a baseline and a center line, which are visually less confusing for children with visual figure-ground deficits.[10] This program was created by an occupational therapist for her son and is very user friendly.

8. Loops and Other Groups

Mary Benbow, 1990, OT Ideas

124 Morris Turnpike
Randolph, NJ 07869
877-768-4332
www.otideas.com

This handwriting curriculum is a kinesthetic program that combines cursive connectors with manuscript letters for a more efficient writing style. The letters are taught in groups that share a common movement pattern. These motor and memory cues are used to help the student visualize and verbalize while experiencing the "feel" of the letters. Mary Benbow is an OT and provides suggestions for handwriting remediation. Her program is very helpful for students in the second grade and higher who have been taught cursive handwriting but have difficulty with letter formation.

9. Palmer Method

King F: Palmer method, Schaumburg, IL, 1976, AN Palmer.

This handwriting program is the traditional one that has been used in schools for many years and has been the foundation for handwriting styles. The program begins with the letter "A" and goes through to "Z." It uses a "ball and stick" method, causing the child to lift the pencil as the letters are created. This program is really not used anymore, but teachers tend to teach the "ball and bat" method anyway.

10. Zaner Bloser Handwriting

2200 W Fifth Ave
Columbus, OH 43215
800-421-3018
www.zaner-bloser.com

This handwriting program is based on the Palmer method but has simplified the material. The program is easier for schools to purchase and has literature and easy-to-use materials to support the handwriting program.

extremity performing irregular rhythms such as R-R-L-R-R-L.

Visual Perception Intervention Activities

- Use worksheets and perceptual motor booklets that are commercially produced to promote proprioception, figure ground, and eye-hand coordination.
- Reproduce designs with variations so that children can learn that a circle is a circle even when it is small or in different locations on the page.
- Use a chalkboard to encourage free movement patterns with resistance, and then allow a transition from the chalkboard (i.e., vertical surface) to paper.
- Trace on a line or roadway with a toy car. This encourages directionality and eye-hand coordination. A handmade mat that is easily transported can be used to trace roadways (Figure 19-7).
- Copy forms and designs (e.g., parquetry, block, pick-up-stick, and pegboard designs) to enhance form perception, matching, and figure completion.
- Construct simple puzzles obtained from pictures that children glue on sturdy paper and then cut apart, or make a prepackaged puzzle. Locating the puzzle pieces on the table is a visual targeting task as well as a figure ground perceptual skill.
- Illustrate stories using crayons, chalk, a felt board, or finger puppets.

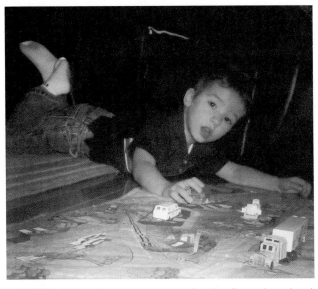

FIGURE 19-7 Tracing encourages directionality and eye-hand coordination.

- Draw a picture, label the items, and write a sentence about the picture.
- Create a book about an event or a family member, or even write a play about his or her day.
- Use the *Box and Dot 7* program, which encourages the child to form letters of the same size, and place the letters inside the box. The program is also helpful if a child reverses letters or needs an idea to establish a starting place for them.

Named Activities

- *Move Your Body.* Have the child lie with his or her back on the floor (for tactile input) and move the feet and arms when requested after hearing different musical rhythms or receiving verbal prompts.
- *Follow Me.* This activity encourages the development of one-handed movements and those crossing the midline of the body. Ask the child to move one leg or arm, providing tactile cues or resistance to the foot or arm that is not moving if necessary. Do imitation patterns of "Angels in the Snow" or Simon Says.
- *Follow Me Directional Skills.* Follow a maze or map or complete an obstacle course following the verbal or written directions for the course.
- *Look at This.* Follow a moving target such as a ball, light, or bubbles. These activities help with visual attention to a task as well as work on visual tracking, pursuit, and targeting skills.
- *Stick Designs.* Copy shapes with toothpicks or coffee stirrers. Increase the difficulty of the task by first copying on top of the picture and then next to the picture and finally copying the hidden picture without looking at it.
- *Create A Name.* Use shapes or putty to write your first name. This is an excellent motor planning as well as perceptual task. See who can create their names the fastest (Figure 19-8).
- *String Art.* Make initials by squeezing the glue and printing the letters. Cut yarn to cover the glue and complete the letters.
- *Write Me Up.* Write in the air to copy the letters or words without resistance.

CONSIDERATIONS FOR HANDWRITING INTERVENTION

Learning Styles

Consideration of the child's learning style is helpful in designing intervention and classroom strategies. Children learn using a variety of senses and learning styles. Some are *tactile/kinesthetic* learners, meaning that they need to physically feel and act out the task to remember the sequence. These children learn or perform a task better when they are allowed to stand up while writing or given the opportunity to move their body through the act. Using proprioceptive input, such as practicing and feeling the letter formation in the air with or without hand-over-hand assistance for additional tactile sensation of the letter shape, supports their learning. They frequently respond well to physical rewards like a pat on the back or running errands to the office.

Children who learn through *auditory* means write better if they hear or verbalize the letters or words while putting them on paper. These children may talk to themselves while writing, saying the letters and verbally describing the letter formation as they write.

Visual learners rely on seeing the written words and directions rather than remembering how to form letters. These learners may have difficulty with comprehension until their reading proficiency improves. They need to see the explanation rather than hear the information. Since the visual learner may have difficulty remembering verbal directions, they will benefit more from a map than verbal instructions. In the area of handwriting, the visual learner might have trouble understanding how to form the letters when given verbal directions without a visual demonstration. It is important to make sure that teachers and OT practitioners capture their visual attention before verbal directions are given, and directions should be repeated if necessary.

Organizational Skills

Organization of the child's workstation and desk is required for successful schoolwork.

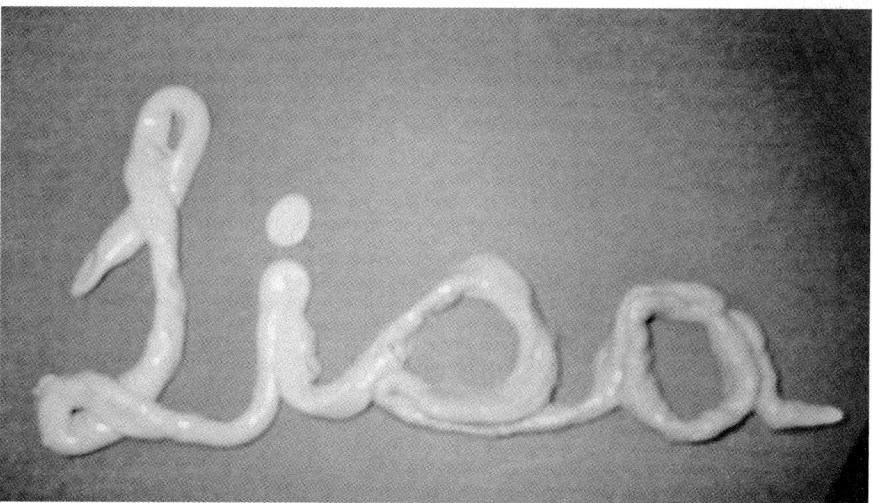

FIGURE 19-8 Using putty to write is an excellent motor planning as well as perceptual task.

Jerome cannot find anything in or on his desk. As a result, he spends too much time looking for papers, folders, or books and misses the lessons. Jerome turns in homework late or loses it in his desk. His papers are torn and wrinkled, resulting in lower grades. The teacher is sometimes unable to make sense of his writing. When he writes Jerome does not know where to start on the paper or does not move to the next line, leading to the letters running together or their superimposition.

Improper placement and orientation of the letters on the line or the spacing between words may indicate organizational difficulties. Children with poor organizational skills may use letters of varying sizes and mix capital and lowercase letters in words.

Some organizational problems are related to poor visual processing, while others are related to poor motor planning or attention. OT practitioners can help determine the root of the organizational problem. For example, visually figuring out how far apart letters should be placed is a perceptual skill, yet moving the fingers to create a letter or form letters counterclockwise requires motor planning.

Organization can be taught to children with frequent reminders and follow-up. Simple systems that the child initiates or helps design are effective.

For example, Scott picked out a Yugihoh day timer to record his assignments. Each week he receives a card if he wrote his assignments. The system works best when the child helps design it.

CLINICAL *Pearl*

Visual learners need to see examples, auditory learners need to hear the steps of the process, and kinesthetic learners need to feel and act out the steps of the process.

CLINICAL *Pearl*

What you see is not always what your brain perceives. Even though the eyes see and ears hear, the brain might not always picture or understand the sensory input.

Organizational intervention

- Keep the child's desk clean and organized so only the important papers are kept.
- Use folders of different colors for different subjects and cover the textbooks with paper of the same color.
- Verbally cue the student and remind the teacher to encourage clearing off the writing surface before starting handwriting assignments.
- Make a bag for the back of the classroom chair to store and make readily available pencils, scissors, and paper.
- Highlight the starting and stopping locations on the paper with a dot or sticker or highlight the lines of the paper.
- Work with the child, parents, and teachers to develop strategies.
- Have two sets of books (at home and school) so that the child does not have to remember to bring them.
- Use a planner to record assignments and have the teacher check to make sure every item is correct.
- Ask the teacher to list homework assignments online (so parents may follow up).

- Provide consequences for late work and bonuses for work on time.

Classroom Accommodations

OT practitioners may help students and teachers by providing classroom accommodations and strategies to encourage success in the classroom. Accommodations or strategies assist with the completion of assignments of written expression. Repetitive rote writing of spelling words or producing multiplication tables does not improve the child's knowledge of the information, nor does it improve their handwriting. Children who fatigue easily may not listen and learn from long writing assignments. Writing repetitively may also reinforce inappropriate letter formation. Accommodations that are appropriate for the individual child should be written on the Individual Education Program (IEP) or the 504 plan to be followed in the classroom.

Strategies for the classroom

- Decrease the amount of written work expected and reduce the redundant written assignments (e.g., completion of 50% of the required work).
- Use a peer buddy to help with journal assignments or written expression. A peer whose handwriting is adequate can write the dictated story of another child and then allow the child to rewrite the story.
- Use a tape recorder so that the child can dictate a story or tape the teacher's lecture.
- Allow preferential seating and optimum positioning of the student in the classroom. Some children need midline positioning because of decreased visual scanning from one side to the other, or there is one-sided neglect. In addition, auditory learners and easily distracted students frequently need to sit near the teacher so that they can be more attentive.
- Use a word processor as a supplemental aid to facilitate written expression. Be careful not to state the name of a specific computer or machine on the child's IEP because if it breaks suddenly or another one is tried, a new IEP would need to be developed immediately to document the change.
- A written list of homework assignments and a checklist of each book or folder that needs to go home will be provided.
- Delegate a packing buddy to help pack up at the end of the day to make sure that all of the necessary papers and books are put in the book bag.
- Allow the child more time to complete written assignments or use an outline format for them.
- Grade and emphasize the content of assignments of written expression and separate the grade from the mechanics of writing.
- Modify testing procedures to maximize student learning (e.g., children with writing difficulties may score poorly on spelling tests due to poor handwriting, so allow oral spelling tests).

COMPENSATORY STRATEGIES

Keyboarding

A word processor is an accommodation or supplemental aid in the classroom for the child with handwriting difficulties. A student could write out his or her rough draft, or "sloppy copy," even if it is not legible, and then type the final draft. If a child is using a word processor, it should be presented to the child as early as possible in his or her educational career. The early provision of a word processor does not allow the handwriting difficulties to interfere with written expression skills. The keyboard would improve legibility and reduce spelling errors in written assignments.[9] Many school districts have computer keyboarding skills in their curriculum; OT practitioners should review what is recommended. Box 19-3 shows the progression of keyboarding development recommended for schools in North Carolina.

Keyboarding requires memorization of where the keys are on the keyboard and how to retrieve the keys and documents. Moreover, to be a touch typist, timing and rhythm as well as bilateral coordination are important. In contrast, keyboarding does not require spatial organization and directionality as in handwriting.[17]

Few studies have been conducted on the use and benefits of word processors in comparison with teaching handwriting. Before recommending a word processor or portable keyboard, the OT practitioner considers the child's ability to organize the work surface. Children who are unable to locate their materials may have difficulty organizing themselves with an additional piece of

BOX 19-3

Summation of the North Carolina Keyboarding Curriculum

Kindergarten: Identify all letters, numbers, and other commonly used keys on the keyboard.

First Grade: Be familiar with the home keys. Fingers should reach keys and correct finger positions should be used while typing spelling words.

Second Grade: Locate and use symbol keys such as **%, ?, Caps Lock, Shift,** and **Esc**.

Third Grade: Be familiar with punctuation marks and practice spelling words and fast written expression. At this time the child should return the hands to the home key promptly after typing.

equipment. The *AlphaSmart* may suffice if more than one child uses the computer. A stand-alone computer is beneficial, but the computer is frequently located along the wall of the classroom, away from the teacher. Laptops have advantages, but the screen interferes with the visibility of the board or teacher. The OT practitioner or assistive technology team should evaluate the use of a word processor in the classroom as well as other settings.

Computer keyboard intervention

- Correct positioning and optimum seating should be provided for the student where the computer is located. Make sure that the screen and keyboard are not too high, the keyboard is aligned at the midline, and there is a steady seat.
- Written instructions about how to use the programs should be placed near the computer so that the staff can refer to it if necessary.
- Reduce eye strain by periodically looking across the room; also take breaks for stretching exercises.[19]
- Encourage the student to use the right hand on the right side of the computer keyboard and the left hand on the left side. Placing color-coded stickers on the fingernails can be a visual reminder. Have the child push the shift key with the little finger and the space bar with the thumb.
- A large mat in QWERTY rather than ABC order can be made for the children to sit on.
- Play keyboard Bingo on laminated copies of the keyboard with Bingo markers. Have the child mark out the spelling words on the laminated keyboard.
- Use a child-sized keyboard, which can be commercially purchased, with keys that are smaller and closer together.
- Use an AlphaSmart, Dreamwriter, Quickpad, or alternative keyboard such as Intellikeys or Big Keys to encourage word processor usage in the classroom. Computer keyboards can be altered with Sticky Keys, Filter Keys, or other choices in the accessibility section of the computer to meet the student's specific needs.
- The team should decide who is responsible for teaching and monitoring keyboarding skills.
- Recommend an assistive technology evaluation to help identify the best equipment or adaptive devices for the specific needs of the student.

One-handed keyboarding technique

A child with hemiplegia (increased muscle tone in one arm) has difficulty with isolated finger movements and should learn the one-hand typing method. The Mathias Corporation offers a program called *Touch Typing with One Hand* that uses FGHJ as the home keys and has the fingers go out from the center of the keyboard.[14] When typing with one hand, the child frequently tries to use the involved hand to assist. The more involved arm and hand tends to get in the way of the keys and can slow the typist down. Instead, the arm should be used to stabilize or support the upper trunk in the optimum position.

Computer mouse

Many of the computer programs used in the school computer labs are mouse driven; that is, the mouse controls most of the action. After the child types his or her name and identification number into the computer, the specific computer lesson comes up. Since many of these programs are mouse driven, the child is required to move the mouse and click on the correct answer. One way to evaluate the proficiency of a preschool to upper elementary school student in using a computer mouse is the *Test of Mouse Proficiency* (TOMP).[13] The TOMP looks at pointing, clicking, dragging, and pursuit tracking with the mouse. Preliminary reliability and validity studies indicate that TOMP is a reliable and valid measure to see how fast and accurate a child is in using the mouse.[12]

Left-handed writers

Children who write left handed may require special accommodations. Writing in a notebook is more difficult for left-handed children because of the placement of the spirals or rings. When writing with the left hand, they find it difficult to see what they have just written because the left hand covers the writing.[3] Left-handed children place their notebooks at a right angle and hook the left wrist in an awkward posture because that is how they were taught to angle the paper (Figure 19-9). Sitting posture is frequently twisted to accommodate the angle of the paper. The left-handed writer tends to push the pencil rather than pull it from left to right.

Left-handed intervention

- Group left-handed children together or at the end of the row so they do not bang hands with right-handers.
- Develop left-to-right directionality. Do exercises on the blackboard to encourage full arm movements and discourage excessive loops and flourishes while writing.
- Teach vertical writing. Do not insist on a right slant. Lefties should write with a left-handed slant and paper at the midline, angling the paper in the same direction as the forearm.
- Cross the letter "t" from right to left so the student is pulling the stroke toward the hand.

SERVICE OPTIONS

Direct Services

Direct therapy for handwriting can be implemented either individually or in a group setting.

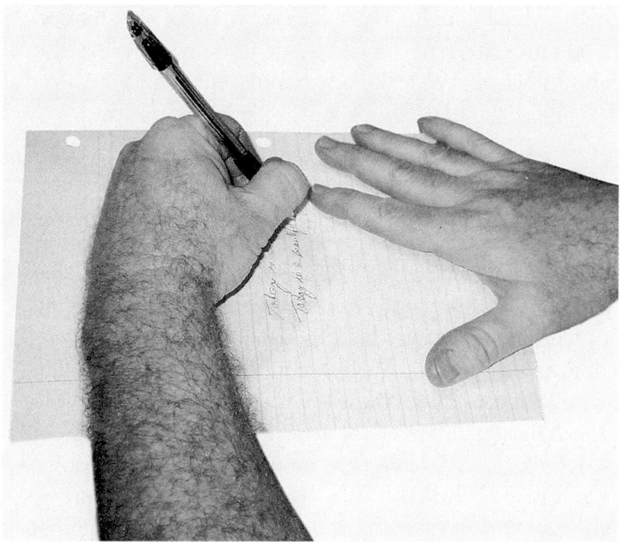

FIGURE 19-9 Left-handed writing is often awkward.

An example of a direct therapy session to improve handwriting ability might include the following sequence of activities.

Begin the session with a whole-body activity such as an obstacle course, which maneuvers around cones and through and under classroom desks. This works on postural control. Eye-hand coordination and visual scanning may be enhanced with a beanbag coordination game. To promote rhythmic movements, these activities can be done with music or a metronome that has a variable beat.

Next, enhance fine motor strength and coordination using Theraputty, clothespins, and wind-up toys or other activities. In-hand manipulation is facilitated by the placement of coins one at a time in a slot made in the lid of an empty frosting container.

Have the student sign in at either the beginning or end of the session. Signing in and the establishment of a signature are activities that are carried out throughout one's life. Signing in also gives the child the opportunity to learn placement, left-to-right sequencing, and alignment; furthermore, it gives the therapist an ongoing example of the progress in the child's handwriting/signature. Sometimes the goal for a student's handwriting is simply his or her signature in a small space allotted on a form. Practicing the signature and decreasing the size of the signature area in each session assist in accomplishing this goal.

Next, use one of the handwriting programs (see Box 19-2) according to the needs and abilities of the child, or create a handwriting sheet with the letters and "wall words" that the children are working on in class. This makes the therapy sessions more individual to the child or group. Work with the teacher to promote the theme or lesson of the classroom and enhance its follow through. Frequently, science topics and lesson plans that the teacher is working on can be easily reworked into a handwriting or cutting activity. Learning about a caterpillar becoming a butterfly is a wonderful lesson that can be made into an obstacle course.

- For the first step, the child crawls on the ground like a caterpillar.
- The child climbs up some step stools purchased from the hardware store to encourage weight shifting and coordination, like a caterpillar climbing a tree.
- The child rolls up in a blanket or climbs through a cloth tube made out of polyester material to become a cocoon.
- The child then opens up the blanket and becomes a beautiful butterfly, flying with open wings (arms) back to his or her seat.

Following the obstacle course, the child practices handwriting by describing the obstacle course and the emergence of the butterfly.

Finish the session with a "cool-down" period such as the in-hand manipulation task with the pennies and containers. If needed, as a positive reward during the session, a penny or sticker could be given for each successful activity.

Sharing and consulting with the teacher about the importance of moving and having the child alert for the task helps the teacher understand how to prepare the child for work. It is important that both the clinician and teacher use clear, concise, and similar words to describe how to draw the strokes and create the letters.[18] Consultation with the teacher and parents on activities including warm-up, perceptual motor worksheets, and letter practice, is essential and promotes carryover.

Data need to be kept to show continuous intervention improvement and progress in handwriting skills during therapy sessions or in the classroom during written expression. Figure 19-10 provides sample goals for handwriting skills.

Monitoring Services

Monitoring services are provided when the therapist is able to create a program for the student that the staff or family can follow. Frequent contact is made so that the program can be updated or altered if necessary. The personnel who follow the program should be well trained and have a clear understanding of the goals of the program. The activities should be simple enough to be followed in a safe manner without the presence of a qualified therapist. Handwriting programs such as *Handwriting Without Tears* include books for teachers

HANDWRITING: HOW DID I DO?

Name: ______________________________ Date: ____________

1. Letter sitting on line									
2. Letters touching top line									
3. Appropriate letter formation									
4. Attention to task									
5. Handwriting organized on page.									

FIGURE 19-10 An example of a data table.

6. Used a capital at the beginning.									
7. Used capitals correctly.									
8. Needed ____ reminders to complete task.									

FIGURE 19-10, cont'd

with ideas of how the program can be integrated into the school day. The OT practitioner monitors the progress and addresses any questions or concerns about using the program.

Consultation Services

Consultation services are provided when the practitioner's expertise is used to help other personnel achieve the child's objectives. Consultation services include adapting task materials or the environment, designing strategies to improve posture and positioning, and demonstrating how to handle a situation that requires ongoing contact with the teacher or caregiver.

One example is setting up a wheelchair desk in the classroom for a child and consulting with the staff on an ongoing basis to make sure the positioning is optimal. Maintaining optimum positioning may achieve the child's goals. Consultation with the staff continues as the child grows and it becomes necessary to alter the desk.

ROLE OF THE CERTIFIED OCCUPATIONAL THERAPY ASSISTANT

The COTA and registered occupational therapist (OTR) work together to assess and provide services to children. The OTR is responsible for interpreting the assessment results.

The COTA may contribute to the evaluation process by completing a handwriting checklist (see Figures 19-1 and 19-2) or standardized assessment to examine the child's skills.

The COTA, under the supervision of the OTR, may also contribute to the evaluation process by working directly with the students to promote motor planning, postural stability, visual-motor integration, grasping patterns, and letter formation for writing. The COTA provides handwriting intervention and may lead handwriting groups. OT practitioners assist children in gaining the skills for handwriting within the classroom curriculum. The OT practitioner is involved in consultation with the caregivers and teacher to provide ideas on remediation and techniques to improve handwriting in the classroom and at home.

References

1. Beery KE, Buktenica NA: *Developmental test of visual motor integration*, rev 3, Parsippany, NJ, 1989, Modern Curriculum Press.
2. Benbow M: Principles and practices of teaching handwriting. In Henderson A, Pehoski C, editors: *Hand function in the child: foundations for remediation*, St Louis, 1995, Mosby.
3. Boardman C: Reasonable answers to commonly asked handwriting questions—the second in the series, *Occup Ther Forum* 19:14, 1994.
4. Bruni M: *Fine motor skills in children with Down syndrome*, Bethesda, Md, 1998, Woodbine House.
5. Case-Smith J: Effectiveness of school-based occupational therapy intervention on handwriting, *Am J Occup Ther* 56:17, 2002.
6. Chandler B: The power of information: school-based practice survey results, *OT Week* 18:24, 1994.
7. Clark-Wentz J: Improving student's handwriting, *OT Practice* 2:29, 1997.
8. Dennison PE, Dennison G: *Brain gym*, Ventura, Calif, 1987, Edu Kinesthetic, Inc.
9. Handley-More D, Deitz J, Billingsley F, et al: Facilitating written work using computer word processing and word prediction, *Am J Occup Ther* 57:139, 2003.
10. Henry D: Henry Occupational Therapy Services, Inc., PO Box 145, Youngtown, AZ 85363, 888-371-1204, www.henryot.com.
11. Koziatek SM, Powell NJ: Pencil grips, legibility, and speed of fourth-graders' writing in cursive, *Am J Occup Ther* 57:284, 2003.
12. Lane A, Dennis S: The test of mouse proficiency (TOMP), Brisbane, 2000, Spectronics.
13. Lane A, Ziviani J: Assessing children's competence in computer interactions: preliminary reliability and validity of the test of motor proficiency, *Occup Ther J Res* 23:18, 2003.
14. Matias Corporation, 600 Rexdale Boulevard, Suite 1204, Toronto, Ontario M9W6T4, Canada, 1-888-663-4263, www.matiascorp.com
15. McHale K, Cermak S: Fine motor activities in elementary school: preliminary findings and provisional implications for children with fine motor problems, *Am J Occup Ther* 46:898, 1992.
16. Phelps J, Stempel L: *The children's handwriting evaluation scale: a new diagnostic tool*, Dallas, 1984, Texas Scottish Rite Hospital for Crippled Children.
17. Preminger F, Weiss P, Weintraub N: Predicting occupational performance: handwriting versus keyboarding, *Am J Occup Ther* 58:193, 2004.
18. Schneck CM, Henderson A: Descriptive analysis of the developmental progression of grip position for pencil and crayon in nondysfunctional children, *Am J Occup Ther* 44:893, 1990.
19. Strup J: Getting it right, *Adv Occup Ther Pract* 19:47, 2003.
20. Tseng MH, Murray EA: Differences in perceptual-motor measures in children with good and poor handwriting, *Occup Ther J Res* 14:19, 1994.
21. Yakimishyn J, Magill-Evans J: Comparisons among tools, surface orientation, and pencil grasp for children 23 months of age, *Am J Occup Ther* 56:564, 2002.

Recommended Reading

Bergmann K: Incidence of atypical pencil grasps among nondysfunctional adults, *Am J Occup Ther* 44:736, 1990.

Berninger V, Graham S: Language by hand: a synthesis of a decade of research on handwriting, *Handwriting Rev* 12:11, 1998.

Boardman C: Teaching printing with the block and dot method, *Occup Ther Forum* 16:4, 1994.

Cornhill H, Case-Smith J: Factors that relate to good and poor handwriting, *Am J Occup Ther* 50:732, 1996.

Fisher A, Murray E, Bundy A: *Sensory integration theory and practice*, Philadelphia, 1991, FA Davis.

Folio MR, Fewell RR: Peabody Developmental Motor Scales–2, Austin, Texas, 2000, Pro-ed.

Schneck CM: Comparison of pencil-grip patterns in first graders with good and poor writing skills, *Am J Occup Ther* 45:701, 1991.

Tseng MH, Chow MK: Perceptual-motor function of school-age children with slow handwriting speed, *Am J Occup Ther* 54:83, 2000.

REVIEW *Questions*

1. Name two ways that motor and sensorimotor factors, developmental delays, and visual perception can impede the ability to perform handwriting.
2. How should the wrist and hand be positioned for optimum handwriting performance?
3. How do motor planning difficulties interfere with the child's ability to learn and perform handwriting?
4. Identify two different learning styles and describe the ways that work can be adjusted to meet the needs of children with these different learning styles.
5. Outline five different remediation techniques and what the benefits of each strategy are.
6. What are the benefits of using a word processor or computer as an accommodation for a child?
7. How should a left-handed student angle his paper, and what other accommodations could be recommended?
8. In what ways does a COTA work with children to improve their handwriting skills?

SUGGESTED *Activities*

1. Observe the variety of pencil grasps that are used. Ask the person if a tight, nondynamic style of grasp is painful or fatiguing.
2. Try to write with your body in a variety of positions and postures to realize how an awkward posture greatly affects handwriting performance.
3. Use your shoulder to write instead of your hand to realize how smooth writing is very dynamic in nature. Evaluate your pencil grasp and writing method.
4. Perform handwriting with the nondominant hand to understand how difficult directionality and letter formation are when the brain is used to a certain direction.
5. Identify which kind of learner you are. Most adults have one learning style that they prefer but are able to use a blend of different styles.
6. Try to type on the word processor with only one hand. A therapist, typing with just one hand because of recent hand surgery, started this chapter, and it was hard!
7. In the classroom, what kind of accommodations would be helpful for you to learn?
8. Observe the grasping patterns of people who write with their left hand. How many left-handed writers angle the paper the same way that right-handed writers do rather than angle the paper in the same direction as the forearm?

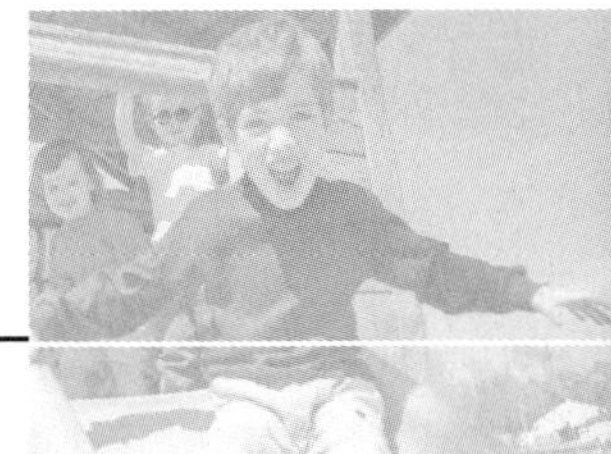

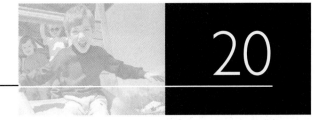

20

Motor Control: Fine Motor Skills

HARRIET G. WILLIAMS

CHAPTER *Objectives*

After studying this chapter, the reader will be able to accomplish the following:

- Outline the nature of fine motor development in typically developing children
- Identify common problems of children with fine motor control deficiencies
- Describe techniques to promote fine motor functioning in children
- Understand basic motor learning principles
- Describe how basic motor learning principles relate to occupational therapy intervention

KEY TERMS

Fine motor development
Construction activities
In-hand manipulation activities
Tool use
Bilateral motor control
Eye movement control
Saccadic eye movements
Pursuit tracking movements
Object manipulation
Power grasp
Precision grasp
Grip reflex

CHAPTER OUTLINE

This chapter addresses two major topics in **fine motor development**: (1) the nature of fine motor development in typically developing children and (2) common problems of children with fine motor control deficiencies. In the first part, we address the following issues: what fine motor development is, why it is important, what the important foundations for developing fine motor skills are, how object manipulation and implement usage skills develop, and some comments and recommendations for the development of writing skills. In the final part of the chapter, we discuss some basic motor learning principles that are important for planning and conducting occupational therapy (OT) sessions to improve fine motor control and facilitate skill acquisition.

Fine motor development is generally defined as the ability to use the eyes, hands, and fingers together in carrying out fine, precise movements that are necessary for performing a variety of daily activities. These movements range from those involved in coloring, drawing, and writing to pasting, cutting, and the manipulation of small objects and implements. Other terms commonly used interchangeably with fine motor development include eye-hand coordination, visuomotor coordination, and distal extremity control.[39-41]

Fine motor control doesn't just happen but rather develops in an orderly, organized fashion and is built on a number of underlying or foundational processes. The development of fine motor skills is an integral part of the overall development of the young child and reflects the increasing capacity of the nervous system to pick up and process visual and proprioceptive information and translate that information into skillful and refined movements. The optimum development of fine motor skills is important in that they are critical components of most of our self-help skills (e.g., eating, dressing, buttoning, zipping), the child's learning environment (e.g., writing, coloring, drawing, cutting, pasting), and other activities of daily living (e.g., typing, turning the pages in a book, threading a needle). They are also integral to successful performance in a number of professions (e.g., surgeons, dentists, musicians, artists, mechanics).

CLINICAL *Pearl*

Children with poor fine motor skills may exhibit the following performance problems:

- Difficulty in cutting and pasting
- Difficulty in manipulating objects
- Lack of smoothness in clapping or tapping rhythmically
- Tendency to hold a pencil awkwardly
- Tenseness in writing and drawing
- Produce strokes that are too heavy or too light

FOUNDATIONS OF FINE MOTOR SKILL DEVELOPMENT

There are several important elements to be aware of in understanding and working with the development of fine motor skills; these elements include bilateral motor control, reaching/grasping, object manipulation, and implement usage.* These elements make up the foundation of fine motor skill development. Bilateral motor control includes large and small (proximal and distal) muscle control; reaching/grasping, another component, is in part an outgrowth of proximal and distal control and is the key component in grasping and the manipulation of objects. Refined object manipulation follows after and is built on the foregoing elements and involves construction and in-hand manipulation activities. **Construction activities** include stacking blocks, putting simple puzzle pieces together, and putting pegs in a pegboard, among others. **In-hand manipulation activities** involve moving objects within the hand and include adjusting a toy or object in the hand, rotating an object in the hand, or picking up multiple objects. Precision grasping and releasing are critical to all of these activities. Finally, **tool use**, or the use of implements, evolves with and in part from earlier experience with object manipulation skills. Overall, the development of fine motor skills is an ongoing, integrated, and complex process. A schema that depicts the relationship among the various elements involved in fine motor development is shown in Figure 20-1 and discussed in more detail below.

Bilateral Motor Control: Large Muscle

Most manipulative activity requires the two arms and hands to work together in adaptive ways; this is referred to as **bilateral motor control**. For example, in cutting, one hand holds and controls the scissors, while the other hand is holding and positioning the paper. Therefore, to cut with precision, both hands must move skillfully and in an appropriate relation to each other.

An initial step in the process of developing fine motor skills is developing control of the large, or

CLINICAL *Pearl*

A wheelbarrow race is a great way to develop shoulder stability in older children. Younger children may enjoy "commando" crawling through tunnels and obstacle courses. Children of all ages enjoy sitting on large therapy balls, which can be tilted to facilitate trunk control. Therapists can easily grade the intensity of these activities.

*References 7, 18, 20, 21, 28, 32, 35, 39, 40, 42.

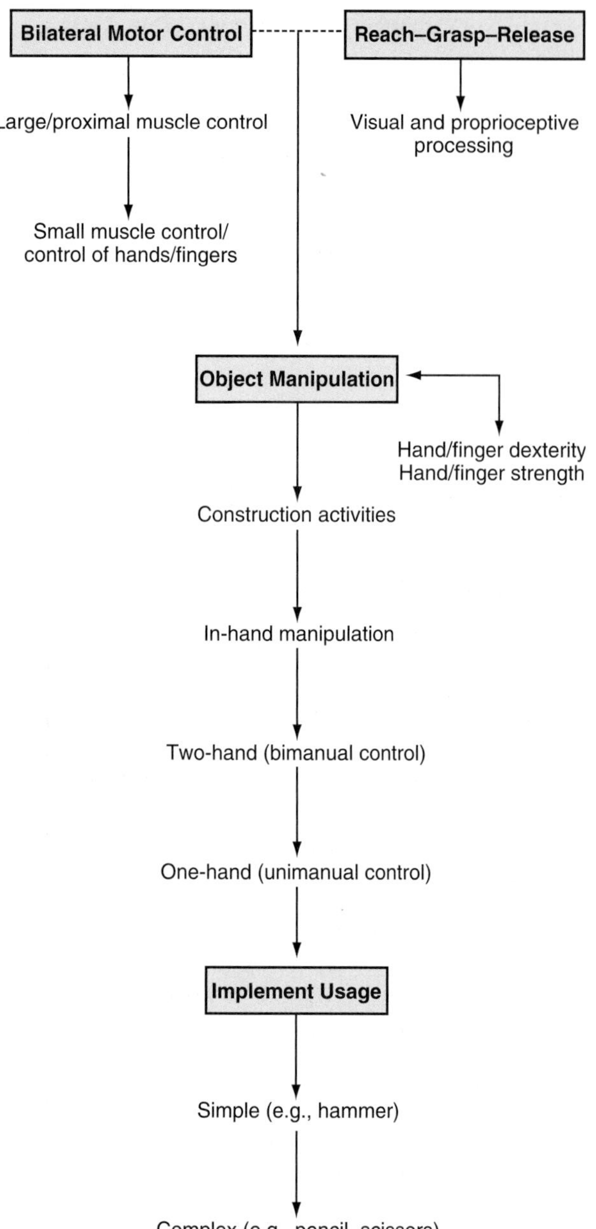

FIGURE 20-1 Foundations of fine motor skill development.

proximal, muscles of the trunk, shoulders, and arms. Control of these muscles frees the arms and allows them to move independent of the trunk, which ultimately provides the hands and fingers with the support needed for independent, intricate, and delicate movements.

There appears to be a general developmental sequence in acquiring large, or proximal, muscle control. First, control of the muscles of the trunk develops; the arms and legs can then be moved independently. This is followed by the capacity to move an arm and a leg on one side of the body independent of the opposite side. This action appears to occur initially on the side with the dominant hand and then on the side with the nondominant one. Finally, control extends to the movement of an arm and a leg on opposite sides of the body, first on the side with the dominant hand and then on the side with the nondominant one. The former movement is known as ipsilateral and the latter as contralateral. Contralateral movements constitute the forerunner of the arm/foot opposition inherent in most locomotor skills. Control of these large, proximal muscles is typically present by 6 years of age; the major developmental changes occur between 4 and 6 years. The examination of bilateral large muscle control can be accomplished at three different levels: (1) by touching the body parts to be moved (concrete, touch-based level), (2) by pointing to the body parts to be moved (less concrete, more visually based level), and (3) by using verbal labels for the body parts to be observed (abstract, language-based level).

The bilateral motor control involved in fine motor development also progresses from crude two-hand (bimanual) movements to one-hand (unimanual) control to refined use of the two hands in lead and assist roles for activities such as buttoning and cutting. Crude bilateral movements represent an initial, possibly inherent, linkage between the two hands and typically involve the two hands working together as one unit, each performing the same action. The processes involved in unimanual control and refined bimanual control (functional asymmetry) are discussed in greater detail below.

Bilateral Motor Control, Small Muscle Control, and Object Manipulation

Small muscle control refers to the control or use of the small muscle masses of the wrist, hands, and fingers to grasp, hold, and manipulate objects. Small muscle, or distal, control typically follows after and builds on the development of a minimum of control of the large, more proximal muscles of the trunk, shoulders, and arms. Small muscle, distal control allows the individual to carry out more precise, adaptive movements that involve intricate manipulation and/or the use of objects and implements. Small muscle control requires adequate hand and finger strength and dexterity; these aspects of hand function should be assessed and included in any rehabilitation activity (Figure 20-2).

The development of unimanual control is associated with the establishment of hand preference or hand dominance. Bimanual control is also intricately linked to small muscle control and hand preference because both optimum unimanual control and hand dominance are integral to the development of lead and assist hands, or bimanual functional asymmetry. All of the foregoing factors are important in acquiring the capacity to

Fine Motor Evaluation

Child's Name: ______________________________

DOB: ______________ DOE: ______________

Diagnosis: ______________________________

Therapist: ______________ COTA: ______________

Reason for Referral:

Background Information (Include the child's grade, developmental history, medications, home situation.):

Physical Structure of the Hand (Note any deformities, contractures, edema, structural integrity of the muscles and joints.):

Muscle Tone (Describe the development of the arches of the hand; very young children and those with low muscle tone exhibit flat hand arches.):

Range of Motion (Examine the wrist, supination/pronation, and all finger and thumb movements.):

Strength (grip strength, pincer strength):

Posture/Balance (Can the child sit, stand, walk independently? What is the quality of his or her movement?):

Postural Adjustments during Fine Motor Tasks (Observe how the child adjusts to changes during fine motor tasks. Does the child move his or her hand/fingers, or whole body?):

Coordination (Are tremors, over reaching, under reaching, or associated reactions noted during activities?):

Attention to Task (Is the child interested in task? Does the child visually attend to task?):

Emotional Reactions to Fine Motor Tasks (Does the child become frustrated easily? Has the child developed compensatory strategies? Does the child attempt to avoid tasks?):

Vision (Does the child get very close to work? Does the child appear to be looking at task? Does the child rely heavily on vision?):

Sensory Reactions to Fine Motor Tasks (Does the child avoid manipulating objects? Does the child under or overreact to touch? Does the child explore objects?):

Development of Fine Motor Skills (Is the child able to grasp, release, manipulate? Use both hands together? Cut? Write? Developmental assessments such as the Hawaii Early Learning Profile provide age ranges.):

Timing and Sequencing:

Quality of Movement (Is the child able to alternate supination/pronation? Release objects precisely?):

Finger Individuation (Is the child able to use one or two fingers alone? Or do all fingers move in the same pattern?):

Pencil Grasp:

Assessment:

FIGURE 20-2 Occupational therapist conducts fine motor assessment with input from the certified occupational therapy assistant (COTA). *DOB*, Date of birth; *DOE*, date of evaluation.

manipulate objects and use implements skillfully. Lead and assist hands, or bimanual functional asymmetry, refer to the use of individual hands in performing different actions involved in a single activity. For example, in the activity of buttoning, one hand manipulates the button and the other manipulates the fabric where the button is to be placed. Two different actions are performed, one by each hand, to accomplish a single goal or task.

The greatest developmental changes in unimanual distal control appear to take place from 4 to 6 years of age, with lesser improvements from 6 to 8 years. Distal control is often assessed through the performance of such actions as repetitive hand patting, alternating hand flexion/extension, alternating arm and hand supination/pronation, and repetitive and successive finger tapping. Hand patting requires the child to tap the whole hand against a surface as quickly as possible, while alternating hand flexion/extension requires the child to move the wrist into and out of flexion/extension as rapidly as possible. Alternating supination/pronation involves moving the hands and forearms in alternating rotation movements (hand palm up to hand palm down repeatedly) as rapidly as possible. Finger movement tasks involve either tapping one finger repeatedly or touching each finger to the thumb in sequence, starting with the index finger; both of these tasks are performed as rapidly as possible. The capacity to perform such movements rapidly and easily is one way to establish the possible presence or absence of deficits in underlying fine motor control processes.

Reaching, Grasping, Releasing, and Fine Motor Development

Reaching, grasping, and releasing are other important components of the development of fine motor skills (both object manipulation and implement or tool usage). For example, to manipulate an object, the individual must first obtain it; this requires that the individual reach for and grasp the object and then use the fingers to move or manipulate it in appropriate ways. Reaching for and grasping an object successfully involve locating the hand in space, locating the object in space, and then acting to bring the two together. It is important that the individual both see and feel the hand in relation to the object to be grasped. In other words, it is important for the child to see and feel the hand and arm as they move toward and grasp the object. This means that the individual must effectively process visual, proprioceptive, and tactile information (seeing and feeling the hand and arm move) and then create and carry out a movement that gets the hand to the object for grasping and manipulation. This process is known as *intersensory* or *sensory-motor integration*. These processes tend to happen naturally and spontaneously during development. When or if they do not, fine motor development is often difficult.

Overall, infants tend to reach out spontaneously for objects that move across their visual field; this reaching tendency is present at birth and is initially visually evoked. In other words, the response appears to be a spontaneous reaction to seeing an object in the environment. Although this early reaching action is crude, it is directed toward the object and will later become a voluntary act that is more precise and better controlled. At this point in his/her development, the child decides when, where, how, and whether to reach for an object and does so skillfully.

Grasping an object is the second step in its manipulation. The early grasping response is reflexive or instinctive in nature and is based largely on proprioceptive and tactile input; later it evolves into a voluntary grasp that relies more on visual information. Vision allows the young child to examine the object (determine its size, shape, location, and other factors) more precisely and then shape the hand and create the force necessary for holding and manipulating the object. Of course, this process is repeated multiple times in many different ways for objects of different sizes, shapes, weights, and uses. Therefore, vision and visual perception become integral factors in the development of fine motor skills. Releasing or letting go of an object is another part of fine motor development and object manipulation. It requires some inhibition of the earlier grasp reflex response because manipulating an object actually involves skillful grasping and releasing of the object in a variety of ways, which allow the individual to explore and/or use the object for a particular purpose (in-hand manipulation).

Eye Movement Control

Visual perception and thus **eye movement control** (how the child or individual moves the eyes to focus on or follow objects in the environment) play an important role in fine motor control and development. There is some evidence that a significant number of children (approximately 78%) with fine motor control problems also exhibit poor saccadic eye movements along with less well developed pursuit eye movements. In **saccadic eye movements** the eye moves rapidly and accurately from item to item (e.g., from point to point in a picture or letter to letter or word to word in reading). In **pursuit tracking movements** the eye moves to follow slow-moving objects, among other things. These eye movements allow the eye and brain to get the information needed to make appropriate decisions about phenomena such as movement, objects, and the content of the written word. Both types of eye movement can be improved with practice and may be worth considering as part of the enrichment activities for improving fine motor control.

CLINICAL *Pearl*

Using black and white infant toys (created to stimulate infants) may improve the eye muscles of children with eye tracking difficulties. Therapists may encourage children to follow the slow-moving (for pursuit tracking movements) or fast-moving (for saccadic movements) object. For older children, black and white pictures or computer games in which the child must point to the object on the screen may be more appropriate.

DEVELOPMENT OF OBJECT MANIPULATION SKILLS

Object manipulation may be thought of as the manual control of objects (i.e., the ability to manipulate or use an object in a variety of desired ways). Object manipulation may involve what some refer to as construction activities and in-hand manipulation activities; both can be bimanual or unimanual. Examples of construction activities include putting puzzles together, building towers out of building blocks, using legos, and putting pegs in a pegboard. Examples of in-hand manipulation activities include turning the lid of a jar, picking up multiple objects, and others in which the thumb plays a prominent role. The skillful manipulation of objects involves in particular the ability to control the actions of individual fingers and groups of fingers (manual dexterity). It also requires that the arm and hand work together to control or use the object (bimanual control); this is often referred to as the arm-hand linkage system and is the basic foundation for the subsequent development of implement usage skills.*

The arm and hand each play different roles in the successful manipulation of objects, the nature of which changes in relation to the goal of the task and the age and developmental level of the child. For example in placing pegs in a pegboard (construction activity), the arm provides support for the hands and fingers to hold the pegs and positions the hand so that the peg can be put in the board. In eating with a spoon (implement or tool usage), the arm positions the hand to hold the spoon; the hand and fingers control the position and movement of the spoon.

Generally, the arm and hand each have three independent functions that are used in different ways to accomplish different tasks. The three functions of the arm are (1) positioning the hand (i.e., getting the hand in an appropriate location or position for grasping the object of interest); (2) supporting the hand (i.e., keeping the arm/hand combination relatively immobile so that the necessary hand and finger movements can be executed properly); and (3) on some occasions producing force, such as that required in pounding a peg or turning a doorknob. The functions of the hand are to pick up the object, hold or grasp the object, and execute the movements needed to manipulate the object or implement. Developmental progressions have been loosely defined for each of these hand functions.

*References 5, 6, 11-15, 19, 22, 28, 29, 39, 40.

Picking Up an Object

In picking up an object, the individual may initially scoop it up with the whole hand, often on the ulnar (little finger) side. Later the child uses individual fingers and finger actions to pick up the object. A pincer grasp that involves finger-thumb opposition, such as the use of the thumb and index finger or index and middle fingers, is usually the most effective way to pick up objects.

Grasping an Object

There are two types of grasps used in holding objects or implements. One is the **power grasp,** in which the handle or object is held tight against the palm and the arm and shoulder produce the movement. A good example of this type of grasp is the use of a hammer in pounding a nail or peg; the hammer is held in a kind of palmar grasp and the arm and shoulder create the force needed to pound the peg. The other is the **precision grasp,** in which the thumb and fingertips are used to change the object's position or move the implement. In contrast to the power grasp, the precision grasp involves wrist and finger action (distal control) to perform the task. More accurate movement is possible with the precision grasp.

Manipulating an Object

As with grasping an object, in manipulating an object the palm or whole hand is used initially; later the fingers and thumb are used to explore, examine, or move the object or implement in intricate ways.

FORCE PRODUCTION AND OBJECT MANIPULATION SKILLS

Generally, adults and children with typical development or function exhibit patterns of force production and modification that allow them to create and apply the force needed to manipulate objects effectively. Therefore, adequate strength along with the ability to produce appropriate force and apply that force when it is needed is integral to fine motor control and development. If the amount of force is inadequate or the application or use of that force is poorly timed, the object may slip or slide, and the skillful and efficient use or manipulation of the object may be hindered. Producing force involves, among other things, the activation of appropriate muscles and the proper timing of the contraction of those muscles to produce the force needed for effective object manipulation. Force production and modification of that force are integral to all types and forms of object manipulation. For example, appropriate levels and timing of force are needed to lift an object; here the amount of force produced should be equal to the weight of the object to be lifted. This requires accurate anticipation of the weight of the object and the ability to plan the movement to produce that force. Another example is the transport or movement of an object from one place to another (e.g., picking up pegs and putting them in a pegboard). This involves upward, downward, and horizontal movements and varying the force as needed. Another important component is the ability to respond appropriately to variables such as changes in object position and slippage of the object; this is referred to as **grip reflex,** or the timing and application of appropriate force to adapt to changes in object position.[16,17,23,38,41]

Typically in development, the force aspects of fine motor control evolve naturally and spontaneously; however, with a number of developmental delays, after trauma, or with certain neurological disorders, these processes are disrupted. In other words, the child is unable to produce or modify the force needed to meet the changing demands inherent in using objects. For example, children with fine motor problems begin to initiate force for lifting objects prematurely (i.e., before that force is really needed). There is also often a delay in the increase in force needed once the object is lifted or moved; therefore, control of the object may become problematic. In addition, the response of these children to slippage or some unexpected change in the position or orientation of the object is slower and more variable than that for typical children. In other words, the initiation of the grasp reflex takes significantly longer and is extremely inconsistent. As a result, for the child who has difficulties with fine motor development, the grip reflex is at times rapid and appropriate; at other times it is slow and maladaptive. The result is often the fumbling, dropping, or awkward handling of objects.

Activities to Promote Strength Development

Adequate muscular strength of the hands and fingers is important to produce the force needed to carry out fine motor tasks with skill and efficiency.[40] The following are some examples of activities that may be helpful in strength development:

- Pinch putty between the thumb and individual fingers in sequence from the index to the little finger and vice versa.
- Push slowly into a putty ball; hold each finger extended.
- Press cookie cutter into Play-Doh or another similar substance.
- Hold putty or soft ball in the palm of the hand and squeeze.
- Squeeze a turkey baster or other plastic item.
- Crumble sheets of paper into a ball.
- Twist or wring putty or other material with palm toward and away from the body.
- Squeeze water out of a sponge or other soft material.
- Hold playing cards between two fingers; try to knock the cards out of the finger grasp
- Holding a weight in one hand, with the palm down and forearm supported, flex and extend the wrist.
- Use rubber bands as resistance to finger and wrist movements.

CLINICAL *Pearl*

Pet squeeze toys are lightweight and easy for infants with poor grip strength to squeeze. These toys provide a successful experience for children and may encourage further activity. Some are also small enough to fit in the tiniest of hands.

For older children, computer typing programs are available that use musical rhythms while teaching keyboarding skills.

One way to assess the ability of the child to consistently produce an appropriate amount of force is the use of tapping activities. Can the child tap consistently for a designated period of time? Variation in tapping can be easily observed, and if a metronome is used, it becomes readily evident. The metronome can be used to help the child improve the consistency of the timing of force production. Children with coordination difficulties generally exhibit an inability to maintain a consistent tapping rate; this is especially true if the period of tapping is a long one. These children become more variable as the time involved in tapping increases. They are the most consistent in the initial 10 seconds of such an activity and become much more variable as the duration increases to 20 or 30 seconds. It is a good idea to use short durations initially and gradually increase them as the child improves.

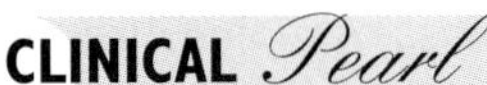

For older children, computer typing programs are available that use musical rhythms while teaching keyboarding skills.

DEVELOPMENTAL PROGRESSION FOR OBJECT MANIPULATION

There are several overlapping trends or dimensions of behavior to consider in looking at the development of fine motor object manipulation skills.[6,14,39,40] They include indicators of the development of hand control (how and for what purpose the child uses the hands), spatial-temporal accuracy (skills that require judging the space and timing of the action of the hands), and self-help skills. Examples of the general developmental sequence of some of these behaviors are given in Box 20-1.

DEVELOPMENT OF IMPLEMENT USAGE SKILLS

Implement usage skills involve the use of tools to accomplish specific goals.[6,8,40] Tools can be used to act on oneself or the environment. Development begins with the use of simple implements such as a hammer or brush or another object and proceeds to the use of more complex and specialized tools such as pencils and scissors. Using an implement involves functional asymmetry, or the use of the lead and assist hands. To use a tool or implement properly, the individual must hold it correctly and maintain the appropriate relationship between the tool and the object on which it is used. For example, in using a hammer, it is important to maintain an appropriate relationship between the hammer and the nail to make successful contact with the nail. The same is true in using scissors for cutting, a pencil for writing, and a wrench for turning a screw. Developmental steps in acquiring the skills of cutting and writing are addressed below.

Cutting

There are several components that constitute part of the development of cutting skills.[31,39,40] They include how the scissors are held (the grasp or prehension of the scissors), the use of the assist hand (lead and assist usage), the relationship between the paper and scissors, and the cutting action. Cutting skill is often assessed by observing and evaluating the child as s/he cuts a straight line, square, and circle. Of the three, the circle is reported to be the most difficult.

BOX 20-1

Examples of General Developmental Sequences for Object Manipulation

HAND CONTROL

Hands fisted: flexion dominates
Hands open: more opportunity for use
Fingers used in play
Picks up cube: uses the whole hand (left and right)
Transfers cube hand to hand: whole hand involved
Transfers cube hand to hand: thumb/finger opposition involved
Reaches unilaterally (one arm)
Builds tower of cubes
Unwraps cube
Turns pages
Holds crayon adaptively
Scribbles spontaneously
Imitates vertical and horizontal strokes

SPATIAL-TEMPORAL ACCURACY

Visually tracks object across midline
Reaches for objects
Plays pat-a-cake
Puts three cubes in a cup
Puts several beads in a box
Puts one peg in pegboard (repeated)
Puts nine cubes in cup
Places round, square, and triangular shapes in form board

SELF-HELP SKILLS

Drinks from cup
Uses spoon; spills a little
Removes clothes
Washes/dries hands
Puts on shoes (does not tie)

Holding the scissors

The mature and preferred grasp of the scissors is with the thumb in the upper handle and the index finger or index and middle fingers in the other, with the other fingers gently flexed. Another early grasp that is also biomechanically efficient for the young child is with the thumb in one handle, the middle finger in the other, and the index finger extended along the scissors for stability. Most children with fine motor difficulties use immature prehension or grasp patterns (82% in cutting a line, 69% in cutting a square, and 77% in cutting a circle). Seventy-three percent to 83% of children with typical development use the mature grasp for cutting shapes and lines.

In developing cutting skills, the scissors are initially held with both hands; each hand holds one handle that moves the blade to cut. A second person holds and moves the paper to assist in cutting. This is usually followed by the child holding the scissors with one hand and using the thumb and fingers to move the scissors, which free the opposite hand to hold or move the paper to accommodate the cutting. At this point the mouth also often moves in concert with the action of the scissors. Ultimately it is primarily the thumb that controls the action of the scissors. When the scissors are grasped with one hand, the thumb is usually placed in the upper handle and the index finger or index and middle fingers in the lower handle.

Using the assist hand

Using the assist hand, or lead and assist usage (also known as *paper strategy*), refers to how the child holds the paper and uses the assist hand. The mature manner of holding the paper is one where the thumb is placed on top and the fingers underneath. Significant percentages of children with fine motor difficulties use immature lead and assist patterns for cutting tasks (59% for the line, 50% for the square, and 65% for the circle). In terms of development, there is no use of the assist hand initially because the child holds the scissors with both hands and a second person holds the paper. The next step involves the use of the assist hand; when it is used, the paper is often held with the fingers on top and the arm in a pronated position. This is a less efficient position for ease and flexibility in cutting. At this time there is considerable inconsistency in how the assist hand is used, and many different combinations of fingers or thumb on top are seen. The last step is to use the assist hand with the thumb on top and the arm in a more supinated position. This position allows for greater freedom in orienting the paper to the scissor action and makes for increased ease and efficiency in cutting.

Paper-scissors relationship

The paper-scissors relationship involves (1) how the paper is maintained in relation to the scissors and (2) where the child holds the paper in relation to the scissor blades. With regard to how the paper is maintained in relation to the scissors, the paper is initially held against the table for support. This is usually related to inadequate stability of the trunk and shoulder girdle. The next step is for the paper to be held in place (the paper is not moved) and the scissors moved to accomplish the cutting task. The biomechanically more efficient approach is seen in the subsequent development of cutting skills and involves the scissors being maintained in a relatively stationary position and the paper moved to accommodate the cutting action.

With regard to where the child holds the paper in relation to the scissor blades, typical patterns include holding the paper in front of the blade, holding it behind the blade, holding it so that it crosses over the scissors, and holding it in multiple positions in relation to the blade. Holding the paper in an inappropriate position in relation to the paper makes it difficult to cut accurately, smoothly, and in an efficient, coordinated fashion. Children with coordination difficulties often use immature patterns in executing the appropriate paper-scissors relationships (41% for the line, 75% for the square, and 65% for the circle).

Cutting action

Cutting action is sometimes referred to as cutting strategy and involves the type of cutting motion and selection of the appropriate place to initiate cutting (i.e., where to start to cut). There are two major types of cutting action. The first is the short, segmented cutting action, or what is referred to as snipping. This type of action appears to be easier to control and therefore is usually seen in the initial steps of cutting. The second is a longer gliding action that is more continuous in nature. This action is present in more skillful cutters. Depending on the nature of the item to be cut, the ultimate skill in cutting requires an appropriate combination of short, segmented cuts integrated with longer gliding actions.

With regard to where to start to cut, some 65% to 69% of children with fine motor control difficulties use inappropriate starting positions; they have to snip, return to the edge of the paper, and restart the cutting task multiple times. Many children with fine motor problems do not use a continuous motion in cutting.

Pencil Usage

Handwriting is one of the most important skills that adults and children alike acquire and use throughout life; for children handwriting is a skill that is critical during the school years. Between 10% and 20% of school-aged children have difficulties with handwriting. Handwriting problems are the most frequent reason that children are referred to OT practitioners working in schools. When handwriting is deficient or problematic, there are often consequences related to academic performance as well as social interaction that can limit participation in basic school and social activities.* What is involved in handwriting? What are some of the major foundational skills that are prerequisites to developing skillful handwriting? The skills in Box 20-2 have been shown to contribute in different ways to speed and/or accuracy in handwriting.

The important elements to consider in examining skill in the use of a pencil can and should include all of

*References 2-4, 6, 9, 10, 25, 30, 31, 33, 34, 36, 37, 42.

BOX 20-2

Foundational Skills Contributing to Handwriting Speed and Accuracy

FINGER FUNCTIONS

Intricate and skillful use of the fingers

- Finger lifting: accuracy in lifting fingers pointed to (related to speed and accuracy)
- Finger recognition: accuracy in lifting fingers touched when vision is not available (related to speed)
- Complex finger opposition: speed and accuracy of touching fingers to thumb rapidly/consistently (related to speed)

VISUAL-MOTOR INTEGRATION

Appropriate use of visual information and ability to integrate vision with movement responses

- Copying forms: design copying (related to speed and accuracy)
- Identifying forms: visual recognition of forms (related to speed)
- General eye-motor coordination: drawing lines accurately (related to speed)

LEFT-RIGHT DISCRIMINATION

Awareness of right-left parts of the body (related to accuracy)

PENCIL EXCURSION

Accuracy of figures drawn without vision (related to speed)

EYE MOVEMENT CONTROL

Appropriate saccadic and pursuit tracking movements (related to speed)

the above. The major motor control issues are the grasp of the pencil and the locus of control for the action of moving it. Examples of the steps in grasping and controlling the pencil are described below.

Palmar grasp

The palmar grasp appears earliest in development. Two types of palmar grasp have been described: the radial cross-palmar and the palmar supinated, with the former preceding the latter developmentally. With the palmar grasp, the writing implement is usually held tightly in the palm, as in a power grip. The hand holds the pencil and the arm and shoulder move it through proximal muscle action. The arm is usually held in the air; neither the wrist nor the elbow touches the writing surface. Approximately 31% of young children with handwriting difficulties tend to use variations of the palmar grasp. These children often move the hand as a single unit, with little or no finger involvement.

CLINICAL *Pearl*

Radial cross-palmar grasp. The pencil tip extends out from the thumb (radial) side of the hand and crosses the thumb.

Palmar supinated grasp. The pencil tip extends out from the little finger (ulnar) side of the hand, with the hand fully fisted in a power-like grasp.

Prestatic tripod: transitional grasps

There are a variety of transitional grasps that occur before the more consistent use of the static tripod. These include the digital pronated, brush, and cross-thumb grasps.

CLINICAL *Pearl*

Digital pronated grasp. This grasp is essentially the same as a palmar supinated grasp, with the index finger extended along the pencil; the arm and shoulder move the pencil.

Brush grasp. The pencil is held with the fingers but is positioned against the palm; the palm is pronated; and the wrist and shoulder move the pencil, with the forearm held in the air.

Cross-thumb grasp. The fingers are tucked loosely in the palm with the pencil held against the index finger with the thumb crossed over the pencil and against the index finger, both wrist and fingers move the pencil, and the forearm is supported against the table.

Static tripod grasp

The static tripod grasp is an important and integral step toward the development of the dynamic tripod. In this grasp the implement is held with the thumb and index and middle fingers. For the first time the thumb is in full opposition to the index finger. The pencil rests in the open web space between the thumb and index finger. The forearm is supported by the table or support surface. The arm and shoulder control the action of the implement, with occasional wrist action. There is little or no finger action (the hand moves as a whole unit). Approximately 19% of young children with writing difficulties use this type of grasp.

Predynamic tripod: transitional and frequently observed grasps

There are several transitional grasps that are observed as the individual moves toward the consistent use of the

CLINICAL *Pearl*

Four-finger grasp. The implement is held with the four fingers and thumb in opposition. The wrist and fingers move the pencil while the forearm is being supported by the table or writing or drawing surface.

Lateral tripod grasp. The implement is stabilized against the radial side of the middle finger; the thumb is abducted and braced along the lateral border of the index finger. The wrist is slightly extended, with the ring and little fingers flexed to help stabilize the grasp. There is some finger and wrist action in making vertical and horizontal strokes. The forearm rests on the table.

Locked grip with thumb wrap. This grasp is also commonly called the white-knuckle grip. The pencil is pressed against the radial side of the middle finger, with the index finger against the pencil; the thumb is wrapped over the index finger and presses it downward. The ring and little fingers flex to help support the pencil. There is little or no digital action in moving the implement.

Locked grip with thumb tuck. This grasp is similar to the thumb wrap except that the thumb is tucked under the index and/or middle fingers. There is little or no use of the fingers in moving the pencil.

Quadruped grasp. The pencil is held against the ring, or fourth, finger by the thumb. The little finger is flexed to help support and stabilize the pencil. The thumb and index and middle fingers hold the pencil securely. The pencil is essentially held in the open web space between the index finger and thumb. This grasp can be either static or dynamic.

dynamic tripod grasp. They include the four-finger grasp, lateral tripod grasp, locked grip with thumb wrap, locked grip with thumb tuck, and quadruped grip.

Dynamic tripod grasp

The dynamic tripod is the preferred mature grasp. The pencil is held between the thumb and index and middle fingers; the index finger is placed on top of the pencil, with the thumb in full opposition. The ring and little fingers are flexed to help stabilize the grasp. The wrist and fingers are used to move the pencil, and there is greater digital control of it. The arm simply positions the hand for the appropriate manipulation of the pencil by the fingers. The dynamic tripod grasp is typically present by 6 to 7 years of age. Approximately 19% of young children with fine motor problems use this mature grasp. Overall, most children, typical or otherwise, use the same hand for cutting and writing. Some of them may use an adapted tripod grasp. The pencil is held between the index and middle fingers, with the thumb pressed against it for stability. The ring and little fingers are flexed to assist in supporting the implement. The action of moving the pencil is similar to that in the dynamic tripod grasp.

DEVELOPMENTAL PROGRESSION OF IMPLEMENT USAGE

The following are simple descriptions of some aspects of the development of pencil usage.[14,39,40] (They may or may not resemble the recovery of similar functions after injury or trauma.)

Scribbling

If given a figure to copy, the young child's reaction is often a spontaneous scribble that bears no relation to the figure or model. In other words, the response does not seem to be influenced by the visual configuration. Later the figure to be copied is given more attention, even though the product may not closely resemble the target figure and is often not reproduced in any detail. Looping is also a common response in scribbling.

Simple Line Drawing

In simple line drawing, the individual draws vertical, horizontal, diagonal, and curved lines. Initially the lines are copied in a large space and in response to a line drawn by another person. With increasing experience and further growth, the individual draws lines independently (i.e., without an example) and can do so in structured areas with more narrow boundaries. Drawing vertical, horizontal, and diagonal lines with increasingly greater precision is an important forerunner of skill in writing letters, numbers, and other conventional symbols.

Tracing

The individual completes simple dot-to-dot line grids that involve vertical, horizontal, diagonal, and curved lines in various combinations and different degrees of complexity.

Freehand Drawing

Freehand drawing involves both copying (i.e., the item is drawn from a model that is provided) and sketching (the figure is drawn from memory). Various types of configurations, ranging from simple geometric figures to more complex, abstract designs, are used. With regard to geometric shapes, the circle is typically the first one to be mastered (3 years); the cross and square are next (4 years). The progression continues to mastery of the triangle and rectangle; the diamond and the star are the last to be acquired. These latter shapes primarily involve the production of diagonal lines and angles and are typically mastered by 6 to 7 years of age. More complex, abstract designs are accomplished later. The ability to draw or copy shapes accurately is strongly related to copying letters legibly in kindergarten and as young children.

PREREQUISITE EXPERIENCES FOR WRITING

Experience and practice are important ingredients in mastering pencil skills; there are a number of foundational experiences that are integral to the effective mastery of pencil usage.[2,3,40,42] They include developmental readiness; balance; shoulder, forearm, and wrist stability; object manipulation; functional asymmetry; grasp of the implement; general prewriting; and coloring activities. Each of these experiences is described briefly below.

Developmental Readiness

The individual must be ready to write!

Balance

At a minimum, the individual must be able to sit independently with good trunk control; this is necessary to free the arms for writing or using an implement. If the balance is poor, the ability to concentrate on writing may be compromised. Therefore, the individual should be placed in the most stable position possible. Different positions should be considered, such as prone, sitting in a chair with support, standing at a board, and kneeling at a low table.

Stability

Stability can and should be addressed in many ways. For shoulder and elbow stability, positions in which the individual leans forward and rests the elbows on the table, holds the upper arms at the sides of the body, and performs the activity in a prone position are techniques for improving stability. For forearm and wrist stability, weights on the wrists; placing the weight of the body on the forearms; or writing, drawing, or copying on a board that is slanted are possible techniques.

Object Manipulation

A wide variety of experiences in using and manipulating objects of various sizes, weights, and shapes are important. Incorporating the gross motor eye-hand coordination skills of throwing, catching, and striking are also helpful.

Functional Asymmetry: Lead-Assist Hand Usage

To develop functional asymmetry, incorporate a variety of bimanual tasks that involve manipulation of objects and implements. If the opposite hand cannot be used, the paper can be attached to the writing surface in different ways (e.g., taped or placed on a clipboard). The assist hand may also be used to hold an object or squeeze a ball, Play-Doh, or other object.

Grasp of Writing Tool

To develop a comfortable and efficient grasp, a wide variety of different implements should be used. Pencil grips, triangular-shaped pens, easy-grip crayons, and talking pens are among other possibilities. The individual should be involved initially in activities that do not require fine or precise control.

General Prewriting

A broad base of prewriting experiences is important in preparing the individual for writing. Writing on different kinds of surfaces (e.g., aluminum foil, waxed paper, sandpaper, paper bags) is important and fun. Tracing around stencils with the finger(s) and around different two- and three-dimensional shapes and using a crayon or other implement (e.g., scented markers, weighted paintbrushes, chalk, toothpick, small stick, thimble on the finger) to trace around different shapes, figures, or objects can be done as well. Writing in the sand, mud, pudding, gelatin, and soap suds are also fun ways to engage in prewriting. Using scarves, paper towels, or magic wands to make lines or shapes in the air adds another dimension that challenges the individual. Remember that the sequence to follow is from the imitation of your drawing to tracing prepared figures to copying lines, shapes, and letters to writing freehand.

Coloring Activities

In developing or recovering implement usage skills, coloring is an important technique for providing experience. The following are some suggestions that may be used to promote progress. Initially use a large space or area for coloring; there is often no real pattern or attention to lines by the person coloring. Proceed to use gradually smaller spaces (e.g., an $8^1/_2 \times 11$ paper) and then a circle, square, or other shape with a 6″ diameter, then a 2″ diameter, and finally smaller designs that are more complex. Each of these steps requires increasingly greater control. The initial response is usually to color with random strokes and go outside the boundaries because of the lack of control. This is followed by a more controlled use of unidirectional strokes and moving the paper to fit the stroke direction. In the final step, multidirectional strokes are used to fit the design to be colored; the strokes are more controlled and remain within the boundaries of the figure.

IMPORTANT MOTOR LEARNING CONCEPTS

There are several motor learning concepts that, if understood and followed by practitioners, can help facilitate the skill learning/acquisition process.[1,24,26,27] Some of the more common and scientifically sound concepts related to skill acquisition are discussed below. They include transfer of learning, selected aspects of feedback, distribution and variability of practice, whole-part practice, and mental practice.

Transfer of Learning

Transfer of learning refers to the influence of the previous practice of or exposure to a skill on the learning or acquisition of a new skill. This concept is important because it helps direct the clinician in determining the protocol(s) to be used with clients; it can and should be used to help determine the sequence in which the skills are practiced. Since the goal of therapy is to assist the child in developing the ability to use the skill(s) acquired in the clinical setting in everyday activities, awareness and use of the concept of transfer of learning is important. The following are basic guidelines for applying this concept.

- Skill experiences need to be presented in a logical progression.
- Simple foundational skills should be practiced before more complex skills.
- Skill practice should include practice in real life and simulated real life settings to enhance transfer.
- Skills with similar components are more likely to show the transfer effect.

Kevin is a 5-year-old boy in kindergarten with developmental delays. His teacher is concerned that he holds a crayon awkwardly. Kevin scribbles spontaneously but does not imitate horizontal or vertical strokes. His mother is concerned that he is not developing the necessary skills for school and also states that Kevin will not practice.

The registered occupational therapist (OTR) evaluated Kevin and identified his grasp pattern as a brush grasp. The team decided that Kevin would receive OT services twice weekly in school to work on improving handwriting skills.

Natasha, the certified occupational therapy assistant (COTA), designed an intervention using the principles of motor learning. She began her treatment session by working on some gross motor activities to ready his posture and attention to fine motor tasks; she presented Kevin with some Legos to build some trucks and move them along so that he could work on his hand strength. Finally, Natasha worked with large crayons and allowed Kevin to scribble at first. She showed him how to hold the crayon with a static tripod grasp and allowed him to scribble this way. She then made a road for the Lego truck by making a line and asking him to make one next to it. Kevin was intrigued with the idea of the line; he asked how to do it. Natasha showed him using a hand-over-hand approach. They made many roads until he could do it on his own. At the end of the session, Natasha played teacher and asked Kevin to draw vertical lines on a sheet of school paper. She will ask the teacher to allow him to use the large crayon, and they will continue to work on his grasp until he is able to hold a regular crayon with a tripod grasp.

Following motor learning principles, Natasha used a logical progression of activities. They practiced simple foundational skills (e.g., posture, hand strength, grasping a large crayon) before the more complex skills. Finally, Natasha simulated school by playing teacher and using school paper. She also asked the teacher to follow through with the work they had done in the session.

Feedback

The use of feedback to inform the learner about his or her progress and about issues that still need to be addressed is integral to developing a skill. There are many forms or types of feedback. Our focus is on some guidelines for using augmented feedback to promote skill development. The term *augmented* refers to the fact that the feedback information is provided by some external source, either a person or the environment. The goal of augmented feedback is twofold: to help the learner achieve the goal of developing a skill and motivate the client to continue to work toward achieving that goal. Several important concepts related to augmented feedback and their roles in improving skill performance are described below.

Modeling or demonstration

This type of feedback involves providing visual information about how to perform a skill or task. It is a common approach to facilitating skill acquisition and has been shown to be an effective technique. The following are principles that have been shown to hold true in using demonstrations to enhance skill learning.

- Demonstrations are best if they are given to the individual before practicing the skill and in the early stages of skill acquisition.
- Demonstrations should be given throughout practice and as frequently as deemed helpful.
- Demonstrations should not be accompanied by verbal commentary because this can reduce attention devoted to important aspects of the skill being demonstrated.
- It is important to direct the individual's attention to the critical cues immediately before the skill is demonstrated.

The case study illustrates these principles; Natasha demonstrated how to hold the pencil and draw the two lines to make a road. During her demonstration she did not provide verbal commentary but did direct Kevin's attention to the critical cues. "See, I started at the top and went to the bottom; nice, straight roads. I will draw one side; you draw the other." Natasha demonstrated one side; Kevin made the other. Natasha did not say anything while they were making the lines. She would periodically stop and look at the roads and say "Start at the top and go to the bottom; nice, straight roads."

Verbal Instruction

The practice of a skill is often preceded or accompanied by verbal instruction or cues. These cues can affect the learning or skill acquisition process in positive ways if organized and used appropriately (Box 20-3).

During Kevin's session, Natasha provided brief verbal cues such as "nice, straight roads." She did not correct him on holding the crayon but only on the quality of his lines. She repeated these verbal cues throughout the session until Kevin was also saying them.

BOX 20-3

Verbal Cues

Verbal cues should be brief, to the point, and involve one to three words.
Verbal cues should be limited in terms of the number of cues given during or after the performance.
Only the major aspect(s) of the skill that is being concentrated on should be cued.
Verbal cues should be carefully timed so that they do not interfere with the performance.
Verbal cues can and should be initially repeated by the performer.

Knowledge of Results

Knowledge of results (KR) involves information provided from an external source about the outcome or end result of the performance of a skill or task. It answers the question of whether the goal was achieved? KR is usually provided by the clinician; however, at other times the clinician may structure the environment or task so that KR can be a natural part of it. For example, if the therapist says that a client completed the task in 45 seconds, s/he is providing information about the outcome of the performance. If the therapist provides a target to throw at, whether the ball or beanbag hits or misses the target, there is immediate KR about the outcome of the performance (i.e., the performer knows if the goal was achieved). This is a result of structuring the environment to provide information about the outcome of the performance.

Natasha provided Kevin with KR by saying that he made a road.

Knowledge of Performance

Knowledge of performance (KP) involves providing information about the nature or characteristics of the movement used to perform the task. In other words, the clinician provides information about how the task is performed; it answers the question, "what did the individual actually do?" or "how did s/he move to carry out the task?" For example, a therapist might say, "I need you to sit up straight with your back against the chair when you place the pegs" or "you should use the thumb, index, and middle fingers to grasp the pegs." Both of these suggestions/directions involve providing information about the movement or performance characteristics of KP. If the therapist also said that a client placed 10 pegs in 20 seconds, s/he has provided KR. There are also nonverbal means of providing KP, such as the use of videotapes of actual performance.

A variety of different combinations of both KR and KP typically help facilitate learning.

- KP error information (information about what the client did incorrectly) may help the performer change important performance characteristics and thus may help facilitate skill acquisition.
- Information about the appropriate or correct aspects of performance helps motivate the person to continue practicing.
- It is important to provide a balance between feedback that is error based and that which is based on appropriate or correct characteristics of the performance.
- KP feedback can also be descriptive (i.e., describing only the error observed in the performance) or

prescriptive (both describing the performance errors and indicating what needs to be done to correct them); prescriptive KP is more helpful than descriptive KP alone in the early or beginning stages of learning.

- KP and KR should be given close in time to but after completion of the task.
- KP and KR should not necessarily be given 100% of the time.
- Learning is enhanced if KR and KP are given at least 50% of the time.
- A frequently used procedure for giving KR and KP is to practice a skill several times and then provide the appropriate feedback.

Natasha asked Kevin which road he liked best, and they drove the truck on that road. This provided him with KP because he was able to see that the road was wide and straight enough for the truck to fit. She emphasized how straight and long the road was, which provides information about the correct aspects of performance. Since they practiced the skill many times, Kevin was provided with lots of KR and KP feedback.

Another approach to providing feedback is to ask for comments and thoughts from the child or client. For example, the therapist or clinician might ask the child, "do you understand what to do?" and "what are two things that you need to think about as you perform the task?" After completion of the task, it is also appropriate to ask the child or client for his or her opinion(s) about how s/he performed the task and whether s/he thought the goal(s) were reached. These comments can and probably should be discussed in preparation for the next practice. This type of interaction with the child or client also provides a way for the clinician to determine if the client understood the task and how s/he is feeling about how they are doing.

Distribution and Variability of Skill Practice

Skills may be practiced in a variety of ways, which include massed practice (a practice schedule in which the rest intervals between practice sessions or trials are very short), distributed practice (a practice schedule in which the rest intervals are longer), and variability of practice (practice experiences in which there are a variety of tasks in different environmental contexts).

- Shorter, more frequent practice sessions are preferable to longer, less frequent practice.
- If a skill or task is complex and/or requires a relatively long time to perform or it requires repetitive movements, relatively short practice trials or sessions with frequent rest periods are preferable.
- If the skill is relatively simple and takes only a brief time to complete, longer practice trials or sessions with less frequent rest periods are preferable.
- It can enhance skill acquisition to practice several tasks in the same session.
- If several tasks are to be practiced, divide the time spent on each and either randomly repeat them or use a sequence that aids the overall practice.
- Providing a number of different environmental contexts in which the skill is practiced appears to facilitate learning.
- With regard to the amount of practice, more is not necessarily always better.
- Clinical judgment should be used to recognize when practice is no longer producing changes; at this time a new or different task could and probably should be introduced.

Delia is a 9-year-old girl with developmental coordination disorder. She exhibits poor hand strength, quality of movement, and coordination. The team decided that Delia must learn to type efficiently so that she can eventually use a laptop for course work. Shauna, the COTA, developed a plan to use a computer typing program daily for 10 minutes at school and 2 nights at home. The typing program is designed for children and has frequent rest breaks embedded in the program. Delia is allowed to repeat the same session if she wishes. She is also encouraged to use the computer in the classroom for assignments. The teacher is aware that it may take her longer at the start.

This plan takes into account the principles and variability of skill practice outlined above. Specifically, Delia will engage in shorter, more frequent sessions (10 minutes 5 days a week and 2 nights at home). Since typing is complex, the program has frequent rest breaks. Furthermore, she will be practicing several typing tasks during the session (e.g., hand position, accuracy, timing, copying). The tasks are practiced at the child's level so that s/he will not get frustrated or overwhelmed. The COTA has designed the session, so Delia practices in school and at home to provide different environmental contexts. Since more practice is not always better, the COTA will pay attention so that she can recognize when Delia needs a new or different task. The computer program also allows for some variability in the tasks.

Whole versus Part Practice

How a skill is practiced is important. In general skills may be practiced as a whole or in parts. There are three major approaches to part practice. First, fractionalization is an approach to part practice that is often used with bimanual skills; each arm/hand is practiced separately before the two are put together to perform the task. The progressive part method is an approach that involves dividing the skill into its component parts; one part is practiced and then another one is added to the first until the whole skill is completed. Simplification is a part approach that involves simplifying the task in a variety of ways. The critical ingredient in any approach to part practice is identifying the appropriate parts.

- Whole practice is better when the skill or task to be performed is simple.
- Part practice may be preferable when the skill is more complex.
- If part practice is used, be sure that the parts practiced are natural units or go together.
- To simplify a task, reduce the nature and/or complexity of the objects to be manipulated (e.g., use a balloon for catching instead of a ball).
- To simplify a task, provide assistance to the learner that helps to reduce attention demands (e.g., provide trunk support during the practice of different eye-hand coordination tasks).
- To simplify a task, provide auditory or rhythmic accompaniment; this may help facilitate learning through assisting the learner in getting the appropriate rhythm of the movement.

Corey is a COTA who is working on improving the ability of 3-year-old Donovan to feed himself with the use of a spoon. Before practicing the task, Corey works with Donovan to be sure that he can sit independently in a supportive chair and hold a spoon (part practice). Once positioned in a supportive high chair, Corey provides finger foods for Donovan, who quickly picks up the food and brings it to his mouth. This is a natural unit for spoon-feeding. Corey then brings out Donovan's favorite pudding. He holds the spoon but has difficulty keeping it upright once it is full of pudding. Corey allows Donovan to spill the pudding and helps correct the grasp of the spoon. Later Corey builds up the tray so that Donovan does not have so far to bring the spoon (i.e., reducing the demands of the task).

Corey has structured the session so that Donovan can complete the task. It is not desirable to bring a spoon halfway to one's mouth; this is not functional. Therefore, Corey adapted the environment so that Corey could achieve the task, which will promote more practice of this skill. Corey may be able to move the tray closer to the original position in the next session.

Mental Practice

Mental practice involves cognitive or mental rehearsal of a skill; it is done without actually moving and typically involves mental imagery (i.e., mentally picturing oneself practicing the skill).

- Mental practice can help facilitate the acquisition of new skills as well as the relearning of old ones.
- Mental practice can help the person prepare to perform a task.
- Mental combined with physical practice works the best.
- For mental practice to be effective, the individual should have some basic ability to use imagery.
- Mental practice should be relatively short, not prolonged.

Children with developmental coordination disorders have at least average intelligence quotients (IQs) and are therefore able to practice the skills mentally. Clinicians can encourage older children to picture themselves completing motor tasks. After the child completes the task, it may be beneficial to review the performance to help him or her develop mental imaging strategies.

SUMMARY

This information provides a brief look at the foundations of fine motor development and the intricacy of how a number of components contribute to and are critical in the development of fine motor skills. The description of the steps involved in the development of object manipulation and implement usage skills provides a simple guideline for use in organizing and planning appropriate sequences for therapeutic activity. Last but not least, a number of simplified motor learning concepts along with some behavioral examples are presented; they are designed to help support the planning of practice for the learning and/or relearning of a wide variety of fine motor skills and should be helpful to the thoughtful and caring clinician.

References

1. Bass-Haugen J, Mathiowetz V, Flinn N: Optimizing motor behavior using the occupational therapy task-oriented approach. In Trombly C, Radomski M, editors: *Occupational therapy for physical dysfunction*, Philadelphia, 2002, Lippincott, Williams & Wilkins.
2. Benbow M: Principles and practices of teaching handwriting. In Henderson A, Pehoski C, editors: *Hand function in the child: foundations for remediation*, St Louis, 1995, Mosby.

3. Benbow M, Hanft B, Marsh D: Handwriting in the classroom: improving written communication. In Royeen CB, editor: AOTA *self-study series: classroom applications for school-based practice*, Rockville, Md, 1992, AOTA.
4. Berninger V, Rutber J: Relationship of finer function to beginning writing: application to diagnosis of writing disabilities, *Dev Med Child Neurol* 34:198, 1992.
5. Case-Smith J: Comparison of in-hand manipulation skills in children with and without fine motor delays, *Occup Ther J Res* 13:87, 1993.
6. Case-Smith J: Hand function and developmental coordination disorder. In Cermak S, Larkin D, editors: *Developmental coordination disorder*, Albany, NY, 2002, Delmar Thomson Learning.
7. Cermak S: Somatodyspraxia. In Fisher A, Murray E, Bundy A, editors: *Sensory integration: theory and practice*, Philadelphia, 1991, FA Davis.
8. Connolly J, Dalgleish M: The emergence of a tool-using skill in infancy, *Dev Psychol* 25:894, 1989.
9. Daly J, Kelley G, Krauss A: Relationship between visual-motor integration and handwriting skills of children in kindergarten: a modified replication study, *Am J Occup Ther* 57:459, 2003.
10. Deuel R: Developmental dysgraphia and motor skill disorders, *J Child Neurol* 10:57, 1995.
11. Eliasson A: Sensorimotor integration of normal and impaired development of precision movement of the hand. In Henderson A, Pehoski C, editors: *Hand function in the child: foundations for remediation*, St. Louis, 1995, Mosby.
12. Exner C: Development of hand skills. In Case-Smith J, editor: *Occupational therapy for children*, ed 5, St Louis, 2005, Mosby.
13. Exner C: In-hand manipulation skills. In Case-Smith J, Pehoski C, editors: *Development of hand skills in the child*, Rockville, Md, 1992, AOTA.
14. Folio R, Fewell R: *Peabody developmental motor scales*, Allen, Texas, 1983, DLM Teaching Resources.
15. Hill E, Wing A: A dyspraxic deficit in specific language impairment and developmental coordination disorder? Evidence from hand and arm movements, *Dev Med Child Neurol* 40:388, 1998.
16. Hill E, Wing A: Coordination of grip force and load force in developmental coordination disorder: a case study, *Neurocase* 5:537, 1999.
17. Hill E, Wing A: Developmental disorders and the use of grip force to compensate for inertial forces during voluntary movement. In Connolly KJ, editor: *Psychobiology of the hand*, London, 1998, Mac Keith Press.
18. Hulme C, Smart A, Moran G, et al: Visual, kinaesthetic and cross-modal development: relationship to motor skill development, *Perception* 12:477, 1983.
19. Jucaite A, Fernell E, Forssberg H, et al: Deficient coordination of associated postural adjustments during a lifting task in children with neurodevelopmental disorders, *Dev Med Child Neurol* 45:731, 2003.
20. Kuhtz-Buschbeck J, Hoppe B, Golge M, et al: Sensorimotor recovery in children after traumatic brain injury: analyses of gait, gross motor, and fine motor skills, *Dev Med Child Neurol* 45:821, 2003.
21. Langaas T, Aadne R, Dahle E, et al: *Clinical assessment of eye movements in children with reading disabilities and with developmental coordination disorder*, 2002, Abstract. http://www.abstractsonline.com
22. Lederman S, Klatzky R: The hand as a perceptual system. In Connolly KJ, editor: *Psychobiology of the hand*, London, 1998, Mac Keith Press.
23. Lundy-Ekman L, Ivery R, Keele S, et al: Timing and force control deficits in clumsy children, *J Cogn Neurosci* 3:367, 1991.
24. Magill R: *Motor learning: concepts and applications*, New York, 2001, McGraw-Hill.
25. Meulenbroek R, van Galen G: Perceptual-motor complexity of printed and cursive letters, *J Exp Educ* 58:95, 1990.
26. Missiuna C, Mandich A: Integrating motor learning theories into practice. In Cermak S, Larkin D, editors: *Developmental coordination disorder*, Albany, NY, 2002, Delmar Thomson Learning.
27. Niemeijer A, Smits-Engelsman B, Reynders K, et al: Verbal actions of physiotherapists to enhance motor learning in children with DCD, *Hum Movement Sci* 22:567, 2003.
28. Pehoski C: Object manipulation in infants and children. In Henderson A, Pehoski C, editors: *Hand function in the child: foundations for remediation*, St Louis, 1995, Mosby.
29. Pitcher T, Piek J, Hay D: Fine and gross motor ability in males with ADHD, *Dev Med Child Neurol* 45:525, 2003.
30. Preminger F, Weiss P, Weintraub N: Predicting occupational performance: handwriting versus keyboarding, *Am J Occup Ther* 58:193, 2004.
31. Rodger S, Ziviani J, Watter P, et al: Motor and functional skills of children with developmental coordination disorder: a pilot investigation of measurement issues, *Hum Movement Sci* 22:461, 2003.
32. Rosblad B, van Hofsten C: Repetitive goal-directed arm movements in children with developmental coordination disorders: role of visual information, *Adapt Phys Activ Quart* 11:190, 1994.
33. Schneck C: Comparison of pencil-grip patterns in first graders with good and poor writing skills, *Am J Occup Ther* 45:701, 1991.
34. Schneck M, Henderson A: Descriptive analysis of the developmental progression of grip position for pencil and crayon control in nondysfunctional children, *Am J Occup Ther* 44:893, 1990.
35. Smits-Engelsman B, Wilson P, Westenberg Y, et al: Fine motor deficiencies in children with developmental coordination disorder and learning disabilities: an underlying open-loop control deficit, *Hum Movement Sci* 2:495, 2003.
36. Thomassen A, Teulings H: The development of handwriting. In Martlew M, editor: *The psychology of written language*, New York, 1983, John Wiley & Sons, Inc.
37. Weil M, Cunningham Amundson S: Relationship between visual motor and handwriting skills of children in kindergarten, *Am J Occup Ther* 48:982, 1994.
38. Williams H: Motor control in children with developmental coordination disorder. In Cermak S, Larkin D, editors: *Developmental coordination disorder*, Albany, NY, 2002, Delmar Thomson Learning.

39. Williams H: *Perceptual and motor development*, Englewood Cliffs, NJ, 1983, Prentice-Hall, Inc.
40. Williams H: *Smart text: fine motor control and development*, Columbia, SC, 2004, University of South Carolina.
41. Williams H, Woollacott M, Ivry R: Timing and motor control in clumsy children, *J Motor Behav* 24:165, 1992.
42. Ziviani J: The development of graphomotor skills. In Henderson A, Pehoski C, editors: *Hand function in the child: foundations for remediation*, St Louis, 1995, Mosby.

Recommended Reading

Benbow M: Hand skills and handwriting. In Cermak S, Larkin D, editors: *Developmental coordination disorder*, Albany, NY, 2001, Delmar Thomson Learning.

Schmidt R: *Motor control and learning: a behavioral emphasis*, ed 4, Chicago, 2005, Human Kinetics Publishers, Inc.

REVIEW *Questions*

1. Define and differentiate between the following terms: motor adaptation, motor control, motor learning, and occupation.
2. Describe an OT session that teaches a child to use both hands together using random practice.
3. Using motor learning principles, describe how you would provide a child feedback and demonstration.
4. Describe how the principles of motor control would be applied to teach a child to button a shirt. Be sure to discuss demonstration, feedback, practice, adaptations, and so on.
5. Describe the progression of fine motor skill development.

SUGGESTED *Activities*

1. Demonstrate an OT activity to improve fine motor skills using random practice, mass practice, and distributed practice. Discuss the benefits of one type of practice over the other.
2. List five principles of motor learning and describe how you would use these to teach a child a new skill.
3. Have each student bring in an item (for each student in the class) that could be used as an activity in a fine motor or gross motor kit. Ask the students to discuss how this item could be used in the clinic, with special emphasis on the client factor it addresses. Students share their items so that everyone leaves with a variety of items that may be useful in the clinic.
4. Require students to visit a website to find activities that would improve fine or gross motor skills in children. Share the activities and websites so that they may be used as a resource.
5. Observe typical children learning a new fine motor or gross motor skill. Which teaching techniques were helpful and why? How could these techniques be used in occupational therapy practice?

21

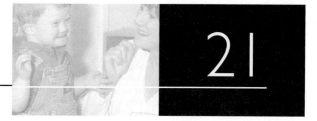

Sensory Processing/ Integration and Occupation

RICARDO C. CARRASCO
SUSAN STALLINGS-SAHLER

CHAPTER *Objectives*

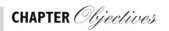

After studying this chapter, the reader will be able to accomplish the following:

- Define the principles of sensory integration treatment
- Understand the role of the certified occupational therapy assistant in working with children who have sensory processing dysfunction
- Define sensory modulation disorder
- Describe sensory modulation intervention strategies
- Understand the types of sensory movement disorder and intervention strategies
- Identify intervention techniques to work with children who have postural-ocular and bilateral integration dysfunction
- Identify intervention techniques to work with children who have developmental dyspraxia

KEY TERMS

Sensory integration
Sensory processing
Sensory modulation disorder
Praxis
Functional support capacities
Postural-ocular and bilateral integration dysfunction
Developmental dyspraxia
Ideation

CHAPTER OUTLINE

Dr. A. Jean Ayres, the originator of **sensory integration** (SI) theory, assessment, and treatment, strongly believed and advocated that the practice of SI by an occupational therapist should take place only at the postgraduate level. SI theory, assessment, and treatment are extremely complex, although the activities appear deceptively easy because they are so playful when effectively implemented by a skilled therapist. However, in settings with close supervision by an appropriately SI-trained and experienced pediatric occupational therapist, the certified occupational therapy assistant (COTA) can contribute effectively to the child's intervention program.

Sensory processing refers to the means by which the brain receives, detects, and integrates incoming sensory information for use in producing adaptive responses to one's environment. Children who have sensory integrative dysfunction have a cluster of symptoms that are believed to reflect dysfunction in central nervous system (CNS) processing of sensory input rather than a primary sensory deficit such as a hearing impairment, blindness, a frank CNS insult such as stroke or traumatic brain injury, or even that which comes from chromosomal or genetic abnormalities such as Down syndrome. The disorder leads to disorganized, maladaptive interaction with people and objects in the environment. Such interaction in turn produces distorted internal sensory feedback, which reinforces the problem.[5]

However, there are several subtypes of sensory processing dysfunction. Whereas individuals with SI dysfunction (or sensory processing dysfunction) share many similarities, they do not all appear alike. Children with the disorder often have a primary diagnosis such as autism, learning disability, or attention deficit disorder or psychogenic comorbidities related to anxiety, panic, or attachment disorder. There is also a range of levels of severity, from mild to quite severe. In some children sensory processing dysfunction may lead to disabling learning problems, causing academic failure.[5] In others it may be reflected in clumsiness and the struggle of the child to acquire everyday occupations that others take for granted. Whereas some children may exhibit impairment in the ability to regulate incoming sensations, others may fail to detect and orient to novel or important sensory information, which is called **sensory modulation disorder.**[5,6,12,62,68]

Some types of sensory processing impairment may lead to poor social adaptation; the inability to form close, intimate relationships; and difficulty in expressing and interpreting socioemotional cues.[43] Led by the pioneering work of the late A. Jean Ayres, PhD, OTR, occupational therapists have examined and developed treatment strategies for sensory integrative dysfunction in the early intervention and school-age child population since the early 1970s.*

The early signs of sensory processing problems can be observed even in infancy[64] (Figure 21-1). Parents often report that they have noticed subtle differences as early as the perinatal period, such as a lack of cuddling behavior, failure to make eye contact, oversensitivity to sounds or touch, difficulty with the oral-motor demands of suckling, and chewing food[44,71] (Figure 21-2). Poor self-regulation of arousal states, irritability, and colic are frequently reported.[1,45,67,71] In the toddler period the motor, social, and self-care milestones may be delayed. The child may lack normal curiosity about the environment. On the other hand, s/he may explore the world in a disorganized and destructive manner, which does not lead to learning and mastery. Figuring out basic whole body movements such as how to climb backwards downstairs or climb onto a riding toy are bewildering and frightening tasks.[62,64]

The preschooler with sensory-based motor planning problems may be unable to organize the body postures and gestures that are appropriate for nonverbal communication, such as the need for affection, to use the toilet, or for a favorite snack.[64] Typically developing preschoolers can seem almost mesmerized with learning the process of dressing and will attempt the donning and doffing of clothes, shoes, and coats seemingly for hours at a time. However, the child with sensory-based motor planning deficits (called dyspraxia) may be dependent on caregivers for assistance and often avoids dressing and hygiene activities altogether. S/he may handle toys and objects ineptly, constantly damaging or breaking them.

As the child attains school age, the heightened challenges of the elementary grades—paying attention in class, reading, listening, using writing and art tools, and interacting with peers—bring sensory processing dysfunction to light even more. During leisure time the child avoids fine manipulative activities or skilled gross motor play, instead preferring more sedentary activities such as watching television, playing video games, looking at books (Figure 21-3). Highly creative and intelligent children may conceal their motor control inadequacies through verbal make-believe play, which emphasizes imagination and social interaction (with a lot of aimless running around) over toy manipulation and body coordination.

Occupational therapy (OT) practitioners need to consider observations such as the above behaviors within the context of the child's family system, cultural expectations and norms, and socioeconomic advantages and limitations. As members of a team of professionals, we also utilize multiple sources of information from our

*References 2, 4, 5, 8, 10, 12, 32, 41, 59, 63, 65, 72.

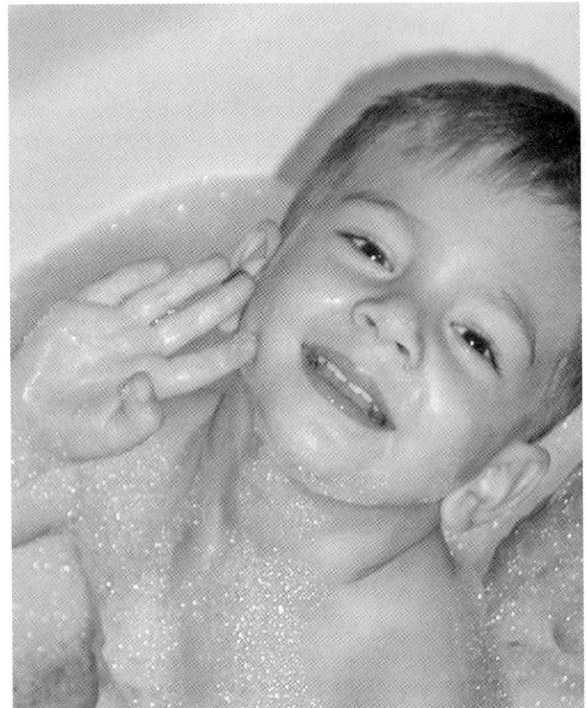
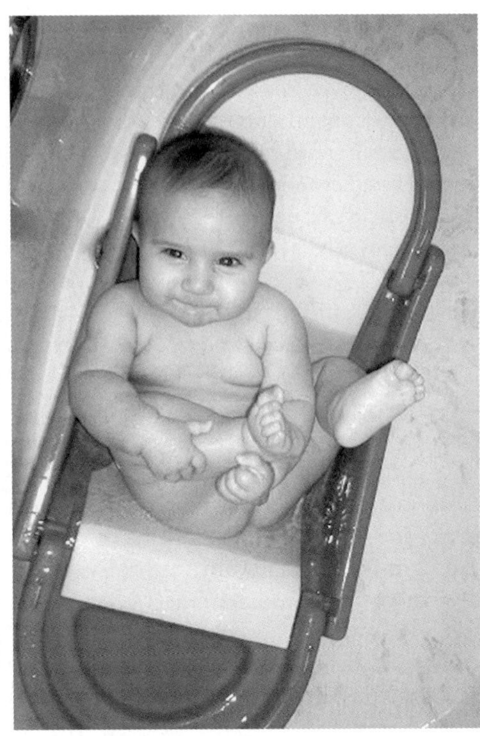

FIGURE 21-1 **A,** Typically developing children enjoy sensory experiences such as bath time. **B,** Typically developing infants enjoy the sensory experience of finding their feet and playing in the bath.

coworkers about the child's cognitive, language, and social development because these areas of function will have significant effects on the quality of the child's adaptive behavior.[29] A child whose sociocultural and socioeconomic environments do not provide adequate opportunities for movement exploration and object play may need environmental enrichment to facilitate the emergence of motor planning skills.

ASSESSMENT OF SENSORY PROCESSING

Initial OT evaluation typically employs a top-down approach; the first tier of focus is the child's daily occupational and role performances.[31,66] However, it may become apparent during the evaluation of occupational performance that sensory processing deficits are major contributors to his or her functional difficulties, although the specific nature of the deficits cannot be delineated without further assessment. The COTA may be trained to administer a number of sensorimotor screening tests and other structured assessments of sensory processing and motor performance. The interpretation of the results should be performed by the OT supervisor (i.e., the registered occupational therapist [OTR]), but the COTA can provide important insights into that process. The COTA and/or his or her OT supervisor will often collect this type of information on the children referred for OT because sensory processing dysfunction frequently interferes with other more typical functional difficulties for which children are referred, such as poor handwriting, trouble with self-care tasks, behavioral problems, and evaluation for adaptive technology.

A very important part of the assessment process includes getting initial data from observations of the child by his or her caregivers, teachers, and/or other therapists. If you are still not sure of the existence of a sensorimotor processing issue, you and your supervisor may then decide to administer a standardized screening test. Based on the results of those two sources, an experienced team of OT practitioners may have enough data to formulate a treatment plan. Otherwise, a decision may be made to pursue more comprehensive evaluation of the child's capacities for SI.[22]

A complete sensory processing evaluation typically covers five major areas: (1) sensory modulation across each sensory system (i.e., tactile, mobile, visual, auditory, olfactory, and taste); (2) perceptual discrimination ability in most of these areas; (3) postural-ocular

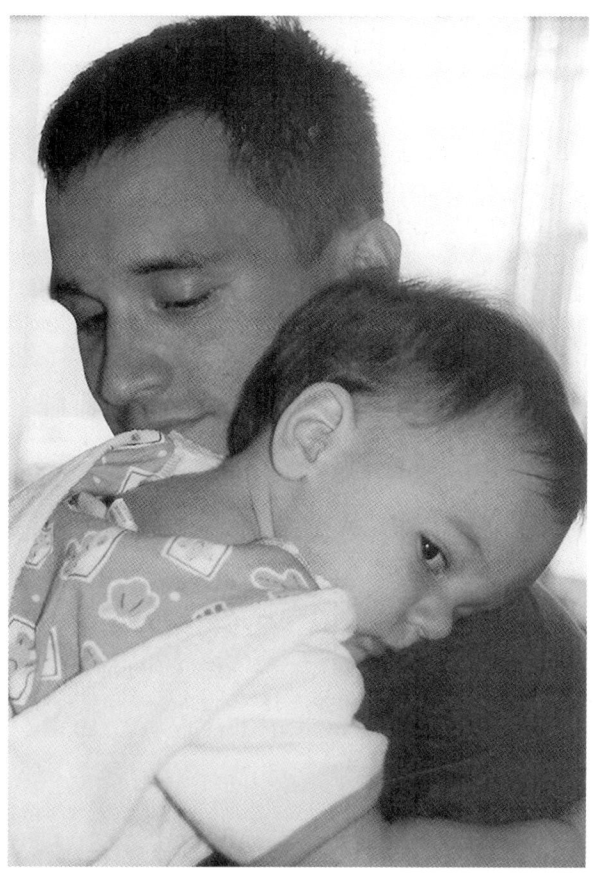

FIGURE 21-2 Whereas typically developing children gain comfort in being held closely by dad, those with sensory processing difficulties may find it discomforting.

function; (4) bilateral motor coordination (including organization at and across the midline of the body); and (5) praxis (the ability to internally visualize and plan skilled movement actions).[6,18] However, the OT supervisor may elect to focus on fewer areas if the initial OT assessment and SI screening indicate that certain areas are not problematic.

Observational and History-Taking Assessment

Observation of the child in his or her natural environment(s) is essential because not only can it show us areas in which there may be sensory issues but it should also demonstrate how those issues affect the child's performance during daily occupational roles and tasks. The main concerns of the child, family, and others usually relate to difficulties with vital age-expected play skills, social activities, capacity for self-regulation, and academic learning that the child must master to grow up successfully. It is to these concerns that we need to direct

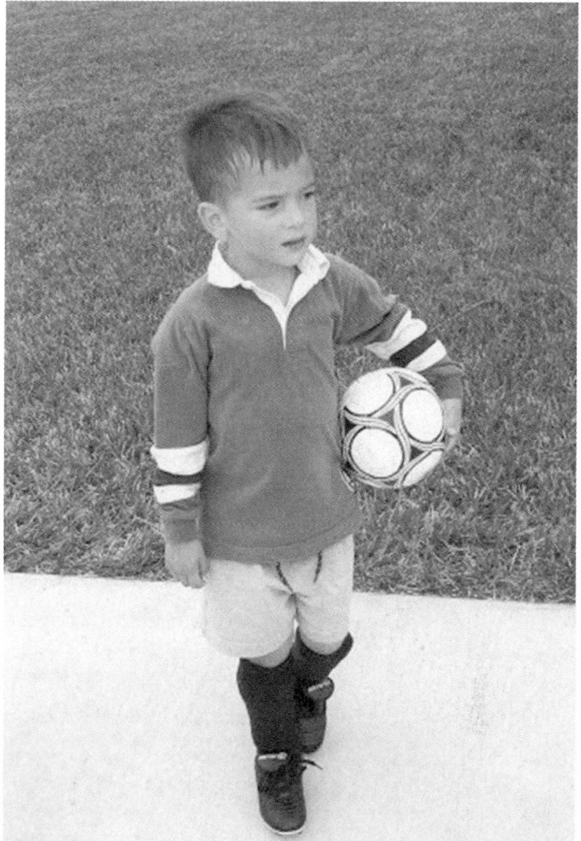

A

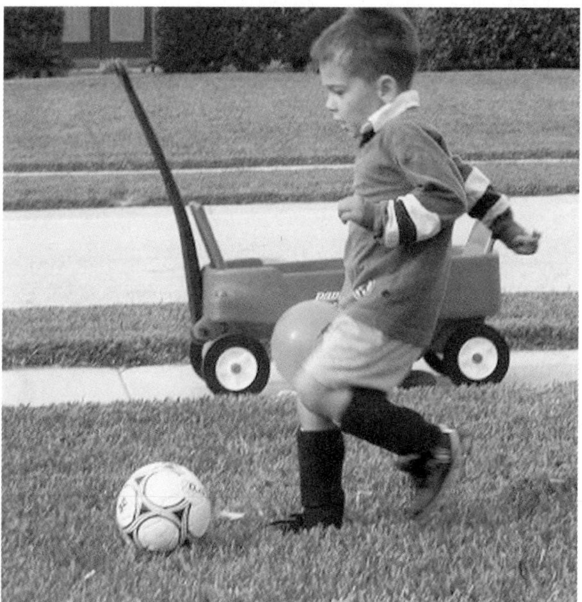

B

FIGURE 21-3 **A,** A child's ability to participate successfully in leisure/play activities such as soccer requires coordination, motor planning, sequencing, timing, and body awareness. **B,** Liam shows adequate coordination, motor planning, sequencing, timing, and body awareness as he kicks the soccer ball in the desired direction.

our attention and then, like peeling away the layers of an onion, begin to probe the "why?" underlying those occupational challenges.

Jason's teacher may report that his letter formation is acceptable, but his handwriting movements are slow and laborious and he presses down so hard that he tears his paper or breaks the pencil lead. He stops frequently to shake or stretch his fingers and complains of pain in his hand. Consequently, Jason fails to complete both classroom and homework written assignments on time, and his grades are suffering. His parents complain that it is a fight each night at home to get Jason to begin and complete his written homework.

In this case, the inability to complete handwritten assignments is the occupational activity that initially brought about the referral. However, assuming that we have ruled out other causes, we can use sensory processing theory to analyze the qualitative nature of Jason's handwriting. From this we hypothesize that Jason is receiving insufficient proprioceptive feedback from the joints and muscles in his fingers, so he must bear down harder on his pencil to obtain it, which assists him in controlling and guiding the pencil. This attempt to respond adaptively to his impairment slows Jason's progress and creates exceptional fatigue and discomfort in his hand and finger joints. This hypothesis must then be tested by means of a sensory processing evaluation of Jason's somatosensory (tactile-pressure sense) system.

The hypothesis about the contribution of sensory processing dysfunction will help shape one aspect of our intervention approach, which will probably include activation of Jason's proprioceptive system before handwriting activities. Therefore, when relating our SI assessment results to caregivers and other members of the team and in planning a course of intervention, the OT supervisor/COTA team must bring their interpretation of sensory processing issues full circle in order to help explain concern about the child's occupational performance, which was the original source of the referral. Furthermore, we would go on to recommend either classroom or direct service interventions to address the underlying sensory processing issues (Figure 21-4).

Multiple observation checklists are available for use.[24] Some can be found in pediatric OT textbooks, whereas others are available for purchase from test publishers. Some checklists are informal and based on SI problem behaviors cited in the clinical literature rather than on norms derived from children of various ages. They can be used to gain informative data from teachers as well as caregivers. Such tools can be helpful if used with the age range intended.[19] Two examples of such tools are the Sensorimotor History Questionnaire[25,28] and the Teacher Questionnaire of Sensory Behavior[27] (see Chapter 21, Appendices A and B).

Formal Assessment Tools

CLINICAL *Pearl*

Informal checklists like the examples given above should never form the entire basis of the conclusions made about a child's sensorimotor functioning.

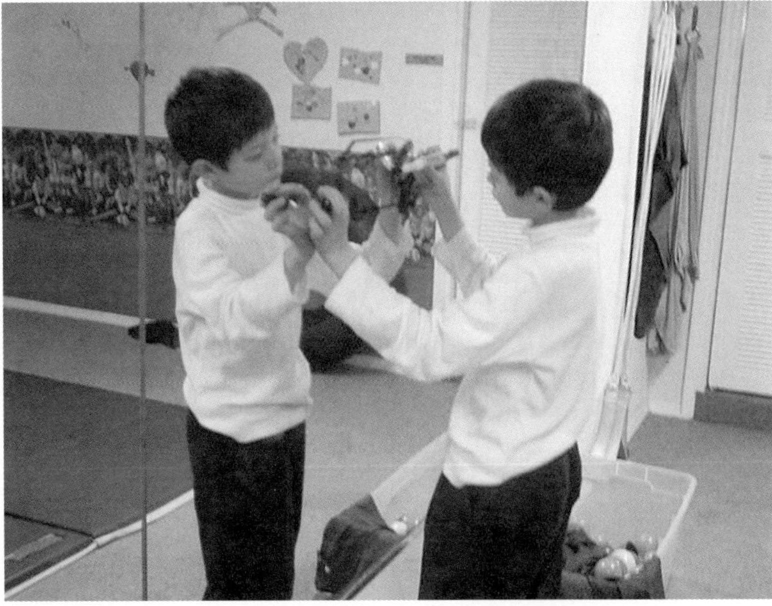

FIGURE 21-4 Children with sensory processing difficulties may experience poor body awareness. Standing while writing may help them become more aware of their bodies and movements. This child writes on a mirror, which also provides visual cues to help him.

Formal rating scales are based on knowledge of a child's developmental history and direct observation, by trained professionals who know the child's behaviors, abilities, and preferences well. Such scales are often well researched and standardized on normative groups and fit into the class of SI screening instruments. A summary of them can be found in the literature,[21] and some are described in Table 21-1.

Comprehensive Evaluation of Sensory Processing/Integration

The most comprehensive standardized test battery of SI functioning for children ages 4 years, 0 months through 8 years, 11 months is the one consisting of the Sensory Integration and Praxis Tests (SIPT).[3] These tests include measures of vestibular, proprioceptive, and somatosensory processing; visual perceptual and visuomotor integration; integration between the two sides of the body; and many of the components of the complex set of abilities known as **praxis.** The praxis tests include measures of postural imitation, motor planning in response to a verbal request, motor sequencing ability, imitation of oral movements, graphic reproduction, and three-dimensional block construction.[2,3,11]

Because of its complexity, only certain licensed rehabilitation professionals with a baccalaureate or graduate degree who have undergone documented rigorous training may administer the SIPT. To become more familiar with the various components of SI

TABLE 21-1

Summary of Screening or Structured Assessments of Sensory Processing and Sensory-Based Motor Dysfunction

NAME OF SCREENING TOOL	STATED PURPOSE	INTENDED AGE RANGE
Test of Sensory Function in Infants[32]	Designed to measure an infant's sensory reactivity and processing to determine the presence and extent of the deficit	4 to 18 months
The Infant/Toddler Sensory Profile[35]	By means of the parents' report, measures infant and toddler reactions to everyday sensory events across all modalities	Birth to 36 months
The Sensory Profile[34]	Measures child's responses to sensory experiences as well as perceived movement competence by means of the parents' report	3 to 10 years
The Short Sensory Profile[50]	A one-page questionnaire with 38 items divided into 7 sections; answers based on a five-point scale	3 to 10 years
The Adolescent/Adult Sensory Profile[39]	Self-report; measures responses of teens through mature adults to sensory events in everyday life	11 to 90 years
The First STEP Screening Test for the Evaluation of Preschoolers (Parent Checklists)[51]	General screening of major developmental areas, including several creative items of bilateral integration and praxis	2 years, 9 months to 6 years, 2 months
The DeGangi-Berk Test of Sensory Integration[33]	A total of 36 items that measure overall sensory integration as well as postural control, bilateral motor integration, and reflex integration	3 to 5 years
The Miller Assessment for Preschoolers[52]	Broad overview of a child's developmental status; several indices assessing key areas of sensory integration performance	2 years, 9 months to 5 years, 8 months
Clinical Observations of Sensory Integration[2] Clinical Observations Based on Sensory Integration Theory[14]	Informal floor assessment primarily assessing a child's postural reactions and oculomotor responses that are included in most neurological screenings of soft neurological signs	Various ages; recommended for ≈ ages 5 through 10 years
Bruininks-Oseretsky Test of Motor Proficiency[17]	Both short screening and long evaluation forms included; measures a variety of gross and fine motor skills; includes many items for assessing bilateral coordination	4.6 to 14.5 years

evaluation, we recommend that pediatric COTAs have a qualified SIPT examiner administer this instrument to them and engage in a reflective discussion of their experiences. This will provide valuable insights about both the process of SI and its assessment.

One of the most challenging aspects of the interpretation of SI and praxis evaluation data is the lack of a concrete one-to-one correspondence between a low score on a particular test and the meaning of that score. Invariably, the SI assessment is about discovering the underlying sensory disorganization that leads to poor performance in one or more "end products." These end products can come in the form of functional motor skills such as riding a bicycle or using tools, academic learning skills such as reading and computation, cognitive abilities such as language and abstract thinking, or psychosocial capacities such as emotional attachment and self-esteem. However, between sensory disorganization and these end products there are also intermediate abilities termed by Kimball **functional support capacities.**[46] Functional support capacities represent secondary neurobehavioral, motor, social-emotional, and cognitive proficiencies that are not functional in the occupational sense but are considered prerequisites for end products to develop normally. A number of these are measured by the SIPT and other tests and include components such as bilateral motor coordination, various types of praxis, postural tone, self-regulatory mechanisms, cognitive sequencing, and the ability to cross the midline of the body. Therefore, numerous patterns of underlying dysfunction are possible; end product impairments are interpreted according to the way in which the test scores cluster.

Two 7-year-old children, Emma and Brian, present with severe handwriting problems along with other fine motor difficulties. However, their SIPT results are distinctly different. Emma's profile displays a low score on copying designs along with many low scores on visual and tactile space perception and low postrotary nystagmus (a vestibular marker), but motor accuracy and praxis tests fall within normal limits. By comparison, Brian's SIPT profile also shows a low score on copying designs, but postrotary nystagmus and visual and tactile space perception scores are in the normal range. However, his motor accuracy performance is poor, a number of praxis tests are low, and he has low scores on finger identification, touch localization, and kinesthetic perception.

Both of these children had similar end product outcomes, yet their SI and praxis evaluations demonstrated sensory processing and functional support pathways different from that outcome. Emma's pattern of scores suggests that her poor handwriting and design reproduction skills are probably attributable to impaired visual space perception resulting from poor integration of vestibular, somatosensory, and visual sensory input. On the other hand, disorganized motor planning, which is attributable to the inefficient processing of upper extremity proprioceptive input and a poor body scheme, is the hypothesized source of Brian's impaired handwriting.

Herein lies the difference between a sensory processing evaluation approach and a direct occupation-based assessment model. The former is based on an attempt to measure the underlying neuromotor and sensory mechanisms that support the function and occupation. The latter documents and describes the nature of the occupational outcomes. Accordingly, OT interventions based on a top-down teaching strategy to address handwriting issues might look very similar for these two children. However, an SI approach would take the differences in underlying sensorimotor organization into consideration, and the SI treatment program for these two children would look quite different.

In summary, research using the SIPTs, as well as Ayres's earlier tests, has demonstrated that (1) various aspects of the components of sensory discrimination, bilateral motor organization, and motor planning tend to group together statistically to form predictable clusters; (2) developmental trends can be identified in most SI constructs; and (3) certain sensory systems integrate with one another to give rise to higher-order capacities in behavior and ability.[3,5,7,9] With regard to the role of the additional neurobehavioral construct of sensory modulation, although Ayres originally identified the phenomenon of sensory registration disorders, which are now called sensory modulation disorders, her life ended before she was able to pursue more objective measurement of them. Research on theory and measurement has contributed significantly to our understanding in this area.*

SENSORY MODULATION DISORDER

When a COTA hears terms such as tactile defensiveness, gravitational insecurity, poor sensory registration, and sensory hypersensitivity, s/he is exposed to some of the clinical language that refers to behaviors representing the class of sensory processing impairments termed sensory modulation disorder. Normal sensory modulation is a regulatory process of the nervous system that controls the perceived intensity of incoming sensations through the raising or lowering of neuronal thresholds to that sensory input. This is achieved by means of adaptive

*References 35, 37-39, 48-50, 53, 54, 56, 57, 69, 71.

balancing of inhibition and excitation at many levels of the CNS. Excitation of a neuron tends to lower its threshold to stimulation, thereby allowing more of the sensory input to be experienced in the nervous system. In contrast, if there is more inhibition, the neuronal thresholds tend to rise, in effect partially or fully blocking the sensory input from being registered in our awareness. Your CNS is regulating sensations in this way as you read this chapter. If it did not, your brain might be so flooded with sensory messages that you would not be able to focus your attention, control your posture, or think about what you are reading. On the other hand, you might have such high sensory thresholds that you overfocus, being unable to hear someone calling you from another room, feel a tap on your shoulder, or sense that your body is about to fall out of a chair.

This is only an imaginary taste of what life is like for people with sensory modulation dysfunction. However, some have sensory experiences that are so distorted that everyday sensations are uncomfortable, painful, frightening, or surreal in nature. A woman with agoraphobia and sensory modulation disorder once told this author that at times she could be walking along a concrete and tile floor in a department store and would suddenly feel as if the floor were soft and her feet were going through the floor rather than striking the hard surface. At other times she had trouble falling asleep because she felt as if bugs were crawling on her. Children commonly manifest sensory modulation irregularities by their intolerance of such stimuli as clothing, food textures, imposed touch, and household noises (e.g., a phone ringing or appliance operation) or, conversely, by not noticing salient stimuli in their environment. Probably the earliest harbinger of SI dysfunction in infancy is unusual overreactivity to touch, taste, or smell. Some forms of gastric reflux in infancy appear to be precipitated not by gastroesophageal abnormalities but by olfactory hypersensitivity, which causes the infant to become nauseous.[65]

Examples of hyper- and hyporeactivity can be identified as you look through the Sensory History Questionnaire (SHQ) shared previously. Research in which *The Sensory Profile*[38] and *The Adolescent and Adult Sensory Profile*[16] were used revealed that children and adults develop behavioral patterns of dealing with their modulation problems, which have been described by Dunn in her model of sensory processing.[15,36] These patterns tend to divide into four quadrants that are bounded by (1) a continuum of sensory avoidance to sensory seeking and (2) a continuum of acting in accordance with threshold to acting to counteract threshold. We all fall within one of these quadrants, but dysfunction lies more at the extreme ends of the continua, where a person's daily life and relationships are more apt to be disrupted by modulatory irregularities. For more information on this, the reader is referred to the work of Dunn, Miller, Wilbarger, and associates.*

SENSORY-BASED MOVEMENT DISORDER

Sensory-based movement disorder refers to both (1) postural system disorganization due to poor vestibular and proprioceptive processing and (2) impairments of complex midbrain or cortically controlled internal visualization and motor planning. Children who are found to have sensory integrative problems leading to **postural-ocular and bilateral integration dysfunction** typically manifest poor vestibular-proprioceptive processing, mild hypotonia, a delay in the development of postural and equilibrium reactions, and problems with midline integration. They may have no or at least an insignificant degree of motor planning deficits. A more motorically involved child will usually exhibit a similar picture of immaturity in postural mechanism development but be compounded by a condition Ayres and others have termed **developmental dyspraxia.** Of these two conditions, the child with dyspraxia is usually identified more readily because of his or her obvious awkwardness and tendency to have more difficulties with play and acquisition of functional skills.

Postural-Ocular and Bilateral Integration Dysfunction

Of the two broad patterns of sensory-based motor dysfunction, this one is milder in severity. It may be identified by a cluster of several sensory, behavioral, and motor characteristics, including poor sensory modulation; low scores on tests of postrotary nystagmus, vestibular response to tilt, and bilateral motor coordination; measures of standing and walking balance; sluggish postural tendencies such as an inclination toward inactive positions and sedentary activities; W sitting; poor balance; difficulty with two-handed tasks; a delay in demonstrating hand preference; and a tendency not to cross the midline of the body after age 5.[3,47,64]

Other concerns frequently noted include poor protective, righting, and equilibrium responses during functional movement or clinical assessment. Also noted may be immature gait patterns such as the use of a wide base, with lateral weight shifting of the lower extremities. To compensate for low extensor muscle tone in the upper body, shoulder girdle positioning may be marked by scapular retraction, shoulder elevation, and high guard arm posturing. These patterns are typical in toddler and early preschool development but usually give way to mature postural organization, smooth bilateral-

*References 34, 36, 51, 57, 59, 60, 63, 71-73.

reciprocal movements, and normal lateral dominance during the period between the ages of 4 and 6.[40,66]

Assessment

Potential problems with postural adaptation can be observed during the performance of certain items from standardized child development or motor proficiency tests. In infancy the items from tests such as the *Bayley Scales of Infant Development–II*,[13] the *Peabody Developmental Motor Scales*,[42] and others are listed in Box 21-1.

For example, the preschooler with low muscle tone and/or difficulties with balance, postural mechanisms, and bilateral coordination as well as symmetry of left/right function may be identified from the items of the *Miller Assessment for Pre-Schoolers*[51] listed in Box 21-2. Three year olds who are at risk for postural and bilateral integration deficits will experience difficulty with the items on the *DeGangi-Berk Test of Sensory Integration*,[33] which are listed in Box 21-3. The *Bruininks-Oseretsky Test of Motor Proficiency*[17] (now being restandardized) contains many good postural-ocular and bilateral coordination items, which are listed in Box 21-4.

Developmental Dyspraxia

This disorder represents the second broad category of sensory-based motor dysfunctions. It is important to realize that children with cognitive impairments will usually have some degree of motor planning difficulty that is part of the diagnosis and is consistent with their development across the board. However, in some cases sensory processing deficits may also play a role along with the inborn condition. There are three major processes

BOX 21-1

Test Items to Observe Postural Adaptation in Infants

- Postural responses while being picked up, held, and handled
- In late toddlers/young preschoolers, more mature postural responses, such as shifting weight in preparation for kicking a ball; positioning the upper body for catching a ball
- Observations of protective, righting, and equilibrium reactions
- Observations of organization of two-sided body/leg movements: early crawling movements, crawling/creeping patterns; stair-climbing patterns; jumping with both feet; hopping; arm thrusts
- Observations of organization of two-sided upper extremity movements: test items examining symmetry/asymmetry; the ability to use the hands together at midline; catching a ball with two hands; hand-to-hand object transfer; all items requiring one hand to hold or stabilize one object while the other hand is moving or placing objects into or on it

BOX 21-2

Test Items to Observe Postural Adaptation in Preschoolers

- Tower
- Sequencing
- Stereognosis
- Finger localization
- Maze
- Romberg
- Stepping
- Kneel/stand
- Walk line
- Rapid alternating movements, depending on the age of the child and normative expectations

BOX 21-3

Test Items to Observe Postural Adaptation in Three Year Olds

- Airplane
- Diadokokinesis
- Drumming
- Jump and turn
- Monkey task
- Prone on elbows; neck cocontraction
- Rolling-pin activity
- Scooter board cocontraction
- Side-sitting cocontraction
- Upper extremity control
- Wheelbarrow walk

BOX 21-4

Test Items to Observe Postural Adaptation for Postural-Ocular and Bilateral Coordination

- Balance items
- Bilateral coordination items
- Visuomotor control items
- Upper limb speed and dexterity items
- Strength (e.g., observations of postural tone during writing or manipulation tests, play)

involved in praxis, and impairment in any of them can lead to dyspraxia. The first and most fundamental process is the ability to register and organize tactile, proprioceptive, vestibular, and visual (and to a lesser extent other sensory) input in order to assemble accurate cognitive constructions of the body scheme as well as the environmental scheme of people and objects with which the body typically interacts. The second process, which is based on these constructions and repeated experiences observing and interacting within the environment, requires one to possess the ability to conceptualize internal representations of purposeful actions, termed **ideation** in the neuropsychological and rehabilitation literature. The third process is the planning of sequences of movements within the temporal and spatial demands of the task and environment, including the ability to anticipate future movements that will be needed to be successful in the execution of the action or task.

Impairment in praxis ability can occur anywhere within this neurodevelopmental chain of events. Children who are the most severely impaired lack even that internal visualization of what could be done with the object. They typically also demonstrate poor registration (i.e., failure to notice) of sensory events. On the other hand, children who have only a planning problem know what could be done, but they can't program the aspect of "how to do it." These children typically do not have poor registration (sensory hyporeactivity); in fact, they may have a sensory modulation disorder in the direction of hyperreactivity or defensiveness. Furthermore, they tend to have poor somatosensory perception for use in motor planning. Ayres named the subtypes of developmental dyspraxia, which is according to the sensory processing dysfunction associated with each one, in research conducted with the use of SIPT[3] as well as previous research with the use of the Southern California Sensory Integration Tests.[9]

The most common subtype of dyspraxia was termed *somatodyspraxia* by Ayres. This disorder refers to dyspraxia deficits that result from the inefficient processing of tactile-kinesthetic, proprioceptive, and/or vestibular sensory input within the body. A second type was termed *visuodyspraxia,* which reflects dyspraxia deficits that result from the poor processing of visuospatial cues and affects one's ability to program movements in performing a visual construction task such as drawing designs, directing a pen along a line accurately, or building a three-dimensional structure with blocks. In some cases the child may have a combination of these two clusters; this condition is termed visuo-somatodyspraxia. A third type is called *dyspraxia on verbal command* and is the result of difficulty with motor planning in response to a verbal command; therefore, it is more language related. For this reason, Ayres proposed that this category of praxis dysfunction is the result of more specific left hemisphere dysfunction and is consequently not a true SI disorder, which is by definition subcortical in origin.[3,30,60]

Assessment

Praxis ability or impairments in it can be observed during many exploratory, play, self-care, school, and physical education activities. Infants may display difficulty and frustration with simple adaptive movement responses that challenge his or her simple problem-solving abilities (i.e., "What do I do?"), such as an inability to figure out how to climb onto a riding toy, removing an irritating clothing item on the head, an inability to imitate simple gestures, and leading grownups to something the child wants done (e.g., opening a door). Children ages 4 to 7 with dyspraxia may struggle to use tools and materials at school properly (e.g., cutting, pasting, coloring); they may actively avoid challenging motor planning tasks such as self-dressing, using eating utensils, and playing with manipulative toys; or they may not participate in gross motor activities and games requiring praxis ability.[60,64]

Besides the praxis tests of the SIPT, other developmental and motor tests have items that directly test praxis or the child's quality of execution can be observed. However, as stated earlier, most other tests cannot provide information on underlying sensory processing. In infants, the *Bayley Scales of Infant Development–II*[13] has the following relevant items:

- Imitates hand movements
- Imitates postures
- Pats toy in imitation

Items on the *Miller Assessment for Preschoolers,*[51] which are used to observe praxis qualities, include the following:

- Imitation of postures
- Items that require the child to follow the demonstration of the examiner (rapid alternating movements, kneel/stand, walk line, stepping)
- Maze
- Tower and block designs (constructional praxis)
- Block tapping (motor sequencing)
- Puzzle (visuoconstructional praxis)

As Ayres says, "The child must organize his own brain; the therapist can only provide the milieu conducive in *[sic]* evoking the drive to do so. Structuring that therapeutic environment demands considerable professional skill."[5]

INTERVENTION

Principles of Sensory Integration Intervention

The central principle of this intervention approach is the provision of controlled sensory input, through activities presented by the therapist, to elicit adaptive responses from the child, thereby bringing about more efficient brain organization (Figure 21-5).[6] This latter result becomes observable in the increased organization of behavior, movement, and affective expression that is seen in the client. Perhaps the most difficult aspect for new or untrained therapists to comprehend is that there is no such thing as an SI protocol or curriculum. (This aspect also needs to be explained carefully to both parents and teachers.) Nor is there a set protocol for treating each of the various types of SI dysfunction, although there are guiding principles. However, the results of our evaluation should provide a sensorimotor developmental road map that shapes the treatment plan.

SI treatment is centered on the child and guided by the practitioner; it is freedom within structure (Figure 21-6). The therapist follows a child's lead, yet s/he does not merely allow the child to run wildly around the clinic. Nor does the OT practitioner present the child with a predetermined list of what they are going to do on a given day. How can this be? How do we reconcile these seemingly opposite concepts?

For example, let's begin with the challenge of a child who is running wildly around a room or area of a clinic, stopping briefly to look at or touch toys and equipment but then charging on to the next room or area. We might think to ourselves, "That's not a 'lead' I should be following." Yes and no. In this situation the client is leading his therapist—or at least communicating to him. The child is telling his therapist, "I am overstimulated, disorganized, and out of control. I don't know how to modulate and organize all of these novel sensations coming into my nervous system. I need you to help me self-regulate." The OT practitioner must then think critically (and quickly) about how to do this. S/he must ask, "What is overstimulating this child? Is the child seeking additional input? What types of sensory input would be calming and organizing to his nervous system? How can I get him to arrest this random running around and convert that energy into meaningful exploration and interaction?"

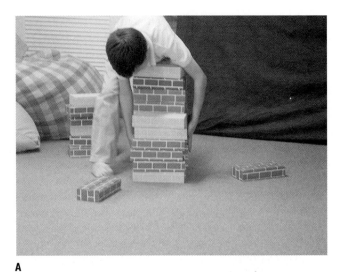

A

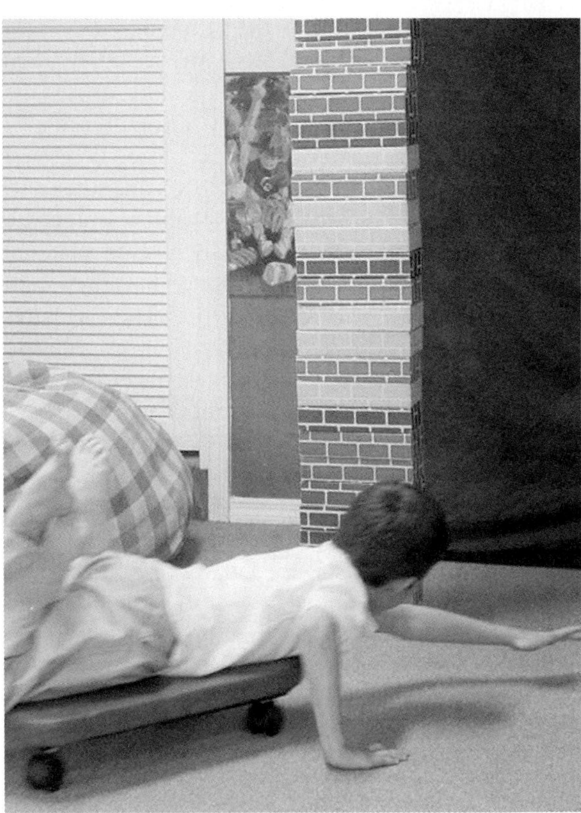

B

FIGURE 21-5 Sensory integration treatment is child directed and initiated. **A,** This child decides to build a block tower. **B,** The child chooses to knock the blocks down while riding a scooter. This activity provides proprioceptive and vestibular input to the child; it is child directed and fun.

Intervention of Sensory Processing Disorder

As mentioned earlier in this chapter, Dr. Ayres strongly believed and advocated that the practice of SI assessment and treatment should be performed by an occupational therapist with postgraduate education. Classic assessment and especially the treatment of sensory processing disorder appear deceptively easy and playful because the therapist is skilled not only in

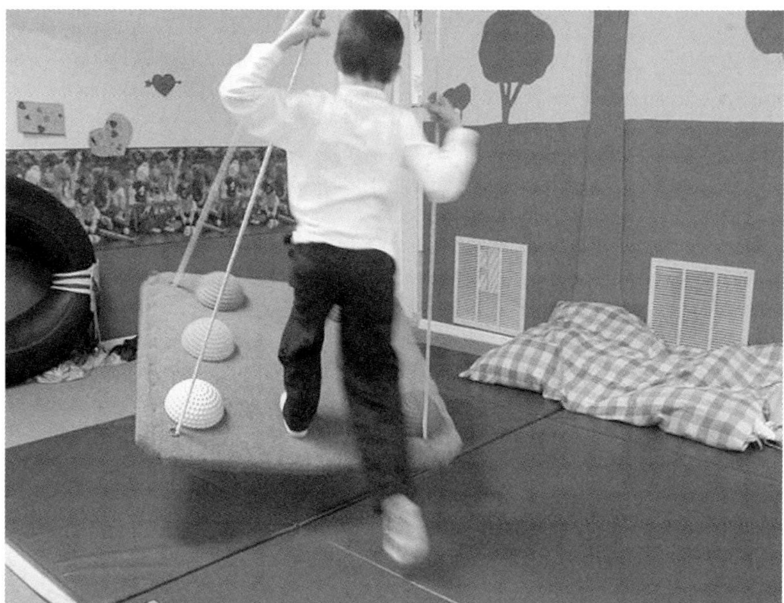

A

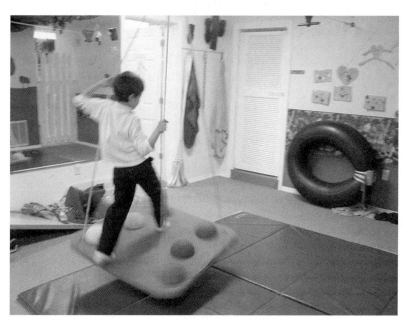

B

FIGURE 21-6 A, This child uses the platform swing to challenge his balance and timing. He pretends that he is on a spaceship and must deflect the meteors by hitting them with a "scientific deflector." Children with sensory integration dysfunction may be very creative. Occupational therapy (OT) practitioners can use this creativity to make intervention sessions fun and interesting. **B,** The OT practitioner is able to provide the "just right" challenge to this activity by controlling the speed of the spaceship (platform swing) and the location of the deflectors (objects to be thrown) and meteors (targets).

administering the test items, which are in themselves challenging to the examiner, but also in directing therapy procedures that are child directed, active, and result in adaptive responses, thereby promoting better brain organization. This ability to go with the client's flow derives from the therapist's knowledge of neurobiology; the capacity to observe when the child is attempting to make an adaptive response to a challenge; and skill in introducing novelty, adjustments, and activity adaptations to make the challenges just right. This therapeutic artistry prevents the child from becoming frustrated if the activity is too difficult on the one hand or bored if the activity is not sufficiently challenging on the other.

These strategies do not necessarily use protocols of assessment and treatment per se, but they consist of

CLINICAL *Pearl*

When an appropriately SI-trained and experienced pediatric occupational therapist is available only on a limited basis (or not at all), the COTA can contribute effectively to promoting sensory processing with practical intervention strategies.

sensorimotor, perceptual motor, and other programs that are repetitive, oriented toward end skills, and many times require a cognitive orientation. However, if utilized properly, these specially selected activities can provide experiences that are rich in sensory processing and be implemented in a variety of settings. Examples of these strategies and treatment activities are shown in Table 21-2, adapted from Carrasco[23] together with the ages and stages of typical development, with corresponding sensory processing levels proposed by Kimball.[46]

PROMOTING DIFFERENT LEVELS OF SENSORY PROCESSING

Facilitating Sensory Modulation

Just like intervention for other types of sensory processing disorder, the treatment of sensory modulation dysfunction (SMD) follows similar guiding principles. Here are some suggestions from Carrasco, which are outlined in Box 21-5.[23]

As soon as the child walks into the room, *determine the arousal level* by observing behaviors that give you clues about whether the child is alert, tired, agitated, sleepy, wired, or some other state. This will give you an idea whether the planned treatment is appropriate. If the child needs excitation, then you would provide activities like jumping; fast movements on the swing, probably more rotational than linear; or a louder and higher-pitched voice. Knowing the arousal level tells you where to start, when to adjust, when to stop, and when to continue a certain activity or use of equipment.

If necessary, *use stimulation protocols* such as the Wilbarger brushing protocol if you are appropriately trained; if not, exercise appropriate supervision, making sure that the protocol is followed up at home. If you are hesitant or unable to pump a selected swing, passively push the swing in the direction you feel would bring about the result of excitation, inhibition, or inclusion in a purposeful activity as needed. When passive activation of the swing is necessary, patiently expect the child to eventually pump the swing actively by himself or herself.

The focus of sensory processing intervention is really aimed toward the organization of multiple sources of sensory input. The focus is also on the lower brain processing of vestibular input in collaboration with proprioceptive and visual input, making it important to *identify the target sensory system(s)*. Pumping a platform swing to move forward and backward while in a circle-sitting position provides not only vestibular input but also integrates proprioception in the neck, trunk, and eyes. This integration of sensations paves the way not only for postural integration but also the conjugate eye movements that are necessary for fine and visuomotor activities. However, some behaviors that suggest SMD are system specific, such as sensitivity to touch, taste, sights, movement, and smells.

Although movement is a commonly observed end product as a result of efficient sensory processing, the COTA should also consider *monitoring cognitive, affective, and physiological responses to sensory processing demands*. Cognitive and emotional responses are also helpful windows through which the child lets you know whether or not the sensory experience is meaningful. Holding on tightly for comfort when placed on a rocking chair or horse is an indication that the child is afraid—of the equipment, a toy, the rocking, perhaps the therapist, or simply being away from the caretaker. Frustration can be the result of the inability to figure out what to do because the task is too difficult and boredom if it is too easy. Sweating, paleness, and other autonomic signs of distress indicate that the sensations are overwhelming and should be monitored, especially when providing passive direct or ambient sensory input.

Behaviors related to hypersensitivity and hyposensitivity to sensory input can vary between what is seen at home and in another setting, such as the school or even the clinic, if not from day to day. Ideally, the response would be similar in all settings, so the sensitivity to food textures would be similar at home and in school during snack time. *Compare the consistency of observed behaviors;* if they are not consistent, consider giving the parents and teachers some tips on how to handle a manipulative child. Sometimes, while looking at family dynamics, sleeping and eating patterns may provide information on how to manage sensory modulation disorder.

The introduction of new toys, sounds, smells, and even movement on a swing prevents habituation and elicits vigilance to new incoming sensations. *Employing novelty* does not necessarily mean changing the equipment (the toy) or, in the case of a writing activity, the pen size, shape, and color or smell of the ink or the sound that the pen makes with pressure.

Whether the threshold is high or low, the goal of intervention is to *influence the threshold level,* or at least bring it to the most functional level. Monitor the behaviors that suggest the need to raise or lower the threshold depending on whether the child or person withdraws from, seeks, or responds slowly to sensations. Provide activities such as swinging a ball or throwing it to a target and sliding down outdoor equipment and ending up in a circle on the sandbox, which provide repetition of similar tasks that require or produce similar

TABLE 21-2

*Intervention Strategies to Promote Sensory Processing and Related Developmental and Occupational Information**

LEVEL OF SENSORY PROCESSING	AGE/STAGE	DEVELOPMENTAL TASK	OCCUPATIONAL CHALLENGES	TREATMENT STRATEGIES FOR CLASSIC TREATMENT OF SENSORY PROCESSING DISORDER
Sensory modulation	First 2 years of life	Physiological homeostasis; self-regulation of arousal and attention Attachment based on self-regulation Primary sensorimotor stage of learning or learning through sensory input Adaptive reflex behavior to purposeful action Exploratory play	Irritability Poor sleep cycles Intolerance to being held or cuddled or exploring objects and people Poor tolerance to positional changes Frequent startling Slow development but usually within normal limits	Use inhibitory* techniques to decrease heightened sensitivity down to levels of functional modulation, with activities rich in one of the following: slow, rhythmical movements; deep proprioceptive input; low-spectrum sounds; dim lighting; minimized environmental sensory input; low-pitched voice and tone. Employ excitatory* techniques to alert the central nervous system, such as fast movements; higher and louder pitch of voice; fast, rhythmical sounds or music; light touch; and different textures and consistency of toys and walking surfaces. *Many individuals with sensory modulation disorder exhibit paradoxical behaviors and responses to treatment. Paradoxical behaviors are manifested when they show hyperresponsiveness to tactile input but hyporesponsiveness to vestibular input; their responses to inhibitory and excitatory strategies may also show such paradoxical behavior, so they respond with excitation when the therapist's intention is for the input to be inhibitory. In such cases, close observation of a pattern of behavior is necessary so that appropriate changes in the strategies can be made as they happen. In such cases, consultation with a supervising therapist trained in sensory integration is warranted.

*See level-specific treatment guidelines in the following sections.

TABLE 21-2

Intervention Strategies to Promote Sensory Processing and Related Developmental and Occupational Information—cont'd*

LEVEL OF SENSORY PROCESSING	AGE/STAGE	DEVELOPMENTAL TASK	OCCUPATIONAL CHALLENGES	TREATMENT STRATEGIES FOR CLASSIC TREATMENT OF SENSORY PROCESSING DISORDER
Continuous sensory modulation	Preschool	Automatic self-regulation Integration of both sides of the body Crossing the midline of the body balance reactions Development of body scheme Development of gross motor planning Imagination expressed through pretend play	Short attention span Clumsiness Poor articulation Overreaction or underreaction to slight injury Fear of playground equipment and some walking surfaces (e.g., sand or plush carpet) Very messy and picky eater No awareness of danger and avoidance of novelty Avoidance of peers; a tendency to play with much older or younger children	While conducting activities that promote sensory modulation (i.e., inhibition and facilitation), include those that promote the foundation for the ocular and bilateral integration, balance reactions, and body scheme. Helpful strategies include the use of controlled sensory input that taps the proximal senses (vestibular and somatosensory, especially deep proprioceptive input that includes those of neck proprioceptors and extraocular muscles), which form the foundation for the work of the more distal senses, such as vision and hearing. These strategies should involve the active participation of the child in gross and fine motor activities that require the use of the entire body or parts thereof while moving through space and playing with a variety of objects that s/he can move, manipulate with the fingers, inspect with the eyes, make sounds with, or use some other sense.
Sensory discrimination	Early school age, 5 to 7 years	Increased skill in differentiating the qualities and characteristics of sensations, such as the intensity, degree, volume, and direction of sensory input Increased fine motor planning Establishment of dominance (lateralization) Flexible social and peer play	Fine motor problems Hyperactivity (often associated with sensory seeking) Impulsiveness Dislike or avoidance of textures in food (lumps), activities (finger painting), and clothing (labels or seams, softness) Difficulty in gross motor activities, with falling or avoidance Accidentally breaks toys or is rough playing with objects or peers	While system-specific sensory input is useful, a strategy that also provides multisensory input is helpful. The novelty and variety of sensory input provide challenges in differentiating and remembering such qualities as sound, distance, texture, color, movement, and taste but also in categorizing and organizing as well as other challenges. Use activities that promote sensory discrimination during but especially at the end of the treatment session.

TABLE 21-2

Intervention Strategies to Promote Sensory Processing and Related Developmental and Occupational Information—cont'd*

LEVEL OF SENSORY PROCESSING	AGE/STAGE	DEVELOPMENTAL TASK	OCCUPATIONAL CHALLENGES	TREATMENT STRATEGIES FOR CLASSIC TREATMENT OF SENSORY PROCESSING DISORDER
Sensory-based movement disorder—postural-ocular and bilateral integration disorder	School age and up (7 years and older) Continued in next age/stage level	Increased abstract thinking Academics More sophisticated tool use Competence in complex skills dependent on previous phases Games with rules and competition	Increased academic problems frequently associated with attention and frustration Poorly or compulsively organized Reversals in writing Continued clumsiness with poor sequencing of tasks Self-esteem problems "Splintered" skills (i.e., lack of generalization ability) Trouble keeping up with peers in activities (especially motor based—slower)	Observe in order to monitor sensory modulation and behavior regulation that may be expressed as inattention or diminished frustration tolerance and endurance. Provide a balance of movement challenges that incorporate flexional, extensional, and rotational components, preferably during activities that require the child to move the whole body or, when seated at a table or the floor, the arms through space. Infuse the session with experiences that require the crossing of one arm across the midline. Also include activities that require the use of both sides of the body, especially but not only the hands with guidance by the eyes and with one side of the body performing independently or in collaboration with the other.
Sensory-based movement disorder—developmental dyspraxia	Starts with previous level and continues into adolescence and adulthood	Continuation of previous level Concern with physical relationships Team sports Establishing identity Career choice Leisure preferences	Organizational problems (e.g., time management) Trouble finishing homework or tasks started Immature physical skills and social relationships Increased dependence Loses or forgets things May be socially isolated Avoids team sports or chooses heavy contact sports	Observe in order to monitor sensory modulation. Provide challenges that require active participation in following verbal, written, or other types of directions for task performance and participation such as the construction of two-dimensional end products (e.g., drawings, written work) or three-dimensional constructions (e.g., block towers, obstacle courses). Provide multiple experiences that require the execution of gross, fine, oral, and visuomotor tasks with projected action sequences or those tasks that require planning of movement to hit targets.

Adapted from Kimball JG: Sensory integration frame of reference. In Kramer P, Hinojosa J, editors: *Frames of reference for pediatric occupational therapy*, Baltimore, Md, 1993, Williams & Wilkins; Carrasco RC, Sahler SS: *Sensorimotor history questionnaire—research edition*, Winter Park, Fla, 2005, FiestaJoy Foundation, Inc.

BOX 21-5

Tips for Facilitating Sensory Modulation

- Determine arousal level.
- If necessary, use stimulation protocols.
- Identify the target sensory system(s).
- Monitor cognitive, affective, and physiological responses to sensory processing demands.
- Compare the consistency of observed behaviors.
- Employ novelty.
- Influence the threshold level.
- Monitor signs of sensory overload or shutdown behaviors.
- Facilitate a balance between seeking and avoiding behaviors and contextual reality.
- Facilitate behavior regulation.
- Prescribe a sensory diet.

sensations. Allow continuation of sensory bombardment with similar activities.

While engaging in the above activities, introduce changes in sequence and other components of the activity to *monitor signs of sensory overload or shutdown behaviors*. This will sustain interest and maintain vigilance during change, thereby influencing attention. Monitor the signs of sensory overload but also shutdown behavior such as purposeless running around, losing track of the end goal of an activity, or simply suddenly becoming quiet and retreating to a corner.

Seeking and avoiding behaviors are considered "normal" at home but negative in school. Communication with teachers, family members, and therapists is essential, especially when recommending adaptations such as pencil grips, seating wedges, "fidget" toys, and quiet break rooms. This communication will help *facilitate a balance between seeking and avoiding behaviors and contextual reality*.

Facilitate behavior regulation by providing different levels of emotional engagement within a session, offering rewards as needed, and progressing from immediate to delayed gratification as needed. Provide experiences in detecting not only changes in verbal intonation of emotion but also nonverbal expressions such as that found in body language and facial expressions either directly through experiences or indirectly through toys or other technology, such as DVDs or CDs. Infuse sessions with experiences to detect changes in one's feelings about what is going on emotionally during the session, and label such feelings.

Prescribe a program of activities that provides sensory experiences on a regular basis (i.e., a *sensory diet*). It may come in the form of a schedule that includes engaging in activities on awakening and bringing down the system to a modulated level when ready for day care or school. The diet can include those activities designed with and/or provided to the school or family to implement. The activities consider the child's sensory needs based on a comprehensive assessment and diagnosis of sensory modulation disorder but should include a variety of experiences to give the child the opportunity to participate as fully as possible without being threatened by them.

BOX 21-6

Tips for Promoting Sensory Discrimination

- Look out for indicators of current or residual modulation disorder.
- Raise modulation level to awareness.
- Identify the sensory "on ramp."
- Infuse activities with controlled novelty.
- Use a variety of materials to infuse novelty.
- Grade complexity of sensory input and adaptive responses.
- Be alert to affective responses.
- Intervene when difficulty comes with diminished visual inspection.
- Keep track of visual dependence and intervene when its presence or absence is observed.
- Select activities that challenge visual discrimination.
- Provide challenging, age-appropriate, fun activities with intrinsic recognition, matching, and categorization of textures, shapes, sizes, or other characteristics of the object.
- Provide opportunities for auditory localization, sequencing, and figure ground.
- Challenge localization of sensations.
- Provide opportunities for discrimination abilities.

Suggestions for Promoting Sensory Discrimination

A summary of suggestions for promoting sensory discrimination can be found in Box 21-6.

Observe the child for indicators or behaviors that suggest difficulty with sensory modulation or indicate *current or residual modulation disorder*, such as dyspraxia or postural-ocular and bilateral integration dysfunction. Even when the goals and activities are designed to promote sensory discrimination, the chances are that unresolved or residual sensory modulation disorder will come to the surface due to several factors, such as the novelty of the activity, stress, the event(s) that happened last night or on the way to the clinic, and health problems. When this happens, aim for functional modulation and proceed with caution toward your sensory discrimination goal.

When appropriate for age, allow the child to be aware of his or her need to seek sensory input (e.g., the reason for the pencil grip, the purpose of the "fidget" toy, the wedge on the chair). By *raising the modulation level to awareness*, the child will hopefully understand and become an active participant in the therapy process.

Although the therapy program may be very specific, *identify the sensory "on ramp,"* such as visual versus tactile discrimination goals. The sensory on ramp, or the sensory system that you access to introduce activities, may differ from the goals prescribed by the therapy program. For example, the child may be in a vestibular seeking mode when your goal is visual. In this case, activities that provide vestibular input such as running or swinging on the playground may be used as a starting point of the therapy session but at the same time provides visual activities that may in themselves have discrimination components to them.

With new sensory input introduced into the sensory experiences, you are able to help promote the detection of new sensations and vigilance for new experiences to come. *Infusing activities with controlled novelty* is similar to the way in which novelty is effective in managing sensory modulation disorder, only this time it is infused with opportunities to refocus on the variety of the qualities and characteristics of sensations. Additionally, approach novel activities with a *variety of materials* but not at the expense of needed continuation as expressed or observed.

Grade the complexity of sensory input and adaptive responses by matching the child's baseline arousal and processing levels with the sensory components of selected activities and the complexity of the responses expected. As necessary, lower or raise the demands of the activity in relation to the equipment used (e.g., a platform rather than a bolster or dual-sling swing) or the complexity of the toys used (e.g., limiting the Jenga game pieces to 20 instead of 45) (Figure 21-7).

Observe the child for changes in affect, which serve as indicators of emotional responses to the sensory environment and include reactions to interaction and task demands, and *be alert to other affective responses*. Observe not only the endurance level but also frustration tolerance, problem solving, and creativity. Adjust as necessary, raising or lowering the bar for challenges accordingly. Refer to the BRAINS (Behavior Regulation through Activities for the Integration of Novel Sensations) approach for infusing sensory processing treatment with socioemotional strategies.[20,26]

Intervene when difficulty comes with diminished visual inspection, especially of items that are manipulated, smelled, tasted, or some other sensation, giving reminders to do so, such as when manipulating zippers, guiding a spoon to the mouth, perceiving when clothing is twisted, finding items such as coins in pockets, or manipulating small objects and tools without vision (e.g., a pencil, spoon, screwdriver). In addition to diminished visual inspection, *keep track of and intervene when visual dependence or a lack thereof is observed*, such as the above, or when identifying which body part has been touched when vision is occluded, differentiating smells and tastes without visual cues, or being alert to what certain smells mean, such as burning or gas leaks.

Activities in which letters can be easily reversed or inverted, such as *p*, *b*, and *q*, can be used as *selective*

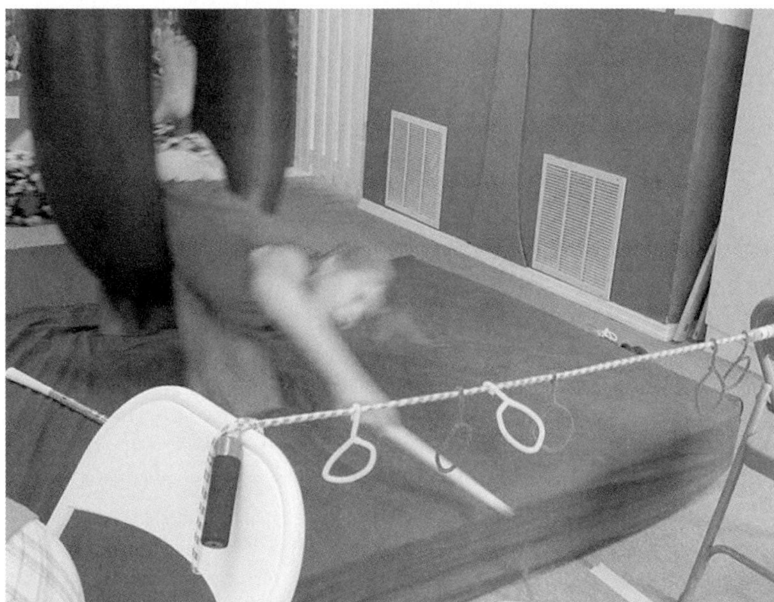

FIGURE 21-7 Swinging on an inner tube provides vestibular and proprioceptive feedback to children. This game requires that the child make adaptive responses in order to hit the rings with the wand. This activity requires timing; sequencing; motor planning; extension through the trunk, shoulder, and elbow; and visual attention.

activities that challenge visual discrimination. Other activities include those that challenge the child to match, recognize, and categorize items according to their qualities, such as color, texture, shape, and size and quickly scanning visual images in sequence, and those that provide challenges to connect dots, write between lines, and play hopscotch, all of which demand visual guidance of fine and gross motor movements.

Provide challenging, age-appropriate, fun activities with intrinsic recognition, matching, and categorization of textures, shapes, sizes, and/or other object characteristics. Likewise, provide experiences that are rich not only in recognizing symbols and gestures and perceiving depth, distance, the location of borders, boundaries, and spaces between objects but also in differentiating foreground from background images, closure of shapes, and pictures.

Challenge the localization of sounds, sights, smells, and other sensations by differentiating and remembering similar words and sounds, such as pat/pack and mitt/meat. Other suggested activities include following instructions with multiple steps and judging the source of a sound, such as turning in the direction of the person calling as well as recognizing the sound of a drum when it competes with the background noise of a toy flute. These activities *provide opportunities for auditory localization, sequencing, and figure ground*.

Provide opportunities during and after the session to *apply discrimination abilities* to ensure their translation into occupations such as maintaining balance while taking a shower with the eyes closed or drying the feet with a towel while standing up, maneuvering the body through tight spaces such as an obstacle course, and writing with appropriate pressure on the paper or chalkboard.

Remediating Sensory-Based Movement Disorder

A summary of remediating sensory-based movement disorder can be found in Box 21-7.

Many children referred for the treatment of sensory-based movement disorder are also referred for reasons other than the sensory processing diagnosis, such as fine motor evaluation, writing problems, and delayed development, but never the underlying sensory processing problems. Our job is to *identify the presenting problem* by linking it to the underlying sensory processing deficit through assessment and historical review. By doing so, foundational intervention, sensorimotor treatment, and environmental adaptation can be designed.

For sensory-based movement disorder, *promote improved somatosensory body scheme organization* with activities such as whole-body playing in a plastic ball bath; using hand cream and rubbing different parts of the body while discussing each one; brushing oneself with a paintbrush or other type of brush; drawing the silhouette of a body on a long sheet of paper; crawling through a lycra fabric "tube" while discussing which parts are passing through it; learning to hop-scotch to a different pattern on the floor; putting on a new article of clothing; and positioning and adjusting the body on a scooter board, a swing, or even a chair.

BOX 21-7

Tips for Remediating Sensory-Based Movement Disorder

- Identify presenting problem(s).
- Promote improved organization of somatosensory body scheme.
- Promote symmetry as well as asymmetry by means of the efficient use of a preferred versus nonpreferred extremity.
- Determine the difficulties and strengths of the practice component(s).
- Infuse the program with constructional activities.
- Infuse the activities with projected action sequences of different types.
- Challenge actions from ideas and images.
- Challenge the ability to learn and smoothly execute new movements.
- Include activities that challenge mouth and tongue movements in coordination with respiration.

Tasks that require bimanual manipulation *promote symmetry as well as asymmetry by means of the efficient use of a preferred versus nonpreferred extremity*. Bimanual or bipedal manipulation encourages the independent as well as cooperative use of two hands or two feet, respectively, such as clapping games, card games, drawing, and sewing. Likewise, watch out for overflow movements in the oral area as well as the opposite side of the body.

Provide challenges to *determine the difficulty and/or strength of the praxis component(s)* by asking "Can you show me a different position to move this swing or a different way to ride on this scooter board?" or "Can you go through the obstacle course backward?" Such challenges indicate whether the praxis components are cognitive or motor. Include manual motor planning activities such as making an origami crane, which requires deciding what to do, what to do first, and how to position and move the fingers and paper to accomplish the task.

Infuse the program with constructional activities in order to determine whether two- or three-dimensional activities such as writing, drawing, and block construction challenge creativity and problem solving by requiring the child to creatively determine how to put together objects and materials for play or leisure activities and school or work projects. *Prepare activities with projected action sequences* of different types, such as the child being required to hit a target with the force of his or her whole body with something that he throws or drawing lines to a target while being aware of their cognitive, motor, and affective abilities when required to do so. Likewise, actively engage the child in organizing a series of actions to produce an intentional movement or figuring out how to do something familiar though different, such as writing with the nondominant hand, writing his or her name, and (more difficult) writing the word *Saskatchewan* spelled backward.

Design activities that *challenge actions from ideas and images* and require performance or the translation of ideas or images into verbal descriptions or interactions as well as products during play, school, or at home (e.g., making a kite from a list of materials). Ask the following question: "How would you 'drive' a bolster swing if it were a school bus, spaceship, race car, fishing boat, or some other mode of transportation." Involve the child in figuring out how to play new games and put things together by organizing a series of actions as needed, asking "How can we use these big blocks to build things like a fort, spaceship docking station, igloo, and Polly Pocket house?"

Fine motor planning can *challenge the ability to learn and smoothly execute new movements.* Ask the child questions such as "Can you swing, let go, and land in the big pillow?" and "Can you ride your elephant over here and roll over into the hay?" Some activities to challenge fine motor planning include movements required in making Mexican "Ojos de Dios" (i.e., "God's Eyes" in English) yarn and stick projects, origami, simple knots of macramé, or cutting pictures for a scrapbook.

Include activities that challenge mouth and tongue movements in coordination with respiration, such as those required when eating different textures of food; when sucking sour candy or popsicles, blowing bubbles, or blowing cotton balls or ping pong balls across the floor while lying prone on a scooter board; and when making appropriate facial gestures during interaction.

SUMMARY

It is hoped that these treatment guidelines and strategies will help OT practitioners understand the basic theory around the model called SI, select appropriate assessment strategies to distinguish typical from atypical sensory processing, and then establish a baseline for intervention that will be meaningful and fulfilling for the child.

References

1. Als H: A synactive model of neonatal behavioral organization: framework for the assessment of neurobehavioral development in the premature infant and for support of infants and parents in the neonatal intensive care environment, *Phys Occup Ther Pediatr* 6:3, 1986.
2. Ayres AJ: *Developmental dyspraxia and adult-onset apraxia,* Torrance, Calif, 1985, Sensory Integration International.
3. Ayres AJ: *Manual: sensory integration and praxis tests,* Los Angeles, 1989, Western Psychological Services.
4. Ayres AJ: Reading—a product of sensory integrative processes. In Henderson A et al, editors: *The development of sensory integrative theory and practice: a collection of the work of A. Jean Ayres,* Dubuque, Iowa, 1974, Kendall/Hunt.
5. Ayres AJ: *Sensory integration and learning disorders,* Los Angeles, 1972, Western Psychological Services.
6. Ayres AJ: *Sensory integration and the child,* Los Angeles, 1979, Western Psychological Services.
7. Ayres AJ: Sensory integrative processes in neuropsychological learning disability. In Henderson A et al, editors: *The development of sensory integrative theory and practice: a collection of the work of A. Jean Ayres,* Dubuque, Iowa, 1974, Kendall/Hunt.
8. Ayres AJ: *Southern California tests of sensory integration tests manual, rev,* Los Angeles, 1980, Western Psychological Services.
9. Ayres AJ: *The effect of sensory integrative theory on learning disabled children: the final report of a research project,* Los Angeles, 1976, University of Southern California.
10. Ayres AJ, Mailloux ZK: Influence of sensory integration procedures on language development, *Am J Occup Ther* 35:383, 1981.
11. Ayres AJ, Mailloux ZK, Wendler CLW: Developmental dyspraxia: is it a unitary function? *Occup Ther J Res* 7:93, 1987.
12. Ayres AJ, Tickle LS: Hyper-responsivity to touch and vestibular stimuli as a predictor of positive response to sensory integration procedures by autistic children, *Am J Occup Ther* 34:375, 1980.
13. Bayley N: *Bayley scales of infant development,* ed 2, San Antonio, Texas, 1993, The Psychological Corporation.
14. Blanche E: *Observations based on sensory integration theory,* Torrance, Calif, 2002, Pediatric Therapy Network.
15. Brown C, Tollefson N, Dunn W, et al: The adult sensory profile: measuring patterns of sensory processing, *Am J Occup Ther* 55:75, 2001.
16. Brown D: *Adolescent/adult sensory profile,* San Antonio, Texas, 2002, The Psychological Corporation.
17. Bruininks RH: *Examiner's manual: Bruininks-Oseretsky test of motor proficiency,* Circle Pines, Minn, 1978, American Guidance Services.
18. Bundy AC, Lane SJ, Murray EA: *Sensory integration: theory and practice,* Philadelphia, 2002, FA Davis.
19. Cammisa KM: Testing difficult children, *Sensory Integration Special Interest Section Newsletter* 14:1, 1991.
20. Carrasco RC: Building brains with sensory integration, *Adv Occup Ther* 19:47, 2003.

21. Carrasco RC: Common test instruments, *Sensory Integration Special Interest Section Newsletter* 14:3, 1991.
22. Carrasco RC: Key components of sensory integration evaluation, *Sensory Integration Special Interest Section Newsletter* 16:5, 1993.
23. Carrasco RC: *Making sense: classical and practical sensory integration testing and treatment for diverse populations and settings—course manuals*, Marietta, Ga, 2005, Advanced Rehabilitation Services.
24. Carrasco RC: *Practical information and useful assessments in sensory integration*, Marietta, Ga, 2001, Advanced Rehabilitation Services.
25. Carrasco RC: Reliability of the Knickerbocker sensorimotor history questionnaire, *Occup Ther J Res* 10:280, 1990.
26. Carrasco RC et al: *BRAINS (Behavior Regulation through Activities for the Integration of Novel Sensations): linking sensory integration and emotions with human performance—infusing sensory integration assessment and treatment with socioemotional intervention*, Marietta, Ga, 2002, Advanced Rehabilitation Services.
27. Carrasco RC, Lee CE: Development of the teacher questionnaire on sensorimotor behavior, *Sensory Integration Special Interest Section Newsletter* 16:1, 1993.
28. Carrasco RC, Sahler SS: *Sensorimotor history questionnaire – research edition*, Winter Park, Fla, 2005, FiestaJoy Foundation, Inc.
29. Case-Smith J: *Occupational therapy for children*, ed 5, St Louis, 2005, Mosby.
30. Cermak SA: Somatodyspraxia. In Fisher A, Murray EA, Bundy AC, editors: *Sensory integration: theory and practice*, Philadelphia, 1991, FA Davis.
31. Coster WJ: Occupation-centered assessment of children, *Am J Occup Ther* 52:337, 1998.
32. DeGangi GA: *Greenspan SI: test of sensory function in infants*, Los Angeles, 1990, Western Psychological Services.
33. DeGangi GA, Berk RA: *DeGangi-Berk test of sensory integration*, Los Angeles, 1983, Western Psychological Services.
34. Dunn WW: *Sensory profile: user's manual*, San Antonio, Texas, 1999, The Psychological Corporation.
35. Dunn WW: *The infant/toddler sensory profile manual*, San Antonio, Texas, 2002, The Psychological Corporation.
36. Dunn WW: The sensations of everyday life: empirical, theoretical and pragmatic considerations, *Am J Occup Ther* 55:608, 2001.
37. Dunn WW: *The sensory profile*, San Antonio, Texas, 1995, The Psychological Corporation.
38. Dunn WW: *The sensory profile: examiner's manual*, San Antonio, Texas, 1999, The Psychological Corporation.
39. Dunn WW, Brown CE: *The adolescent and adult sensory profile*, San Antonio, Texas, 2003, The Psychological Corporation.
40. Fisher AG, Bundy AC: The interpretation process. In Fisher AG, Murray EA, Bundy AC, editors: *Sensory integration: theory and practice*, Philadelphia, 1991, FA Davis.
41. Fisher AG, Murray EA, Bundy AC: *Sensory integration: theory and practice*, Philadelphia, 1991, FA Davis.
42. Folio MR, Fewell RR: *Peabody developmental motor scales*, ed 2, Chicago, 1984, Riverside Publishing Co.
43. Greenspan SI, Weider S: *The child with special needs*, Reading, Pa, 1998, Addison-Wesley.
44. Harris MB: Oral-motor management of the high-risk neonate, *Phys Occup Ther Pediatr* 6:231, 1986.
45. Jirgal D, Bouma K: Sensory integration interview guide for infants, *Sensory Integration Special Interest Section Newsletter* 12:5, 1989.
46. Kimball JG: Sensory integration frame of reference. In Kramer P, Hinojosa J, editors: *Frames of reference for pediatric occupational therapy*, ed 2, Baltimore, Md, 1999, Williams & Wilkins.
47. Mailloux Z, Parham LD: Sensory integration. In Case-Smith J, editor: *Occupational therapy for children*, ed 5, St Louis, 2005, Mosby.
48. Mangeot SD, Miller LJ, McIntosh DN, et al: Sensory modulation dysfunction in children with attention deficit hyperactivity disorder, *Dev Med Child Neurol* 43:399, 2001.
49. McIntosh DN, Miller LJ, Shyu V, Dunn W: Overview of the Short Sensory Profile (SSP). In Dunn W, editor: *The sensory profile: examiner's manual*, San Antonio, Texas, 1999, The Psychological Corporation.
50. McIntosh DN, Miller LJ, Shyu V, et al: Sensory-modulation disruption, electrodermal responses, and functional behaviors, *Dev Med Child Neurol* 41:608, 1999.
51. Miller LJ: *Manual: the FirstSTEP screening test for evaluating preschoolers*, San Antonio, Texas, 1993, The Psychological Corporation.
52. Miller LJ: *Manual: the Miller assessment for preschoolers*, San Antonio, Texas, 1982, The Psychological Corporation.
53. Miller LJ, Brett-Green B, Dickinson M, James K: *Effectiveness of occupational therapy for children with sensory processing impairments: a pilot study*, (in process).
54. Miller LJ, Lane SJ: Toward a consensus in terminology in sensory integration and practice: Part I: taxonomy of neurophysiological processes, *Sensory Integration Special Interest Section Quart* 23:1, 2000.
55. Miller LJ, Lane AE, James K: *Defining the behavioral phenotype of sensory processing dysfunction*, Estes Park, Colo, 2002. Paper presented at the University of Colorado Health Sciences Center Developmental Psychobiology Research Group 12th Biennial Retreat, "Behavioral phenotypes in developmental disabilities."
56. Miller LJ, McIntosh DN, McGrath J, et al: Electrodermal responses to sensory stimuli in individuals with fragile X syndrome: a preliminary report, *Am J Med Genet* 83:268, 1999.
57. Miller LJ, Reisman J, McIntosh DN, et al: An ecological model of sensory modulation: performance of children with fragile X syndrome, autism, attention deficit/hyperactivity disorder, and sensory modulation dysfunction. In Roley SS, Blanche EI, Schaaf RC, editors: *Understanding the nature of sensory integration with diverse populations*, San Antonio, Texas, 2001, Therapy Skill Builders.
58. Miller LJ, Wilbarger JL, Stackhouse TM, et al: Use of clinical reasoning in occupational therapy: the STEP-SI model of treatment of sensory modulation dysfunction. In

Bundy AC, Lane SJ, Murray EA, editors: *Sensory integration: theory and practice*, ed 2, Philadelphia, 2002, FA Davis.

59. Parham DL: Evaluation of praxis in preschoolers, *Occup Ther Health Care* 4:28, 1987.
60. Reeves G, Cermak S: Disorders of praxis. In Bundy AC, Lane S, Murray EA: *Sensory integration: theory and practice*, ed 2, Philadelphia, 2002, FA Davis.
61. Royeen L: Tactile processing and sensory defensiveness. In Fisher AE, Murray EA, Bundy AC, editors: *Sensory integration: theory and practice*, Philadelphia, 1991, FA Davis.
62. Stallings-Sahler S: Case presentation: child with gastro-esophageal reflux and severe sensory modulation disorder, *Sens Integr Int Quart* pp1-2; spring/summer, 2000.
63. Stallings-Sahler S: Case report: report of an occupational therapy evaluation of sensory integration and praxis, *Am J Occup Ther* 44:650, 1990.
64. Stallings-Sahler S: Sensory integration assessment and intervention. In Case-Smith J, editor: *Pediatric occupational therapy and early intervention*, ed 2, St Louis, 1998, Elsevier/Butterworth-Heinemann.
65. Stallings-Sahler S: Sensory integration: creating a challenging environment, *Occup Ther Week* 5:10, 16, 1991.
66. Stewart S: *The relationship between children's intellectual abilities and their socio-emotional presentation in a clinically referred sample*. Atlanta, April 2004. Paper presented at the Society for Research in Child Development.
67. Turkewitz G, Kenny PA: The role of developmental limitations of sensory input on sensory/perceptual organization, *Dev Behav Pediatr* 6:302, 1985.
68. Wilbarger J, Stackhouse TM: *Sensory modulation: a review of the literature*, Sensory Integration Resource Center website, May 1989.
69. Wilbarger P: Planning an adequate sensory diet: application of sensory processing theory during the first year of life, *Zero to Three* 5:7, 1984.
70. Wilbarger P: The sensory diet: activity programs based on sensory processing theory, *Sensory Integration Special Interest Section Newsletter* 18:1, 1995.
71. Wilbarger P, Wilbarger J: *Sensory defensiveness in children aged 2-12: an intervention guide for parents and other caregivers*, Denver, 1991, Avanti Educational Programs.
72. Williamson GG, Anzalone ME: *Sensory integration and self-regulation in infants and toddlers: helping very young children interact with their environment*, Washington, DC, 2001, Zero to Three National Center for Clinical Infant Programs.

REVIEW *Questions*

1. What is sensory integration?
2. Define and describe sensory modulation disorder.
3. Define developmental dyspraxia and provide intervention techniques.
4. What are functional support capacities?
5. How does sensory processing affect movement in children?
6. Describe the principles of sensory integration intervention.
7. Identify intervention techniques to work with children who have postural-ocular and bilateral integration dysfunction.

SUGGESTED *Activities*

1. Administer a sensory questionnaire to parents of typically developing children. Discuss the results in class.
2. Go to a specialized SI clinic and observe typically developing children playing on the equipment. Describe the motor planning and activity levels of the children.
3. Go to a specialized SI clinic and use the equipment for play activities. Note the intensity level of the experience. How did the activity feel to you?
4. Go through a catalog, such as the one for Southpaw Enterprises, Inc, and develop a list of games and activities for each piece of equipment. Make a notebook of these activities for future use.
5. Observe an SI session with a child and take notes of examples of how the therapist used the principles of SI treatment (e.g., child initiated, use of suspended equipment, adaptive responses, controlled sensory input).
6. Observe an SI session with a child either in person or by means of videotape. Describe the type of sensory input and the adaptive responses required. How would you modify the activity?

CHAPTER 21 APPENDIX A

Example of Informal Checklist for Parent/Caregiver

Sensorimotor History Questionnaire
Adapted by Ricardo C. Carrasco and Susan Stallings-Sahler, 2005

Child's Name: ______________________________
Completed by ______________________

Birthdate: ____ - ____ - ____ Today's Date: ____ - ____ - ____
Chronological Age: ___________

Please respond to the following statements concerning your child's past and present behaviors and abilities. What do you recall as being different from other children? Were there times when his or her behavior was difficult for the family to cope with? What solutions have you found for any of these behavior issues?

These questions are asked to help us assemble a more complete picture of your child's development across time. Some questions may apply to children who are older than your child. In these cases, you may cross out the verb tense that does not apply. Check the choice that applies: **Yes, No,** or **N/A** (i.e., not old enough yet, not applicable). Add any comments that provide information you feel would be important for us to know about.

1.0 RESPONSES TO VISUAL AND LIGHT STIMULI IN THE ENVIRONMENT

#	Which of the following statements describes your child either currently or in the past?	Yes: Currently	Yes: In the past	Seldom or never	Further explanation or N/A
1.1	Is highly distracted; stressed by too many surrounding visual stimuli				
1.2	Does not visually orient to people and objects in environment				
1.3	Avoids making eye contact; looks away from face				
1.4	Seems overly sensitive to light; prefers to sit in dark room				
1.5	Seems driven to visually inspect the details of objects closely				

2.0 RESPONSES TO SOUNDS IN THE ENVIRONMENT (AUDITORY)

#	Which of the following statements describes your child either currently or in the past?	Yes: Currently	Yes: In the past	Seldom or never	Further explanation or N/A
2.1	Has an actual hearing loss (please explain if mild, moderate, severe, or profound)				
2.2	Has been diagnosed with childhood auditory processing disorder				
2.3	Often fails to listen or pay attention to what is said				
2.4	Often fails to follow through or act on verbal requests to do something; forgets or misunderstands instructions				
2.5	Is very distracted by sounds; seems to hear faint sounds that go unnoticed by others				
2.6	Talks excessively, almost compulsively				
2.7	Is stimulated to be overly verbal when others talk				
2.8	Puts hands over ears even when others are speaking only at a conversational level				
2.9	Has difficulty understanding the teacher when there is background noise in the classroom				
2.10	Sounds such as vacuum cleaner and blender perceived as noxious and painful to hear				
2.11	Is distracted by environmental sounds such as air conditioner fan, refrigerator, and fluorescent light bulbs				
2.12	Speech difficult to understand; contains sound reversals and substitutions (e.g., "callerpitter," "W" instead of "L" or "R")				
2.13	Responds with "Huh?" when spoken to, but after a delay of 1 to 3 seconds displays comprehension of what was said				

3.0 RESPONSES TO MOVEMENT SENSATIONS (VESTIBULAR)

#	Which of the following statements describes your child either currently or in the past?	Yes: Currently	Yes: In the past	Seldom or never	Further explanation or N/A
3.1	Late in pregnancy or at birth, infant presented in the breech position (feet first)			No	
3.2	Placed on back for sleeping 75% to 100% of the time after age 3 months				
3.3	Placed on back for awake play time for 75% to 100% of the time after 4 months				
3.4	Very low tolerance for being placed on stomach for awake play time after 4 months				
3.5	Not motivated to move from one spot, even toward a new toy or family member				
3.6	Seemed to have ability to stand and walk at normal age but was fearful and hesitant about doing so				
3.7	Dislike of being moved in space or tossed up in the air during play				
3.8	Unable to fall asleep without rhythmic movement (e.g., rocking, riding in car, putting infant seat on running washing machine)				
3.9	Seems more active than most infants of same age				
3.10	Becomes anxious and fearful when feet are not touching the floor				
3.11	Becomes car-sick frequently/easily.				
3.12	Becomes dizzy or nauseous easily from circling movements on rides or playground				
3.13	Craves being in high places; climbs up to unusual heights but without fear				
3.14	Extremely afraid of heights (e.g., going up a ladder, walking down a flight of stairs)				
3.15	Seems to crave substantial or intense movement (e.g., being swung through the air, whirling/spinning)				
3.16	History of chronic middle ear infections				Since age_____ Tubes?_____

4.0 RESPONSES TO SMELLS AND TASTES (OLFACTORY/GUSTATORY)

#	Which of the following statements describes your child either currently or in the past?	Yes: Currently	Yes: In the past	Seldom or never	Further explanation or N/A
4.1	Wants to smell almost everything; explores new environments by smelling				
4.2	Seems unaware of smells or tastes; uninterested in food				
4.3	Becomes nauseous when exposed to many common food smells				
4.4	Craves ingesting unusual or non-nutritive tastes and substances (e.g., glue, dirt, soap)				
4.5	Tolerates only very bland foods (e.g., vanilla pudding, white bread, mashed potatoes)				
4.6	Has a history of chronic gastric reflux				
4.7	Prefers extremely spicy, hot, sour, or sweet tastes (circle those that apply)				
4.8	Has a history of food allergies and/or lactose intolerance				

5.0 RESPONSES TO TOUCH, PRESSURE, TEMPERATURE, AND PAIN (SOMATOSENSORY)

#	Which of the following statements describes your child either currently or in the past?	Yes: Currently	Yes: In the past	Seldom or never	Further explanation or N/A
5.1	Was picky about shape of bottle or pacifier nipples as an infant				
5.2	Dislikes being fed or eating with metal utensils; prefers to finger-feed				
5.3	Rejects food that has too much texture, lumps, or different-sized pieces in it				
5.4	Seems overly sensitive to certain textures of clothing, bedding, or other material in contact with skin				
5.5	Seemed to dislike being cuddled or held as an infant				
5.6	During toilet training seemed not to notice when bladder was full, causing "accidents."				

5.7	Seems excessively ticklish; panics or becomes combative when tickled				
5.8	Seems easily irritated or enraged when touched by siblings or playmates				
5.9	Gets into fights at school, such as standing in line at water fountain or engaged in activities on the playground				
5.10	Has strong need to touch objects and people				
5.11	Unusually afraid of dogs and pets that move quickly and/or jump up				
5.12	Seems to lack normal awareness of cold outdoor temperatures; goes out in winter without appropriate clothing				
5.13	Overdresses; seems to be unaware of excessive summer outdoor heat				
5.14	Seems to feel room temperature in marked contrast to what others find comfortable ("too hot" or "too cold")				
5.15	Seems overly sensitive to warm water temperature for a bath, wants it to be noticeably cool				
5.16	Overly sensitive to food temperature; wants it to be cool				
5.17	Strong dislike for taking showers or placing hands under a spray faucet to wash				
5.18	Seems almost unaware of painful experiences such as falling on hard surfaces; doesn't cry or complain				
5.19	Has/Had difficulty learning to put clothes on the correct parts of the body; needs to be able to see own body in order to dress				
5.20	Stomps feet very hard on steps when going up stairs				
5.21	Likes roughhouse play on the floor, such as being thrown down or "crashing" play				
5.22	Bears down extremely hard on crayons or pencils to the point of breaking them				

5.23	Cried as a toddler with normal weight bearing during creeping or standing				
5.24	Dislikes being handled or held in a firm manner				
5.25	Interprets deep pressure on skin (e.g., rubbing and massaging) as ticklish				
5.26	Resists having hair washed or cut or having fingernails trimmed				

6.0 SELF-REGULATORY CAPACITIES (AROUSAL, ATTENTION, AFFECT, ACTION)

#	Which of the following statements describes your child either currently or in the past?	Yes: Currently	Yes: In the past	Seldom or never	Further explanation or N/A
6.1	Seldom sleeps through the night				
6.2	Other sleep "issues" (explain)				
6.3	Is an early riser; wakes easily and becomes alert fairly quickly				
6.4	Very difficult to wake up in the morning; takes a long time to "get going"				
6.5	Rapidly went from sleeping, to awake, to frantic crying during infancy				
6.6	Has difficulty experiencing the transition from one activity or environment to another				
6.7	Gets "wound up" easily and then is very difficult to calm down				
6.8	Uses a favorite self-regulatory strategy to calm down or go to sleep (e.g., sucking thumb, holding blanket)				
6.9	Has "meltdowns" in late afternoon (overwhelmed by day at school or day care)				
6.10	Seeks out enclosed spaces to play in at home or school (e.g., under table, in bed under canopy, in a corner)				
6.11	Struggles to pay attention at school, at music or dance lessons, in church, or in other environments				

6.12	Takes medication to improve attention or reduce hyperactivity				
6.13	Seems unusually shy or clinging; anxious around strangers				
6.14	Seldom smiles or laughs; has a limited range of emotions; seems "flat"				
6.15	Loses control of laughter and becomes overly silly if laughed at or someone says something funny				
6.16	Does things impulsively; blurts out comments in class; has difficulty waiting turn				
6.17	Overattends to activities to the exclusion of other stimuli (e.g., teacher calling name, activity of others signaling a change, bell ringing at school)				
6.18	Seems hyperactive; unable to stop random running around; squirms in seat at school				

7.0 GROSS MOTOR (LARGE MUSCLE) MOVEMENTS AND SKILLS

#	Which of the following statements describes your child either currently or in the past?	Yes: Currently	Yes: In the past	Seldom or never	Further explanation or N/A
7.1	As an infant or toddler, was difficult to hold and carry because of being "floppy"				
7.2	As an infant/toddler, was difficult to hold and carry because of stiffness and arching				
7.3	As an infant, was difficult to hold for feeding; needed to use infant carrier to feed				
7.4	Stage of crawling on stomach was brief or skipped				
7.5	Stage of creeping on all fours was brief or skipped				
7.6	Sat up, stood, or walked independently earlier than others of same age				
7.7	Sat up, stood, or walked later than others of same age				
7.8	Could creep up stairs but was unable to come back down				
7.9	Engages in unusual movements such as walking on toes, flapping arms, and repeated rocking				

7.10	Late in learning how to hop and skip				
7.11	Late in learning to ride a bicycle				
7.12	Movement appears slow, plodding, or sluggish				
7.13	Seems hyperactive; in constant motion for most of the day				
7.14	Prefers sedentary activities (TV, reading, video games) and positions (lying down, partially reclined) instead of active play at >4 years of age				
7.15	More frequent falls and other accidents than other kids of same age				
7.16	Trouble with learning new movement skills such as those involved in skating, dancing, and sports				
7.17	Seems clumsier than others of same age				
7.18	Runs into other people, furniture, or side of door for unknown reasons				
7.19	Misunderstands verbal instructions to move a certain way				
7.20	Plays with toys and/or other children immature for his age				
7.21	Dislikes playing with manipulative toys (e.g., blocks, puzzles, Legos, transformers)				
7.22	Undresses dolls or stuffed animals but is unable to put clothes back on				
7.23	Has difficulty engaging in any prolonged play activity at home; constantly complains of being bored even though toys are available and there are activities to participate in				
7.24	Seems overly destructive with toys; breaks things a lot				
7.25	Has trouble with handling clothing fasteners (e.g., zippers, buttons, shoelaces)				
7.26	Experiences difficulty with handling school, art, or construction tools and materials correctly (e.g., scissors, paintbrush, stapler, glue, tape, hammer)				

8.0 SCHOOL PERFORMANCE QUESTIONS (Omit items that are not age appropriate; teachers' reports and conferences from previous years would be helpful as well as discussions with the teachers about some of the following.)

#	Which of the following statements describes your child either currently or in the past?	Yes: Currently	Yes: In the past	Seldom or never	Further explanation or N/A
8.1	Does significantly better one on one for school assignments than in a group				
8.2	Frequently slouches, props head on hand, or lies down on arm while reading or writing at desk				
8.3	Hand dominance still unclear after age 4; switches hands frequently				
8.4	Gets confused when putting on shoes (which one goes on which foot)				
8.5	Makes top-bottom inversions when writing numbers or letters (they appear upside down)				
8.6	Prints letters or numbers backward				
8.7	Confuses similar letters when reading, such as *b* and *d* and *m* and *w*				
8.8	Reverses sequential order when reading or writing "teens" (e.g., "41" instead of "14")				
8.9	Confuses reversible words, such as *dog* and *god* and *saw* and *was*				
8.10	Has great difficulty writing and looking at and listening to the teacher simultaneously				
8.11	(For children studying Hebrew) The problem of reversal in letters and words in English reappears after having been mastered earlier				
8.12	Shows an unusual amount of confusion in recognizing letters in Hebrew that are very similar in form				
8.13	Experiences significant problems in coping with written instructions during laboratory sessions, cooking class, or shop work				
8.14	Regards gym and participation in sports in general as distasteful or too hard				
8.15	Please cite any additional information about performances that teachers indicate are problems at school, either academically or behaviorally.				

9.0 SOCIAL ADJUSTMENT

#	Which of the following statements describes your child either currently or in the past?	Yes: Currently	Yes: In the past	Seldom or never	Further explanation or N/A
9.1	Finds it hard to make friends with peers				
9.2	Prefers the company of adults or older children, who allow more room for mistakes				
9.3	Has difficulty reading body language and other nonverbal social cues from others				
9.4	Tends to play with children who are a year or two younger.				
9.5	Is picked on by other children; tends to be a "loner"				
9.6	Expresses feelings of low self-esteem				
9.7	Tends to be bossy and dominating in play with peers				
9.8	Frequently expresses feelings of failure and frustration				
9.9	Seems discouraged and depressed				

OTHER PROFESSIONAL REPORTS: Evaluations from the following sources are available and will be forwarded.

Physician

Psychologist

Other Physical or Occupational Therapists

Teacher(s)

ADDITIONAL COMMENTS:

Adapted from Knickerbocker BM: *A holistic approach to the treatment of learning disorders*, Thorofare, NJ, 1980, CB Slack.

CHAPTER 21 APPENDIX B

Example of Informal Checklist for a Child's Teacher: Teacher Questionnaire on Sensorimotor Behavior

RICARDO C. CARRASCO

The Teacher Questionnaire on Sensorimotor Behavior (TQSB) was designed as a screening tool for either the occupational therapy (OT) practitioner or the teacher so that children with behaviors that are suspect or at risk for learning and relational behaviors can be referred for further OT screening or a more comprehensive evaluation. The results are useful in refuting or supporting historical, contextual, and other data in an impression or sensory integration dysfunction (DSI). Information on internal, concurrent, and construct validity and reliability is published in the literature and available through the author.

ADMINISTRATION AND SCORING INSTRUCTIONS

The item behaviors in this questionnaire were selected to investigate your student's performance at school. They are divided into sections, namely Motor Organization, Somatosensory System, Form/Space Perception and Visuoconstruction, Auditory/Language, Olfactory and Gustatory Systems, and Social Adjustment. Most of the items address behaviors that can be readily observed in the classroom. However, there are some that may require additional observations during library or lunch time, recess, or outdoor equipment use or on arrival at school from either the bus or private transportation. Completing the questionnaire will assist in compiling a comprehensive and descriptive picture of the child's sensorimotor function but more importantly in determining how such function affects the daily activities that comprise his or her daily occupations.

1. Put a check or an X mark under the Yes or No column as appropriate. If the behavior does not apply, please put N/A under Yes.
2. Use the column under Comments or Sample Behaviors to describe or give examples of behaviors for that particular item (e.g., for item 1.63—especially when printing letters but not when drawing figures).
3. After completing the questionnaire, total the number of Yes responses in each section and record the total at the bottom of that section.
4. Convert the section total score to Normal, Suspect, or High based on the ranges of scores specified in the conversion table below.

Conversion Table

SECTION	NORMAL	SUSPECT	HIGH
Motor Organization	0 to 4	5 to 15	15 or higher
Somatosensory System	0 to 3	4 to 11	12 or higher
Form/Space Perception and Visuoconstruction	0 to 2	3 to 10	11 or higher
Auditory/Language	0 to 1	2 to 5	6 or higher
Olfactory and Gustatory	0	1	2 or higher
Social Adjustment	0	1 to 2	3 or higher

A predominance of Suspect scores suggests further screening at the discretion of the professional; Predominantly High scores warrant further professional evaluation. The Interpretation Key can be used by the OT practitioner or other qualified professional and is available from the author.

Child's Name: ______________________ Date of Birth: ___ - ___ - ___

DOT: ___ - ___ - ___ Chronological Age: ___ ___ ___

1.00 Motor Organization: Vestibular, Proprioceptive, and Visual Senses

ITEM #	YES	NO	ITEM BEHAVIORS	COMMENTS OR SAMPLE BEHAVIORS
1.00			Performs school tasks with slow, deliberate movements	
1.20			Falls when attempting to hop on one foot	
1.21			Falls when attempting to skip	
1.30			Finds gym or outdoor play equipment distasteful	
1.31			Often feels sick on disembarking from school bus or car	
1.32			Gets sick and vomits from movement experiences, e.g., games, turning around	
1.33			Does not adequately inform others of these feelings	
1.34			Twirls on piano stools, swivel chairs, or similar equipment more than other children	
1.35			Seeks stimulation on school playground equipment, e.g., seesaw, merry-go-round, more than other children	
1.36			Hangs upside down on jungle gym	
1.37			Dislikes climbing on playground equipment	
1.38			Hesitates when going up or down stairs or stepping on or off curbs	
1.39			Avoids balancing activities	
1.40			Tires easily	
1.41			Stands with shoulders forward or swayed back	
1.42			Muscles seem tight	
1.43			Muscles seem flabby	
1.50			Poor rhythm walking	
1.51			Shuffles feet when walking	
1.52			Drops toes when walking	
1.63			Needs reminders to hold paper for writing	
1.70			Persistently gets confused over which hand or foot is left or right	

1.71			Gets confused easily about crossover patterns to find the right side of a person facing him	
1.72			Prints numbers or letters backwards	
1.80			Appears to be accident prone, e.g., spills milk, drops pencils or books, trips over or bumps into furniture	
1.90			Continues movements or mannerisms after it is time to stop	
1.91			While writing or working with dominant hand, other hand looks tense or mirrors dominant hand	
1.92			Inconsistent use of left or right hand	
1.93			Complains of hand or back fatigue or pain during pencil tasks	
1.94			Makes holes in paper while trying to erase or write	
1.95			Shakes or stretches hand during long periods of writing	

Motor Organization: Total __ Conversion: Normal __ Suspect __ High __

2.00 Somatosensory System: Touch and Proprioception

ITEM #	YES	NO	ITEM BEHAVIORS	COMMENTS OR SAMPLE BEHAVIORS
2.10			Dislikes being held or cuddled	
2.11			Dislikes being barefoot	
2.12			Has changed from disliking to liking being held or cuddled	
2.13			Seems excessively ticklish	
2.14			Pulls away or is easily irritated when touched by classmates or school staff	
2.15			Picks fights at school, e.g., standing in line on the playground, in the lunchroom, in the library	
2.20			Fidgets, pushes or pulls fingers with other hand, repeatedly touches various parts of the body, or puts hands or objects in mouth	
2.21			Has a strong need to touch objects and people	
2.30			Lacks typical awareness of being touched by classmates or school staff	

2.31			Lacks awareness of cold outdoor temperature	
2.32			Overdresses, seemingly unaware of excessive summer heat	
2.33			Underdresses, seemingly unaware of excessive winter cold	
2.34			Feels room temperature in marked or some contrast to what others feel comfortable	
2.35			Often seems unaware of bruises, cuts, and bleeding gashes until informed by others	
2.40			Clumsy when playing with toys	
2.41			Volitionally engages in prolonged manipulative tasks, e.g., puzzles, mazes	
2.42			Engages but needs prompting in prolonged manipulative tasks given by teacher or aide	
2.43			Has trouble paying attention to classroom task at hand	
2.44			Overly destructive with classroom desk or materials, e.g., books, workbooks, toys	
2.50			Difficulty in manipulating tools with hands, e.g., spoons, pencils	
2.51			Cannot push blades of scissors together	
2.52			Holds pencil too tight	
2.53			Holds pencil too loose	
2.54			Grasps pencil without use of thumb and index and middle fingers	
2.56			Constantly changes pencil grasp while writing	
2.57			Pencil pressure on paper too heavy	
2.58			Pencil pressure on paper too light	

Somatosensory System: Total___ Conversion: Normal ___ Suspect ___ High ___

3.00 Form/Space Perception and Visuoconstruction

ITEM #	YES	NO	ITEM BEHAVIORS	COMMENTS OR SAMPLE BEHAVIORS
3.10			Highly distracted by visual stimuli	
3.11			Concentrates better when desk is not cluttered	
3.12			Functions significantly better in a one-on-one relationship in class	
3.19			Reads letters or numbers backward	
3.21			Reverses sequential order of "teen" numbers e.g., forming a 4 and then placing the 1 in front of it	
3.22			Gets confused when reading reversible letters such as *b* and *d*	
3.23			Gets confused when reading reversible words such as *dog* and *god* and *saw* and *was*	
3.30			Moves head rather than eyes only when reading sentences from a book	
3.31			Uses fingers or a line guide to prevent losing place while reading	
3.40			Blinks eyes, places hands over face, or ducks while playing ball	
3.50			Has trouble finding way from one place to another and gets lost easily	
3.60			Has trouble recognizing similarities and differences in patterns or designs	
3.70			Cannot make letters and numbers stay between lines or spaces	
3.71			Often overshoots or undershoots targets, e.g., placing pencils or crayons in a box	
3.80			Has difficulty putting parts of a toy or puzzle together	
3.81			Frequently supports head with hand while reading or writing at desk	
3.90			Difficulty copying from blackboard or chalkboard	
3.91			Cannot adequately draw forms or shapes	
3.92			Holds head close to paper while writing	
3.93			Rotates paper more than 45 degrees when writing	
3.94			Does not leave adequate space between words or letters	
3.95			Tips head to one side during activities, as if using only one eye	

Form/Space Perception and Visuoconstruction: Total __ Conversion: Normal __ Suspect __ High __

4.00 Auditory/Language

ITEM #	YES	NO	ITEM BEHAVIORS	COMMENTS OR SAMPLE BEHAVIORS
4.10			Gets distracted by sounds; hears sounds that go unnoticed by others	
4.12			Gets distracted by sounds in the classroom, e.g., music, classmates talking	
4.13			Gets distracted by sounds, e.g., fluorescent light bulbs, heaters, refrigerators	
4.20			Often fails to listen or pay attention to what is said	
4.21			Often fails to follow through or act on requests to do something	
4.22			Is unable to function if two or three steps of instructions are given at once	
4.23			Talks excessively	
4.24			Talking by others becomes stimulus to be overly verbal	
4.25			Talking interferes with ability to listen	
4.26			Has difficulty remembering sequence of numbers heard	
4.27			Has difficulty remembering sequence of words heard	
4.30			Reverses sequence of words or numbers heard	
4.31			Misunderstands the meanings of words used in relation to movement, e.g., push/pull, go left/right, up/down	

Auditory/Language: Total ___ Conversion: Normal ___ Suspect ___ High ___

5.00 Olfactory and Gustatory Systems

ITEM #	YES	NO	ITEM BEHAVIORS	COMMENTS OR SAMPLE BEHAVIORS
5.10			Highly sensitive to scents and odors	
5.20			Seems to lack typical awareness of odors easily perceived by others	
5.30			Expresses strong like or dislike of food smells (explain)	
5.40			Expresses strong dislike of other scents (explain)	

5.50			Shows strong reaction to otherwise common food tastes, e.g., salty, sweet, sour	
5.51			Desires excessive flavor in or condiments for food, e.g., salt, ketchup, mustard	

Olfactory and Gustatory: Total __ Conversion: Normal __ Suspect __ High __

6.00 Social Adjustment

ITEM #	YES	NO	ITEM BEHAVIORS	COMMENTS OR SAMPLE BEHAVIORS
6.10			Finds it hard to make friends with peers	
6.11			Prefers company of adults or older children	
6.12			Tends to play with children a year or two younger	
6.20			Is a loner	
6.30			Expresses feelings of low self-esteem	
6.40			Expresses feelings of failure	
6.50			Gets frustrated easily	
6.51			Seems discouraged or depressed	
6.60			Is more emotionally sensitive; feelings get easily hurt	
6.70			Cannot tolerate changes in plans or expectations	

Social Adjustment: Total __ Conversion: Normal __ Suspect __ High __

Additional Information

____

Teacher's Name and Signature

Adapted from the Sensorimotor History Questionnaire and other unpublished sensorimotor behavior questionnaires by Ricardo C. Carrasco.

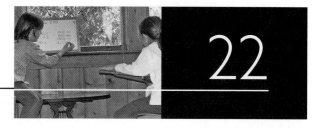

22

Assistive Technology

GILSON J. CAPILOUTO

CHAPTER *Objectives*

After studying this chapter, the reader will be able to accomplish the following:

- Describe the terms, concepts, legislation, and trends in the use of assistive technology in pediatric rehabilitation
- Demonstrate an understanding of the specific classes of assistive technology available to children with disabilities
- Discuss the role of the certified occupational therapy assistant as it relates to the successful evaluation and implementation of assistive technology services
- Describe the best practice strategies required for successful evaluation and implementation of assistive technology services
- Demonstrate an understanding of the characteristics of assistive technology and its relative importance in making technology decisions
- Compare and contrast assistive, rehabilitative, educational, and medical technologies
- Provide examples of switch technology and the ways in which it might be used to assist a child in achieving a goal
- Describe the characteristics of switches and specific considerations when selecting a switch for an individual user
- Describe the ways in which environmental control units operate and how environmental control unit (ECU) technology might be used for a child with a disability
- Discuss the role of simple communication technologies for children who are unable to communicate verbally

KEY TERMS

Assistive technology
Assistive technology services
Assistive technology team
Rehabilitative technology
Educational technology
Medical technology
Low technology
High technology
Assistive appliance
Assistive tool
Access
Control site
Direct selection
Indirect selection
Switch
Environmental control unit
Communication technologies

CHAPTER OUTLINE

In the past decade, technology has changed all of our lives considerably. We now have daily dependence on a variety of technologies, which include computers, cell phones, and personal digital assistants (PDAs). Each of these technologies has the potential to make our lives a little easier and more comfortable by helping us be more productive and efficient. For people with disabilities, technology is especially important because it can mean the difference between being able to accomplish a task alone and being forced to depend on someone else. In fact, technology has been described as the great equalizer for people with disabilities because it provides an important vehicle for maximizing capability.[6,10] Congress acknowledged the crucial role of technology in the lives of people with disabilities when they passed Public Law (PL) 100-407, titled the Technology-Related Assistance for Individuals with Disabilities Act of 1988.[11,13] In the preamble to PL 100-407, Congress described four major benefits of assistive technology (AT) for individuals with disabilities: greater control over their individual lives, increased participation in their daily lives, more widespread interaction with non-disabled individuals, and the capacity to benefit from the opportunities that non-disabled individuals frequently take for granted.

The Tech Act, as it is commonly referred to, allocated financial resources to support states' efforts to increase awareness of the benefits of technology for people with disabilities, increase funding for the provision of AT devices and services, increase the number of personnel trained to provide such services, and increase coordination among state agencies and public and private entities to deliver AT devices and services.[7]

DEFINITIONS

The formal definition of **assistive technology** is, according to the federal government, "Any item, piece of equipment, or product system, whether acquired commercially off the shelf, modified, or customized, that is used to increase or improve functional capabilities of individuals with disabilities."[13] The important thing to remember about this definition is the fact that *anything* that helps a person be more functional is considered AT. The term *assistive technology* naturally makes us think that AT has to be commercially manufactured and expensive. This is not true! In addition, of particular importance to us as therapists is the fact that the law includes a focus on **assistive technology services** in addition to the aids and devices themselves. According to the law, AT services include "any service that directly assists an individual with a disability in the selection, acquisition, or use of an assistive technology device."[13] The fact that the legislation defines AT services means that its authors recognized that equipment alone is not enough; professional services are also required to evaluate AT and train personnel in its use.

Why should we consider the use of AT in the care of individuals with disabilities? A brief look at a distinction made by the World Health Organization among the terms *impairment*, *disability*, and *handicap* illustrates the importance of AT.[14] Let's say a child is born without his upper extremities (the impairment), so he is unable to perform the basic activities of daily living (ADLs) (the disability). If this child is prevented from participating in a local drawing class because of this impairment/disability, then he is handicapped. AT addresses the *disability* aspect of the individual (the individual-environment interface) and minimizes *handicap* because when we identify an aid or device that allows the individual to meet the goal of drawing, s/he can assume his or her role in society (e.g., a young child who wants to draw), thereby minimizing the disability.

CLINICAL *Pearl*

AT refers to anything that helps a person be more functional in his or her daily life.

ASSISTIVE TECHNOLOGY TEAM

Interdisciplinary teamwork is considered the cornerstone of effective rehabilitation.[2] The need for teamwork is particularly crucial as it relates to the use of AT. The disciplines that are represented as part of the **assistive technology team** may vary according to the needs of the client and the disabling impairment or condition (Box 22-1). For example, a physical therapy practitioner provides important information about gross motor strength and function as well as positioning for function and mobility. The occupational therapy (OT) practitioner provides valuable information on fine motor function, participation in ADLs, and positioning for access. The speech-language pathologist is concerned with overall communication ability as well as specific strengths related to language comprehension and expression. The user as well as the parents, guardians, or caregivers of a child who has special needs are always central members of the team and should be involved in all aspects of decision making concerning equipment and/or implementation. Additional team members could include a rehabilitation engineer, who is charged with designing and fabricating aids or devices; an equipment vendor, who provides medical equipment supplies; and a teacher, who is concerned with using technology to assist students in meeting their educational potential and achieving their educational goals. Regardless of which

BOX 22-1

Potential Members of the Pediatric Assistive Technology Team

- Child
- Family members/caregivers/guardians
- Teacher in regular and/or special education
- Classroom assistants
- Daycare workers
- Physical therapist
- Occupational therapist
- Speech-language pathologist
- Vision specialist
- Audiologist (hearing specialist)
- Physician
- Case worker and/or social worker
- Rehabilitation engineer
- Vendor (assistive technology supplier)

professionals make up an individual's team, it is the responsibility of all the AT team members to work together to decide on the technology that will be of benefit to an individual user, how it will be used, how the equipment will be maintained, and how the impact of the technology will be measured.[4]

CLINICAL *Pearl*

A team approach is necessary for successful AT service delivery.

ROLE OF THE CERTIFIED OCCUPATIONAL THERAPY ASSISTANT

AT services vary depending on the setting and the experience of the individuals constituting the AT team. As such, the role of the certified occupational therapy assistant (COTA) will also vary according to the setting and experience. The registered occupational therapist (OTR) and COTA are important members of the AT team; they are involved in its evaluation and service provision.

At one time or another, the OTR and COTA may also be involved in securing the necessary funding for AT, supervising the use of equipment, measuring the outcomes related to equipment use, and equipment fabrication and/or adaptation. Additional roles of the COTA might include client and family education or instruction in the use of AT for other team members, including regular and special educators and classroom assistants.

CHARACTERISTICS OF ASSISTIVE TECHNOLOGY

The term *assistive technology* is used to describe a broad range of assistive aids and devices that include but are not limited to the following: aids for daily living, seating and positioning aids, communication aids and devices, environmental control units, aids for persons with visual impairments, and assistive listening devices. As a group these technologies share some common characteristics, which are important to consider in delivering quality AT services (Table 22-1). First, and most important, is to understand the distinction between AT and rehabilitative, educational, or medical technology.[5] The term *assistive technology* should be used to refer to only the aids and devices that are used *daily* to complete a given task. The terms **rehabilitative technology** or **educational technology** should be used when referring to the use of technology as only one aspect of an overall rehabilitation or education program. **Medical technology** refers to the use of technology to support or improve life functions. The following case studies illustrate why this distinction is so important.

TJ has chronic Guillain-Barré syndrome and as a result is unable to use either of his upper extremities and is nonambulatory. He uses an electric wheelchair for mobility and operates it by means of a series of switches mounted on his headrest. Because of his upper extremity impairment, TJ cannot independently play with age-appropriate toys. To eliminate this handicap and minimize his disability, his OT practitioner has adapted a commercially available, battery-operated toy so that it turns on when a switch is activated. The OT practitioner wants TJ to use switches so that he can play independently. To use the switch and adapted toy as AT, we would want to place the switch in a location that would be the most convenient for TJ's current abilities. This might mean mounting the switch on the headrest of his wheelchair because his head appears to be the fastest, most energy-efficient control site he currently has.

Maria has a developmental disability characterized by gross and fine motor delay. Currently, she does not maintain her head in an upright position for any length of time. Her OT practitioner is trying to devise activities that will encourage her to maintain head control, thereby strengthening the muscles required to develop this skill. The OT practitioner has decided that introducing a switch-operated toy may motivate Maria to maintain an upright head position for increasingly longer periods of time. In this case, we might

TABLE 22–1

Characteristics, Definitions, and Examples of Assistive Technology

CHARACTERISTIC	DEFINITION	EXAMPLE
Assistive technology	Technology used daily to improve function	Communication aid
Rehabilitative or educational technology	Technology only one aspect of rehabilitative or educational program	Software program for teaching ABCs
Medical technology	Technology used to sustain life	Respirator
Low technology	Easy to obtain and use	Reacher
High technology	Difficult to obtain and use	Electric feeding machine
Assistive appliance	Beneficial without skill development	Foot orthotics
Assistive tool	Requires skill development to be useful	Switch-adapted toy

consider mounting the switch so that it is activated only when the head is upright. The same technology that was used for TJ assistively is now being used for Maria rehabilitatively.

Recall that our definition of AT emphasizes function, not disability. Since Maria has to work very hard to activate the toy and this is only one of many activities she is engaged in to increase independent head control, the use of the toy and switch would be considered rehabilitative technology.

CLINICAL *Pearl*

AT targets function, while rehabilitative and educational technology target dysfunction.

You might still be confused about why this distinction is so important. In the case study of TJ, our goal is to make technology *easy* to access. But in the case study of Maria, the technology is actually *hard* to access. We would certainly not want an individual to work as hard as Maria if our goal were daily independent play. This distinction is important for more practical reasons as well. For example, whether we use something daily (like TJ) or temporarily (like Maria) has a direct impact on the necessary durability of the device, the degree of cost we will consider, and the level of difficulty required to operate it. If we are going to use a device only a few times to develop a particular skill, we do not want to spend a significant amount of money on an aid that will require a substantial amount of time to develop operational competence. Instead we should focus on an aid or device that is relatively inexpensive and quick and easy to learn. This distinction between AT and rehabilitative or educational technology is also very important for setting technology-related goals as well as gauging ur expectations for technology use (i.e., whether we expect AT to be used daily or over a long period).

AT can also be characterized as **low technology** or **high technology**.[5] This distinction is somewhat self-explanatory. Low technology is easy to obtain, easy to use, and relatively low in cost. In contrast, high technology is more difficult to obtain, requires greater skill to use, and is frequently more costly. We consider these factors when weighing the options for individual users. For example, if we are working with an individual who we know to be technophobic, then we would probably want to keep our AT options toward the low technology end. At the same time, we don't want to make AT decisions based simply on the fact that someone enjoys and is comfortable with technology. My motto is simple: Never buy a Jaguar when a Volkswagen will do! To be safe, we should always make sure our decisions about technology are based on the goals and abilities of the patient.[7]

The last characteristic of AT that we need to consider is the distinction between *tools* and *appliances*.[5] An **assistive appliance** includes any aid or device that provides benefit to the user with little or no training or skill development. This could include items such as eyeglasses and orthotics. On the other hand, an **assistive tool** requires the development of skill in order to be of value to the user. Some examples of assistive tools include feeding machines, communication aids and devices, and mobility aids. This distinction is especially important when speaking with users and caregivers about their expectations for AT. A good example is in the selection of a communication aid or device. Too often there is the misconception that if we "just find the right thing," the user will be able to communicate instantaneously. It is important for everyone to be clear about the fact that any communication aid or device is an assistive tool and as such requires a certain degree of training before it can be of benefit to the user.

CLINICAL *Pearl*

Assistive appliances such as eyeglasses provide benefit to the user without skill development.

CLINICAL *Pearl*

Assistive tools such as communication technologies require skill development to be of benefit to the user.

MYTHS AND REALITIES OF ASSISTIVE TECHNOLOGY

In their book on assistive technology, Jan Galvin and Marcia Scherer describe a number of myths and realities with respect to AT, many of which are important to share before moving forward.[7] As you have already seen, AT does not need to be expensive or complicated. A simple pad and pencil can be the perfect communication aid. Moreover, keep in mind that people with the same disability do not necessarily require the same devices. For example, we do not recommend the same wheelchair for every person needing one! It is especially important for you to keep in mind that assessment, as it relates to AT, is an ongoing process. It is simply not possible for us to know everything about an individual user in the course of three or even four encounters. Additionally, as users develop and improve their skills as a result of treatment, reassessment of AT needs is warranted. We will discuss this further when we talk about the assessment process. Finally, it is important for us to be open to multiple sources of information about AT. The field of AT is changing at a remarkably rapid pace, and it is very difficult for any single professional to be familiar with everything that is available. Consequently, consumers, family members, and even vendors can provide us with valuable input about appropriate technology for individual users.

ASSISTIVE TECHNOLOGY ASSESSMENT

Like so many aspects of rehabilitation, AT assessment is a team endeavor. Although as a COTA you will not be conducting evaluations yourself, it is critical that you understand the process of evaluation so that the clinical information you share with the OT can be valuable in making adjustments to AT goals and treatment procedures for individual users. There are numerous approaches to decision making for AT. The one discussed here is adapted from a model rooted in the field of human factor engineering,[5] which is a field of study devoted to the interface between humans and machines. It is well suited for application to the field of AT. As you read this section, it will be helpful to refer to the schematic of the assessment process shown in Figure 22-1.

In the rehabilitation field, we frequently begin the assessment process by administering standardized tests and criterion-referenced measures in an attempt to answer the question, "What *can't* the individual do?" However, remember that AT targets function rather than dysfunction, so knowing what an individual can't do is not very helpful when trying to determine whether technology would be of benefit. Instead, when considering technology, the rehabilitation specialist asks, "What is it the user wants to do?" and/or "What is it the user needs to be able to do?" With these questions as the focus, the AT assessment process begins where it should, with the *goals for the user*.

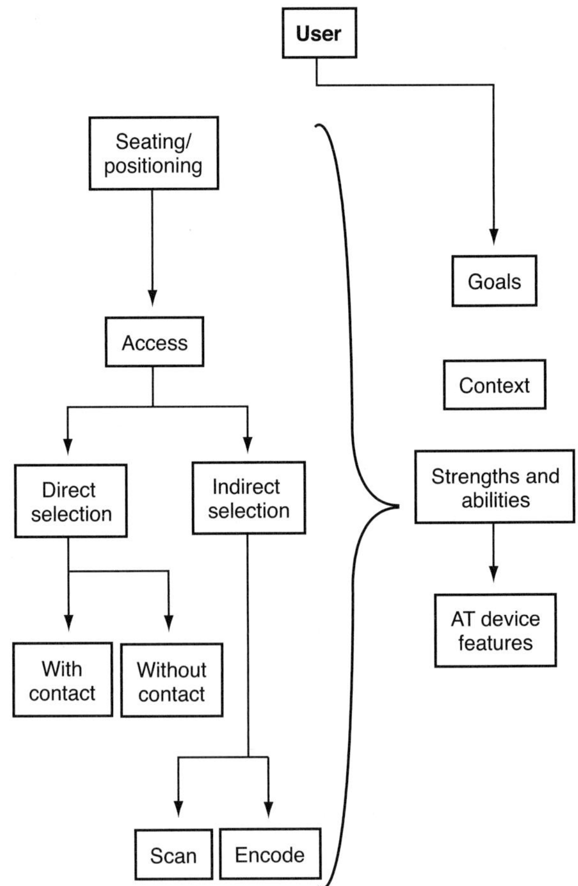

FIGURE 22-1 A schematic model of the assessment process for assistive technology (AT) adapted from human factor engineering.

When establishing goals for individual users, therapists consider the following:

1. Is this goal rehabilitative or functional?
2. Is this goal shared by the student or user, the family, and other members of the team?
3. Does the goal make sense; is it logical?

You will recall that the distinction between goals that are assistive and those that are rehabilitative has an impact on how we set up equipment (i.e., the conservation of effort and energy as much as possible [assistive] or as a motor challenge [rehabilitative]) and the type of equipment we might consider (i.e., since rehabilitative technology would most likely be used for a comparatively shorter time than AT, the learning time and cost are viewed somewhat differently). Also, when equipment is being considered, treatment goals should be discussed with everyone who has a vested interest in the user because assistive devices frequently require the support of caregivers and other team members for training and maintenance. For example, the OT practitioner, along with the physical therapist, may want to increase a student's exposure to powered wheelchairs as part of a goal focused on independent mobility. However, his or her family is committed to emphasizing the use of a walker, so they do not want to consider a powered wheelchair. Since the caregivers do not share the goal of powered mobility, it may be best not to pursue it at this time.

Finally, when establishing goals, it is important to consider whether we are asking the user to do something that you and I could or would do. For example, if we have a goal which states that the user will attend to an activity for 30 minutes, we have to ask ourselves whether or not *we* would attend to the same activity for that length of time! As we develop goals for individuals, we begin to ask ourselves whether or not the client's ability to achieve certain goals would be enhanced by the use of assistive equipment.

After establishing goals, our next question becomes "Where and with whom will the goal(s) be addressed?" This question focuses on the setting for each of the client's goals, such as the home, school, or community. Each of them can potentially affect device decisions. For example, if the context for a goal is the home, school, and community, one of the device features we would be concerned with would be portability. The question of context also includes the social contexts for a given goal. For example, will the goal be addressed with familiar or unfamiliar peers, familiar or unfamiliar adults, all of the above, or alone? Let's say that a client's goal included communication with unfamiliar peers. In such cases it would be important for any communication system to include messages of introduction. Finally, context takes into account the physical environment of a goal, including temperature (impact of excessive heat or cold), sound (ambient noise), and light (ambient light). The impact of these factors is fairly obvious. For example, any goal that includes the playground as a setting would need to account for outside elements as well as changes in light (natural versus unnatural).

The third primary component of assessment involves the specific strengths and abilities of the user. This is where information from specific team members becomes critical. The areas of strength and ability include familial, gross motor, fine motor, cognitive, communicative, and sensory. In Figure 22-1 we can see that seating and positioning issues as well as those of access are superimposed on this aspect of the assessment model. **Access** refers to the point of contact between the user and whatever it is they want to control. For example, you and I access the computer by means of a keyboard and/or mouse. We access room lights by means of an on/off switch. For the purposes of AT, it is important for us to keep in mind that an individual's muscle tone (e.g., hypertonia and/or hypotonia) as well as the presence of primitive reflexes, skeletal deformities, and/or movement disorders will influence functional access to equipment. Seating and positioning become critical in minimizing the influence of these characteristics on access options. See Chapter 13 for specific information regarding the best practice principles of seating and positioning.

A number of decisions must be made when determining how an individual will access a potential aid or device. Among the issues that must be resolved is the identification of a particular **control site** (i.e., location on the body that can be used to operate it).[5] Potential sites for controlling aids or devices include the hands and fingers, arms, head, eyes, legs, and feet. Ultimately, the site and movement chosen should represent the fastest, most energy-efficient, and most reliable ones available.

There are two options available for making a choice with a control interface: **direct selection** and **indirect selection.**[3,5,7] In direct selection, an individual simply identifies a target and goes directly to it with or without physical contact. A user can indicate a choice by using his or her fingers or hands (i.e., with physical contact) or movements of the head or eyes (i.e., without physical contact). When direct selection is not possible, indirect selection is used.[3,7] The most common forms of indirect selection utilize scanning and/or encoding devices.[5] In the former, users are required to scan through a selection set; when the element they wish to select is presented, they generate a signal by means of a control interface such as a switch or switch array. In the latter, an individual uses multiple signals that together specify a selection (e.g., Morse code).

Physically, direct selection is considered to be more difficult than indirect selection because it requires more refined, controlled movements.[5] However, because all of the elements in the selection set are equally available and do not need to be scanned, direct selection is considered the faster form of device control.[3] It is also considered to be less cognitively complex than indirect selection because it is more intuitive.[1] For these reasons, direct forms of device control are considered better options than indirect forms.

CLINICAL *Pearl*

Because indirect selection is slower and more cognitively complex than direct selection, we should exhaust all possible direct selection options before considering indirect.

As information is gathered by various team members, the necessary features of any aid or device become apparent. For example, if in the course of team conferencing we learn that a client has decreased visual acuity, then any aid or device we consider should include features that account for that ability, such as bright colors, tactile discrimination, auditory feedback, and/or magnification options. The next section describes some of the more common classes of AT tools used among the pediatric population.

ASSISTIVE TECHNOLOGY FOR PEDIATRICS

A number of classes of AT tools should be considered when working with pediatric clients. In this chapter, we focus on technology for leisure activities and environmental control and simple communication technologies. Although our focus is primarily on simple technology solutions, it is important to remember that in many instances high-tech approaches may be required for individual users.

Technology for Leisure Activities

For very young children, leisure activities mean play. It is important to keep in mind the definition of play because it is easy for us to turn play into therapy. Play is an intrinsic activity engaged in for its own sake rather than a means of achieving a specific end.[9] It should be fun, spontaneous, and voluntary. Adapted play refers to the fact that toys are modified to enable children with disabilities to participate and learning is intentionally incorporated into play activities.[9]

Greenstein[9] suggests that simply observing a child with a particular toy can tell us much about what we need to know before considering adapted toys. First, we should ask ourselves whether a child is playing with a toy because s/he wants to (intrinsic motivation) or someone else wants them to (extrinsic motivation). This is important because research suggests that using rewards to encourage a child to engage in an activity will decrease the child's subsequent interest in the activity. It reminds us that children should be playing because *they* want to. When we observe that a child with a disability is not playing with a toy, Angelo[1] suggests three possible reasons that should be considered: (1) they are not interested in the toy (lack of motivation); (2) frequent failure in playing with toys has reduced their motivation to try (learned helplessness); and (3) the child wants to play but is physically unable to. It is for this last reason that we investigate how adapted play can facilitate participation.

The first consideration in adapting play materials for individuals with disabilities is whether the materials simply need to be stabilized.[8] Children with physical disabilities frequently need a stable surface on which to play so that the objects will not move. For example, lining a tray with indoor/outdoor carpet and then attaching hook or loop Velcro to the base of books, baby dolls, and trucks can serve to hold the objects in a stable position and encourage play.

A second strategy, suggested by Glennen and Church,[8] is to enlarge materials, which serves to enhance visual perception and decrease reliance on fine motor skills. Simple solutions include attaching handles to puzzle pieces and pop-up boxes and putting brushes, markers, and utensils in foam to make them easier to hold. Finally, toys can be attached to trays and/or children with elastic so that if they fall out of reach they can be easily retrieved.

A third strategy, suggested by Musselwhite,[11] includes ensuring that all play materials are accessible; as much as possible, children should be able to physically select and choose their own toys and activities. For example, for children in wheelchairs, toys should be attached at chair height on a wall with Velcro or in nets hung from the ceiling. For children who are physically unable to retrieve their own toys, the items should be arranged so that they can be easily obtained by means of a gross reach or point. An alternative could be to develop simple picture or object displays that would allow children to indicate the toy or game they want to play (e.g., a strip of hard-backed poster board with actual objects or large photographs from which to choose). Keep in mind that the choices should be spaced far enough apart to allow children to select a picture of the activity or toy by using either a gross upper extremity movement or their eyes (Figure 22-2).

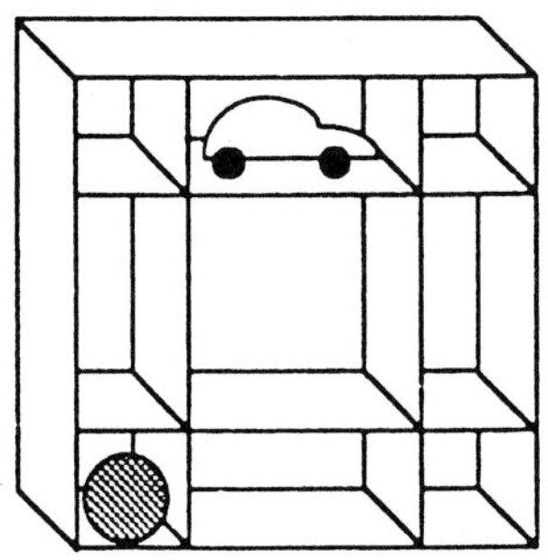
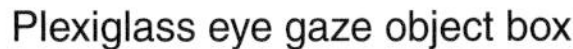

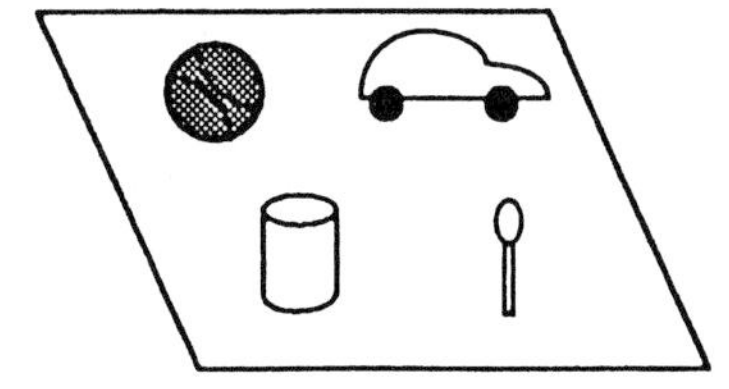

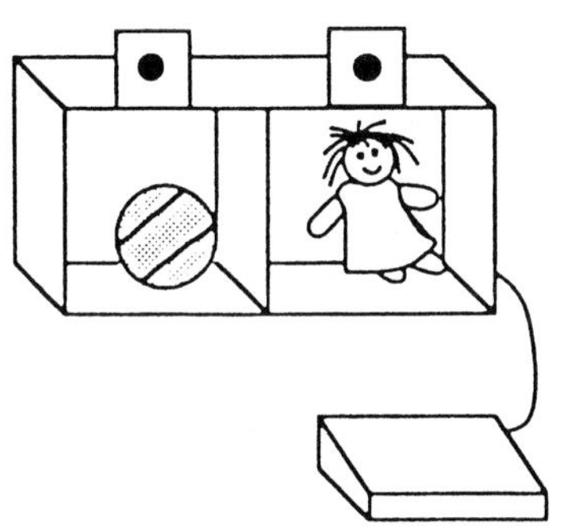

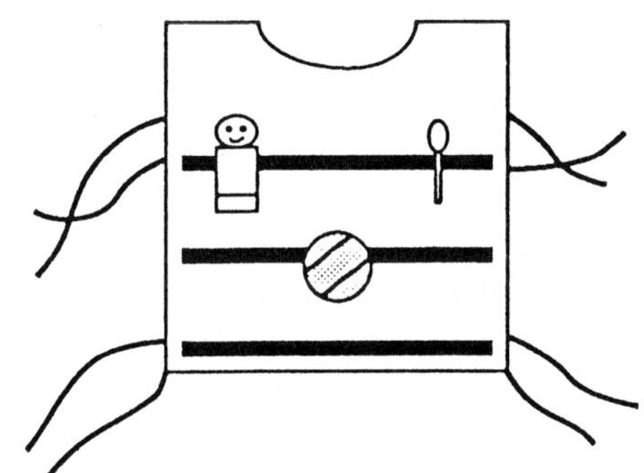

FIGURE 22-2 Play activity choice boards. (From Glennen S, Church G: Adaptive toys and environmental controls. In Church G, Glennen S, editors: *The handbook of assistive technology,* San Diego, 1992, Singular Publishing Group.)

Switch-activated toys

Employing switches to play with toys and use appliances is another form of adapted play. Such adaptations allow children with physical limitations to engage in independent exploration and interaction with the environment. Moreover, using switches with toys can be considered a preliminary activity that serves to develop the skills needed to control a wheelchair or operate a communication device. **Switches** open and close a circuit, so they operate in the same way as many of the appliances you use daily, such as the television, light switch, CD player, and toaster (Figure 22-3).[1] Switches give a person with a physical limitation the option of controlling toys and appliances that they would otherwise be physically unable to manage.

Switches come in all shapes and sizes with varying visual, auditory, and other sensory features. When selecting a switch for an individual user, we must consider the following questions.

1. What is/are the potential control site(s) for a switch (e.g., head, hand, arm, foot)?
2. What is/are the functional range(s) of motion of the potential site(s)?
3. Does the user have any special sensory needs that should be considered?
4. What mounting issues need to be considered?

In fact, just looking at a given switch should tell you a lot about its intended user. Keep in mind that manufacturers design switches for very specific reasons; it is not a random process. For instance, ask yourself the following questions. Does the size of the activation surface suggest a person who uses more gross or fine motor movements? Is the switch intended for foot/hand, cheek/chin, or head/thumb activation? Do the physical characteristics of the switch suggest an appeal to a child or an adult? Do the physical characteristics of the switch suggest anything about vision or cognition? What about the strength requirements for operating the switch? Remember that our task is to match a user's skills and abilities to the features of a switch. As an example of the process, consider the following case study:

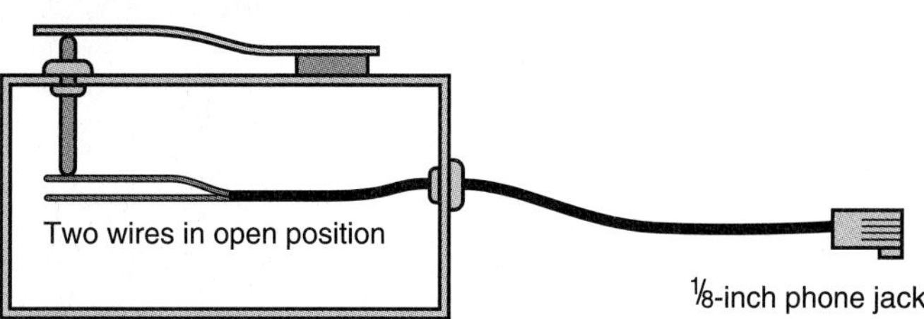

FIGURE 22-3 Anatomy of a switch.

Jeremy is a 12-year-old boy with a diagnosis of cerebral palsy with spastic quadriplegia. He has also been diagnosed as having visual impairment, although the degree of visual loss is not known. He uses a manual wheelchair for mobility but he does not use it independently. Although it is difficult to determine precisely his abilities from standardized tests, his teachers feel that he is responsive to communication and laughs and smiles appropriately when others direct attention to him. He uses multiple nonsymbolic forms of communication that include postural changes associated with excitement and anticipation, swiping at unwanted items with his right upper extremity, and vocalizing to express pleasure or displeasure. The members of his professional team think he is a good candidate for running an appliance operated by a switch.

Using the Switch Analysis Worksheet (Figure 22-4), note the descriptions of each of the pictured switches. Of those presented, which one offers features you believe are the best match for Jeremy's described strengths and abilities? If you picked switch #1, you are correct. The Lighted Signal Switch offers a relatively large surface area that complements Jeremy's gross motor approach to tasks. It addition, it offers sensory features that are well suited to accommodate his visual handicap, including the fact that it lights up and provides auditory feedback on activation. Finally, the ribbed surface offers Jeremy tactile stimulation as well.

The preceding case study reiterates the importance of selecting switches based on individual needs. Using a worksheet such as the one provided here can assist you in analyzing the characteristics of various switches. If we are not careful in selecting the appropriate switch, we run the risk of drawing conclusions about a student's ability to use a switch, which may or may not be correct. For example, if we had only switch #2 available for our use, Jeremy would most likely be unsuccessful due to its small size and minimum feedback. As a result of his performance, we might deduce that he is not capable of using a switch when in fact the switch we selected did not accommodate his specific needs.

Once we have selected a specific switch for trial use, we turn our attention to developing an activity for introducing the switch. The activity we choose should be age appropriate and motivating to the user. It is also important to be precise in the placement of the switch and appliance or toy in relation to the user and to duplicate that placement each time the user engages in switch-activated play. Moreover, trial use of a switch should be carefully monitored before altering the switch or its placement. Users need the opportunity to practice using a switch across a variety of activities before changes are considered. This is because switches are considered assistive tools and thus require some skill development before they can be of benefit and before we can draw conclusions about success or the need for program adjustments.

As stated previously, there are a number of potential adapted play options, depending on the goals for an individual user. Adaptive switches can be used to operate a variety of battery-run or electronic toys and appliances.[8] Switches attach to toys or appliances by means of cables. More often than not, switches will come with a cable attached. At the end of the cable will be a miniature plug (Figure 22-5, *A*). Toys or appliances that have already been developed for the switch user will come equipped with a cable receptor in the form of a switch interface jack (Figure 22-5, *B*). Alternatively, one can use a battery adapter designed for use with commercially available battery-operated toys and appliances. Battery adapters have a cable receptor with a female phone jack at one end and a copper plate at the other. The copper plate is sized to fit the specific battery (e.g., AAA, C, D) and is placed between the battery and one of the metal battery contacts, thus interrupting the on/off circuitry[8] (Figure 22-5, C). When the toy or appliance is placed in the 'on' position, it will not operate until the switch is activated. The difficulty in using both adapted toys and battery adapters is that different manufacturers use different-sized cable jacks and receptors, so it is frequently necessary to use adapters to convert between female- and male-sized

Switch	Picture	Access	Control Site(s)	Sensory Features	Other
1. Lighted Signal Switch ($62.95) Enabling Devices 385 Warburton Avenue Hastings-on-Hudson, NY 10706 http://enablingdevices.com/	5" diameter	Gross access	Upper Extremities; fisted or open hand; foot	Ribbed surface for tactile stimulation; activation feedback; lighted	Angled presentation; Suction cup feet
2. Specs Switch ($49.00) **AbleNet, Inc.** 2808 Fairview Avenue Roseville, MN 55113-1308 http://enablingdevices.com/	1 3/8" diameter	Fine access	Single digit; head; cheek	Activation feedback; bright colors	Various mounting options-velcro strap
3. Pal Pad ($27.00) **Adaptivation, Inc.** 2225 W. 50th Street, Suite 100 Sioux Falls, SD 57105 http://www.adaptivation.com/	2.5 x 4 x .1 "	Gross access	Open hand; foot; elbow	Bright color	Completely flat
4. Plate Switch ($32.95) **Enabling Devices** 385 Warburton Avenue Hastings-on-Hudson, NY http://enablingdevices.com/	5" x 8"	Gross access	Open hand; foot	Activation feedback; bright color	Angled presentation; Suction cup feet

FIGURE 22-4 Sample switch analysis worksheet.

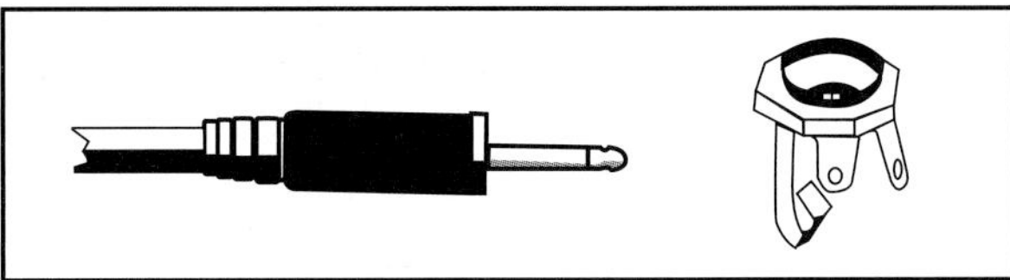

A

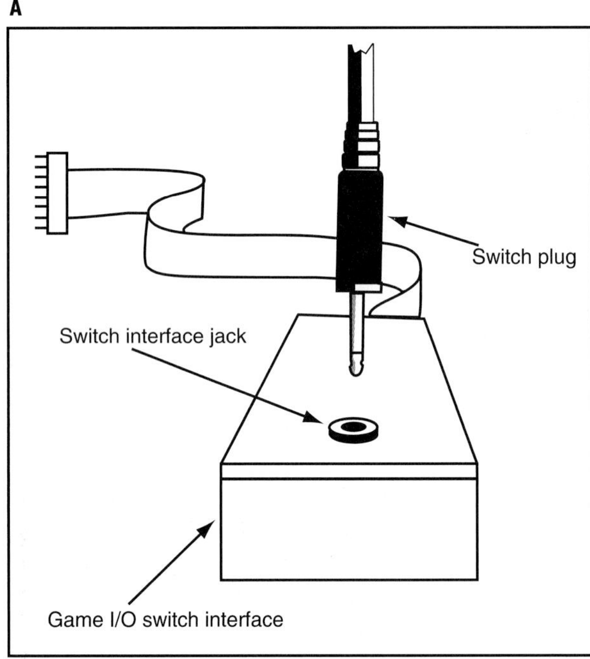

B

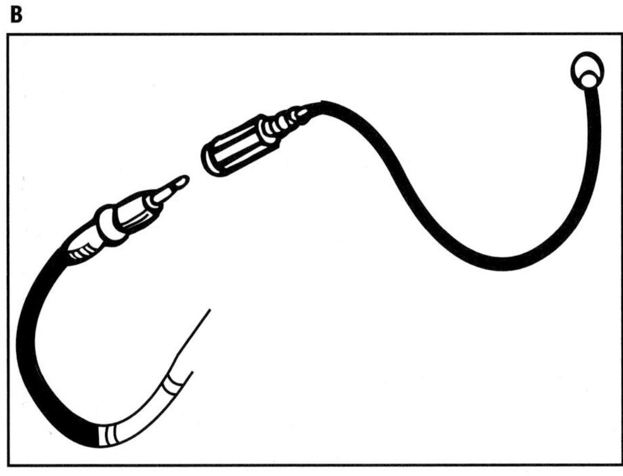

C

FIGURE 22-5 **A,** Miniature plug: typical sizes 1/8, 1/4, and 1/2 inch. **B,** Switch plug and switch interface jack. *I/O,* Input/output. (From Glennen S, Church G: Adaptive toys and environmental controls. In Church G, Glennen S, editors: *The handbook of assistive technology,* San Diego, 1992, Singular Publishing Group.) **C,** Sample battery adapter. (From Adaptivation Incorporated: *Recipes for success,* Sioux Falls, SD, 1999, Adaptivation.)

jacks. Resources for battery adapters and cable adapters are included at the end of this chapter.

Finally, it is important to understand the three modes of operation available when using switch technology with individual users. In momentary or continuous mode, the user must maintain pressure on the switch in order to keep the toy or appliance operating.[1] This is also referred to as the direct mode. Unfortunately, this is not particularly functional. Think about how often you would watch TV or listen to music if you had to continually press the 'on' button to do it! Switch-latch timers are devices designed to eliminate this need.[1] To operate, the switch is plugged into one part of the switch-latch timer while the device to be operated is plugged into another part (Figure 22-6). When set in the latched mode, activation of the switch turns the device on and reactivation turns it off. This is a very functional setting for activities such as making milk shakes in a blender or listening to the radio and watching TV. In the timed mode, activation of the switch turns the device on and it stays on for the amount of time you specify, which could be seconds, minutes, or hours. This mode is particularly helpful when you want to determine whether an individual understands that the switch is being used to operate something. For example, with a tape recorder and a switch-latch timer, activation of the switch would result in music being played. When the music stopped, you could look for signs that the user understood that the switch and tape recorder were somehow related. For example, did s/he reach for the switch, reach for the tape-recorder, look at the switch, or look at the tape recorder? These are all signs that the user understands the relationship between the switch and what is being controlled and thus can be taught to control appliances and toys with switches.

Environmental Controls

Environmental control units (ECUs) provide individuals with disabilities to control over their environment. An ECU consists of an input device, a throughput method, and some form of output (see Table 22-1). There are three common transmission methods that can be used to purposefully manipulate and interact with the environment (Figure 22-7). ECUs offer a motivating option for increasing the functional independence of children with disabilities. ECUs constitute an important class of AT tools to keep in mind when considering user goals because they represent an option frequently overshadowed by adapted-play and communication technologies. It is essential to keep in mind that infants as young as 9 months old will reach for the remote control and proceed to aim it at the television!

Angelo[1] suggests a number of questions that should be considered when making decisions about ECU options for clients. These include asking what the user wants to be able to do, what the user's strengths and

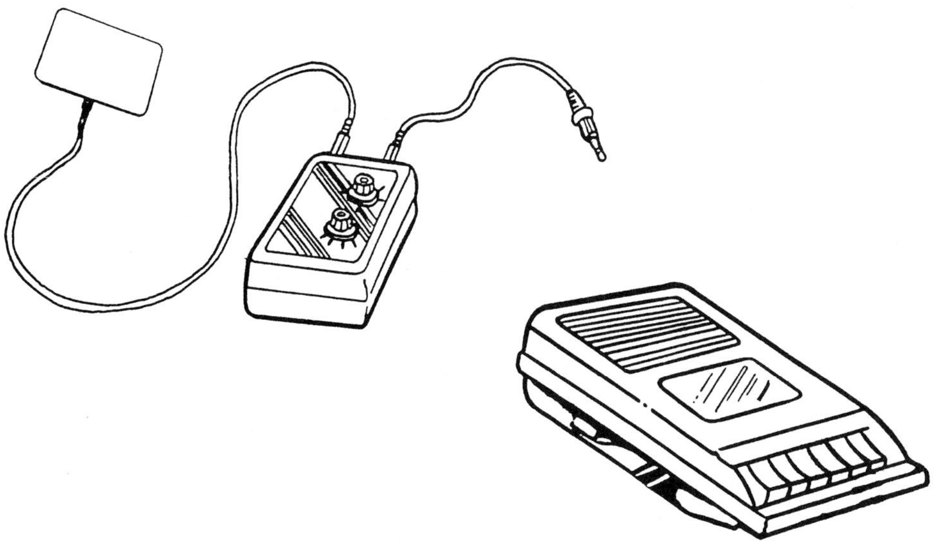

FIGURE 22-6 Switch-latch timer with switch *(left)* and toy (tape recorder *[right]*). (From Adaptivation Incorporated: *Recipes for success*, Sioux Falls, SD, 1999, Adaptivation.)

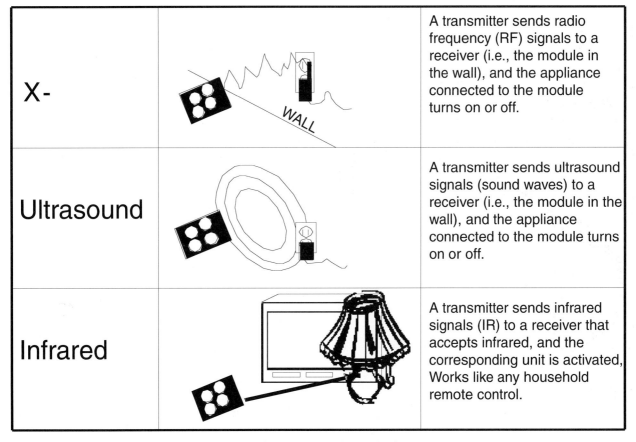

X-	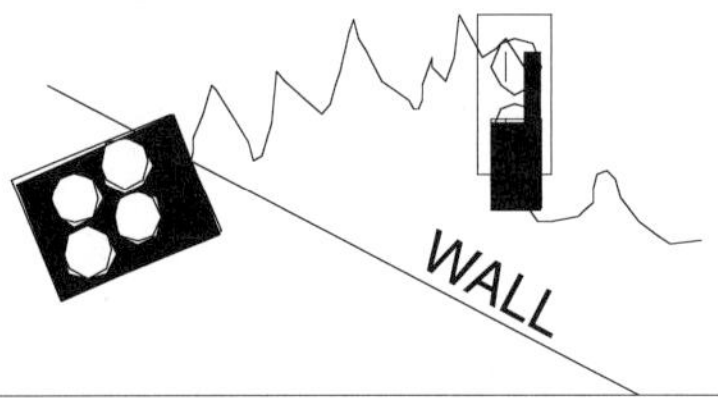 WALL	A transmitter sends radio frequency (RF) signals to a receiver (i.e., the module in the wall), and the appliance connected to the module turns on or off.
Ultrasound	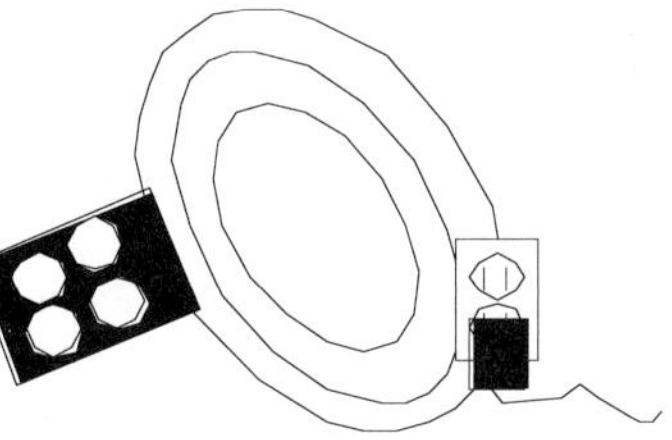	A transmitter sends ultrasound signals (sound waves) to a receiver (i.e., the module in the wall), and the appliance connected to the module turns on or off.
Infrared	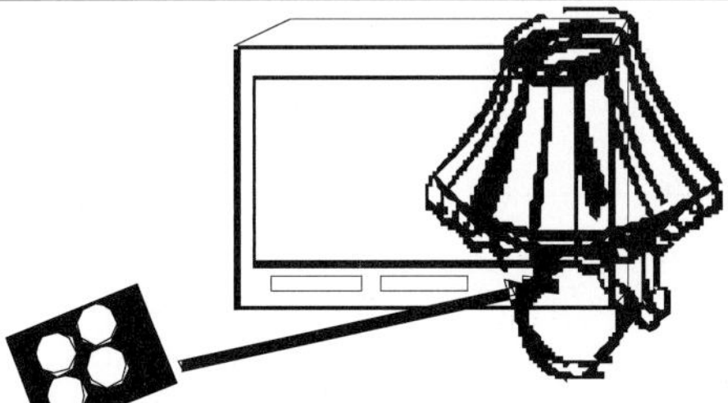	A transmitter sends infrared signals (IR) to a receiver that accepts infrared, and the corresponding unit is activated, Works like any household remote control.

FIGURE 22-7 Three common transmission methods for environmental control units.

abilities are, the context(s) for the ECU, and the type of feedback needed by the user. As you can see, these questions are essentially the same as the ones we used in our assessment model. Consequently, such a model has merit regardless of the class of AT tools under consideration. The following case study should be helpful in understanding the role of ECU options for pediatric clients with disabilities.

TABLE 22–2

Control Sequence for Environmental Control Units

INPUT	THROUGHPUT	OUTPUT
Activates system by sending a signal	Receives and transmits signal	Signal received and output given
Examples include voice signal, switch activation, and button depression	Examples include radiofrequency, ultrasound, and infrared transmission.	Examples include lights turned on or off, volume turned up or down, and CD player turned on.

Sandy is a 4 year old with cerebral palsy characterized by spastic quadriplegia. She loves to listen to music and recently received a CD player for her birthday. Her practitioner is interested in giving Sandy the option of controlling her CD player when she is in her bedroom because that is where she plays her music. Sandy uses primarily a gross swipe toward objects. She has some difficulties with visual acuity but has demonstrated the ability to discriminate line drawings of 3 square inches. The OT practitioner decides to try the Cordless Big Red from Ablenet, Inc. It comes in a variety of bright colors and has a 5-inch-diameter activation surface. It operates by radiofrequency and thus comes with a receiver module. The large surface area of the Cordless Big Red can accommodate a 3-inch-square line drawing of a CD player to help Sandy associate the ECU with the device it operates. With four modes of control (i.e., direct, timed-second, timed-minute, and latched), the Cordless Big Red offers control flexibility. The practitioner decides to introduce the ECU using the timed-minute mode, and once Sandy has the idea, she switches over to latched mode, giving Sandy complete control.

In summary, ECUs for young children are generally straightforward and simple to operate.

Simple Communication Technologies

Communication technologies (augmentative and alternative communication [AAC]) focus on an area of clinical practice that attempts to compensate (either temporarily or permanently) for a person's difficulty using speech as a primary means of communication. It is important to understand that an AAC device is only *one* aspect of an individual's communication *system*, which also includes gestures, facial expressions, body language, and other nonsymbolic forms of communication.

A certified, licensed speech-language pathologist makes decisions about specific aids and devices for individual users. However, it is critical that all team members provide input regarding the specific strengths and abilities of a given user so that the speech-language pathologist can make an informed decision. Moreover, it goes without saying that all persons involved in the care of an individual using AAC would need to understand how the system operates as well as how to interact with an individual using an AAC aid or device.

In this chapter, we focus on simple AAC. It comprises systems that are either manual (i.e., have no electronic components) or simple electronic devices (i.e., use household batteries for operation). Referring back to our assessment model, the speech-language pathologist looks to various team members to provide input regarding optimum seating and positioning for access to AAC as well as a user's strengths and abilities relative to direct or indirect selection options and mounting needs. With that said, the remaining decisions deal specifically with what is referred to as the language options for AAC. They include how language will be represented (symbol type), the specific words or phrases that need to be available to the user (vocabulary selection), what the user will see when s/he looks at the aid or device (display organization), and finally how messages will be stored and retrieved.

For very young children, simple AAC tends to be activity based; that is, children use specific displays to engage in the context of a specific activity, such as playing with Play-Doh, blowing bubbles, or completing puzzles. Displays tend to include simple line drawings arranged in a row-column format that include anywhere from two to 32 vocabulary items, depending on a client's language ability. Manual displays might be presented by means of a vest, eye gaze frame, or single sheet display, depending on individual motor abilities (Figure 22-8).

A number of simple battery-operated AAC systems take advantage of human recorded speech to transmit messages. The motivation of hearing a spoken message cannot be underestimated for young children for whom speech is difficult. Single-message devices can give children an opportunity to request attention ("Please come here"), request assistance ("Can you help me?"), express a desire ("Please leave me alone!"), request recurrence ("Let's do it again!"), or even that favorite

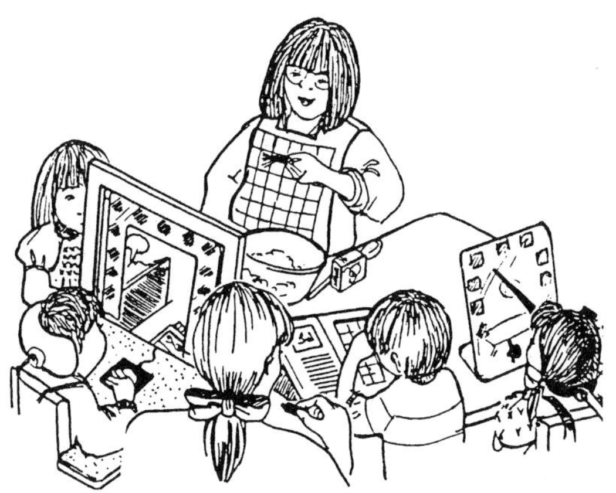

FIGURE 22-8 Options for a manual communication board display. In the figure, shadow light cuing is performed by a second facilitator. (From Goossens C, Crain, SS, Elder PS: *Engineering the preschool environment for interactive symboli communication: 18 months to 5 years developmentally,* ed 2, Birmingham, Ala, 1994, Southeast Augmentative Communication Publications, Clinician Series.)

toddler expression "NO!" Devices designed to present a series of messages (e.g., Step-by-Step Communicator by Ablenet, Inc; Sequencer by Adaptivation, Inc) can give the student the opportunity to actively participate in story time ("He huffed and he puffed and he blew the house down!"), serve as the leader of an activity ("Ready, set, go!"), or tell Mom and Dad what happened at school that day ("I had pizza for lunch," "We played musical chairs," "I sat next to Billy on the bus").

Simple battery-operated devices also come in more complex displays ranging from two to sixteen possible messages. When using devices with limited messaging capability, speech-language pathologists make an effort to program messages that have applicability across a variety of contexts as opposed to those that are limited in use. For example, messages such as "I want a drink" and "I want to eat" are limited in scope. Mealtime and snack time are generally built into one's school day, so the need to request food or drink becomes superfluous. More powerful messages such as "my turn," "finished," "more," and "come here" are useful across a variety of activities and thus give the student an opportunity to use his or her AAC device multiple times throughout the course of the day.

AAC devices place special cognitive, motor, perceptual, and learning requirements on those who use them *and* on their communication partners. It is for this reason that the successful use of communication technologies involves a coordinated team approach focused on interactive communication and motivating activities. Careful planning and training is required for children to be competent users of AAC systems. Remember that our goal is to reinforce and facilitate *any* attempt at communication because it is more important *what* children have to say than *how* they say it!

FUNDING FOR ASSISTIVE TECHNOLOGY

Federal legislation provides the foundation for funding of AT. In other words, lawmakers (senators and legislators) design bills (laws), using input from advocates (in this case persons with disabilities, their caregivers, and professionals), that are designed to ensure "BY LAW" that people have access to the equipment they need.

Before the 1970s, very little legislation addressed the needs of persons with disabilities (pwds). Therefore, pwds and their families relied on private and religious charities, fended for themselves, or just went without. The rehabilitation act of 1973 (referred to as sec-tion 504) was the first major piece of legislation affecting pwds. It established the ideas of reasonable accommodation (RA) and least restrictive environment (LRE).

RA refers to the fact that the needs of persons with disabilities must be accommodated in order to not exclude them from the same experiences and opportunities as those of non-disabled individuals. RA was written very vaguely and is essentially determined by the courts (i.e., lawsuits). LRE refers to the degree of modification in a job or academic program that is acceptable. The Rehabilitation Act was patterned after civil rights legislation. Simply stated, it became unlawful to discriminate against individuals because of their disabilities. No handicapped person could be excluded from employment or secondary education solely on the basis of his or her handicap. It mandated that employers and institutions of higher education receiving federal funds accommodate the needs of PWDs.

In 1975 Congress enacted another major piece of legislation, also patterned after civil rights legislation, this time protecting the rights of children with disabilities. The Education for All Handicapped Children Act, PL 94-142, later became known as the Individuals with Disabilities Act (IDEA).[12] In this legislation, handicapped children were acknowledged as people endowed with certain inalienable rights, which are outlined in Box 22-2.

As it pertains to AT, IDEA mandated that public schools (1) provide evaluation for AT; (2) purchase, lease, or by other means provide for the acquisition of the aid or device; (3) select, design, fit, customize, adapt, repair, and/or replace the aid or device; (4) coordinate and use other services with AT; (5) train the child and family, and (6) train professionals.

Private insurance coverage for AT is dependent on individual policies. Often you will not see a specific

BOX 22-2

Assistive Technology Mandated by the Individuals with Disabilities Act for Children with Disabilities

A free and appropriate education regardless of the handicapping condition
Provision of educational services to the maximum extent appropriate in the least restrictive environment
The participation of parents in the educational process
Due process procedures
The right to related services to benefit from special education instruction
The development of an Individual Education Plan—what we are going to do, who is going to do it, where it will be done, when it will be done, and how we will know it is complete (functional outcome)

service such as AT or rehabilitative technology but rather a provision for durable medical equipment, which may or may not include the specific AT device or service that you want to recommend. Historically, private insurers have followed the lead of Medicare/Medicaid in detailing coverage for specific classes of AT tools. Service clubs, foundations, volunteer organizations, and low-interest bank loans should also be considered potential sources of full or supplemental funding for AT. Regardless of the source of funding, AT should be described in terms of the medical benefit to the client, which could include the prevention of secondary disability as well as the impact on quality of life. Specific details regarding expected outcomes and how they will be measured and documented should always be included in a request for funding.

SUMMARY

AT appliances and tools constitute an integral part of OT practice. AT fosters functional independence in persons with disabilities. The use of AT in pediatrics can motivate children with disabilities early on and, in so doing, ward off the negative impact of a lack of motivation and learned helplessness. Because the range of AT products and devices is constantly changing, this chapter focused on the best practice of AT-related principles, which will serve the OT practitioner regardless of the specific aid or device in question. Furthermore, because of the dynamic nature of this field, it is imperative that the OT practitioner view his or her role as a member of a *team* of professionals that always includes family members and equipment manufacturers as potential sources of information about the complex and advancing field of AT aids and devices.

References

1. Angelo J: *Assistive technology for rehabilitation specialists*, Philadelphia, 1997, FA Davis.
2. Capilouto G: Rehabilitation settings. In Kumar S, editor: *Multidisciplinary approach to rehabilitation*, Boston, 2000, Butterworth Heinemann.
3. Church G, Glennen S: *The handbook of assistive technology*, San Diego, 1992, Singular Publishing Group.
4. Clayton K, Mathena CT: Assistive technology. In Solomon J, editor: *Pediatric skills for occupational therapy assistants*, ed 1, St Louis, 2000, Mosby.
5. Cook A, Hussey S: *Assistive technologies: principles and practices*, ed 2, St Louis, 2002, Mosby.
6. Fallon M, Wann J: Incorporating computer technology into activity-based thematic units for young children with disabilities, *Infants Young Child* 6:4, 1994.
7. Galvin J, Scherer M: *Evaluating, selecting and using appropriate assistive technology*, San Diego, 1996, Singular Publishing Group.
8. Glennen S, Church G: Adaptive toys and environmental controls. In Church G, Glennen S, editors: *The handbook of assistive technology*, San Diego, 1992, Singular Publishing Group.
9. Greenstein DB: It's child's play. In Galvin J, Scherer M: *Evaluating, selecting and using appropriate assistive technology*, San Diego, 1996, Singular Publishing Group.
10. Hollingsworth M: Computer technologies: a cornerstone for educational and employment equity, *Can J Higher Ed* 22:1, 1992.
11. Musselwhite C: *Adaptive play for special needs children*, San Diego, 1986, College-Hill Press.
12. PL 94-142: Individuals with Disabilities Act, 1975, US Congress.
13. PL 100-407: Technology-Related Assistance for Individuals with Disabilities Act, 1988, US Congress.
14. World Health Organization: *International classification of functioning, disability and health (ICF)*. Retrieved December 30, 2004, from http://www.who.int/classifications/icf/en/.

Internet Resources

States Funded Under the Assistive Technology Act of 1998 (PL 105-394)
http://www.resna.org/taproject/at/statecontacts.html
Rehabilitation Engineering and Assistive Technology Society of North America
http://www.resna.org/
Orcca Technology, Inc; The Assistive Technology Exploration Center
http://www.orcca.com/
Ideas for Assistive Technology Activities with Ablenet Products
http://www.ablenetinc.com/productIdeas.asp
Handouts and Documents: Ideas for Assistive Technology Activities from Adaptivation
http://www.adaptivation.com/
Information on Switch Technology
http://www.abilityhub.com/switch/index.htm
A not-for-profit charitable organization dedicated to the most effective communication for people who rely on augmentative and alternative communication
http://www.aacinstitute.org/
Resource on Adapted Play
http://www.ataccess.org/resources/wcp/enswitches/endefault.html
Information on Environmental control units
http://cat.buffalo.edu/newsletters/ecu.php
Assistive Technology and the Individual Education Plan
http://www.katsnet.org/fact4.html
Family Guide to Assistive Technology
http://www.pluk.org/AT1.html
Guidelines for Assistive Technology
http://www.birth23.org/Publications/assistivetech.pdf

REVIEW *Questions*

1. Define AT and its services and discuss their importance in the field of OT.
2. Describe potential members of the AT team and why a team approach is critical.
3. Define and give examples of assistive, rehabilitative, educational, and medical technologies.
4. Compare and contrast high and low technology.
5. Describe the difference between an assistive tool and an assistive appliance, and state why the distinction is important.
6. Using Figure 22-1, describe the various components of AT assessment.
7. Define adapted play and give two examples of adapted play activities.
8. What are three things one must think about when considering switch selection for an individual user?
9. Name and describe the three modes of operation available for switch technology and the function of a switch-latch timer.
10. Describe the three common modes of transmission for ECUs.
11. State the difference between manual and simple electronic communication technologies, and describe three simple communication technologies commonly used in pediatrics.
12. Name five potential funding sources for AT in pediatrics.

SUGGESTED *Activities*

1. Contact the Tech-Act program in your state and find out what services they provide.
2. Interview a person who uses AT to determine the selection process, their satisfaction with AT, and the funding process.
3. Visit a local AT supplier and see what products they have available and their relative costs.
4. Contact OT practitioners in a local school system, children's hospital, and rehabilitation center to see the ways in which AT is used in different settings.
5. Volunteer to fabricate a low-tech recreational aid or device for a youngster in the public school system.
6. Review the websites listed in the resources section of this chapter for specific information on AT products, services, and activities.
7. Contact ORCCA Technology for information on their virtual reality exploration centers in assistive technology.

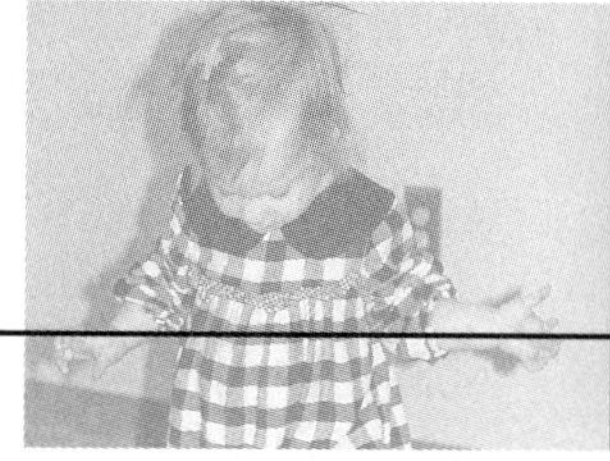

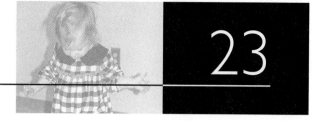

23

Splinting for the Child and Adolescent

MELISSA A. FULLERTON
ALLYSON LACHANCE
MELISSA A. MAILHOT*

CHAPTER *Objectives*

After studying this chapter, the reader will be able to accomplish the following:

- Explain how splints have an impact on children's and adolescents' occupational performance
- Recognize important general considerations with regard to splinting
- Understand the goals for splinting in the pediatric population
- Understand common pediatric upper extremity problems and splinting options
- Understand common pediatric lower extremity problems and splinting options
- Understand intervention techniques within the pediatric population with regard to splinting
- Understand the role of a certified occupational therapy assistant in occupational therapy treatment for children and adolescents with orthoses.
- Explain various strategies that might increase compliance with splinting- or brace-wearing schedule and use

*The authors wrote this chapter as an elective assignment to fulfill requirements for the Masters of Science degree in occupational therapy from the University of New England under the guidance of Jean Solomon and Jane O'Brien.

KEY TERMS

Splints
Orthosis
Static splint
Dynamic splint
Exploration stage
Competency stage
Achievement stage
Contractures
Decubitus ulcers

CHAPTER OUTLINE

The primary outcomes of pediatric occupational therapy (OT) are to promote independence and optimum occupational performance for children and adolescents who have special needs. For those who have disabilities or impairments that cause decreased upper or lower extremity function because of abnormal tone, decreased mobility, or decreased functional skills, splinting may help achieve more functional independence. Both the registered occupational therapist (OTR) and certified occupational therapy assistant (COTA) have important roles in the fabrication and application of splints for children and adolescents receiving OT services.

DEFINITION

Splints are devices that immobilize, restrain, or support a part of the body.[5] The term **orthosis**, or orthotic device, is sometimes used in place of the word *splint*. A splint is often temporary, while an orthotic device usually refers to one that is more permanent.[5] It should be noted that in some of the literature and in this chapter, the terms are used interchangeably.[10]

Splints may be used for interventions involving the upper extremity, lower extremity, and trunk. There are several types of splints, and they may be classified as static or dynamic. **Static splints** prevent movement and often promote functional position. They are used to prevent deformity. They can be made from several materials and are molded around a joint or other part of the body, often including fasteners such as Velcro to hold them in place. **Dynamic splints** assist an individual with movements and may include pulleys, springs, screws, hooks, elastics, and other outriggers to assist with the desired motions.

The purpose of a splint is to protect, correct, or assist a joint, limb, or muscle in order to increase functional performance.[10] For example, a splint might protect an injured wrist from increased pain while a child or adolescent is playing or prevent deformity during sleep.

GENERAL CONSIDERATIONS

The primary goal for an OT practitioner providing intervention to children and adolescents who have disabilities is to promote participation in daily activities by choosing activities that are meaningful to the person. OT focuses on improving one's physical, emotional, and social abilities by facilitating the interaction among the child or adolescent, the family members, and the environment.[8] By encompassing all of these dimensions of a person and considering the various contexts (e.g., cultural, social, physical, spiritual, temporal, personal), the OT practitioner can facilitate positive health outcomes.[1,4] Identifying important occupations during childhood or adolescence is then necessary to enhance participation and engagement in the intervention sessions.

Play/leisure activities are important occupations for all people. Play is the occupation of children and adolescents. Through play a child or adolescent explores his or her environment while learning the cognitive, social, emotional, and physical skills needed to be a healthy adult. Splints can help stabilize body parts of children and adolescents so that they may effectively use their hands for play.

At one time or another, we can all remember a time when we participated in a game or activity that caused pain or injury. One may recall stories of events that resulted in a cast, stitches, or Band-Aids. In many cases, children's and adolescents' injuries are predictable due to the fact that most of the injuries sustained during childhood and adolescence can be linked to age and developmental level.[9] Table 23-1 illustrates the most common injuries sustained during childhood.[9] Keep in mind that a child does not need to have special needs to have these injuries, and other injuries may be sustained during childhood and adolescence.

CLINICAL *Pearl*

Accidental head injury during recreational or play activities is the leading cause of death in children.[11] There are 900 documented cases of head injuries related to bicycle accidents in the United States each year.[11] When they are worn correctly, helmets can reduce the possibility of head injury. The following guidelines help to ensure that a helmet properly fits a child or adolescent (Figure 23-1).

The helmet should rest just above the child's or adolescent's eyebrows.

The straps must be snug and secure.

The helmet should fit snugly on the head. It should not move excessively on the head while the child or adolescent is playing.[11]

COMMON INJURIES

Child and adolescent injuries most often consist of fractures of the elbow, wrist, and carpal bones.[9] Extremity fractures can take place at any age; however, the occurrence of upper extremity fractures increases when children and adolescents become more independent.[9] Extremity fractures account for approximately 10% to 15% of all injuries sustained during childhood or adolescence.[9] Upper extremity fractures in pediatrics are challenging to address because of common errors associated

TABLE 23-1

Common Injuries of Childhood

AGE AND CHARACTERISTICS	COMMON INJURIES
The infancy or early childhood stage (0 to 2 years) is considered the **exploration stage.** Children at this stage explore the self and environment by manipulating toys and seeking pleasure from tactile stimulation. Children of this age have some control over bodily functions, enabling them to walk and control bowel and bladder functions.	Choking Extremity fractures Head injuries Toxic ingestion
The **competency stage** is referred to as the toddler or middle childhood stage (2 to 6 years). Children begin to identify roles, make decisions, and have greater independence; however, they still need caregivers for support. During this stage, children facilitate pregames, engage in fantasy play, refine necessary skills, and begin to distinguish from right and wrong, thus developing a conscience.	Extremity fractures/injuries Falls Bicycle accidents
The late childhood stage (6 to 11 years) is considered the **achievement stage.** Children enter the student role. They become aware of consequences of activities. Social interaction with peers and separation from the family environment occur during this stage.	Extremity fractures/injuries Athletic injuries Head injuries Bicycle injuries

Adpated from Thomas DO: Quick *Reference to Pediatric Emergency Nursing,* 1991, Aspen Publishers.

CLINICAL *Pearl*

The most common types of child and adolescent upper extremity fractures are supracondylar, lateral condylar, medial epicondylar, radial neck, transphyseal, and miscellaneous fractures of the T-condylar, Monteggia, and olecranon processes of the elbow[3] (Figure 23-2).

with intervention and management of the injury.[14] OT practitioners can fabricate a splint that follows casting, aiding in protection and healing of the injury.[14] In many clinical cases, the OT practitioner may receive a referral for a client late, when the fracture is healing improperly and in a nonfunctional position. In these cases, treatment adaptations may be necessary. The OT practitioner can

TABLE 23-2

Pediatric Upper Extremity Gross and Fine Motor Skills

AGE SKILL APPEARS, MO	UPPER EXTREMITY GROSS AND FINE MOTOR SKILLS
0 to 2	Physiologic flexion
2	Grasp reflex
3	Hands together on chest in supine position
4	Grasp reflex diminishing; objects held in both hands at midline; in supine position bears weight on forearm, with more weight on the ulnar than the radial side; pats sides of bottle with hands
5	Two-handed approach to objects, but grasp is unilateral; bilateral transfer; extended-arm weight bearing in prone position; places two hands on bottle, with some forearm supination
6	Weight shifts on extended arms in prone position; sits with a straight back; elbows fully extend when reaching
7	First purposeful release; pulls self to stand
8	Crawls on hands and knees
9	Active forearm supination when reaching
10	Pokes with index finger
12	Uses hands in coordinated manner in which one hand stabilizes and the other manipulates; begins to scribble
15	Releases a pellet with wrist extension and precision

Adapted from Jacobs ML, Austin N: *Splinting the hand and upper extremity: principles and process,* Baltimore, Md, 2003, Lippincott Williams & Wilkins.

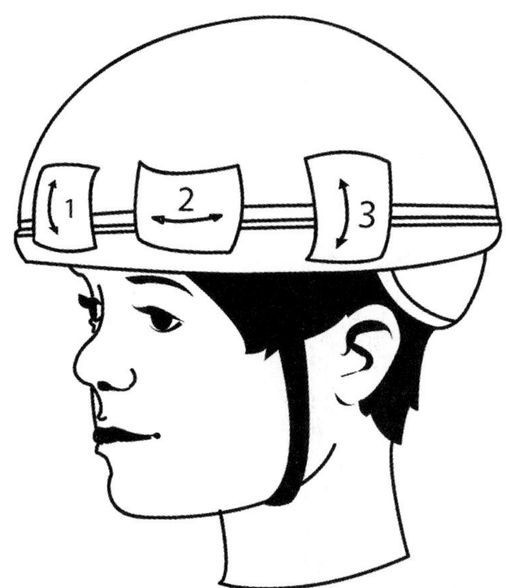

FIGURE 23-1 Proper helmet fit.

fabricate and apply a splint that sets the fracture in the proper position and facilitates healing in that functional position.

GOALS OF SPLINTING

OT practitioners must consider splinting fundamentals and normal child and adolescent development, including gross and fine motor skill development, when fabricating a splint. (See Table 23-2 for a description of gross and fine motor skill development.) Because the goal of OT is to promote function, an awareness of the development of hand skills is important. Practitioners consider the skills required for the age and use splinting as a technique to develop or assist the child. For example, when splinting an 8 month old, the OT practitioner considers that at this age children crawl on the hands and knees. Therefore, the practitioner will want to promote hand function while allowing the child to crawl. It may be possible to fabricate a splint that protects the wrist and allows the child to bear weight on the palms.

There are four main reasons for splinting an extremity: to improve function, prevent further injury, improve hygiene, and prevent skin breakdown.

Splints are customized to fit any individual and meet his or her occupational needs.[5,6,14] By placing an injured limb or joint in a functional position, children and adolescents may engage in meaningful occupations, such as play and activities of daily living (ADLs), that mirror their habits and daily routines.

Splinting for Function

Jane is a 4-year-old girl with cerebral palsy (CP). She has decreased wrist stability, which causes difficulty in holding utensils. She is able to sit at a table but has poor coordination and is continuously dropping her spoon. A wrist cock-up splint was fabricated for Jane to help her hold her spoon (Figure 23-3).

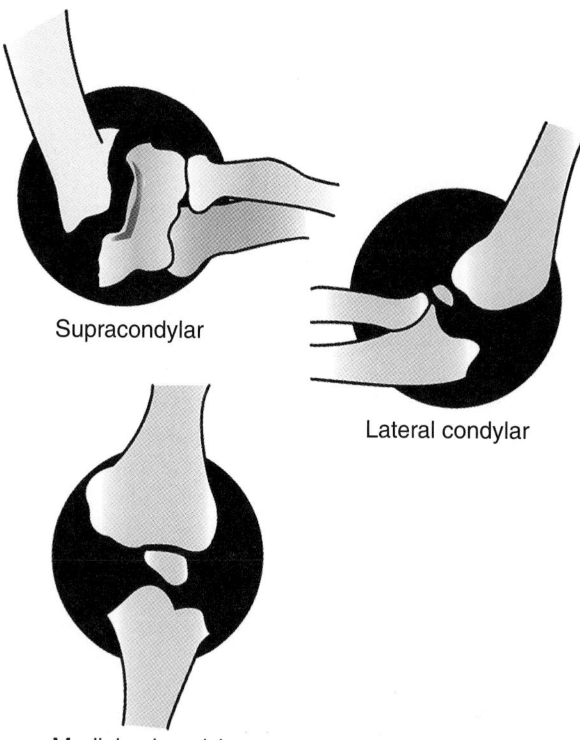

FIGURE 23-2 Common elbow fractures.

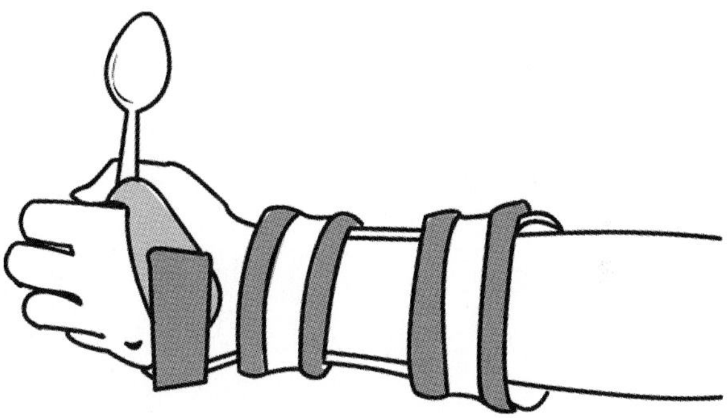

FIGURE 23-3 Functional splint—wrist cock-up splint with spoon attached. (Redrawn from Armstrong J: Splinting the pediatric patient. In Fess EE, Gettle KS, Philips CA, et al: *Hand and upper extremity splinting: principles and methods*, ed 3, St Louis, 2005, Mosby.)

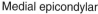

A splint can be used to supplement existing function. A functional splint can substitute for weak or absent muscles, which may be caused by peripheral nerve dysfunction, neuromuscular disorders (e.g., CP), or spinal cord injuries.[5,7] One can be designed to hold a pencil, toy, or eating utensil.

A supported wrist splint was designed for Jane to wear while eating. This splint will provide Jane with the wrist support she needs to increase hand control and allow her to be successful in this important daily occupation. OT practitioners need to remember that proximal stability leads to distal mobility. Creating stability around the wrist or elbow with a splint may promote hand functioning.

Splinting for Position

Timmy is an 8-year-old boy who is developing ***contractures*** *(limitations in movement caused by soft tissue shortening, which may result in a "stiff" or fused joint that is unable to move) in his hands secondary to juvenile rheumatoid arthritis (JRA). His wrists are beginning to deviate in an ulnar direction; there is redness and swelling surrounding the joints. If a joint remains in an abnormal position, the risk of fusion (bony deformity) increases, which may ultimately lead to an inability to maintain functional use of the hands. Thus, splinting the joint early may be beneficial because the splint will apply a continuous stretch to the shortened tissues and promote the ability to perform daily occupations.*

A positional splint can do the following:

- It can decrease or prevent contractures by maximizing range of motion (ROM), thus preventing soft tissue shortening through immobilization.
- A mobilization splint can aid in elongating soft tissue over an extended period of time, thus decreasing an existing contracture.
- It can provide stability to an unstable joint. A splint can provide external support to a joint or series of joints, thereby improving the biomechanical functioning of the hand.
- It can improve joint alignment and prevent the progression of deformity. A splint may place the child's or adolescent's hand in the proper anatomical position, which helps prevent deformity of the bony structures and surrounding tissue.
- It can provide rest for the affected structures, which is an integral part of the healing process. A splint will hold the hand in proper anatomical alignment allowing the soft tissues to heal and edema and inflammation to diminish.[7]

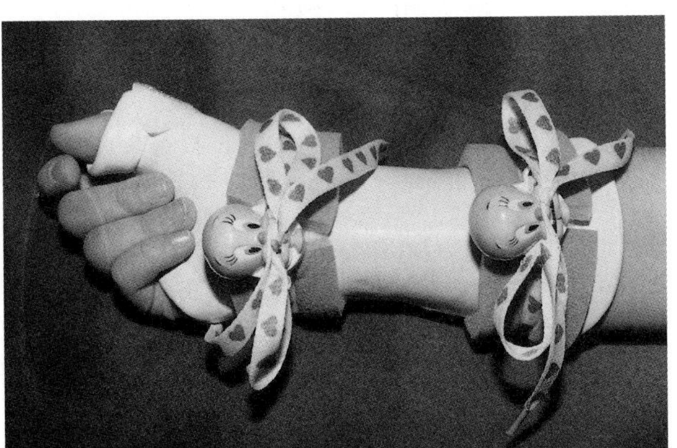

A

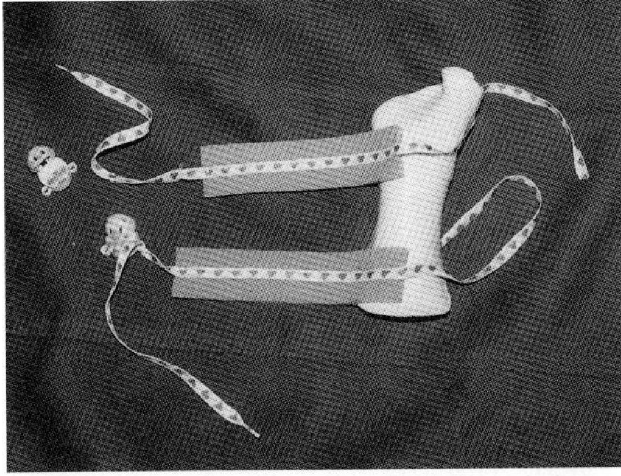

B

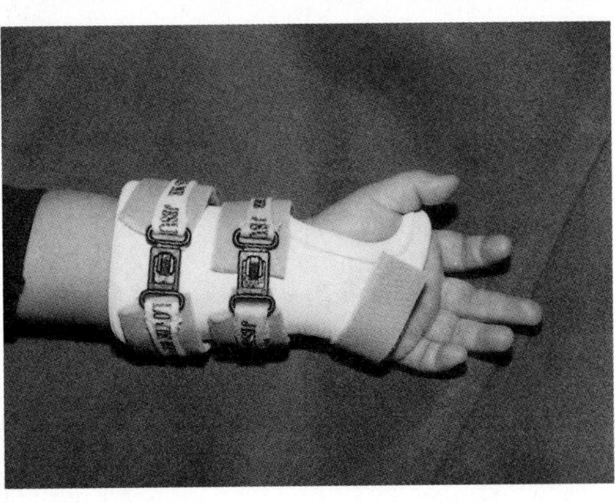

C

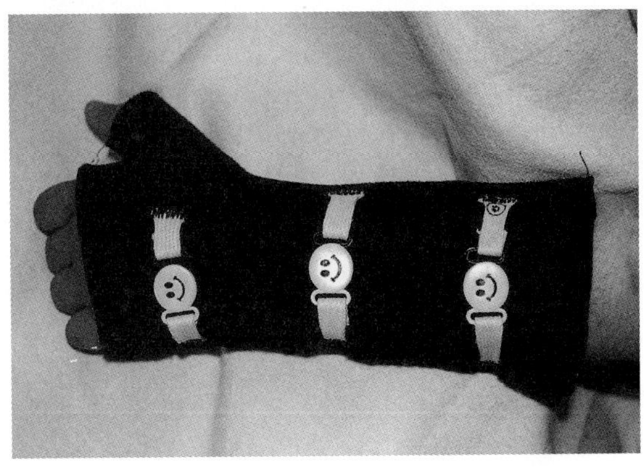

D

FIGURE 23-4 A-D, Splinting for position—wrist cock-up splints with ulnar deviation block. (From Armstrong J: Splinting the pediatric patient. In Fess EE, Gettle KS, Philips CA, et al: *Hand and upper extremity splinting: principles and methods*, ed 3, St Louis, 2005, Mosby.)

TABLE 23-3

Common Pediatric Diagnoses Utilizing Splinting Interventions

DIAGNOSIS	SPLINTING INTERVENTIONS
Cerebral palsy Hemiplegia – involvement on one side of the body	Functional splints that facilitate proper positions of arms, such as wrist/hand immobilization splints, neoprene splints, Joe Cool splints, and thumb abduction splints
Quadriplegia – all four extremities involved	Wrist/hand immobilization splints, antispasticity ball splints, neoprene splints, Carrot splints, Pucci splints, and Cone splints
Duchenne muscular dystrophy	Functional splints that promote stability in weak joints for increased function, such as wrist/hand immobilization splints and ring splints
Rett syndrome	Splints designed to protect clients from self-abusive behaviors such as elbow sleeve
Osteogenesis imperfecta	Splints designed to protect clients from frequent fractures due to decreased stability and structure of the bones, such as nonarticular humerus splints and wrist/hand immobilization splints for infants
Arthrogryposis	Functional splints fabricated to promote engagement in functional activities and prevent further contractures, such as wrist/hand immobilization splints, neoprene splints, and elbow extension mobilization splints
Brachial plexus palsy	Functional splints fabricated to inhibit stretching and facilitate protection of the muscles and nerves, such as wrist/hand immobilization splints, elbow extension immobilization splints, neoprene splints, and shoulder abduction immobilization splints
Juvenile rheumatoid arthritis	Functional splints fabricated to promote ROM for engagement in functional activities and for protection and to decrease deformities, such as wrist/hand immobilization splints, ring splints, neoprene wrist splints, MP joint extension mobilization splints, and Dynasplints

Adapted from Jacobs ML, Austin N: *Splinting the hand and upper extremity: principles and process*, Baltimore, Md, 2003, Lippincott Williams & Wilkins.
MP, Metacarpal phalanges; *ROM*, range of motion.

After evaluation of Timmy's hand and related needs, the COTA and OTR designed a wrist cock-up hand splint with ulnar deviation block for him (Figure 23-4). See Table 23-3 for other splinting options. The wrist cock-up splint held Timmy's hand in slight wrist extension while allowing for a passive stretch to prevent joint fusion. He wore his resting hand splint for 2-hour increments to eliminate joint stiffness. See Figure 23-5 for Timmy's splint schedule.

Splinting for Hygiene

Alex is a 10-year-old boy with spastic CP. He has a fisted left hand with an in-dwelling thumb. His parents and teachers are concerned with his sweaty, smelly hand, which is caused by the continuous fisting. Alex's hand is also flaking and collecting food. His fingernails are long and digging into his palm. Furthermore, when ranging Alex's hand, his palm is red and bleeds. A hygiene splint can be used to protect the palm from long or jagged fingernails.

A splint can help prevent or improve hygiene problems.[5-7] For example, a spastic hand that remains fisted is at a high risk for skin breakdown. The inability to extend the fingers makes nail clipping difficult, and long or sharp fingernails can cut the skin and may lead to infection. Splints are frequently fabricated to protect the palm and decrease the risk of skin breakdown (Figure 23-6).

The COTA and OTR collaborated to design a palm protector splint for Alex in order to improve hygiene and prevent his fingernails from cutting into his palm. He wore the splint during waking hours, taking it off only for bathing and grooming. At night Alex's hands were sufficiently relaxed and open, so he did not require a night splint.

Name: Timmy Smith
Splint: Wrist cock up with ulnar deviation block

Schedule: 2 Hours ON, 2 Hours OFF
Purpose: Keep hand in a healthy position; stop stiffness and pain

I wear my splint for 2 hours.

Then, I keep it OFF for 2 hours. Then I put it back ON.

My splint helps my arthritis feel better.

My schedule helps me and my OT know when I am wearing my splint.

I stop wearing my splint if I see any red areas or if it hurts.

	SUN.	MON.	TUES.	WED.	THURS.	FRI.	SAT.
8 - 10 am	ON ★	ON	★ ON	ON	ON ★	ON	ON
10 - 12 pm	OFF	OFF ✋	OFF ★	OFF ★	OFF ✋	OFF ★	OFF
12 - 2 pm	ON ★	ON	ON	ON ★	ON	ON	ON
2 - 4 pm	OFF	OFF	OFF	OFF	★ OFF	OFF	OFF
4 - 6 pm	ON ★	★ ON	ON	ON	★ ON	★ ON	✋ ON
6 - 8 pm	OFF	OFF	OFF	✋ OFF	OFF ★	OFF	OFF
Bedtime	OFF						

★ = YES, I followed my schedule ✋ = NO, I did not follow the schedule

FIGURE 23-5 Sample splint-wearing schedule.

Splinting for Protection

Sammy is a 12-year-old girl with attention deficit hyperactivity disorder (ADHD) who is very impulsive. She receives OT services within the school system. She just had

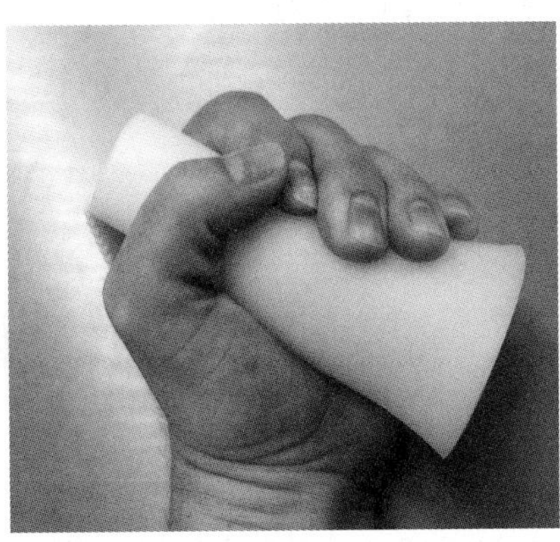

A

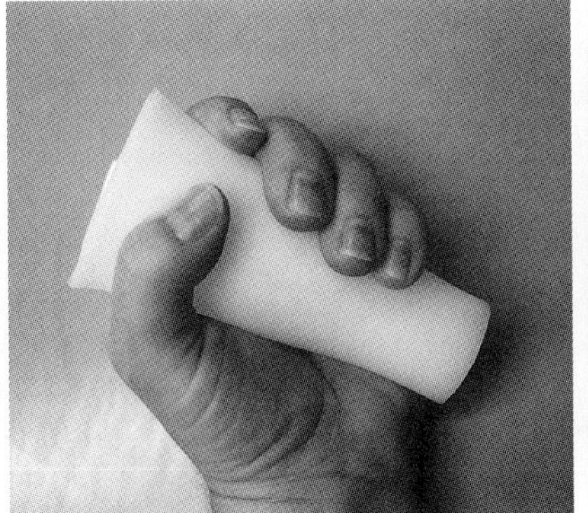

B

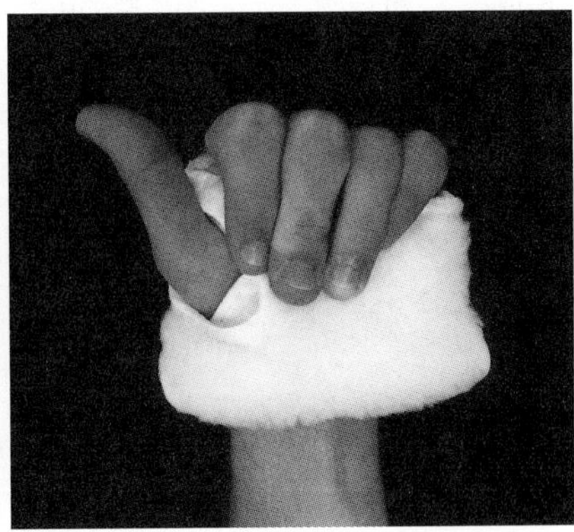

C

FIGURE 23-6 A-C, Splinting for hygiene. (From Fess EE, Gettle KS, Philips CA, et al: *Hand and upper extremity splinting: principles and methods*, ed 3, St Louis, 2005, Mosby.)

her cast removed following a radial fracture. Because Sammy is active and impulsive, her parents are concerned that she may fracture her arm again. Her teachers are hesitant for her to play on the playground for fear of refracture. A splint can be used to protect the bones and joints as they continue to heal. Splints can be used for active children and adolescents who are at risk of reinjury.

Splinting for protection may be used either after a surgical procedure or to prevent a child or adolescent from self-abuse or interfering behaviors.[5-7] A splint can protect a postoperative area after the cast has been removed but before complete healing has occurred.

Sammy's COTA made a radial gutter splint to wear in order to protect the bone and joints as they continue to heal (Figure 23-7). This splint allows Sammy to continue her occupations and allows her to play on the playground without the risk of reinjury.

Matt is a 10-year-old boy with pervasive developmental disorder (PDD). He continually picks at his scabs, increasing the risk of infection. Since his scabs are not able to heal and bleed continuously, they are beginning to scar. A splint is needed to protect Matt's fragile skin.

The OTR working with Matt decided on a protective covering. His COTA, under the supervision of the OTR, fabricated a covering made of stockinette and terry cloth to provide comfort but also cover the existing scabs. However, after several weeks it became apparent that Matt was able to pick and bite through the covering. After collaboration with the OTR, the COTA applied splinting material over the stockinette so that he would be unable to pick at his scabs (Figure 23-8).

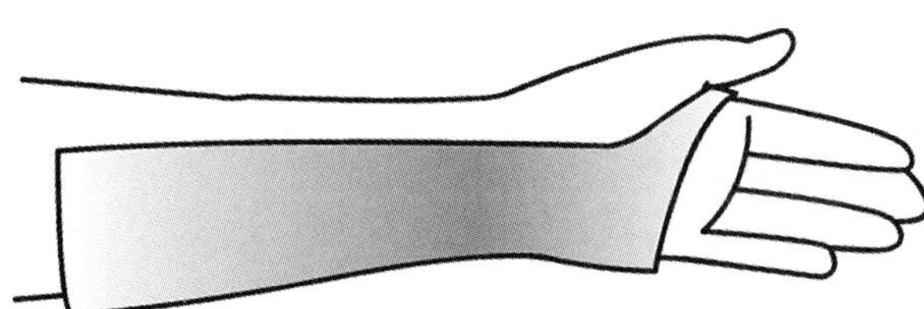

FIGURE 23-7 Splinting for protection—Sammy's radial gutter splint.

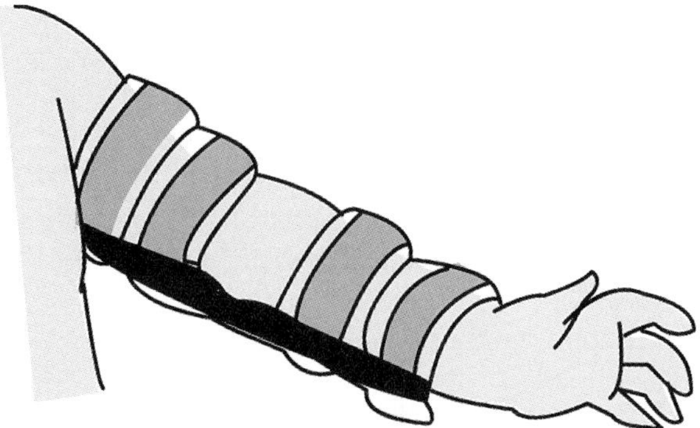

FIGURE 23-8 Splinting for protection—elbow extension splint.

ISSUES SPECIFIC TO PEDIATRIC SPLINTING

There are several considerations that an OT practitioner must take into account when using splints as an intervention in therapy. They include the child's or adolescent's motivation to wear a splint, his or her developmental and functional levels, skin integrity, edema, and the ability to don and doff the splint.

Compliance

Motivation is a key component of the splinting process and includes whether or not a child or adolescent can tolerate a splint. For those who have the cognitive ability to understand, in simple terms, why a splint is being used, time should be taken to educate them. For children and adolescents who are unable to understand and may attempt to remove the splint, additional precautions must be taken to ensure that the splint is being worn as prescribed. For some children and adolescents, splints may be seen as something that sets them apart from their peers; they may feel as though the splints make them "stand out." These individuals may not follow the splinting protocol because of social factors. Therefore, education is critical to the success of the intervention. Compliance with the splinting protocol may be increased by following these guidelines:

- Provide the child or adolescent and caregiver with education regarding the purpose and goals of the splint.[5] S/he may be more apt to wear the splint if s/he understands why it is necessary. For example, if a child or adolescent understands that wearing the splint will help him play video games with his or her friends, s/he might be more likely to wear it.
- Provide simple written, verbal, and pictorial instructions. Keeping the instructions clear will serve as a point of reference for the child or adolescent and caregivers.

- Use positive reinforcement for following the splinting protocol.[5] This may include verbal praise, stickers, and completion of a splint schedule checklist.
- Include the concerns of the child or adolescent and caregiver regarding the splint and make the necessary adjustments to it.[5] This is particularly important for feelings of discomfort and even those regarding how it looks.
- Demonstrate the proper splint application to a child or adolescent and caregiver.[5] The demonstration should be an integral part of the splinting process and easy to follow at home.
- In a hospital setting, correlate the splint-wearing schedule with staff shift changes.[5] Incorporate issues of the splint-wearing schedule and hygiene into the child's or adolescent's hospital care plan.
- To assist in application, label the splint clearly. Color coding or using a number system to show the child or adolescent and caregiver how to don a splint might prove helpful.[5]

Skin Integrity

Splinting can lead to skin breakdown. Therefore, children and adolescents and caregivers must know what signs to look for in checking for skin breakdown. These signs include redness, soreness, and broken skin. Skin breakdown can lead to pressure sores, or **decubitus ulcers** (Box 23-1), which can develop relatively quickly when the skin is compromised. Poor skin integrity may lead to serious health issues and decreased use of the splint.

To prevent skin breakdown from a splint, the OT practitioner notes the location of a bony prominence (e.g., the ulnar styloid process) and takes care to ensure that there is sufficient padding around that area or that it is not in contact with the splinting material.[10] The padding may include self-sticking foam or gel padding. Applying the padding to the prominences during the fab-

CLINICAL *Pearl*

An OT practitioner can take several avenues to increase compliance. Involving the child or adolescent in the splinting process is crucial. This may include allowing the child or adolescent, when applicable, to choose the color of the splint or strapping. Feedback from him or her and the caregiver on how a splint feels and looks should be encouraged. Children and adolescents may be more likely to wear splints that they find either aesthetically pleasing or functional. They may like the splint better if it is personalized. Personalizing a splint may include allowing the child or adolescent to attach stickers or write, draw, or paint on the splint. See Figure 23-9, which shows a festive Halloween drawing. Directions for putting on and taking off the splint should be kept simple, and a splint-wearing schedule may assist him or her in doing so independently. For some children and adolescents, behavioral strategies such as reward systems may be helpful.

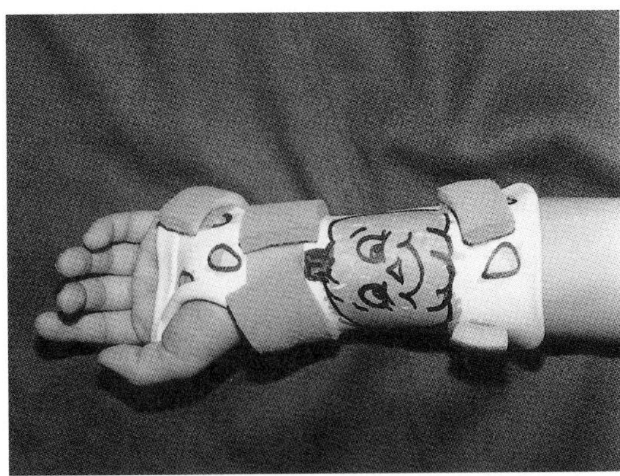

FIGURE 23-9 Wrist cock-up splint with festive drawing. (From Armstrong J: Splinting the pediatric patient. In Fess EE, Gettle KS, Philips CA, et al: *Hand and upper extremity splinting: principles and methods*, ed 3, St Louis, 2005, Mosby.)

BOX 23-1

Decubitus Ulcers

Decubitus ulcers are sores that result from pressure on the skin over a bony prominence, or as the result of continuous pressure on any area. While these ulcers can occur on any area of the body, some common ones are the buttocks, heels, and hips. They can also occur as a result of splints that are not properly fitted or are worn for long periods of time. Decubitus ulcers occur in four stages.[2,15]

1. Stage 1 is characterized by redness of the skin.
2. Stage 2 is characterized by skin loss involving the top two layers of the skin—the epidermis and the dermis. A Stage 2 decubitus ulcer may appear as a blister or a small, open sore.
3. Stage 3 involves damage to the epidermis and dermis but also the deeper tissue.
4. Stage 4 extends down into the muscle and bone.

Moisture, impaired sensory perception, low levels of physical activity, decreased mobility, inadequate nutrition, and poor overall skin care may increase the likelihood of decubitus ulcers.[15]

CLINICAL *Pearl*

Padding can actually create pressure points in other places. OT practitioners need to carefully and frequently inspect all areas of the skin for redness as well as inform caregivers on how to inspect the skin.

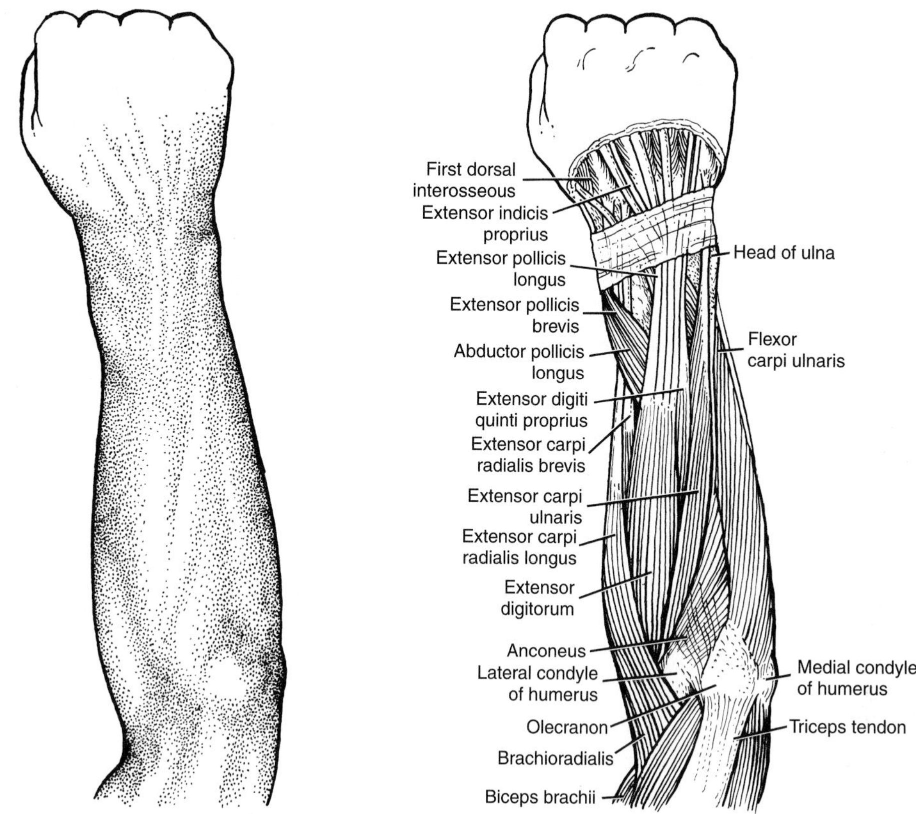

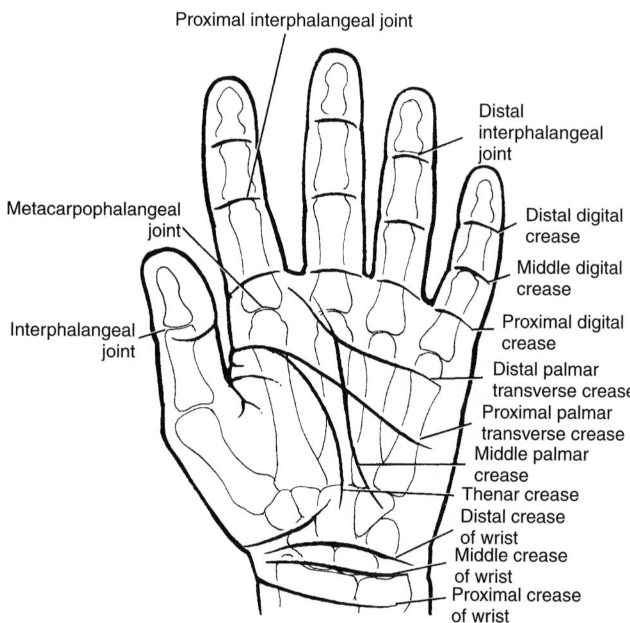

FIGURE 23-10 Anatomical structures of the hand and forearm. (From Fess EE, Gettle KS, Philips CA, et al: *Hand and upper extremity splinting: principles and methods*, ed 3, St Louis, 2005, Mosby.)

rication of the splint helps to protect them. Stockinette can also be used to protect the integrity of the skin.

Additional care should be taken to prevent pressure sores for a child or adolescent who has decreased sensation or decreased ability to communicate. Careful inspection of the skin by both caregivers and OT practitioners is necessary.

Splinting Evaluation

The OT receives the referral and assesses the need for and determines the type of splint that will serve as an adjunctive approach to assist the client in achieving the goals for the OT intervention. The role of the COTA is dependent on his or her level of experience, with the ultimate responsibility falling on the OTR. The OT practitioner must determine the type of splint to be used as well as the functional goal of splinting before proceeding to the intervention. Because the practitioner works on increasing engagement in occupations, the splint should lead to an increase in these two objectives. When evaluating a child or adolescent with a neurological condition, the practitioner must pay special attention to muscle tone and how it may affect the splinting process. The OTR will evaluate and design a splint that provides a mix of function, protection, hygiene, and position. Because children and adolescents are constantly growing and factors such as muscle tone can frequently change, splints must be adjusted regularly. Once the goal of the splint has been identified, the following factors must be considered.

- *Anatomical structures.* The OT practitioner examines hand structures to determine if deformities or abnormalities are present. Children and adolescents with congenital hand anomalies have unusual anatomy that will change the splint plan (Figure 23-10).
- *Abnormal tone.* Because various levels of spasticity may influence different types of splints in different ways, the effect of a splint on tone must be constantly assessed. For example, they can be applied to single joints but may normalize the tone affecting other joints of that extremity.[6]
- *Time frames for healing.* Healing rates are different between adults and children or adolescents. Children tend to heal more quickly but will remain in a cast or splint for longer periods of time. Some children and adolescents have a difficult time adhering to their splinting protocol, which may have an impact on healing time.

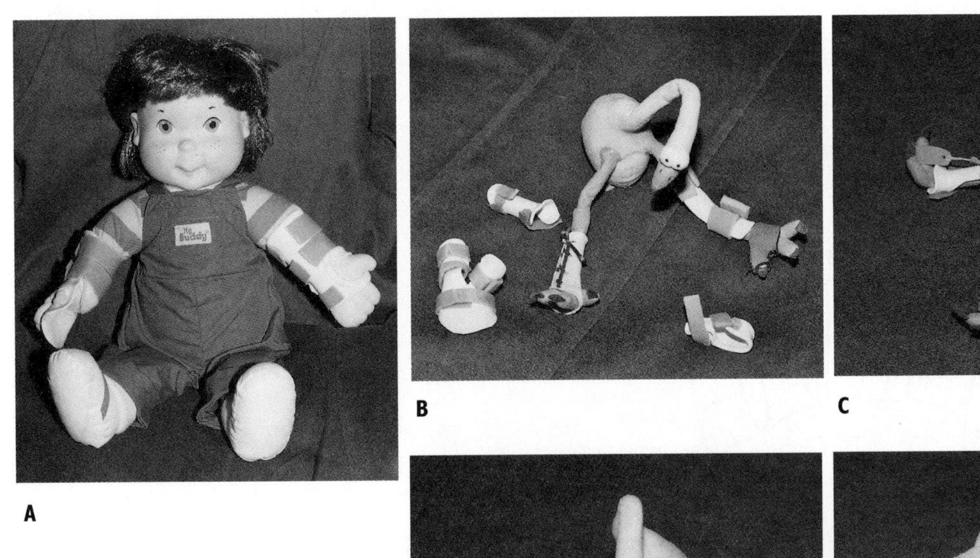

A B C

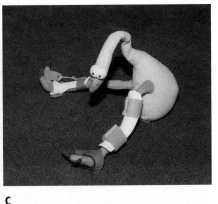

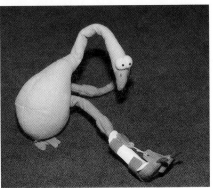

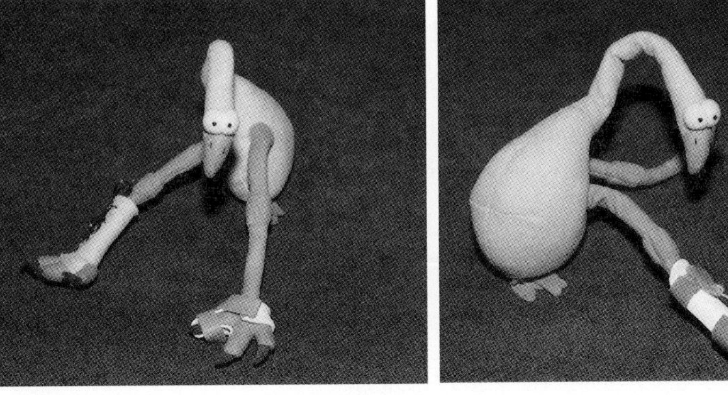

D E

FIGURE 23-11 A-E, Playing with splint material to increase compliance. (From Armstrong J: Splinting the pediatric patient. In Fess EE, Gettle KS, Philips CA, et al: *Hand and upper extremity splinting: principles and methods*, ed 3, St Louis, 2005, Mosby.)

- *Swelling.* Managing edema (swelling) remains the same for children, adolescents, and adults (e.g., ice, elevation, compression). Careful observation and management by caregivers are very important. Splints may need to be remolded or refitted if a client develops edema, which may cause the skin to be more sensitive to pressure and lead to decubitus ulcers.
- *Compliance.* Compliance can affect the length of time a splint needs to be prescribed and may also affect treatment planning and goal setting. See Figure 23-11 for creative ideas to help with compliance while working with children and adolescents.
- *Sensory factors.* Some children and adolescents are hypersensitive to touch and may not be able to tolerate a splint. Those who are nonverbal may not be able to verbalize that they are in pain or discomfort. Padding around bony prominences, the use of a stockinette, and careful monitoring can prevent skin breakdown.
- *Cognition and developmental age.* The child's or adolescent's age will affect the fabrication of the splint. For example, if a child is still mouthing objects, the splint should not have small pieces or contain glue or adhesive that is toxic.
- *Latex allergies and precautions.* Many children and adolescents with special needs develop latex allergies. Some splinting materials or attachments (rubber bands) may contain latex. Practitioners need to be aware of these potential reactions and may use alternative splinting materials.
- *Home environment.* Children or adolescents who live in geographic areas with warm climates may need to use perforated thermoplastic material to allow airflow, decrease sweating, and prevent melting of the splinting material.

BOX 23-2

Specific Splinting Fabrication Tips

1. If a child or adolescent does not like to be touched or is in pain but remains cooperative, the therapist may use a drapable plastic-like material. In order to minimize contact with the client's skin, double-sided tape can be used to stabilize the position of the forearm trough until the splint cools and hardens. Before fabricating the splint the arm can be positioned in supination, with the wrist in extension over the edge of a splinting wedge. In this position, gravity helps maintain the wrist in the desired position during splint fabrication.
2. For a child or adolescent who is squirming around during splint fabrication but not in pain, a more forgiving material, such as one in the rubber category, which allows the therapist to hold on to the splint and the limb with more force while molding, can be used.
3. A perforated material should be used with a child or adolescent who tends to perspire excessively or in climates that are hot and humid. A stockinette sleeve/glove may help absorb the moisture from the perspiration.
4. With few exceptions, outriggers and splint attachments are not recommended for children because they tend to have small pieces that may become detached and consequently be a choking hazard and could also cause injury to the eyes, ears, and other areas of the body if the child is running and falls on the splint.

FABRICATION TIPS

The OTR is responsible for determining the type of splint that would be the most beneficial for the client. The most appropriate splint might be one that is fabricated from a pattern/protocol, one that is fabricated with modifications to the pattern/protocol, one that is of a design unique to the client, or one that is prefabricated. The type of material that the OTR decides to use will depend on the client's age, muscle tone, level of cooperation, and level of pain.[5] The OTR and the COTA often assist each other during the fabrication of pediatric splints because of the special issues with this population. Box 23-2 provides the reader with more specific tips that might be helpful during the pediatric splinting process.

Splinting Material

The weight of the splinting material needs to be taken into consideration, especially with very young child or adolescent with weak muscles. The thinner materials ($^1/_{16}''$ to $^3/_{32}''$) often provide adequate positioning while minimizing weight. They also allow for better conformability to smaller hands.[7,13]

Neoprene splints may be more comfortable for children or adolescents with contractures because of the soft nature of the material (Figure 23-12). Severe spasticity and rigid deformity cannot be controlled with neoprene.[7,13]

Questions to Ask When Fabricating a Splint

The following are good questions to ask when fabricating a splint[12]:

1. What is the desired outcome of using the splint?
2. How will the splint have an impact on the client's ability to engage in occupations?
    - Will the splint improve the client's ability to perform?

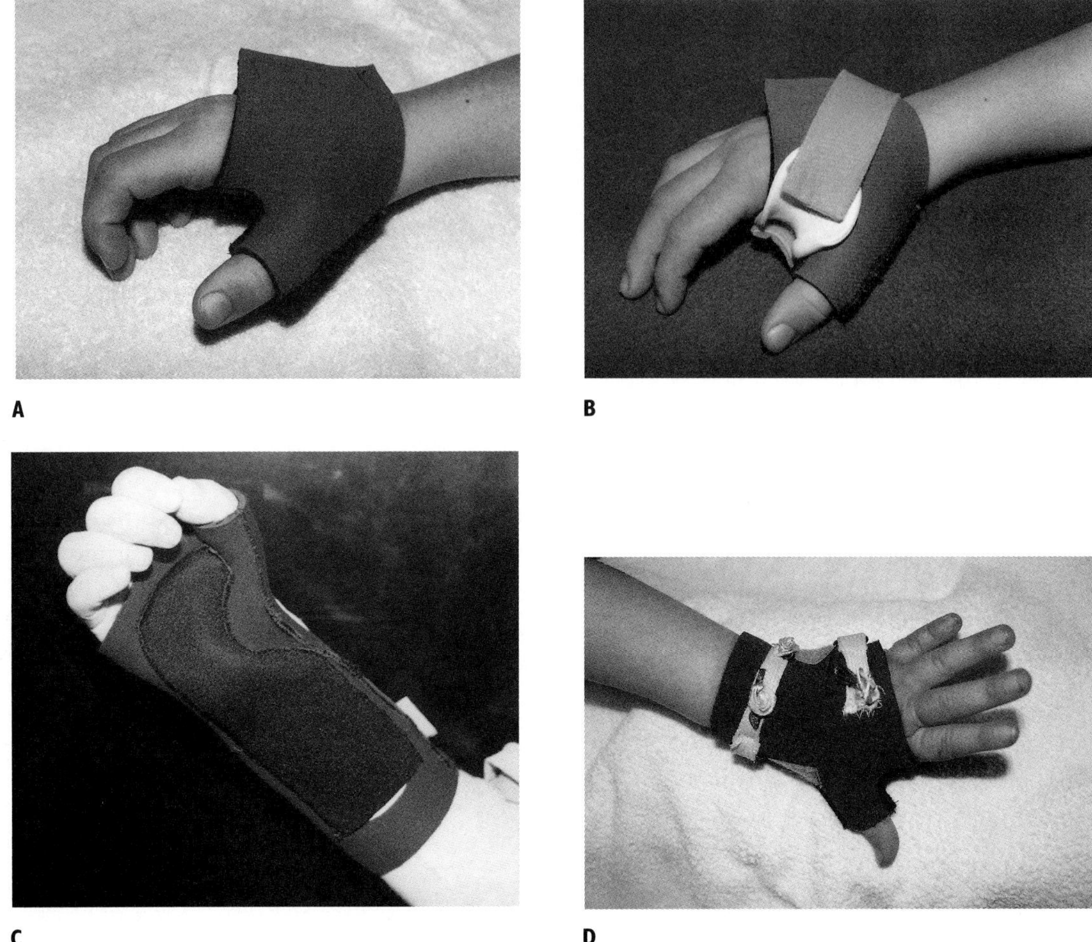

FIGURE 23-12 Neoprene splint. (From Armstrong J: Splinting the pediatric patient. In Fess EE, Gettle KS, Philips CA, et al: *Hand and upper extremity splinting: principles and methods*, ed 3, St Louis, 2005, Mosby.)

3. What are the client's or family's habits and routines? How will this have an impact on the splint-wearing schedule and its use?
4. Will the splint "fit" within the context(s) of the client (e.g., physical, personal, social, cultural)? Are there any modifications that may make it a better fit (e.g., wear splint only at home)?
   - Will the splint be worn?
5. What are the client's primary, secondary, and associated problems?
   - How does the client feel about the splint?
   - Are there any associated sensory needs?
   - What are the client's physical needs?
6. How will the associated problems affect the splint?
   - What are the biomechanical principles being addressed by the splinting process (e.g., stretch, position, alignment, stability)?
7. What splint design will best address the child's or adolescent's needs?
   - Should the splint be static or dynamic?
   - Should the base be dorsal or volar?
8. What splint components are integral to correction of the problem?
   - What joints should be included in the splint?
   - Is the splint easy to don and doff?

Table 23-3 is a representation of common pediatric diagnoses for which splinting interventions are used.

For more extensive pediatric problems and splinting options see the appendix at the end of this chapter.

CONGENITAL HAND DIFFERENCES

Some children and adolescents are born with deformities of the hand or upper extremity, known as congenital hand differences. For some of them, these congenital hand differences may have little impact on occupational performance. The child or adolescent may have learned to

TABLE 23-4

Common Pediatric Congenital Hand Differences

SPECIFIC DIAGNOSIS	TYPES	DESCRIPTIONS	DEVELOPMENTAL ISSUES	SPLINTING OPTIONS
Camptodactyly	Infant	Congenital flexion of PIP	Lack of full finger opening	Serial splinting
	Adolescent	Nontraumatic PIP flexion contracture		
	Syndromic	Congenital flexion of PIP		
Syndactyly	Simple	Only skin is involved	Limited finger use	Postoperative splinting
	Complex	Fusion of bone and skin	Limited grasp	
Radial ray deficiencies: hypoplastic thumbs	1st Degree	Slim thumb	May avoid use of thumb	Soft neoprene splint
	2nd Degree	Poor thenars Unstable MP Tight web		Soft or rigid splint Postoperative protective splinting
	3rd Degree	Absent thenars Unstable MP	Uses scissor grasp	Rigid splint Postoperative protective splinting
	4th Degree	Floating thumb	Nonfunctional thumb Uses scissor grasp	Postoperative protective splinting
	5th Degree	Absent thumb	Uses scissor grasp	Protective splinting
Radial ray deficiencies: radial club hands	Type 1	Short radius Hypoplastic thumbs	Normal use except thumbs	Splinting as needed for thumbs
	Type 2	Hypoplastic radius	Lack of crawling Difficulty weight bearing	Radial- or ulnar-based splint Postoperative protective and night splinting
	Type 3	Absent distal radius	Little finger prehension	Radial- or ulnar-based splint Postoperative protective and night splinting
	Type 4	Aplastic radius	Little finger prehension	Radial- or ulnar-based splint Postoperative protective and night splinting
Thumb-in-palm deformity	Type 1	Extensor pollicis brevis and longus deficiencies	Poor prehension	Soft splint for day Rigid splint for night
	Type 2	Extensor pollicis brevis and longus deficiencies Contractures	Poor prehension	Soft splint for day Rigid splint for night Postoperative protective splinting
	Type 3	MP instability	Minimum thumb use	Soft splint for day Rigid splint for night Postoperative protective splinting
	Type 4	Miscellaneous deformities	Minimum thumb use	Splinting as needed
Trigger thumb/fingers		Triggering/crepitus Palpable nodule	May resist use due to pain Limited grasp and release	Splinting as needed
Arthrogryposis	Distal	Flexed, webbed, and overlapping fingers MP joints in ulnar deviation Adducted thumbs	Limited grasp/release Poor prehension	Static progressive splint Postoperative protective and night splinting

TABLE 23-4

Common Pediatric Congenital Hand Differences—cont'd

SPECIFIC DIAGNOSIS	TYPES	DESCRIPTIONS	DEVELOPMENTAL ISSUES	SPLINTING OPTIONS
	Amyoplasia	Absent muscle mass Internally rotated shoulders Extended elbows Flexed wrists	Limited grasp/release Difficulty with self-feeding Poor weight bearing Limited mobility and ADLs	Serial casting Static progressive splint Postoperative protective splinting

Adapted from Peck-Murray J, Gibson G: *Rising to the challenge: children with congenital hand differences,* Presentation at the American Occupational Therapy Association Annual Conference and Expo, Long Beach, Calif, May 13, 2005.
ADLs, Activities of daily living; *MP*, metacarpophalangeal; *PIP*, proximal interphalangeal.

TABLE 23-5

Common Lower Extremity Splints

TYPE OF DEVICE	OBJECTIVES	INDICATIONS
Posterior ankle-foot orthosis	To rest the ankle in order to relieve pain To immobilize the ankle To correct or prevent contractures	For non-weight bearing situations including the following Mild to moderate spastic hemiparesis Injuries to distal tibia/fibula or ankle Clients at risk of developing ankle flexion contractures Congenital foot differences Cerebral palsy Acute burns Nerve injuries Flaccid hemiparesis
Static hip-stabilizing orthosis for hip dysplasia	To maintain proper position of a displaced hip in order to allow for hip stabilization	Unilateral or bilateral hip dysplasia
Spiral dynamic hip-knee-ankle-foot strap	To promote proper positioning of lower extremity To improve gait pattern To normalize tone To stabilize the head of the femur in the acetabulum	Head injury Spina bifida Cerebral palsy Lower extremity paralysis
Posterior knee orthosis	To prevent or reduce knee flexion contracture To stabilize the knee during ambulation To rest the knee	Burns Knee fracture Flexion contracture
Circumferential tibia-stabilizing orthosis	To stabilize a tibia fracture For protection	Midshaft tibial fractures Osteogenesis imperfecta

Data from McKee P, Morgan L: *Orthotics in rehabilitation: splinting the hand and body*, Philadelphia, 1998, FA Davis.

adapt and function without the use of a splint or prosthetic device. For others the impact may be more severe. An OT practitioner may receive a referral for an infant who has a congenital hand difference or may see an older child or adolescent for whom the difference is now posing a problem in his or her functioning. It is imperative that the practitioner take into account the child's development and have an accurate picture of how s/he is currently functioning when considering splinting options. See Table 23-4 for descriptions of common pediatric congenital hand differences and common splinting options for such conditions.

SPLINTING OF THE LOWER EXTREMITY

OT practitioners often work in therapy with children and adolescents who require the use of splints for the lower extremity. For these clients in particular, communication and collaboration with the physical therapist are necessary. Generally the OT practitioner has greater knowledge of the process of fabrication and application of most orthoses; however, the physical therapist is the expert in the areas of lower extremity anatomy, kinesiology, and gait. Communication and collaboration between the two disciplines promotes a successful intervention program.

Children and adolescents with abnormal tone, burns, fractures, or other injuries or conditions affecting the lower extremity may benefit from splinting of the lower extremity. See Table 23-5 for descriptions of common lower extremity splints.

The same precautions and considerations that are taken with splinting the upper extremity must also be applied to splinting the lower extremity.

SUMMARY

Pediatric splinting can be an important part of the OT process. Splinting a child or adolescent presents unique challenges. S/he may be distractible and respond negatively to the splint. The OT practitioner must use creative problem solving and clinical judgment and have the knowledge of all the resources available to apply pediatric splints. The practitioner must also have a strong foundation of knowledge in the anatomy of the upper extremity, the development of upper extremity function, and how hand function affects participation in occupations for children and adolescents.

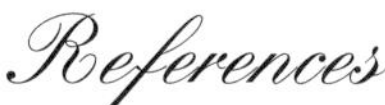

1. American Occupational Therapy Association: *Occupational therapy practice framework: domain and process*, Bethesda, Md, 2002, The Association.
2. Batshaw ML: *Children with disabilities*, ed 4, Baltimore, Md, 1997, Paul H Brooks Publishing Co, Inc.
3. Canale ST, Beaty JH: *Operative pediatric orthopaedics*, St Louis, 1991, Mosby.
4. Britto MT, DeVellis RF, Mhornug RW, et al: Health care preferences and priorities of adolescents with chronic illness, *Pediatrics* 114:1272, 2004.
5. Coppard BM, Lohman H: *Introduction to splinting: a critical-thinking and problem-solving approach*, ed 2, St Louis, 2001, Mosby.
6. Fess EE, Gettle KS, Philips CA, et al: *Hand and upper extremity splinting: principles and methods*, ed 3, St Louis, 2005, Mosby.
7. Jacobs M, Austin N: *Splinting the hand and upper extremity*, Baltimore, Md, 2003, Lippincott Williams & Wilkins.
8. Law M, Finkleman S, Hurley P, et al: Participation of children with physical disabilities: relationships with diagnosis, physical function, and demographic variables, *Scand J Occup Ther* 11:156, 2004.
9. Lewis AM: Managing common pediatric emergencies, *Nursing* 29:33, 1999.
10. McKee P, Morgan L: *Orthotics in rehabilitation: splinting the hand and body*, Philadelphia, 1998, FA Davis.
11. Parkinson GW, Hike KE: Bicycle helmet assessment during well visits reveals severe shortcomings in condition and fit, *Pediatrics* 112:320, 2003.
12. Shurr DG, Cook TM: *Prosthetics and orthotics*, East Norwalk, Conn, 1990, Appleton & Lange.
13. Teplicky R, Law M, Russell D: The effectiveness of casts, orthoses, and splints for children with neurological disorders, *Infant Young Child Adolesc* 15:42, 2002.
14. Townsend DJ, Bassett GS: Common elbow fractures in children, *Am Fam Phys* 53:2031, 1996.
15. United States Department of Health and Human Services, Agency for Health Care Policy and Research: Pressure ulcers in adults: prediction and prevention. Clinical practice guideline, 1992. Retrieved May 23, 2005, from http://0-tpdweb.umi.com.lilac.une.edu/tpweb?Did=1993173836&Fmt=1&Mtd=1&Idx=4&Sid=4&RQT=836&TS=1116857908

REVIEW *Questions*

1. Review the principles of splinting a child or adolescent.
2. What is the role(s) of the COTA in splinting children and adolescents?
3. How does abnormal tone affect an OT practitioner's ability to fabricate a splint?
4. How does abnormal tone affect donning and doffing a splint?
5. How can an OT practitioner improve the compliance rate of a child or adolescent who uses a splint?
6. Why is it necessary to be familiar with the different splinting materials when applying splints to children and adolescents?

SUGGESTED *Activities*

1. Fabricate a splint for protection, hygiene, position, and function.
2. Locate the bony prominences on the elbow, wrist, and hand.
3. Demonstrate the anatomical positions of the elbow, wrist, and hand.
4. Create a splint-wearing schedule for an adolescent.
5. Ask a child or adolescent about his or her preferences regarding a splint.

CHAPTER 23 APPENDIX

Common Pediatric Problems and Associated Splinting Options

Elbow Splints

Problem: Elbow Flexion

ESCS	COMMON NAME
Elbow extension mobilization splint—type 0 (1)	Elbow extension (volar) Elbow extension (circumferential) Elbow extension (bivalve) Air splint Turnbuckle elbow extension
Elbow extension mobilization splint—type 0 (1)	Orthokinetic cuff

Forearm Splints

Problem: Limited Supination

ESCS	COMMON NAME
Forearm supination, wrist extension, thumb CMC palmar abduction mobilization splint—type 0 (3)	Long serpentine (proximal neoprene strap)
Forearm supination, wrist extension, thumb CMC radial abduction and MP extension mobilization splint—type 0 (4)	Long neoprene thumb abduction with serpentine strap
Elbow flexion, forearm supination, wrist extension mobilization splint—type 0 (3)	Long arm (positioned in elbow flexion and supination)

Wrist Splints

Problem: Wrist Flexion

ESCS	COMMON NAME
Wrist extension, index–small finger extension, thumb CMC palmar abduction and MP-IP extension mobilization splint—type 0 (16)	Resting hand (used serially if contractures have formed)
Wrist extension mobilization splint—type 0 (1)	Radial bar wrist cock-up (volar) Radial bar wrist cock-up (dorsal) Wrist cock-up (thumb hole) Wrist cock-up (palmar support only) Wrist cock-up (circumferential thumb hole) Long neoprene (volar or dorsal stay)
Wrist extension, thumb CMC radial abduction and MP extension mobilization splint—type 0 (3)	Long neoprene thumb abduction (volar or dorsal stay)
Forearm supination, wrist extension, thumb CMC palmar abduction mobilization splint—type 0 (3)	Long serpentine (if only mildly involved)
Wrist extension, index, ring–small finger MP abduction, index–small finger extension, thumb CMC palmar abduction and MP-IP extension mobilization splint—type 0 (16)	Antispasticity
Wrist extension mobilization splint—type 0 (1)	Orthokinetic cuff

Problem: Wrist Ulnar Deviation

ESCS	COMMON NAME
Wrist extension mobilization/wrist ulnar deviation restriction splint—type 0 (1)	Ulnar gutter Wrist cock-up with ulnar side support
Wrist extension, thumb CMC radial abduction and MP extension mobilization/wrist ulnar deviation restriction splint—type 0 (3)	Long neoprene thumb abduction with ulnar gutter insert

Problem: Wrist Radial Deviation

ESCS	COMMON NAME
Wrist extension, thumb CMC palmar abduction and MP extension/wrist radial deviation restriction splint—type 0 (3)	Long thumb spica Long thumb opponens
Wrist extension, thumb CMC palmar abduction mobilization/wrist radial deviation restriction splint—type 0 (2)	Dorsal radial bar wrist cock-up with thumb C-bar (splint to increase web space)

Hand Splints

Problem: Thumb-in-Palm Positioning

ESCS	COMMON NAME
Thumb CMC radial abduction and MP extension mobilization splint—type 0 (2)	Neoprene thumb abduction Short thumb opponens Short thumb spica
Thumb CMC radial abduction mobilization splint—type 0 (1)	Thumb loop
Wrist extension, thumb CMC radial abduction and MP extension mobilization splint—type 0 (3)	Long thumb opponens Long thumb spica Wrist cock-up with thumb loop
Wrist extension, thumb CMC palmar abduction mobilization splint—type 0 (2)	Serpentine (short)
Thumb CMC palmar abduction mobilization splint—type 0 (1)	Thumb C-bar
Forearm supination, wrist extension, thumb CMC palmar abduction mobilization splint—type 0 (3)	Serpentine
Forearm supination, wrist extension, thumb CMC palmar abduction and MP-IP extension mobilization splint—type 0 (5)	Serpentine with thumb piece

Problem: Hand Fisting

ESCS	COMMON NAME
Wrist extension, index–small finger MP abduction, index–small finger extension, thumb CMC radial abduction and MP-IP extension mobilization splint—type 0 (16)	Antispasticity ball Antispasticity (dorsal) with finger pan (volar) Resting hand (can add finger spacers)
Wrist extension, index–small finger MP extension mobilization splint—type 0 (5)	MacKinnon
Index–small finger extension, thumb CMC radial abduction and MP-IP extension mobilization splint—type 0 (15)	Cone

Problem: Difficulty with Weight Bearing

ESCS	COMMON NAME
Wrist extension, index–small finger MP extension and IP flexion, thumb CMC radial abduction and MP-IP extension mobilization splint—type 0 (16)	Weight bearing
Elbow extension mobilization splint—type 0 (1)	Elbow extension Elbow air (water wings)

Problem: Inability to Maintain Grasp

ESCS	COMMON NAME
Wrist extension mobilization splint—type 0 (1)	Wrist cock-up Neoprene grasp assist
Thumb CMC radial abduction and MP extension mobilization splint—type 0 (2)	Thumb abduction with sewn neoprene grasp assist Neoprene thumb abduction with sewn elastic pocket

Problem: Difficulty with Finger Isolation for Task Performance

ESCS	COMMON NAME
Wrist extension, index finger MP flexion and IP extension, thumb CMC radial abduction and MP extension mobilization splint—type 0 (6)	Long thumb opponens with index finger included Long neoprene thumb abduction with index finger included

From Fess EE, Gettle KS, Philips CA, et al: *Hand and upper extremity splinting: principles and methods*, ed 3, St Louis, 2005, Mosby.
CMC, Carpometacarpal; *ESCS*, Expanded Splint Classification System; *IP*, interphalange; *MP*, metacarpophalangeal.

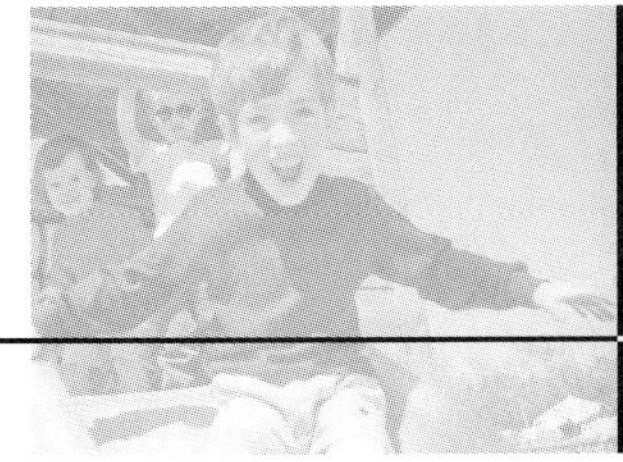

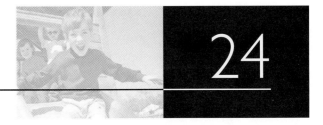

24

Animal-Assisted Services

JEAN W. SOLOMON
JANE CLIFFORD O'BRIEN

CHAPTER *Objectives*

After studying this chapter, the reader will be able to accomplish the following:

- Identify organizations that promote animal and human interaction
- Define and distinguish between animal-assisted activities and animal-assisted therapy
- Describe the types of small and large animals that might be used during animal-assisted activities and animal-assisted therapy
- Define and distinguish between therapeutic horseback riding and hippotherapy
- Describe the mission and function of the North American Riding for the Handicapped Association
- Discuss incorporating animals into pediatric occupational therapy practice

KEY TERMS

Animal-assisted activities

Animal-assisted therapy

Hippotherapy

CHAPTER OUTLINE

Do you have a pet? If so, take a moment to think about how your pet makes you feel. What is the first pet that you remember having? I had a lightening bug that I kept in a vented jar by my bed. The light from this little bug helped me go to sleep at night. It gave me a sense of security.

Research supports the conclusion that animals can reduce social stress, increase motivation, and offer unconditional love (Box 24-1).[1] The focus of this chapter is on animal-assisted services. There are two types of animal-assisted services that will be discussed. These services are animal-assisted activities and animal-assisted therapy.

SELECTED ORGANIZATIONS

There are numerous national and international organizations concerned with the interaction between animals and humans and animal-assisted services. The International Association of Human-Animal Interaction Organizations (IAHAIO), the Delta Society, and Assistance Dogs International (ADI) will be discussed (see Resources at the end of this chapter for a list of organizations).

The IAHAIO was founded in 1990 to provide a forum for national and international associations or related organizations interested in understanding and appreciating human-animal interaction. The primary purpose of the organization is to coordinate its structure nationally and internationally. Its mission is to promote research, education, and the sharing of information regarding the role of animals in human health and quality of life. The activities of the IAHAIO include sponsoring workshops, publishing information that adds to the body of knowledge on human-animal interaction, and influencing public policies that promote the integration of animals into human society.

The Delta Society is concerned with the human-animal health condition. It publishes guidelines for developing animal-assisted therapy programs, professional standards for dog trainers, and information regarding service dogs. It offers workshops and home study courses for registering clinicians who use animals during therapy. According to the Delta Society, there are approximately 2000 animal-assisted therapy programs in the United States. Dogs are the animals most often used during physical rehabilitation intervention.[4]

ADI is a coalition of nonprofit organizations dedicated to training, placing, and using assistance dogs. The organization publishes a newsletter to educate the public on the benefits of assistance dogs.

BOX 24-1

Positive Effects That Animals Have on Humans

Decrease social stress, thus improving social interaction
Improve quality of life by increasing self-competence and control over the environment
Improve cardiovascular health
Increase trust
Offer unconditional love

ANIMAL-ASSISTED ACTIVITIES

Animal-assisted activities are those activities that involve human and animal interaction. Examples of animal-assisted activities include the use of assistance dogs, cats that visit residents in a nursing home, fish in a kindergarten classroom, and participation in a therapeutic horseback riding class (Figure 24-1). These activities offer opportunities for children and adolescents to care for as well as to interact with animals while grooming, feeding, and petting them. During therapeutic horseback riding, the child or adolescent learns to ride and care for the horse.

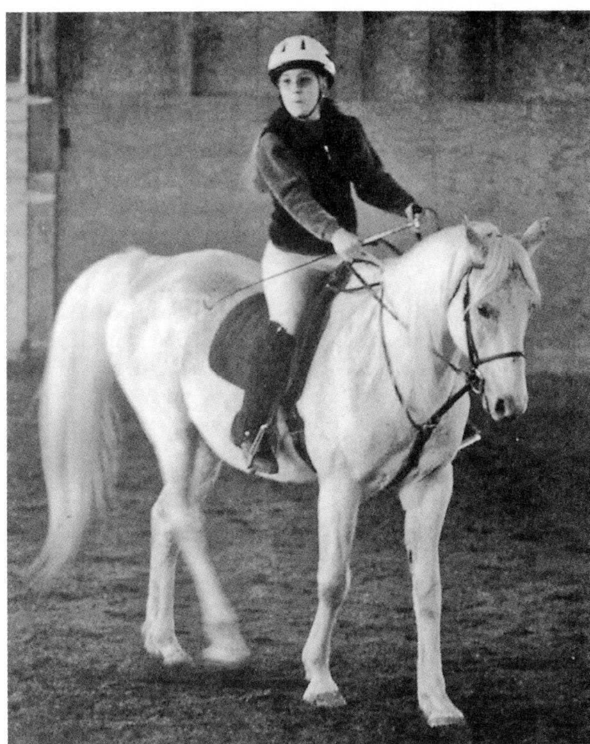

FIGURE 24-1 Amy, riding Magic, is having a riding lesson. (Photo by Donald W. Smith; from Crawford JJ, Pomerinke KA: *Therapy pets: the animal-human healing partnership,* Amherst, NY, 2003, Prometheus Books.)

CLINICAL *Pearl*

The movement of a horse can help a child gain balance. Successful interaction with the horse promotes self-confidence. Its disposition is critical to positive interaction.

ANIMAL-ASSISTED THERAPY

Animal-assisted therapy uses animals to improve the medical, developmental, physical, and mental conditions of children or adolescents. **Hippotherapy,** or therapy using horses, is one of the most popular types of animal-assisted therapy. Dogs are also frequently involved in animal-assisted therapy (Figure 24-2).[4] Animal-assisted therapy is carried out by a qualified occupational therapy (OT) practitioner. This type of therapy includes the evaluation of the child's body functions and structure, the design and implementation of an intervention plan, documentation of goals and progress as well as reevaluation, and planning for the discontinuation of services. In both animal-assisted activities and animal-assisted therapy, the welfare and safety of people and animals are priorities.

Henry is a 6-year-old child who has spastic quadriplegia cerebral palsy. He attends hippotherapy sessions on a weekly basis during the spring and fall seasons. Cletis, the OT practitioner, has set the following goals or anticipated outcomes for this intervention (Figure 24-3).

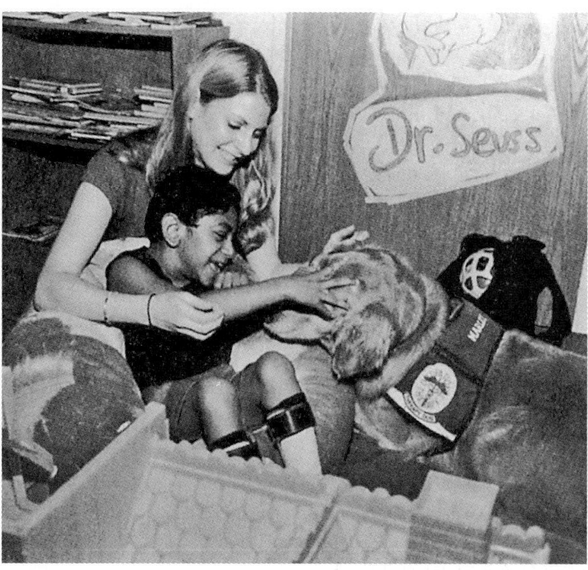

FIGURE 24-2 Marley, the dog, provides the incentive for Jaison to stretch tight muscles. (Photo by Dick Dressel; from Crawford JJ, Pomerinke KA: *Therapy pets: the animal-human healing partnership,* Amherst, NY, 2003, Prometheus Books.)

Long-term goals

- *Henry will demonstrate functional trunk control while sitting during leisure time.*
- *Henry will reach for objects while sitting to perform occupations for activities of daily living (ADLs).*

Short-term goals

- *Henry will maintain an upright position while sitting on the horse for 2 minutes.*
- *Henry will maintain his sitting balance as the horse walks one fourth of the distance of the riding arena.*
- *Henry will touch the horse's ears with each hand, alternating individually and simultaneously (unilaterally and bilaterally), in three out of four sequence trials.*

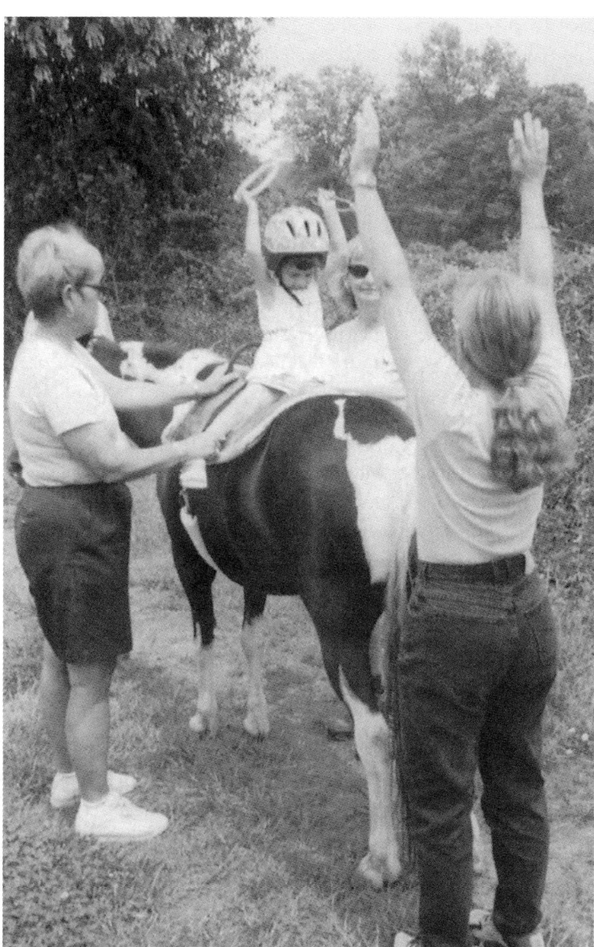

FIGURE 24-3 A hippotherapy session with Chessie participating in balance activities while she is sitting on Sparky. (Photo by Nicholas McIntosh; from Crawford JJ, Pomerinke KA: *Therapy pets: the animal-human healing partnership,* Amherst, NY, 2003, Prometheus Books.)

During Henry's hippotherapy session, Cletis engages him in stretching activities while Henry is seated bareback and backwards on the horse. Cletis assists Henry as Henry is reaching for the horse's ears and hindquarters. While Cletis is assisting Henry with his arms, Becki, a physical therapist assistant, stabilizes his trunk and legs. After the stretching activities, two volunteers join the team to serve as helpers as the horse begins to move under the direction of the trainer/instructor. Cletis facilitates upper trunk and arm control as Becki facilitates pelvic mobility with leg stability. Located in each of the four corners of the riding arena are therapeutic activities: (1) a pressure switch that activates a tape playing Henry's favorite music, (2) a beanbag toss, (3) a punching bag to encourage arm and leg movement, and (4) a ring tree game. Cletis, Becki, and Henry work together at each of the stations as the volunteers manage the horse and offer an extra hand as needed.

Galen lives on a farm, where his family regularly ride horses (Figure 24-4). He is a 7-year-old child with spastic quadriplegia cerebral palsy. The OT practitioner recommended a therapeutic riding program and has set the following goals and objectives for intervention.

Long-term goals

- *Given adaptive equipment for safety, Galen will ride a horse for 20 minutes on trails.*
- *Galen will be able to mount his horse with moderate physical assistance.*

Short-term goals

- *Galen will maintain an upright position while sitting on the horse for 5 minutes.*
- *Galen will maintain an upright position while sitting on the horse as the horse walks one fourth of the distance of the riding arena.*

In this scenario, the OT intervention is similar to Henry's; however, the goals of Galen's and Henry's sessions differ. The goal of Galen's sessions is for him to be a competent rider so that he can participate in the occupations of his family. The goal of Henry's sessions is for him to gain skills that may be used in other occupations (e.g., improved sitting balance, improved reaching). Therapeutic riding often becomes a leisure activity for children, allowing the intervention to become occupation based.

SMALL ANIMALS

Small animals are those that typically weigh less than 40 pounds. Dogs, which are mammals, are one type of small animal. Other types include reptiles, such as snakes; amphibians, such as frogs and fish; and invertebrates, such as hermit crabs and worms (Table 24-1). The different types of small animals will be discussed, with special attention devoted to dogs.

Mammals are animals that have a backbone and are characterized by hair on the skin and mammary glands

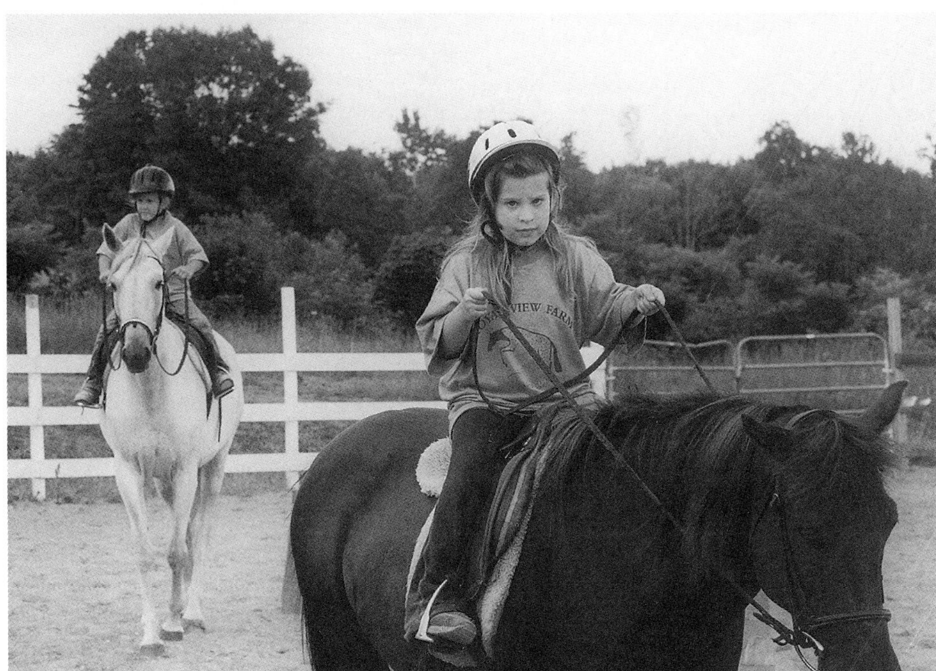

FIGURE 24-4 Alison and Shelby enjoy learning to ride horses at summer camp. For some children, riding is an occupation. (Courtesy Cheryl Joyce.)

A

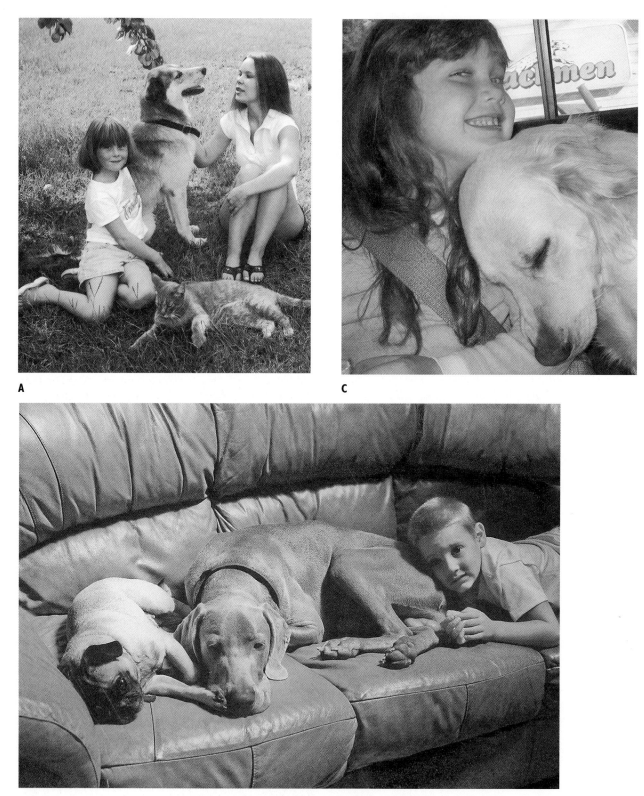

C

B

FIGURE 24-5 **A,** Logan and Alex relax in the shade with their pets Rhett and Wolf. **B,** Max relaxes with his pets. **C,** Caitlin cuddles with Arlo. (**A** Courtesy Susan Gentry. **B** Courtesy Cheryl Joyce. **C** Courtesy Debbie Dewitt.)

TABLE 24-1

Types of Small Animals

CLASSIFICATION	DEFINITION	EXAMPLES
Mammal	Warm blooded with backbone	Dog, cat, rabbit, guinea pig
Reptile	Cold blooded with horny or scaly skin	Snake
Amphibian	Cold blooded with smooth skin	Frog, toad, salamander
Fish	Cold blooded with fins and gills	Goldfish, beta fish
Invertebrate	Cold blooded without backbone	Worm, snail, hermit crab

that produce milk in females. They are warm-blooded animals that maintain a relatively warm body temperature independent of the environmental temperature. Examples of animals that are classified as mammals are dogs, cats, rabbits, and guinea pigs. The following is a discussion of the use of dogs for animal-assisted activities and therapy.

Dogs are one of the most popular pets and the most frequently used small mammal for animal-assisted services (Figure 24-5). They offer a large variety of choices. Dogs are small, medium, or large in size and purebred or a mix of breeds. Examples of small dogs that are purebred are dachshunds, Chihuahuas, and cocker spaniels. Examples of large dogs that are purebred include chows, German shepherds, and standard poodles. Those that are a mix of breeds are often called mutts; they can be small, medium, or large.

The characteristics of a breed and the individual personality of the dog are both considered when selecting a dog for animal-assisted services or for a pet. One aspect of a dog's personality is temperament, which is its natural or instinctive behavior. A dog's temperament manifests the way in which it is expected to respond when stressed. For example, chows are known to respond aggressively under stress.

Training involves teaching a dog to follow commands while being controlled by a person. Although a dog can be trained to be obedient, the temperaments of certain breeds may override their training during stressful situations. For example, in crowds of people with lots of noise and movement, chows tend to growl and become "snappy."

A service dog is one that assists people who have physical or sensory disabilities.[3] According to ADI, there are three types of service dogs: guide dogs, hearing dogs, and medical alert dogs (Box 24-2). A guide dog is one that assists a person who has a visual impairment or is blind. A hearing dog is one that assists a person who has a hearing loss or is deaf. A medical alert dog is one that assists a person in a medical emergency by detecting specific physiological changes and locating assistance during medical emergencies.[3]

BOX 24-2

Types of Service Dogs

- A *guide dog* is one that assists a person who has a visual impairment or is blind.
- A *hearing dog* is one that assists a person who has a hearing loss or is deaf.
- A *medical alert dog* is one that assists a person in a medical emergency by detecting specific physiological changes and locating assistance during medical emergencies.

CLINICAL *Pearl*

Cats are the most suitable as institutional pets because of their lifestyles (eating and toileting habits, exercise requirements) and independence (Figure 24-6).

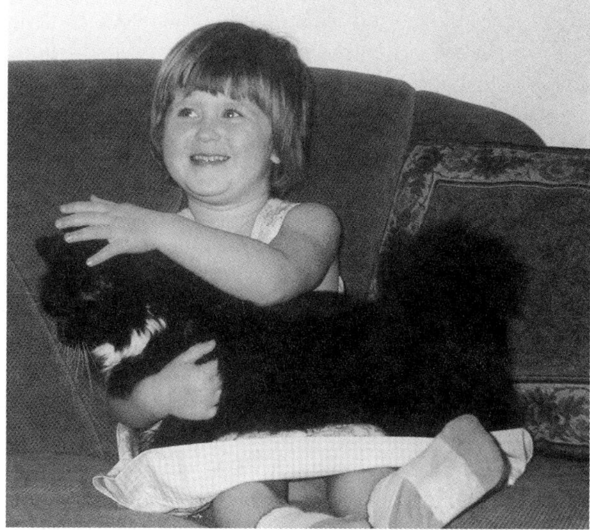

FIGURE 24-6 Marlena enjoys her soft cat. (Courtesy Jan Froehlich.)

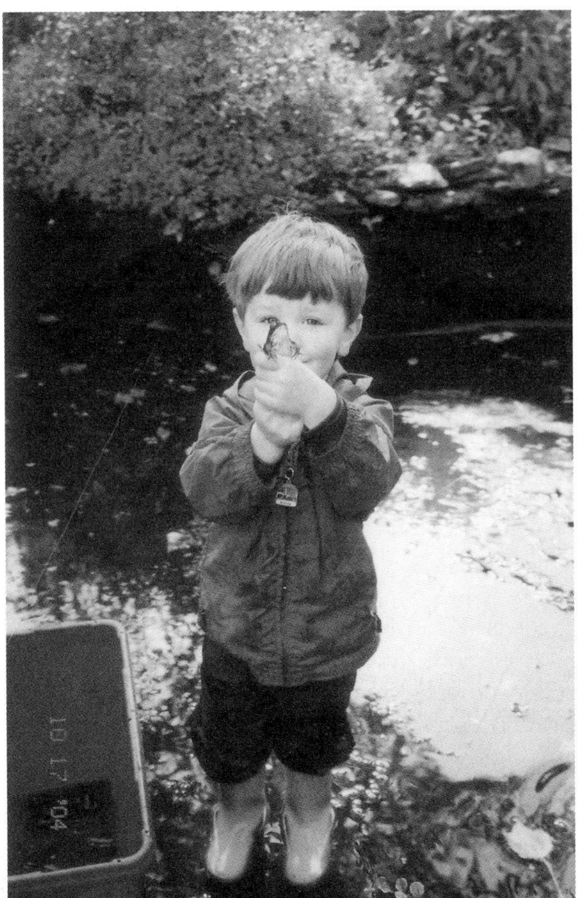

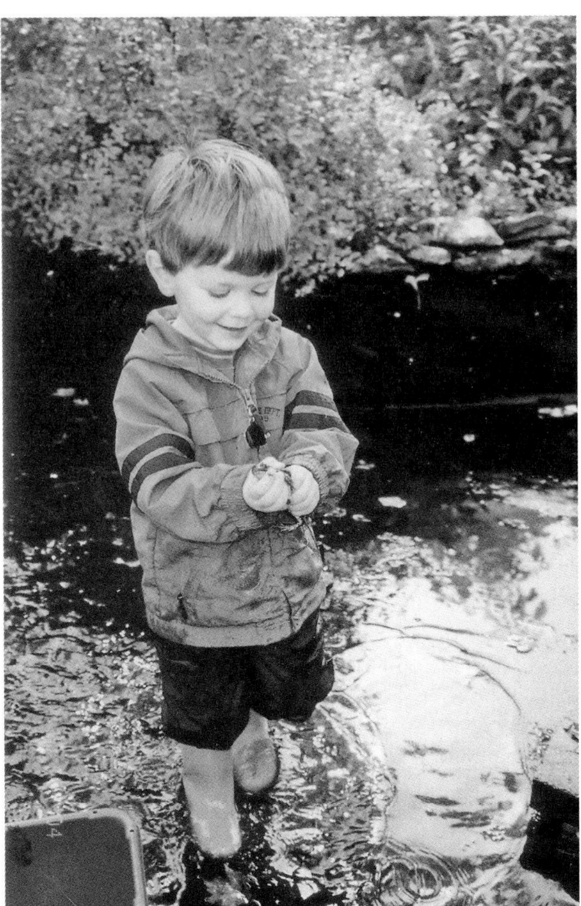

FIGURE 24-7 A little boy catches and holds onto a frog! (Courtesy Michelle Stone.)

Another way to categorize dogs is as a companion or pet. They can be personal or institutional pets. A personal pet is one that lives with an individual or family and is a part of that individual's or family's life. An institutional pet is one that resides in a facility or institution, such as a skilled nursing facility.

Reptiles are animals that have a backbone and horny or scaly skin. Reptiles have lungs to breathe. They are cold-blooded animals that do not have a constant body temperature. Legless lizards and turtles are examples of reptiles that intrigue children. There is a wide range of nonpoisonous snakes that may serve as pets or social companions. Reptilian pets tend to require less human attention and care than other small animals. They require less frequent feeding and handling, which is a consideration in choosing the best animal to be used for animal-assisted services.

Amphibians are cold-blooded animals that have a backbone and smooth skin. All amphibians have gills because at some point in their development an aquatic environment is required. Amphibians lay eggs to reproduce. Examples of amphibians are frogs, toads, and salamanders.

Children and adolescents are usually fascinated by amphibians in their natural environment. Catching, trapping, and releasing frogs or other amphibians in their natural environment require problem-solving and precise motor skills (Figure 24-7).

Fish are cold-blooded animals with backbones, fins for mobility, and gills for breathing. They live in water and are pets that require minimum human attention and interaction. Popular fish for home and classroom pets include goldfish, beta fish, and kissing fish. Animal-assisted activities involving fish might include increasing independence in instrumental ADLs (IADLs) through caring for them. Fish are not an appropriate choice for animal-assisted therapy, although decorating a fish tank and caring for them make a nice activity. Furthermore, many children enjoy the occupation of fishing.

Invertebrates are animals that do not have a backbone. Examples of invertebrates are worms, snails, insects, and hermit crabs (Figure 24-8). My first pet, a lightening bug, is another example of this type of animal. Children who live in rural areas have wonderful opportunities to interact with invertebrates. Hermit crabs and snails are

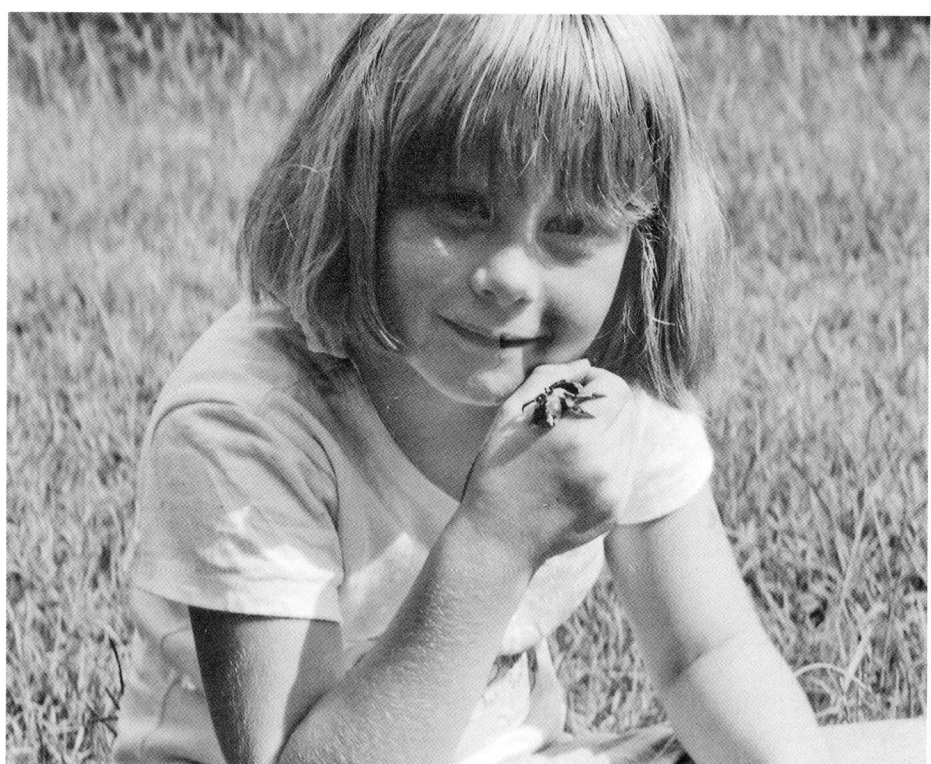

FIGURE 24-8 Logan plays with Kermie, her pet hermit crab. (Courtesy Susan Gentry.)

favorites among this class of animal for pets at home or in a classroom setting.

LARGE ANIMALS

Large animals are those that typically weigh more than 40 pounds. Horses are one of the most frequently used large animals in animal-assisted services. Other large animals that might be considered for human-animal interaction include farm animals, exotic animals, and marine mammals.

Most farm animals are large and live on a tract of land that is being cultivated for food for human consumption. Examples of large farm animals are horses or mules, pigs, goats, cows, and sheep. Farm animals have a monetary value to the person caring for them. A special relationship of mutual respect is obvious between the animal and the human caregiver (Figure 24-9).

CLINICAL *Pearl*

Goldfish in a horse's 75- to 100-gallon water tank can help control the algae, especially during the hot months. Horses and goldfish coexist well in this situation. The goldfish require minimum or no care, especially if the water tank has an automatic system to refill it to the maximum water level.

Exotic animals are those that are considered foreign to or from another part of the world than the United States. Examples of exotic animals are llamas, peacocks, and emus. There is a growing interest in raising exotic animals in many areas of the United States. The potential to incorporate exotic animals into animal-assisted activities and therapy has not been realized.

Marine mammals are warm-blooded animals that live in salt or brackish water. Examples of marine mammals

CLINICAL *Pearl*

Horses will often lick before they bite another horse or human. Cows also enjoy licking the salt from a human's hand. Cows do not have upper teeth and so have no inclination to bite. A horse's tongue is smooth, whereas a cow's tongue is lumpy and coarse.

CLINICAL *Pearl*

Pigs can be taught to come and sit as one would train a dog. Young pigs may be trained by using a harness and leading them. Just like other animals, a pig's temperament varies, although most pigs are typically not mean. Pigs will bite to the side if provoked.

A

B

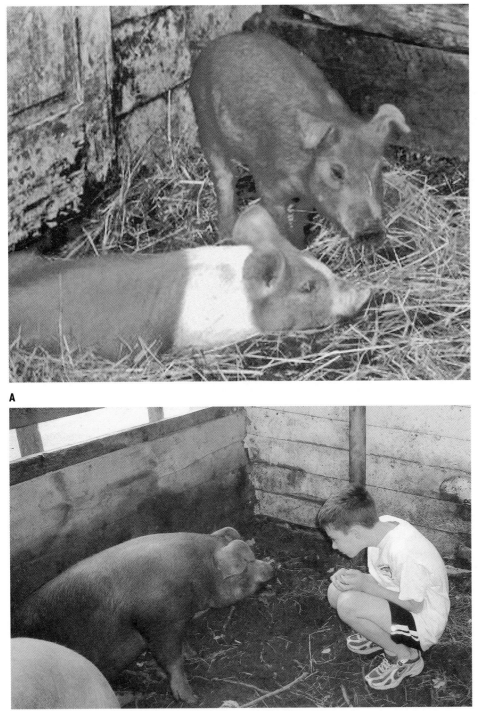

FIGURE 24-9 **A,** The piglets Thunder and Lightning allow children to learn responsibility. **B,** Scott learns how to care for and train Thunder, his pet pig. (**A** Courtesy Cheryl Joyce. **B** Courtesy Mike O'Brien.)

CLINICAL *Pearl*

Llamas regurgitate like cows. Be careful with your children at petting zoos.

CLINICAL *Pearl*

Be careful while collecting eggs because all birds are protective of their nests. If a bird is not nesting, gathering the eggs is much less of a threat or challenge.

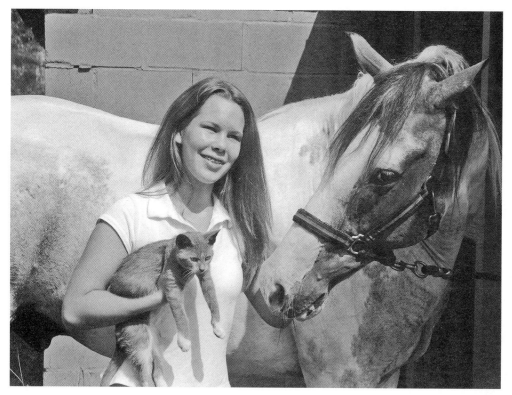

FIGURE 24-10 While preparing Prince for an afternoon ride, Alex is distracted by Ashes. (Courtesy Susan Gentry.)

are dolphins, whales, and seals. Although they are available for animal-assisted activities (enjoyment/play) on a commercial basis, there are no known programs incorporating them into animal-assisted therapy.

Horses are one of the most widely used large animals for animal-assisted services. According to the American Hippotherapy Association (AHA), therapeutic horseback riding is an animal-assisted activity for humans who have physical, emotional, and/or mental disabilities. Hippotherapy is animal-assisted therapy when a clinician or therapist uses the movement of a horse as an intervention tool to improve body function. The horse's walk is rhythmic and repetitive, similar to the pattern of movement in the human pelvis during walking (AHA). In addition to the input from the movement of the horse, the human-horse interaction offers a wide range of sensory experiences that have an impact on the tactile, olfactory, visual, and vestibular sensory systems.

As previously stated, therapeutic horseback riding encompasses a variety of horse-related activities in which people that have disabilities participate. An example of an adolescent engaged in therapeutic horseback riding is described below (Figure 24-10).

Julia is a 12-year-old girl who has osteoporosis of unknown etiology. Her mother Peg takes her to the local stable to ride Scotty, her favorite horse, as a result of the recommendation from her OT practitioner that Julia would benefit from therapeutic horseback riding. She has been involved in this program for 18 months. On their arrival at the barn they are greeted by Toni, who is the barn manager, riding instructor, and trail guide. Toni assists Julia with haltering Scotty and leading him to the tack area, and Peg gets Ace and leads him there also. Once Scotty's and Ace's lead ropes are secured, both are groomed and their hooves picked. The benefits for Scotty and Ace are obvious. The benefits for Julia include weight bearing while shifting weight with the use of a wide range of movements with both arms as she reaches to the top of his hindquarters and the peaks of his ears. The resistance of the tangles in his mane, forelocks, and tail represent strengthening exercises for Julia's arms and a challenge to her trunk balance and leg stability.

After the riders tack their horses, everyone mounts and the trail ride begins. The horse is now doing the work by carrying its rider on its back. The rider and instructor/guide have a mutual responsibility to ensure the safety and well-being of the rider and the horse. The trail ride lasts for an hour, during which time the group encounters narrow paths in the woods to negotiate and small trees to maneuver under and around. The therapeutic benefits for Julia include lower extremity resistive exercise while maintaining trunk and upper extremity stability to keep seated on the horse while reining and steering Scotty.

BOX 24-3

Sample Objectives for Hippotherapy Outcomes

Improve functioning in all areas of occupation by developing the following:

- Muscle tone for improved motor control
- Balance and equilibrium responses
- Gross and fine motor coordination
- Symmetry of motor functions
- Postural control
- Speech and language skills
- Self-efficacy and self-concept
- Body awareness
- Emotional well-being
- Regulation of behavior
- Sense of success

BOX 24-4

Sample Objectives for Hippotherapy Outcomes Based on Occupation

- Improve the child's ability to engage in the occupations involved in the care and maintenance of horses.
- Participate in riding sessions
- Groom and care for the horse
- Participate in social activities (e.g., 4-H)

As stated previously, hippotherapy is performed by a licensed medical professional who incorporates a horse into the therapy session as an intervention tool. Children and adolescents who have pediatric health disorders involving the neuromusculoskeletal system benefit from hippotherapy. Examples of specific conditions include cerebral palsy, developmental delay, and pervasive developmental delay or autism. Box 24-3 lists objectives for the outcomes of hippotherapy and Box 24-4 lists objectives for hippotherapy as an occupation.

The North American Riding for the Handicapped Association (NARHA) is a membership organization that promotes safe, professional, ethical, and therapeutic horse activities through education, communication, standards (Box 24-4), and research for people with and without disabilities.[2] NARHA has certification from the American Hippotherapy Association (AHA) to ensure the professionalism of practicing clinicians and detailed standards to keep participating clients safe.[2] Selecting and training horses for hippotherapy is one purpose of NARHA-certified centers (Box 24-5). These centers also offer opportunities for hippotherapy education and research.

In hippotherapy, a licensed physical, occupational, or speech/language therapist uses the movement of the horse to improve an individual's body function and structure. The goals and objectives of each discipline differ. A therapeutic riding instructor (TRI) often participates in hippotherapy sessions. The TRI will have goals and objectives that concentrate on teaching a child or adolescent to ride a horse. The goals and objectives of the physical therapist will emphasize improving his or her overall mobility and quality of movement. The speech/language pathologist will focus on communication skills. The OT practitioner will concentrate on the underlying performance skills necessary for a child or adolescent to successfully participate in daily occupations. The following case study describes the roles, goals, and objectives of the OT practitioner in hippotherapy.

BOX 24-5

Selected Standards or Guidelines in Choosing a Horse for Animal-Assisted Services

- At least 8 years of age
- Extensive training and riding time (quantified in miles)
- Good conditioning
- Good performance skills (i.e., symmetrical and balanced movement, voice trained [obedient to the trainer's or therapist's voice], tolerant of the rider's unexpected behaviors)
- Excellent temperament

Juan is a 6-year-old child who has a medical diagnosis of autism. He receives OT services through the local school district. He also receives outpatient OT services through a private practice located in the community. For 6 months of the year Juan and Rita, the certified occupational therapy assistant (COTA) assigned to his case, participate in weekly hippotherapy sessions.

Juan's long-term OT goal is that he will ride a horse for 20 minutes as a leisure activity, with stand-by assistance. For his short-term goals, he will hold onto the reigns with both hands while receiving verbal cuing and follow verbal one-step commands while riding the horse.

The physical therapist participates in the session on alternative weeks. The goal of physical therapy is to improve body functions (e.g., improve bilateral coordination, strength, and endurance for riding). The goal of speech therapy is to improve the communication required while riding a horse. The unique nature of OT is shown by the goal of improving the child's ability to engage in the riding session. The OT practitioner may make accommodations to assist the child in being successful at riding. In addition, s/he may consult with and educate the riding staff to optimize Juan's time and success on the horse.

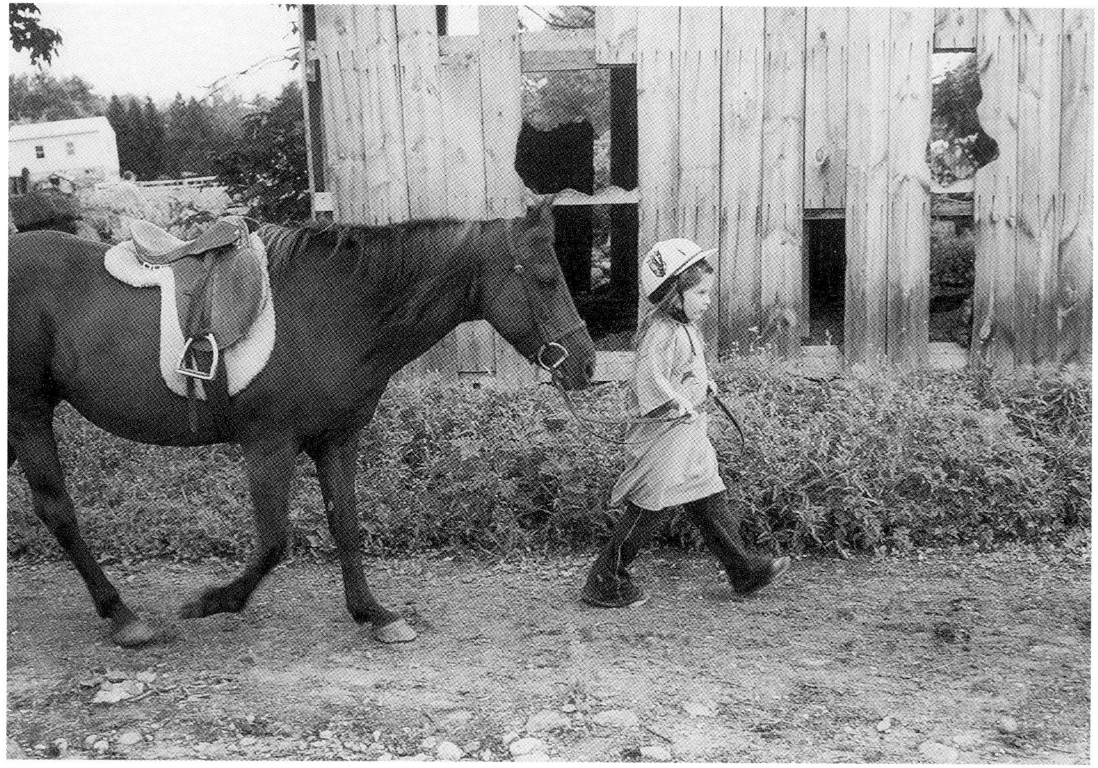

A

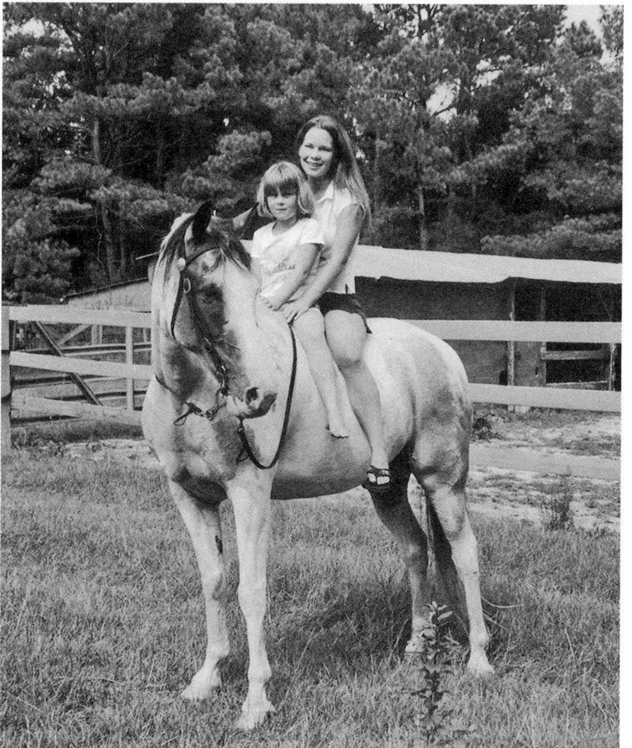

B

FIGURE 24-11 **A,** Alison brings Amber back to her stall. **B,** Prince stands patiently as Logan and Alex pose for a picture. (**A** Courtesy Cheryl Joyce. **B** Courtesy Susan Gentry.)

INCORPORATING ANIMALS INTO PEDIATRIC OCCUPATIONAL THERAPY PRACTICE

Incorporating animals into the OT process involves several areas of occupation or life activities in which individuals participate (Figure 24-11). IADLs such as the care of pets, health management and maintenance, safety procedures, and informal personal education participation might be the outcomes of animal-assisted activities and animal-assisted therapy. The OT practitioner needs to consider the cultural, physical, spiritual, and virtual contexts when incorporating animals into activities and therapy. The activity demands and individual client factors will have an impact on the decision-making process. Some guiding questions might include the following.

- Who are your clients?
- Where will the animal-assisted services be provided?
- Are you considering a large or small animal for these services?
- What characteristics are you looking for in the animal?

A

B

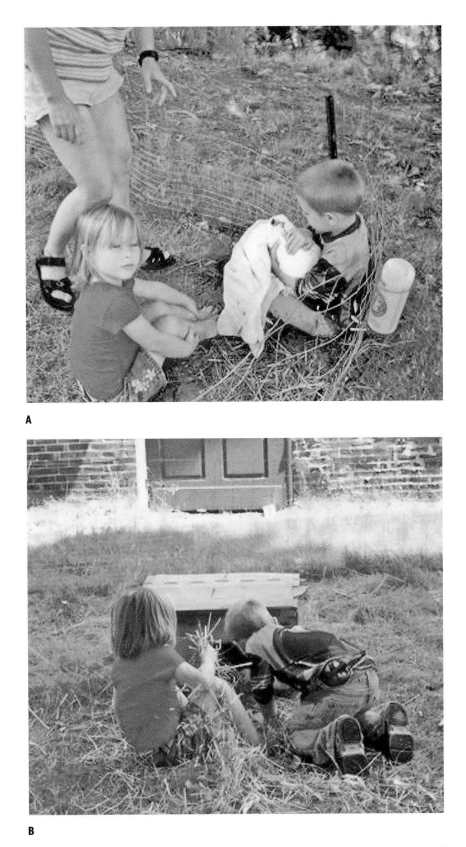

FIGURE 24-12 **A** and **B,** Max and Molly care for their bunnies Bellerina and Lucky as part of their daily chores. (Courtesy Cheryl Joyce.)

- What type of human-animal interaction will be involved?
- What are the potential health hazards?
- What pets or other animals are at home? Does the child have access to them?
- What are the goals of incorporating an animal into the therapy sessions?
- What is the best fit between the animal and child or adolescent?

Intervention Planning

Animals can be used in therapy as a modality (i.e., the animal is the tool to improve the skill) or as the goal itself (i.e., caring for the animal is the occupation that the person is trying to master) (Figure 24-12). Either way, the OT practitioner must carefully analyze the tasks required for participation in the activity in order to use the animal effectively in therapy sessions. Once the practitioner has established the goals of the therapy session, a decision on the type of animal activity is required.

For example, George is a 5-year-old boy who has limited use of his right arm. He loves animals and has a pet cat that he has been unable to see since his hospitalization. The OT practitioner decides to surprise George in the therapy session and bring in a cat for him to brush with the use of both arms and hands. The practitioner positions the cat so that George will have to reach for and hold it. This is a natural activity for him because it demonstrates his love of animals. The goal of the session is to help George improve motor skills (e.g., the use of his right hand). Therefore, throughout the session the OT practitioner skillfully adapts the activity so that George must use his right arm. In this example, brushing the cat is an activity to promote right arm movement.

Brushing the cat could also be considered the goal of the session (e.g., the occupation itself is the goal) in this scenario because George has a cat at home. Therefore, if one of his chores is to brush his cat, the OT practitioner may want to focus the session on how he will be able to do this despite limited movement in his right arm. In this case, the OT practitioner would position the cat so that George would be successful in the task. This would help George adapt and compensate for the limited use of his right arm so that he could effectively fulfil his role as pet caretaker.

The OT practitioner may decide to help children explore their environments in visual, auditory, and/or tactile modalities through animals. Exploration of the environment helps children develop sensory and problem-solving skills.

Seth, a 2-year-old boy with developmental delays, lives in the inner city. The OT practitioner discussed the use of insects and animals in a therapy session. The parents smiled and stated that Seth had never explored a sandbox or the ground like his older brother. Because of his delays, the parents did not realize that he had never felt the ground or grass. The OT practitioner planned a session using sand, worms, ants, and plants. Seth was able to play as his mother was showing him the various objects. The OT practitioner also placed small toys in the sand and allowed Seth to determine whether or not each toy was an animal. Seth smiled and laughed when he picked up a worm and observed its movement. His mother enjoyed teaching her son about the animals and insects and told him stories about when she was a child. This session empowered the mother and reminded her in a subtle way of how children of all levels of ability value exploration. Furthermore, Seth was able to experience typical sensations, although they were somewhat different from those of his inner city environment.

Animal-assisted therapy can help children with emotional and/or behavioral difficulties. They have a calming effect and are responsive to humans. Therefore, children can be taught to read the cues of the animals, which may transfer to reading the cues of other people. Caring for animals can be satisfying to children, and teaching them to perform simple commands is rewarding. The bond between a child and pet is beneficial to those children who experience behavioral and/or emotional difficulties. The feeling of acceptance and the nurturing nature of animals help children. The OT practitioner may need to model the appropriate touching of an animal and help the child bond with it. The session may focus on reading the animal's cues, caring for it, or teaching it to do a trick. Through these sessions the child must show patience, understanding, timing, caring, and perseverance. Caring for animals requires consistency in performance and organization.

Animals may be used as a modality to improve the social participation of children. A child may show friends his or her pet, meet other children with the same type of pet, or join clubs that discuss the care of animals (e.g., a 4-H club, riding organization, fair). These groups help children learn about and gain interest in their pets and develop a sense of belonging. The OT practitioner can help the child with special needs participate in these groups by helping him or her adapt or compensate as needed.

These activities are just a few of the many possibilities that animal-assisted therapy offers to children and OT practitioners. Intervention must be centered on the child's and family's needs. OT practitioners should understand the family's culture and attitude toward animals. There are many activities that can be tailored to meet the needs of the child.

SUMMARY

Animals can be a creative and interesting modality for OT intervention. Furthermore, many children participate in occupations involving animals, making this a natural fit for the OT practitioner. Children of all ages enjoy interaction with animals and occupations that involve them. We urge OT practitioners to continue to explore this area.

References

1. Crawford JJ, Pomerinke KA: *Therapy pets: the animal-human healing partnership*, Amherst, NY, 2003, Prometheus Books.
2. Sheier-Silkwood D: The difference lies in the perspective, NARHAS, *Strides* 9:14, 2003.
3. Occupational Therapy Practice Framework: domain and process, *Am J Occup Ther* 56:609, 2002.
4. Winkle M: Dogs in practice: beyond pet therapy, *OT Practice* 8:12, 2003.

Recommended Reading

Britton W: *William N. Britton's the legend of rainbow bridge*, Morrison, Colo, 1994, Savannah Publishing. (Age 8 to adult.)

Brown M: *The dead bird*, New York, 1983, Harper Collins. (Ages 4 to 7.)

Calmenson S: *Rosie, a visiting dog story*, New York, 1994, Clarion Books. (Ages 4 to 10.)

Coudert J: *The good shepherd: a special dog's gift of healing*, Salt Lake City, Utah, 1998, Andrews McMeel Publishing. (Age 12 to adult.)

Curtis P: *Animal partners: training animals to help people*, New York, 1982, EP Dutton. (Age 8 to adult.)

Curtis P: *Cindy, a hearing-ear dog*, New York, 1981, EP Dutton. (Ages 4 to 10.)

Davis C: *For every dog an angel: the forever dog*, Portland, Ore, 1997, Lighthearted Press. (Age 4 to adult.)

Disalvo-Ryan D: *A dog like Jack*, New York, 1999, Holiday House. (Ages 4 to 8.)

Duncan S: *Joey Moses*, Seattle, Wash, 1998, Storytellers Ink. (Age 10 to adult.)

Fine A: *Handbook on animal-assisted therapy: theoretical foundations and guidelines for practice*, New York, 2000, Academic Press.

Golder S: *Buffy's orange leash*, Washington, DC, 1988, Kendell Green Publications. (Ages 4 to 8.)

Garfield J: *Follow my leader*, New York, 1994, Puffin. (Ages 9 to 12.)

Hocken S: *Emma and I*, New York, 1978, EP Dutton. (Age 10 to adult.)

Hubbard C: *One golden year: a story of a golden retriever*, New York, 1999, Apple. (Ages 9 to 12.)

Kennedy P, Christie R: *Through Otis' eyes: lessons from a guide dog puppy*, New York, 1998, Howell Book House. (Ages 3 to 7.)

Kerswell J: *The complete book of horses*, Avenel, NJ, 1993, Crescent Books.

McGinty AB: *Guide dogs: seeing for people who can't*, New York, 1999, PowerKids Press. (Ages 8 to 10.)

Mooney S: *A snowflake in my hand*, New York, 1983, Delacorte. (Age 12 to adult.)

Moore E: *Buddy, the first seeing-eye dog* (Hello Reader! Level 4), New York, 1996, Scholastic. (Ages 4 to 8.)

Morehead D: *A special place for Charlee: a child's companion through pet loss*, Broomfield, Colo, 1996, Partners in Publishing. (Ages 3 to 6.)

Nieburg H: *Pet loss: a thoughtful guide for adults and children*, New York, 1982, Harper & Row. (Age 10 to adult.)

Ogden PW: *Chelsea: the story of a signal dog*, Boston, 1992, Little, Brown & Co (Age 12 to adult.)

Okimoto JD: *A place for Grace*, Seattle, Wash, 1993, Sasquatch Books. (Ages 4 to 8.)

Osofsky A: *My buddy*, New York, 1992, Henry Holt & Co. (Ages 4 to 8.)

Rogers F: *When a pet dies*, New York, 1988, GP Putnam's Sons. (Ages 3 to 5.)

Rossite NP: *Rugby and Rosie*, New York, 1997, Dutton/Penguin. (Ages 5 to 9.)

Rylant C: *Dog heaven*, New York, 1995, Scholastic. (Ages 4 to 8.)

Rylant C: *Cat heaven*, New York, 1997, Scholastic. (Ages 4 to 8.)

Sibbitt S: *"Oh, where has my pet gone?": A pet loss memory book*, Wayzata, Minn, 1991, B Libby, Press. (Ages 3 to 103.)

Siegel ME, Koplin HM: *More than a friend: dogs with a purpose*, New York, 1984, Walker and Co. (Age 10 to adult.)

Smith ES: *A service dog goes to school*, New York, 1988, Morrow Junior Books. (Ages 4 to 8.)

Vinocur T: *Dogs helping kids with feelings*, New York, 1999, PowerKids Press.

Viorst J: *The tenth good thing about Barney*, New York, 1971, Macmillan. (Ages 4 to 8.)

White B, Sullivan T: *The leading lady: Dinah's story*, New York, 1991, Bantam Books. (Age 12 to adult.)

Wilhelm H: *I'll always love you*, New York, 1985, Crown Publishing Group. (Ages 4 to 8.)

Wilson MS: *No ordinary dog*, Claremont, Calif, 1995, Wilson Publishing. (Ages 8 to 12.)

Yates E: *Sound friendships: the story of Willa and her hearing-ear dog*, Woodstock, Vt, 1987, Countryman Press. (Age 10 to adult.)

This bibliography is formerly part of catalog item PET400. Other parts of PET400 are available: Pet Loss and Bereavement Bibliography and Healthy Reasons to Have a Pet.

RESOURCES

Assistance Dogs International
http://www.adionline.org

The Delta Society
www.deltasociety.org
c/o Delta Society, USA
580 Naches Avenue SW, No. 101
Renton, WA 98055-2297

Human-Animal Interaction for Children
www.deltasociety.org

International Association of Human-Animal Interaction Organizations
www.iahaio.org

PAWS for Health
www.vcu.edu/paws/benefit.htm

RESOURCES FOR GAMES AND ACTIVITIES DURING HIPPOTHERAPY SESSIONS

- Adapted Physical Education catalogs at http://www.flaghouse.com
- Educational catalogs such as Nasco at http://www.nascofa.com
- Freedom Riders at http://www.freedomrider.com
- Lorrie Renker at http://www.educationequine.com
- Sportsmark by Signam at http://www.sportsmark.co.uk

REVIEW *Questions*

1. List specific organizations and associations concerned with the positive effects of human-animal interaction.
2. What is an animal-assisted activity?
3. What is animal-assisted therapy?

SUGGESTED *Activities*

1. Volunteer at your local Society for the Prevention of Cruelty to Animals (SPCA).
2. Volunteer with a therapeutic horseback riding and/or hippotherapy program.
3. Visit a local zoo and, using tables, list and categorize the animals that you see. Describe their behaviors in terms of the humans who are observing them.
4. Go camping on a river or lake. Record and categorize the animals that you interact with.
5. Develop a list of activities involving pets that could be used in practice. Use the OTPF to analyze the client factors and activity demands.

Glossary

abduction Movement away from the midline of the body or body part that is identified as the middle point of reference (e.g., spreading the fingers apart or moving the arm away from the side of the body)

achievement stage The late childhood stage (6 to 11 years of age) in which children successfully accomplish movements and skills

acknowledgment Providing feedback to individuals that assures them that they have been "heard"

acquired condition; acquired disorder An illness or state of health that is not inherited and interferes with an individual's ability to be functionally independent

acquired immunodeficiency syndrome (AIDS) A severe immunological disorder caused by the retrovirus HIV (human immunodeficiency virus) that is characterized by increased susceptibility to infections and certain rare cancers; transmitted primarily through body fluids

activities of daily living (ADLs) Self-maintenance activities such as dressing and feeding

activity Specified pursuit in which an individual participates

activity analysis A tool that helps occupational therapy practitioners prioritize, plan, and implement effective treatment; involves identifying every characteristic of a task and examining each client factor, performance component, performance area, and performance context

activity configuration The process of selecting specific activities to use during an intervention

activity demands Those things which are needed to carry out an activity

activity synthesis Modifying, grading, and/or changing the structure or steps of an activity into a whole; includes adapting, grading, and reconfiguring activities

acute Extremely severe symptoms or conditions; having a rapid onset and following a short but severe course

adaptation Adjustment or change to suit a situation

adapting activities Modifying or changing a task or using adaptive equipment to make a task easier

addiction An intense psychological and physiological craving

adduction Movement toward the midline of the body or body part that has been identified as the middle point of reference (e.g., moving the fingers together or moving the arm toward the side of the body)

alignment To move toward a straight line; posturally, to keep body segment bones and joints correctly oriented toward each other, particularly in the proximal areas of the head, neck, trunk, and pelvis

amputation The loss of a body part, often all or part of an arm or leg

anxiety A state of uneasiness, apprehension, uncertainty, and fear resulting from the anticipation of a threatening event or situation

American Occupational Therapy Association's uniform terminology for occupational therapy Standard terminology for occupational therapy practitioners that has been replaced by the Occupational Therapy Practice Framework (OTPF)

areas of occupation Different kinds of activities in which people engage, including activities of daily living (ADLs), instrumental activities of daily living (IADLs), education, work, play, leisure, and social participation

arthrogryposis A congenital disorder marked by generalized stiffness of the joints; often accompanied by nerve and muscle degeneration, resulting in impaired mobility

assistive technology (AT) A concept that encompasses the process by which an individual with disabilities acquires or sustains independence by using assistive technology devices

assistive technology device (AT device) A piece of equipment that assists individuals with disabilities in performing occupations or daily activities

assistive technology service (AT service) Any service that directly assists an individual with disabilities in the selection, acquisition, and/or use of an assistive technology device

assistive technology team (AT team) A group of professionals who make recommendations and carry out the training of an individual with a disability by using an assistive technology device

ataxia Abnormal fluctuation of muscle from normal to hypertonic (increased muscle tone); loss of the ability to coordinate muscular movement

athetosis A type of cerebral palsy characterized by involuntary writhing movements, particularly of the hands and feet

attention deficit hyperactivity disorder (ADHD) A neurobehavioral disorder characterized by difficulty with attention, hyperactivity, distractibility, and impulsivity

autism A disorder characterized by severe and complex impairments in reciprocal social interaction; communication skills; and the presence of stereotypical behavior, interests, and activities

backward chaining A way to grade an activity in which an individual learns the last step first; begins with the individual completing the last step after watching the occupational therapy practitioner perform the first few steps and progresses to the individual learning the next to the last step (and so on) until the whole sequence is independently performed

bathing and showering Typical skills involving soaping, rinsing, and drying the body that are learned in early childhood

bilateral motor control Both sides of the body working together during an activity

biomechanical frame of reference An evaluation and intervention that focuses on range of motion, strength, endurance, and preventing contractures and deformities; used primarily with orthopedic disorders

body image An attitude toward one's own body

burn An injury to body tissue caused by thermal, electrical, chemical, or radioactive agents

cardiac disorders Conditions that involve the heart and/or vessels

care of others Refers to the physical upkeep and nurturing of pets or other human beings

cerebral palsy (CP) A motor function disorder caused by a permanent, nonprogressive brain defect or lesion; characterized by a disruption in the volitional control of posture and movement; produces atypical muscle tone and unusual ways of moving

client-centered An approach to treatment whereby the therapist includes the client in every part of the evaluation and intervention program, including the decision of what plan of action to choose

client factors Aspects of activities specific to each client that may affect performance

cognition The mental processes of the construction, acquisition, and use of knowledge as well as perception, memory, and the use of symbolism and language

cognitive memory Recall of thought

collaboration Working cooperatively with others to achieve a mutual goal

communication/interaction skill A performance skill involving language and psychosocial skills

community mobility Mobility in the community outside the home

competency stage The toddler or middle childhood stage (2 to 6 years of age) in which children learn basic motor and performance skills

consultation The act or process of providing advice or information

context Conditions surrounding the client that influence performance, including personal, temporal, social, cultural, and virtual

contracture A limitation in movement caused by soft tissue shortening that may result in a "stiff" or fused joint that is unable to move

contusion An injury that does not disrupt the integrity of the skin and is characterized by swelling, discoloration, and pain

cri-du-chat syndrome A rare genetic condition caused by the absence of part of chromosome 5; also known as *cat's cry syndrome* because it is recognized at birth by a kitten-like cry

crush wound A break in the external surface of the bone caused by severe force applied against tissues

cultural considerations Thoughtful contemplation of the client's customs, beliefs, and expectations, which may be part of the larger society to which the individual belongs

decubitus ulcers Sores that result from pressure on the skin over a bony prominence or as the result of continuous pressure on any area

development The act or process of growth and/or maturation

developmental coordination disorder (DCD) Characterized by motor coordination that is markedly below chronological age and intellectual ability and significantly interferes with activities of daily living

developmental disorder A mental and/or physical disability that arises before adulthood and lasts throughout one's life

developmental dyspraxia Difficulty with motor planning that is the result of sensory processing problems

developmental frame of reference Approaches intervention at the level at which the child is currently functioning and requires that the clinician provide a slightly advanced challenge

diplegia A term describing the distribution of affected muscles in individuals with CP in which the musculature of the lower extremities is more affected than that of the upper extremities

dislocation Displacement of the normal relationship of bones at a joint

disruptive behavior disorder A mental disorder characterized by socially disruptive behavior that is typically more distressing to others than to the individual with the disorder

domain A sphere of knowledge, influence, or activity

Down syndrome A genetic disorder caused by the presence of an extra 21st chromosome, which results in mental and motor delays

dressing and undressing Essential, basic self-care skills learned in infancy and early childhood

Duchenne muscular dystrophy The most common form of muscular dystrophy; characterized by pseudohypertrophy, especially of the calf muscles; seen in males

due process Parents' ability to take legal action against a school if their child's educational rights are violated; derived from the words *due*—owed or owing as a natural or moral right—and *process*—to proceed against by law

dynamic splint A splint that assists an individual with movements

eating The ability to keep food and fluids in the mouth, move them around inside the mouth, and swallow them

eating disorder A mental disorder characterized by a disturbance in eating behavior

educational activities Those tasks that promote learning, especially in academic areas such as reading, writing, and math

environmental control unit (ECU) A system that allows an individual with limited motor control to operate electrical devices such as telephones, room lights, and televisions

environmentally induced disorder An atypical condition that results from an environmental toxin (such as lead)

equifinality The inability to predict how a given situation or event in the present will develop in the future

equilibrium reactions; equilibrium responses Automatic, reflexive, compensatory movements of body parts that restore and maintain the center of gravity over the base of support when either the center of gravity or the supporting surface is displaced; complex postural reactions that involve righting reactions with rotation and diagonal patterns and are essential for volitional movement and mobility; responses that begin at 6 months and persist throughout one's life

evaluation The process of using formal and informal measures to quantify an individual's performance in areas of occupation

exceptional educational need (EEN) The determination that a disability or handicapping condition exists and interferes with the child's or adolescent's ability to participate in an educational program

exploration stage The infancy or early childhood stage (0 to 2 years of age) in which the child seeks out stimuli; the child is just beginning to move and perform skills

fading assistance A method of grading an activity by gradually reducing the level of assistance given until the individual performs the activity independently

facilitation Planned, graded physical guidance techniques used to improve movement coordination by increasing inadequate muscle tone, altering sensory responsiveness, and/or altering behavioral states (e.g., hands-on facilitation techniques that are targeted at key postural points such as the shoulders, trunk, and hips)

feeding The process of bringing food and fluids to the mouth from containers such as plates, bowls, and cups

fetal alcohol syndrome A disorder that occurs as a result of excess alcohol consumption by the mother during pregnancy; includes birth defects such as cardiac, cranial, facial, and neural abnormalities, with associated delays in physical and mental growth

fine motor skill The ability to use the small muscles of the body, especially those of the hands, to perform tasks

forward chaining A way to grade an activity in which an individual learns each step from the beginning; begins with the individual starting the sequence and ends with the occupational therapy practitioner finishing what the individual has not yet learned

fracture A break, rupture, or crack in bone or cartilage

fragile X syndrome A reproductive disorder characterized by a nearly broken X chromosome; the signs and symptoms may include an elongated face, prominent jaw and forehead, hypermobile or lax joints, flat feet, and mental retardation

frame of reference Framework that helps the occupational therapy practitioner identify problems, evaluate, develop intervention, and measure outcomes

free, appropriate public education (FAPE) Free public education that is mandated for all children, adolescents, and young adults who have disabilities and are between 3 and 21 years of age

freedom to suspend reality The ability to participate in "make-believe" or activities in which the participants pretend; the ability to create new play situations and interact with materials, space, and people in ways that are fluid, flexible, and not bound to the constraints of real life

functional support capacities Represent secondary neurobehavioral, motor, social-emotional, and/or cognitive proficiencies that are not functional in the occupational sense but are considered prerequisites for the end products to develop normally

fussy baby syndrome Condition in which the infant is easily upset and given to bouts of ill temper; associated with infants who have sensory regulatory disorders

general sensory disorganization Disorders in which sensory systems are providing inaccurate information; may be associated with impairments in the tactile, vestibular, and/or auditory systems; also associated with infants who are characterized as "fussy babies"

genetic conditions Disorders that occur as a result of abnormal or absent genes

global mental functions Refers to consciousness, orientation, sleep, temperament and personality, and energy and drive

gradation A systematic progression of activities

grading activities Changing one or more aspects of a task (usually by increasing or decreasing demands) to make it easier or harder to perform; modifying activities

gross motor skills Activities that require the use of the larger body muscles (e.g., shoulders, hips, and knees)

growth Development; increase in size

handling Methods of providing specific sensory input to individuals with atypical muscle tone, posture, and movement

hearing impairment A disorder in the auditory system that may be a sensorineural or conductive disorder; there are relationships among hearing impairments and the vestibular system, balance, and chronic otitis

hemiplegia A term describing the distribution of affected muscles in individuals with CP in which only the musculature on one side of the body is affected

high technology Technology that is expensive and not readily available, such as computers, environmental control units, and powered wheelchairs

home care An agency that contracts with nurses and practitioners to provide home-based services

home management activities Tasks that are necessary to obtain and maintain personal and household possessions

hypertonicity Abnormally increased muscle tone associated with atypical postural alignment and decreased range of motion at joints; also known as *high tone* or *spasticity*

hypotonicity Abnormally decreased muscle tone associated with atypical postural alignment and excessive range of motion at joints; also known as *low tone* or *flaccidity*

ideation The ability to conceptualize internal representations of purposeful actions

identity The individual and contextual factors that constitute self-perception

inclusion Models that are based on the premise that students with special needs should be educated in a regular classroom (instead of a self-contained classroom), with support personnel or services provided in that classroom (instead of pull-out services)

individual education program (IEP) The written educational plan developed by the IEP team that includes the student's strengths and weaknesses as well as annual goals with short-term objectives

individual education program team The team of parents, teachers, special educators, occupational therapy clinicians, and others that determines a student's need for services

individual family service plan (IFSP) The written intervention plan that is developed by the IFSP team and has as its focus family priorities and resources

Individuals with Disabilities Act (IDEA) Encourages occupational therapy practitioners to work with children in their classroom environments and provide support to the regular education teacher (integration) and encourages schools to allow students with disabilities to meet the same educational standards as their peers

in-hand manipulation Moving objects with the hand

inhibition Planned, graded physical guidance techniques used to reduce excessive muscle tone, calm overly excited behavioral states, and decrease sensory hypersensitivity

instrumental activities of daily living (IADLs) The complex activities of daily living that are needed to function independently in the home, at school, and in the community

intellectual disability Below-average cognitive functioning that causes developmental delays and impairments in multiple areas of occupation, including social participation, education, ADL and IADL skills, and play/leisure

intelligence quotient (IQ) A ratio of tested mental age to chronological age that is usually expressed as a quotient (i.e., the result of dividing one number by another) and multiplied by 100; determined by using a standardized test that measures an individual's ability to form concepts, solve problems, acquire information, reason, and learn

internal control The extent to which individuals are in charge of their own actions and the outcome of an activity

intervention plan A detailed description of the goals, methods, and expected outcomes of therapy

intrinsic motivation A prompt to action that comes from within the individual; drive to action that is rewarded by doing the activity itself rather than deriving some external reward from it

juvenile rheumatoid arthritis A chronic disorder that begins in childhood and is characterized by stiffness and inflammation of the joints, weakness, loss of mobility, and deformity

key points of control Selected body locations that provide therapeutic sensory input

least restrictive environment (LRE) A classroom setting with minimum limitations; associated with the premise that children with disabilities have the right to be with non-disabled children

legitimate tools Instruments that are in accordance with the established and accepted standards of a profession or discipline

leisure Freedom from the demands of work; engaging in a nonobligatory activity that is intrinsically motivating during free time

leisure activities Activities that are not associated with time-consuming duties and responsibilities

leukemia A group of pediatric health conditions involving various acute and chronic tumor disorders of the bone marrow

level of arousal The amount of alertness and attention needed for an activity; must be at the optimum level for learning to take place

levels of supervision Refers to the amount of oversight required for the OT practitioner to perform job duties

life cycle The events that typically occur during one's life

long-term care Care that is provided in a residential facility when a family or primary caregiver is unable meet an individual's medical needs; includes the goals of providing appropriate medical care and therapeutic intervention

low technology Technology that is inexpensive, easy to obtain, and simple to produce

media An intervening substance through which something else is transmitted or carried on; an agency by which something is accomplished, conveyed, or transferred

method A means or manner of procedure, especially a regular and systematic way of accomplishing something

mild mental retardation A category of intellectual disability in which an individual has a below-average IQ (ranging from 55 to 69) and typically requires intermittent support; generally allows the individual to master academic skills ranging from the third to the seventh grade, though more slowly than others

model of practice Framework that helps occupational therapy practitioners organize their thinking

moderate mental retardation A category of mental retardation in which an individual has a below-average IQ (ranging from 40 to 54) and typically requires some level of support as adults; generally allows the individual to master academic skills at the second-grade level, though significantly more slowly than others

mood disorder A mental disorder characterized by a disturbance in mood

morphogenetic principle The theory that systems tend to evolve and adapt to the larger environment

morphostatic principle The theory that systems tend to maintain the status quo (i.e., stay the same)

motor control frame of reference Follows a task-oriented approach that encourages the repetition of desired movements in a variety of settings and circumstances

motor memory Recall of action patterns within body structures like muscles and joints

motor plan A multitude of sequenced steps

motor skill A performance skill involving objects; includes gross and fine motor skills

multidisciplinary Relating to multiple fields of study involved in the care of clients; suggests that although the various disciplines are working in collaboration, they are also working in parallel, with each distinct discipline being accountable and responsible for its tasks and functions regarding client care

muscle tone The degree of tension in muscle fibers while a muscle is at rest; the degree of elasticity and contractility in the muscle tissue; the resting state of a muscle in response to gravity and emotion

neurological conditions Congenital or acquired disorders, such as spina bifida and Erb's palsy, that affect the central or peripheral nervous system

No Child Left Behind Established in 2001 to increase the standards for teaching and improve the results of student learning; supports the use of scientifically based practices by professionals working in the educational setting

non-normative life cycle events The unanticipated events of life, such as the frequent hospitalization of a young child or premature death of a child or parent

normal Occurring naturally; not deviating from the standard

normative life cycle events The usual and expected events of life, such as birth, starting school, and adolescence

obesity Excessively increased body weight caused by an accumulation of adipose tissue or fat

occupation An activity that has unique meaning and purpose for a person

occupational therapy intervention process model (OTIPM) A model for occupational therapy evaluation and intervention in which a client-centered, top-down, occupation-based approach is used

Occupational Therapy Practice Framework Terminology developed to assist practitioners in defining the process and domains of occupational therapy

oral defensiveness Aversion to harmless oral sensations

oral hygiene Typical skills that are learned in early childhood, such as brushing the teeth

oral-motor development Maturation of the oral-motor structures

orthopedic condition A disorder that involves the skeletal system and associated muscles (i.e., joints and ligaments)

orthosis An orthotic device; a term used interchangeably with *splint*; a bracing system designed to control, correct, and/or compensate for bony deformities or muscle imbalance

pediatric medical care system A group of individuals (professional, paraprofessional, and nonprofessional) who form a complex and unified whole dedicated to caring for children who are ill

perceptual coping strategies Defining events, situations, and crises in ways that promote adaptation

performance skills The observable elements of action, including motor skills, process skills, and communication/interaction skills

periods of development Specific developmental stages categorized by age; they include infancy, early childhood, middle childhood, adolescence, and adulthood

personal hygiene and grooming skills Typical skills such as face washing, hand washing, and hair care that are learned in early childhood

pervasive developmental disorders A group of pediatric health conditions affecting a variety of body functions and structures with a wide range of severity

pica behavior Craving and eating inedible items such as plaster and dirt

play Any spontaneous or organized activity that provides enjoyment, entertainment, amusement, and/or diversion; an experience that involves intrinsic motivation, with emphasis on the process rather than product and internal rather than external control; a make-believe experience that takes place in a safe, nonthreatening environment

play adaptations Changes in materials or activities to promote successful play for children who have disabilities

play assessment Observations of children during play by the occupational therapy practitioner

play environment The setting in which the occupational therapy practitioner assesses children at play; consists of child-friendly toys and materials

play goals Outcomes of play during the occupational therapy process

playfulness Abstract noun derived from the adjective *playful;* a behavioral or personality trait characterized by flexibility, manifest joy, and spontaneity

positioning Specific ways of placing an individual to maintain postural alignment, provide postural stability, facilitate normal patterns of movement, and increase interaction with the environment; can include the use of adaptive equipment

postural mechanism Automatic, involuntary movement actions

postural-ocular and bilateral integration dysfunction Sensory-based motor dysfunction identified by a cluster of several sensory, behavioral, and motor characteristics

postural stability The ability to maintain equilibrium and balance or return to the original position after displacement from that position

Prader-Willi syndrome A genetic health disorder that involves chromosome 15; characterized by varying degrees of intellectual disability, overeating habits, and self-mutilating behavior

praxis The ability to conceptualize, organize, and execute nonhabitual, novel motor tasks

prescriptive The role of the therapist in working with a child in a directive manner, providing the family and child with a plan

pretend play Play that involves symbolic games, imagination, and suspension of reality

primitive reflexes A group of reflexive movement patterns that begin emerging at birth and continue until approximately 4 to 6 months of age; reflexes that are controlled primarily by the lower brain centers; reflexes that enable the body to respond to influences such as head or body position mechanically and automatically with a change in muscle tone; reflexes that provide the developing infant with numerous consistent posture and movement patterns for early interaction with the environment

principles of development Refers to the guidelines and general progression of growth and performance skill attainment

process skill A performance attribute involving cognition

profound mental retardation A category of intellectual disability in which an individual has a below-average IQ (25 or lower) and requires pervasive support throughout life and extensive assistance with ADLs; physical disorders generally accompany cognitive limitations

proprioception A sensory system having receptors in the muscles, joints, and other internal tissues that provide internal awareness about the positions of body parts

proprioceptive feedback Muscle-joint input

protective extension reactions Postural responses that are used to stop a fall or prevent injury when equilibrium reactions cannot do so; responses that involve straightening of the arms and/or legs toward a supporting surface

psychosocial occupational therapy The area of clinical practice that provides services to children and adolescents with mental health problems

psychosocial skills Performance components that refer to an individual's ability to interact in society and process emotions; include psychological, social, and self-management skills

quadriplegia A term describing the distribution of affected muscles in individuals with CP in which the musculature of all four extremities is affected; may also affect the musculature of the neck and facial areas

range of motion (ROM) The amount of movement available at a specified joint; measured with a goniometer by occupational therapy practitioners

readiness skills Those abilities in the performance components and areas that are necessary for engaging in activities related to education, home management, care of others, and vocation

reading the child in context A moment-to-moment observation and analysis of a child's relationship to the social and physical environments and the child's responses to the therapeutic process; a tool that helps occupational therapy practitioners plan and implement treatment

referral A request for a screening or evaluation to determine whether one would benefit from occupational therapy services

resources Support in the form of time, money, friends, and family; supplies, equipment, and personnel that provide support

righting reactions Postural reactions that occur in response to a change in the position of the head and body in space; reactions that bring the head and trunk back into an upright position in space; involve extension, flexion, abduction, adduction, and lateral flexion; begin to emerge between 6 and 9 months of age and persist throughout life

role delineation The clear separation of responsibilities between the registered occupational therapist and the certified occupational therapy assistant

rote learning The acquisition of behaviors that become routine, though not always fully understood or carried out with sincerity; learning that usually occurs through memorization and repetition

RUMBA criteria Method of writing and evaluating goals; RUMBA stands for *r*elevant, *u*nderstandable, *m*easurable, *b*ehavioral, and *a*chievable

screening An informal or formal measure that determines an individual's need for occupational therapy evaluation and intervention

seizure A condition in which an individual has sudden convulsions, as in individuals with epilepsy

self-concept The total person that the child or adolescent envisions himself or herself to be

self-efficacy The individual's perception of his/her own capabilities

self-esteem Pride in oneself; self-respect

sensorimotor frame of reference An intervention approach that focuses on using sensory input to change muscle tone or movement patterns; used with children and adolescents who have disorders of the central nervous system

sensory input The basic sensations of touch, sound, and movement that influence the parts of the central nervous system that govern and produce skilled, automatic movements

sensory integration (SI) The organization of sensory input to produce an adaptive response

sensory integration frame of reference An approach to intervention developed by AJ Ayres that utilizes suspended equipment and child-directed activity to facilitate adaptive responses and thereby improve central nervous system processing

sensory modulation disorder Impairment in the ability to regulate incoming sensations or failure to detect and orient to novel or important sensory information

sensory processing The means by which the brain receives, detects, and integrates incoming sensory information for use in producing adaptive responses to one's environment

sensory system conditions Diseases, impairments, or deficits in visual, auditory, vestibular, gustatory/olfactory, or tactile functioning

service competency The process ensuring that two individual occupational therapy practitioners will obtain equivalent results (i.e., replication) when administering a specific assessment or providing intervention

severe mental retardation A category of intellectual disability in which an individual has a below-average IQ (ranging from 25 to 39) and typically requires extensive support throughout life; generally allows individuals to learn basic self-care skills, although they are unable to live independently as adults

shaken baby syndrome A cluster of impairments resulting from an infant being jerked violently back and forth

SOAP note A method of documentation that contains the following subject areas: *s*ubjective (thoughts, feelings, and verbalizations), *o*bjective (session goal and what occurred), *a*ssessment (summary of objectives), and *p*lan (future objectives and session goals)

social participation Associated with the organized patterns of behavior that are expected of a child interacting with others within a given social system, such as the family, peers, or community

soft tissue injury Damage to muscles, nerves, skin, and/or connective tissue

spasticity Increased muscle tone; hypertonicity; often occurs when a stretch reflex is activated in a muscle

specific mental functions Factors that refer to attention, memory, perception, thought, higher-level cognition, language, calculation, sequencing complex movements, psychomotor capacity, emotion, and experience of self and time

spina bifida Split spine (a common disorder seen by the occupational therapy practitioner); comprises three types: occulta, meningocele, and myelomeningocele; common to treat children with myelomeningocele-type spina bifida because of its associated sensory and motor deficits

splint A device that immobilizes, restrains, or supports a part of the body

splinter skill A specific, often complex task mastered by a child who lacks the underlying developmental capabilities to perform it; usually attained through compensatory methods and practice rather than by remediating the underlying developmental components

spontaneity Acting without effort or premeditation; driven by internal forces

sprain A traumatic injury to the tendons, muscle, or ligaments around a joint and characterized by pain, swelling, and discoloration

static splint A splint that prevents movement

stereognosis The ability to identify objects through touch

subacute Conditions present in a person with no symptoms of them

substance abuse A pattern of behavior in which the use of substances has adverse consequences

substance dependence A pattern of behavior in which substances continue to be used despite serious cognitive, behavioral, and physiological symptoms

substance-related disorder A mental disorder resulting from the inappropriate use of drugs, medications, or toxins

suck-swallow-breathe (s-s-b) synchrony A skill used continuously throughout life that allows an individual to breathe while simultaneously and unconsciously sucking in and swallowing food, drink, and saliva; its disruption can interfere profoundly with development

switch A device used to break or open an electric circuit; an item that connects, disconnects, or diverts an electric current; used with children who have disabilities to promote successful interaction with computers, battery-operated toys, and powered mobility systems

symmetry Alignment of the body in such a way that the head is in the midline position, the trunk is straight, and the weight is distributed equally on both sides of the body

teratogen Anything that causes the development of abnormal structures in an embryo and results in a severely deformed fetus

therapeutic media Activities that are meaningful and motivating to clients and address their goals

tic disorder A mental disorder characterized by tics (involuntary muscle contractions)

toilet hygiene Typical skills that are learned in early childhood such as clothing management, maintaining toileting position, transferring to and from toileting, and cleaning the body

tongue thrust A movement in which the tongue extends outside the lips, interferes with swallowing, and causes food to be pushed outside the mouth; often seen in individuals with CP or Down syndrome

top-down approach Focuses on occupations as the means and ends and emphasizing client-centered care

transdisciplinary Refers to "across" disciplines; this approach involves a variety of professionals who work closely with children and may in fact share roles. Team members may work on goals of another profession

traumatic brain injury (TBI) A serious injury to the brain

typical exhibiting qualities, traits, or characteristics that identify a group; not deviating from the standard or norm

visuomotor skills Coordination of the eyes with the hands or other body parts in such a way that the eyes guide precisely controlled movements; also referred to as *visuomotor integration skills* and *eye-hand* or *eye-foot skills*

visual perception The ability to interpret and use what is being or has been seen

vision impairment A condition of decreased visual acuity or impaired processing of visual input

vocational activities Work-related activities that typically have a monetary incentive or salary

whole skills Those occupations or activities that can be done automatically (i.e., without thinking)

work An area of occupation that includes employment and volunteer activities

Index

Page numbers followed by f indicate figures; t, tables; and b, boxes.

D

G

H

I

N

O

T